Tumor Angiogenesis and Microcirculation

BASIC AND CLINICAL ONCOLOGY

Editor

Bruce D. Cheson, M.D.

National Cancer Institute
National Institutes of Health
Bethesda, Maryland

1. Chronic Lymphocytic Leukemia: Scientific Advances and Clinical Developments, *edited by Bruce D. Cheson*
2. Therapeutic Applications of Interleukin-2, *edited by Michael B. Atkins and James W. Mier*
3. Cancer of the Prostate, *edited by Sakti Das and E. David Crawford*
4. Retinoids in Oncology, *edited by Waun Ki Hong and Reuben Lotan*
5. Filgrastim (r-metHuG-CSF) in Clinical Practice, *edited by George Morstyn and T. Michael Dexter*
6. Cancer Prevention and Control, *edited by Peter Greenwald, Barnett S. Kramer, and Douglas L. Weed*
7. Handbook of Supportive Care in Cancer, *edited by Jean Klastersky, Stephen C. Schimpff, and Hans-Jörg Senn*
8. Paclitaxel in Cancer Treatment, *edited by William P. McGuire and Eric K. Rowinsky*
9. Principles of Antineoplastic Drug Development and Pharmacology, *edited by Richard L. Schilsky, Gérard A. Milano, and Mark J. Ratain*
10. Gene Therapy in Cancer, *edited by Malcolm K. Brenner and Robert C. Moen*
11. Expert Consultations in Gynecological Cancers, *edited by Maurie Markman and Jerome L. Belinson*
12. Nucleoside Analogs in Cancer Therapy, *edited by Bruce D. Cheson, Michael J. Keating, and William Plunkett*
13. Drug Resistance in Oncology, *edited by Samuel D. Bernal*
14. Medical Management of Hematological Malignant Diseases, *edited by Emil J Freireich and Hagop M. Kantarjian*
15. Monoclonal Antibody-Based Therapy of Cancer, *edited by Michael L. Grossbard*
16. Medical Management of Chronic Myelogenous Leukemia, *edited by Moshe Talpaz and Hagop M. Kantarjian*
17. Expert Consultations in Breast Cancer: Critical Pathways and Clinical Decision Making, *edited by William N. Hait, David A. August, and Bruce G. Haffty*
18. Cancer Screening: Theory and Practice, *edited by Barnett S. Kramer, John K. Gohagan, and Philip C. Prorok*

19. Supportive Care in Cancer: A Handbook for Oncologists: Second Edition, Revised and Expanded, *edited by Jean Klastersky, Stephen C. Schimpff, and Hans-Jörg Senn*
20. Integrated Cancer Management: Surgery, Medical Oncology, and Radiation Oncology, *edited by Michael H. Torosian*
21. AIDS-Related Cancers and Their Treatment, *edited by Ellen G. Feigal, Alexandra M. Levine, and Robert J. Biggar*
22. Allogeneic Immunotherapy for Malignant Diseases, *edited by John Barrett and Yin-Zheng Jiang*
23. Cancer in the Elderly, *edited by Carrie P. Hunter, Karen A. Johnson, and Hyman B. Muss*
24. Tumor Angiogenesis and Microcirculation, *edited by Emile E. Voest and Patricia A. D'Amore*
25. Controversies in Lung Cancer: A Multidisciplinary Approach, *edited by Benjamin Movsas, Corey J. Langer, and Melvyn Goldberg*
26. Chronic Lymphoid Leukemias, Second Edition, Revised and Expanded, *edited by Bruce D. Cheson*

ADDITIONAL VOLUMES IN PREPARATION

Tumor Angiogenesis and Microcirculation

edited by

Emile E. Voest

University Medical Center Utrecht
Utrecht, The Netherlands

Patricia A. D'Amore

Schepens Eye Research Institute
Harvard Medical School
Boston, Massachusetts

MARCEL DEKKER, INC. NEW YORK • BASEL

ISBN: 0-8247-0264-6

This book is printed on acid-free paper.

Headquarters
Marcel Dekker, Inc.
270 Madison Avenue, New York, NY 10016
tel: 212-696-9000; fax: 212-685-4540

Eastern Hemisphere Distribution
Marcel Dekker AG
Hutgasse 4, Postfach 812, CH-4001 Basel, Switzerland
tel: 41-61-261-8482; fax: 41-61-261-8896

World Wide Web
http://www.dekker.com

The publisher offers discounts on this book when ordered in bulk quantities. For more information, write to Special Sales/Professional Marketing at the headquarters address above.

Current printing (last digit):
10 9 8 7 6 5 4 3 2 1

PRINTED IN THE UNITED STATES OF AMERICA

Series Introduction

Tumor Angiogenesis and Microcirculation is Volume 24 in the Basic and Clinical Oncology series. Many of the advances in oncology have resulted from close interaction between the basic scientist and the clinical researcher. The current volume follows, expands on, and illustrates the success of this relationship as demonstrated by new therapies and promising areas for scientific research.

As editor of the series, my goal has been to recruit volume editors who not only have established reputations based on their outstanding contributions to oncology, but also have an appreciation for the dynamic interface between the laboratory and the clinic. To date, the series has consisted of monographs on topics such as chronic lymphocytic leukemia, nucleoside analogs in cancer therapy, therapeutic applications of interleukin-2, retinoids in oncology, gene therapy of cancer, principles of antineoplastic drug development and pharmacology, and AIDS-related malignancies. *Tumor Angiogenesis and Microcirculation* is certainly a most important addition to the series.

Volumes in progress include works on secondary malignancies, chronic lymphoid leukemias, and controversies in gynecologic oncology. I anticipate that these volumes will provide a valuable contribution to the oncology literature.

Bruce D. Cheson, M.D.

Preface

In previous decades, it was recognized that the development of new blood vessels is crucial to support the growth of tumors and metastases. Starting with the hypothesis of Dr. Judah Folkman that tumor growth is angiogenesis dependent, this area of research now has a solid scientific foundation. Insight into the mechanisms through which tumors regulate angiogenesis and gain access to the circulation has led to the development of treatment strategies targeted against the tumor vasculature. These strategies are based mostly on the observation that newly formed blood vessels have specific characteristics that allow discrimination from mature, resting blood vessels.

To use antiangiogenic therapy effectively requires a significant adjustment of the conventional line of thinking about treating cancer patients. Whereas conventional chemotherapy, radiotherapy, and immunotherapy are directed against tumor cells, antiangiogenic therapy is aimed at the vasculature of a tumor and will either cause total tumor regression or keep tumors in a state of dormancy. This approach has a significant benefit over other treatment modalities in that it is applicable to tumor growth in general and is not dependent on specific tumor characteristics.

Because several of these antiangiogenic and antimetastatic approaches have now reached a stage where they are being tested in clinical trials, we feel that there is a need to highlight the current developments in this research field. The aims of this book are therefore: a) to provide a well-balanced overview of the current biological principles of angiogenesis and microcirculation, b) to outline the methods involved in discovering angiogenesis stimulators and inhibitors,

c) to review promising preclinical modulators of angiogenesis, and d) to show the recent clinical achievements and possible future applications.

We have attempted to create a book that will be of benefit not only to basic scientists working in this field but also to clinicians (pathologists; surgeons; medical, radiation, and hemato-oncologists; and internists) who will perform future clinical studies with angiogenesis inhibitors.

Emile E. Voest
Patricia A. D'Amore

Contents

II Assays to Study Angiogenesis

III Angiogenic Factors

Contributors

Kari Alitalo, M.D., Ph.D. Research Professor of the Finnish Academy of Sciences Molecular/Cancer Biology Laboratory, Haartman Institute, University of Helsinki, Finland

Bela Anand-Apte, M.B.B.S., Ph.D. Staff Scientist, Ophthalmic Research and Cell Biology, Cole Eye Institute, Cleveland Clinic Foundation, Cleveland, Ohio

Robert Auerbach, Ph.D. Harold R. Wolfe Professor, Department of Zoology, University of Wisconsin, Madison, Wisconsin

Wanda Auerbach, M.S. Reference Librarian, Department of Zoology, University of Wisconsin, Madison, Wisconsin

Teresa A. Bennett, Ph.D. Laboratory of Pathology, National Cancer Institute, National Institutes of Health, Bethesda, Maryland

Geert H. Blijham, M.D., Ph.D. Professor of Medicine and Chairman, University Medical Center Utrecht, Utrecht, The Netherlands

Henry Brem, M.D. Harvey Cushing Professor of Neurosurgery, Oncology, and Ophthalmology, and Chairman, Department of Neurosurgery, Johns Hopkins University School of Medicine, Baltimore, Maryland

Peter D. Brown, D. Phil. Project Director, Development, British Biotech Pharmaceuticals Ltd., Oxford, England

David A. Cheresh, Ph.D. Professor, Department of Immunology and Vascular Biology, The Scripps Research Institute, La Jolla, California

Robert J. D'Amato, M.D., Ph.D. Assistant Professor, Department of Ophthalmology, Harvard Medical School, Boston, Massachusetts

Patricia A. D'Amore, Ph.D. Senior Scientist, Department of Ophthalmology, Schepens Eye Research Institute, and Professor of Ophthalmology/Pathology, Harvard Medical School, Boston, Massachusetts

Diane C. Darland, Ph.D. Research Fellow, Schepens Eye Research Institute, Harvard Medical School, Boston, Massachusetts

Juliana Denekamp, B.Sc., Ph.D., D.Sc. Professor, Translation Research Unit, Department of Radiation Sciences, Umeå University, Umeå, Sweden

Brian P. Eliceiri, Ph.D. Research Associate, Departments of Immunology and Vascular Biology, The Scripps Research Institute, La Jolla, California

Berndt Enholm, B.M. Molecular/Cancer Biology Laboratory, Haartman Institute, University of Helsinki, Helsinki, Finland

Matthew G. Ewend, M.D. Assistant Professor of Neurosurgery, University of North Carolina, Chapel Hill, North Carolina

Napoleone Ferrara, M.D. Staff Scientist, Department of Cardiovascular Research, Genentech, Inc., South San Francisco, California

Isaiah J. Fidler, D.V.M., Ph.D. Professor and Chairman, Department of Cancer Biology, The University of Texas M.D. Anderson Cancer Center, Houston, Texas

Martijn F. B. G. Gebbink, Ph.D. Laboratory of Medical Oncology, Department of Internal Medicine, University Medical Center Utrecht, Utrecht, The Netherlands

Arjan W. Griffioen Laboratory of Angiogenesis Research, Department of Internal Medicine, University Hospital Maastricht, Maastricht, The Netherlands

Gerard Groenewegen, M.D., Ph.D. Department of Internal Medicine and Oncology, University Hospital Utrecht, Utrecht, The Netherlands

Yuji Gunji, M.D., Ph.D. Molecular/Cancer Biology Laboratory, Haartman Institute, University of Helsinki, Helsinki, Finland*

Kristiina Iljin, M.Sc. Molecular/Cancer Biology Laboratory, Haartman Institute, University of Helsinki, Helsinki, Finland

Raghu Kalluri, Ph.D. Assistant Professor, Department of Medicine, Harvard Medical School, and Nephrology Division, Department of Medicine, Beth Israel Deaconess Medical Center, Boston, Massachusetts

Arja Kapainen, M.D., Ph.D. Molecular/Cancer Biology Laboratory, Haartman Institute, University of Helsinki, Helsinki, Finland

Robert S. Kerbel, Ph.D. Director, Biological Sciences Program and Division of Cancer Biology Research, Sunnybrook and Women's College Health Science Centre, University of Toronto, Toronto, Ontario, Canada

Olaf A. J. Kerckhaert Department of Internal Medicine, Laboratory of Medical Oncology, University Medical Center Utrecht, Utrecht, The Netherlands

Eli Keshet, Ph.D. Professor, Department of Molecular Biology, The Hebrew University–Hadassah Medical School, Jerusalem, Israel

Eija Korpelainen Molecular/Cancer Biology Laboratory, Haartman Institute, University of Helsinki, Helsinki, Finland

Eola Kukk-Valdre, M.D. Molecular/Cancer Biology Laboratory, Haartman Institute, University of Helsinki, Helsinki, Finland

Rakesh Kumar Department of Cell Biology, The University of Texas M.D. Anderson Cancer Center, Houston, Texas

Michael Leunig, M.D. Attending Physician, Department of Orthopedic Surgery, University of Berne, Berne, Switzerland

Maartje Los, M.D. Department of Internal Medicine, Laboratory of Medical Oncology, University Medical Center Utrecht, Utrecht, The Netherlands

---

* *Current affiliation*: Assistant Professor, Department of Pediatrics, Jichi Medical School, Tochigi, Japan.

Joseph A. Madri, Ph.D., M.D. Professor, Department of Pathology, Yale University School of Medicine, New Haven, Connecticut

Konrad Messmer, M.D. Professor of Experimental Surgery, Institute for Surgical Research, Ludwig-Maximilians-University of Munich, Munich, Germany

Deborah M. Milkowski, Ph.D. Senior Research Investigator, Metabolism and Pharmacology, TAP Pharmaceutical Products Inc., Lake Forest, Illinois

Roberto Montesano, M.D. Professor, Department of Morphology, University of Geneva Medical Center, Geneva, Switzerland

David A. Moscatelli, Ph.D. Research Professor, Department of Cell Biology, New York University School of Medicine, New York, New York

Marsha A. Moses, Ph.D. Associate Professor, Department of Surgery, Children's Hospital and Harvard Medical School, Boston, Massachusetts

Futosha Okada, Ph.D. Instructor, Laboratory of Pathology, Cancer Institute, Hokkaido University School of Medicine, Sapporo, Hokkaido, Japan

Michael S. Pepper, M.D., Ph.D. Department of Morphology, University of Geneva Medical Center, Geneva, Switzerland

Peter J. Polverini, D.D.S., D.M.Sc. Professor and Dean, Department of Pathology, University of Minnesota School of Dentistry, Minneapolis, Minnesota

Janusz Rak, M.D., Ph.D. Assistant Professor, Department of Medicine, Hamilton Civil Hospitals Research Centre, McMaster University, Hamilton, Ontario, Canada

Sophia Ran, Ph.D. Research Assistant Professor of Pharmacology, Simmons Comprehensive Cancer Center, The University of Texas Southwestern Medical Center, Dallas, Texas

Jaap C. Reijneveld, M.D. Department of Neurology, University Medical Center Utrecht, Utrecht, The Netherlands

Laurence D. Rhines, M.D. Assistant Professor, Department of Neurosurgery, The University of Texas M.D. Anderson Cancer Center, Houston, Texas

Daniel B. Rifkin, Ph.D. Professor, Department of Cell Biology, New York University School of Medicine, New York, New York

Donald R. Senger, Ph.D. Department of Pathology, Beth Israel Deaconess Medical Center, Boston, Massachusetts

Ilan Stein Department of Molecular Biology, The Hebrew University–Hadassah Medical School, Jerusalem, Israel

William G. Stetler-Stevenson, M.D., Ph.D. Senior Investigator, Section Chief, Extracellular Matrix Pathology Section, Laboratory of Pathology, National Cancer Institute, National Institutes of Health, Bethesda, Maryland

Robert M. Strieter University of Michigan Medical School, Ann Arbor, Michigan

Vikas P. Sukhatme, M.D., Ph.D. Professor, Department of Medicine, Harvard Medical School, and Chief, Nephrology Division, Department of Medicine, Beth Israel Deaconess Medical Center, Boston, Massachusetts

Beverly A. Teicher, Ph.D. Research Advisor, Cancer Drug Discovery, Lilly Research Laboratories, Indianapolis, Indiana

Philip E. Thorpe, Ph.D. Professor of Pharmacology, Simmons Comprehensive Cancer Center, The University of Texas Southwestern Medical Center, Dallas, Texas

Alicia Viloria-Petit, M.Sc. Graduate student (Ph.D.), Department of Medical Biophysics, Sunnybrook and Women's College Health Science Centre, University of Toronto, Toronto, Ontario, Canada

Emile E. Voest, M.D., Ph.D. Professor of Medical Oncology, Department of Internal Medicine, University Medical Center Utrecht, Utrecht, The Netherlands

Noel Weidner, M.D. Professor and Director of Anatomic Pathology, University of California, San Diego, San Diego, California

Rachelle Weiss, Ph.D. Assistant Director, Clinical Development, TAP Pharmaceutical Products Inc., Lake Forest, Illinois

Inmin Wu, Ph.D. Research Fellow, Department of Surgery, Children's Hospital and Harvard Medical School, Boston, Massachusetts

Li Yan, M.D., Ph.D. Research Fellow, Department of Surgery, Children's Hospital and Harvard Medical School, Boston, Massachusetts

Bruce R. Zetter, Ph.D. Professor of Surgery, Children's Hospital and Harvard Medical School, Boston, Massachusetts

Tumor Angiogenesis and Microcirculation

1

Endothelial Cells and Pericytes in Tumor Vasculature

Diane C. Darland and Patricia A. D'Amore
Schepens Eye Research Institute, Harvard Medical School, Boston, Massachusetts

I. ANGIOGENESIS IS A REQUIREMENT FOR TUMOR GROWTH

In the course of examining tumor establishment, growth, and metastasis, it is important to consider one vital component in this process—the vasculature. It is now well accepted that tumor growth and metastasis require vascularization to provide both nourishment and a route for tumor cell extravasation (1). The basic premise is that tumors less than 1 mm^3 have their metabolic needs met by diffusion. Beyond that size, a more elaborate system for distributing nutrients and removing toxins and metabolites is needed to support tumor growth.

It is not entirely clear how tumor and vessel growth are temporally interconnected. Does tumor growth in the absence of sufficient vascular support create relative local hypoxia and trigger hypoxia-dependent neovascularization? Or does the presence of the tumor lead to changes in the microenvironment, including locally elevated levels of growth factor(s) that, in turn, promote neovascularization to allow continued growth of the tumor (2)? In addition, can the tumor cells ''co-opt'' adjacent vessels to obtain support for tumor growth (3, 4)? Are tumors and their vasculatures connected by mechanisms that vary according to tumor type and location?

Regardless of which mechanism or combination of mechanisms is at play, it is readily apparent that the vascularization of tumors is an integral component of tumor growth. This fact makes angiogenesis a viable target for antitumor therapy (5). Angiogenesis promotion or inhibition in a tumor can be likened to a rheostat, a device that regulates current flow with a series of resistors (Fig. 1A).

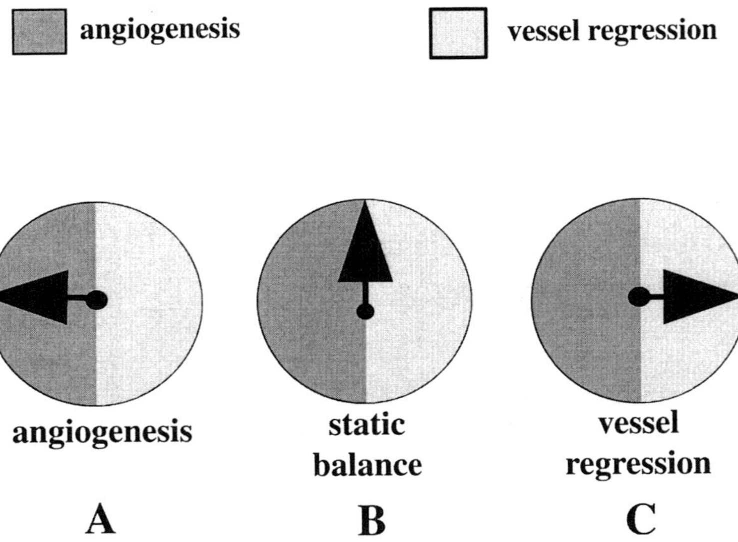

Figure 1 Rheostat model of tumor angiogenesis. When the microenvironment of the tumor vasculature is in the angiogenesis phase, vessel production is favored and the tumor volume is increased (**A**). When angiogenesis is inhibited, vessel regression predominates and the tumor volume is reduced (**C**). When there is a balance between the cycles of angiogenesis and vessel regression, the tumor volume remains relatively static (**B**). Tumor vasculature can be targeted with agents that promote vessel regression by treating with inhibitors of angiogenesis, thereby shifting the direction of the ''angiogenesis rheostat'' and decreasing tumor volume as indicated (**C**).

When growth factor production, cell-cell and cell-matrix interactions are aligned to promote vessel formation, angiogenesis proceeds. When conditions, microenvironmental and otherwise, prohibit new vessel growth, there is a net regression in tumor vasculature and subsequently in tumor volume (Fig. 1C). When both angiogenesis and vessel regression occur, there is no net increase in the tumor vasculature, and the tumor is static in size (Fig. 1B). To examine tumor angiogenesis and its impact on tumor growth, it is imperative to understand the roles of, and the factors that control, the cell types that form the vessels.

II. ENDOTHELIAL CELLS IN TUMOR VASCULATURE

The endothelial cell (EC) is the primary cell type involved in angiogenesis. Endothelial cells form the lumens of blood vessels, function in a variety of local roles including the immune response and the maintenance of a non thrombogenic surface, and participate in nutrient and gas exchange. Endothelial cells of mature, quiescent vessels have characteristically low proliferative rates with estimated turnover times measured in years. The rate of EC proliferation increases dramatically during neovascularization as occurs in wound healing or in the rapidly growing tumor vasculature. For instance, assessment of endothelial proliferation in a Lewis lung carcinoma model of tumor growth revealed a labeling index of 40%, which reflects a rapid cell turnover (3). Similarly, a survey of turnover times calculated from labeling indices among a variety of experimental tumors revealed turnover times ranging from 1 day to about 10 days. This is in contrast to EC of vessels in normal tissues in which turnover ranged from about 80 days in the lung to about 8000 days in the brain (6). Once the nascent vessel structure has become stabilized, EC proliferation is reduced and the EC transition to a quiescent state occurs.

Thus, EC of tumor vessels are distinct from those of the normal vasculature, particularly with regard to their proliferation rate. Endothelial cells in some regions of the tumor vasculature are characterized by a constant high rate of proliferation, reflecting the neovascularization that accompanies increases in tumor volume, whereas EC in other regions of the tumor are undergoing apoptosis in parallel with tumor necrosis and vessel regression (4). Tumor vessel EC can thus be viewed as a heterogeneous population, with the common trait of instability to unite them. The cellular and molecular basis of tumor vessel instability is not entirely clear. The absence or paucity of perivascular cells and the dramatically altered microenvironment with altered levels of proteases, growth factors, and matrix components all appear to contribute to this unstable phenotype. We use the term ''pseudostable'' to characterize the tumor vasculature. Tumor vessels are functional at the level of tumor support but inherently unstable, and therefore are distinct from normal, established vessels.

Endothelial cells of tumor vessels also differ from those of normal vessels in other ways, including the profile and level of cell adhesion molecules that they express. During angiogenesis, EC go through a phase of proliferation and migration during which attachment of cells to one another and to the extracellular matrix is greatly reduced. A number of adhesion molecules have been identified as candidates to mediate EC-EC interactions, as well as EC interactions with the microenvironment (7). As these topics will be covered in greater detail in later chapters, only a few specific proteins will be mentioned here.

One example of a protein likely to be involved in interendothelial cell interactions is vascular endothelial-cadherin (VE-cadherin/cadherin 5). Vascular endothelial cadherin is expressed at high levels on stable vessels where it is localized at cell-cell junctions. Vascular endothelial cadherin is poorly expressed or is absent in nonjunctional locations as well as in vessels of hemangiomas and angiosarcomas (8). These observations suggest that loss (or absence) of VE-cadherin results in vessel destabilization and may lead to abnormal remodeling. There is also considerable evidence for an involvement of the integrin αvβ3 in EC-extracellular matrix interactions as well as EC-platelet interactions. αvβ3, a cell surface receptor that can bind to fibronectin, fibrinogen, and von Willebrand factor, is highly expressed in new vessels in wounds (9) in comparison with quiescent vessels. Tumors treated with antagonists of αvβ3 exhibit increased apoptosis and vessel regression (9). These results indicate that αvβ3 is an integral component of the angiogenic process. At least one aspect of αvβ3's role in the tumor vasculature is that it mediates tumor EC adhesion to ECM molecules. In fact, cell anchoring has been clearly shown to be required for EC survival (for review see [10]).

In contrast to the EC of quiescent vessels, EC of tumor vessels show a marked dependence on growth factors for survival. One of the earliest experimental demonstrations of this fact dates back to early observations of vessels induced in the rabbit corneal pocket assay by tumor cells (11). Implantation of a tumor fragment induced new vessels that arose from the limbal vessels. Removal of the tumor, however, led to rapid vessel regression. Although the cellular and molecular basis for the instability of these vessels was unknown, it was clear that the new vessels were somehow dependent on the presence of the tumor.

Insight into the mechanism underlying this phenomenon became possible once factors involved in tumor vessel growth were identified. A large body of data has indicated a central role for vascular endothelial growth factor (VEGF) in the induction of host vessels into the growing tumor (12). Dependence on the continued presence of VEGF was demonstrated in an experimental model using a C6 glioma with tetracycline-regulated VEGF expression in which turning off VEGF expression led to vascular collapse and tumor necrosis (13). Furthermore, not all of the vessels in this glioma regressed. Instead, variable stability among the tumor vessels was correlated with the extent of pericyte association with the vessels (14) (See below for a discussion of pericytes in tumor vessels.)

Another area in which tumor vessels differ from normal vessels is in the degree of vessel integrity, which depends on the association between the EC. Tumor vessels are distinguished from nontumor vessels in their degree of permeability. At least some of the "leakiness" of tumor vessels is due to the generally high levels of VEGF in tumors. Vascular endothelial growth factor causes transient increases in permeability of normal vessels (15). The mechanisms underlying the increased leakiness are not known but have been suggested to include decreased interendothelial connections (16), stimulation of transcellular transport (17), and formation of fenestrations (18, 19).

III. PERICYTES IN TUMOR VASCULATURE

Interestingly, the greatest area of exchange across the EC in normal vessels is at the level of the microvasculature that has the lowest level of perivascular cells or pericytes. It is also the microvasculature that is the initiation site for angiogenesis. Undoubtedly, this is not a coincidence and leads to consideration of the other major cell type in the vasculature, the pericyte. Pericytes are perivascular cells that are thought to surround and stabilize new vessels. They are smooth musclelike cells that are associated with the microvasculature and are sparsely distributed along the length of the vessel (20). Pericytes extend thin processes around and along the length of the microvascular tubes and have areas of direct contact with EC. This is in contrast to the vascular smooth muscle cells that associate with larger vessels and completely surround the vessel. There is a layer of continuous basement membrane between the smooth muscle cells and the EC, with points of contact in regions where smooth muscle (SM) cell processes have breached the membrane to establish direct contact with the EC (21, 22). There is a positive correlation with vessel size and the complexity of the pericyte/SM cell layer that surrounds the vessel (22), although some of the functional differences remain unclear.

Limited information is available as to the role of pericytes in tumor vasculature. Although it is generally commented that tumor vessels have a paucity of vessel wall cells (pericytes and SM cells), few studies have examined this issue systematically. Only recently have investigators begun to recognize the possible role of the pericyte in tumor vessel stabilization (23). In the tetracycline-regulated VEGF tumor model described above, vessel injury and regression were evident only in vessels devoid of α-smooth muscle actin (SM-actin)-positive cells (e.g., pericytes) (14). Similar analyses were conducted in archival sections of human prostate tumors in which it was observed that only 40% of vessels larger than capillaries had associated SM-actin-containing cells. This was in comparison to human glioblastomas in which only 25% of the vessels larger than capillaries had SM-positive cells. This difference was of interest, in that prostate tumors are considered to be slow-growing tumors, whereas glioblastomas grow rapidly.

One recent study has assessed pericyte association with vessels of renal cell, colon, mammary, lung, and prostate carcinomas, as well as with glioblastomas (24). Assessment of pericyte association with vessels was accomplished by immunohistochemical staining for SM-actin to identify the pericytes and CD34 to localize the EC. These analyses revealed a large degree of heterogeneity among the vasculatures of these tumors. For example, 12.7 ± 7.9% of microvessels in glioblastoma had both pericytes and EC, whereas 67.3 ± 4.2% of vessels in mammary tumors had vessels with associated pericytes. On the other hand, some tumors are reported to have significant numbers of pericytes (25).

Most of the information on pericytes that has been accrued to date is derived from analysis of pericytes in normal vasculature, in wound healing, and in diabetic retinopathy (26). In normal angiogenesis, EC recruit and induce the proliferation of surrounding mesenchymal cells (23). Upon contact with the EC, the mesenchymal cells are induced toward a pericyte lineage (27). Association of the pericyte with the nascent EC tube is thought to initiate a transition toward vessel stability. There appears to be a window of sensitivity during angiogenesis in which vessels are sensitive to regression. A recent study in glioma and prostate tumors showed that vessels lacking periendothelial cells were vulnerable to growth factor withdrawal and underwent apoptosis, but those with associated pericytes were resistant (14). The role of perivascular cells in vessel stabilization in vitro and in vivo reflect the importance of pericyte association with vessels in promoting normal vessel pruning and stabilization.

IV. PERICYTES AND TUMOR VESSEL STABILITY

We propose that the presence of pericytes is one component of vessel heterogeneity, with the association of pericytes with tumor vessels leading to vessel stabilization and absence of pericytes leading to vessel destabilization. Regions of the tumor vasculature that have associated pericytes can be called *pseudostable*. The term ''pseudostabilization'' refers to vessels that are not currently undergoing neovascularization, but by their nature as tumor vessels do not achieve stability characteristic of normal vessels. Areas of the vasculature lacking pericytes represent areas of potential flux. Either vessels can regress because instability or be invested with pericytes and subsequently stabilized. Where vessels are sparse, there is resultant relative hypoxia. Angiogenesis is initiated in these areas with the early phase of EC proliferation from a pre-existing vessel. The growth of the tumor depends in part on the balance of the vasculature overall, as suggested by the rheostat model (Fig. 1). A greater percentage of vessels undergoing angiogenesis relative to the pseudostable and regressing areas will result in increased tumor vasculature. This hypothesis is a new perspective on tumor vessel stability for which there is increasing supporting data (14, 24). However, the hypothesis of pericyte investment regulating tumor vasculature stability has yet to be thoroughly tested as a mechanism for controlling tumor angiogenesis.

Cumulatively, these and other data indicate that there are distinct parallels between angiogenesis in tumor vessels and angiogenesis in an injury response. The similarities are close enough to suggest that tumor vasculature represents a chronic wound situation, unable to cycle through to stasis—an idea that has been proposed by Dvorak and coworkers in their examination of tumor angiogenesis (2, 28). This perspective indicates a theoretical avenue for inhibiting tumor angiogenesis through stabilizing the tumor vasculature and preventing further tumor expansion, although whether the vessel can remain stable in the face of elevated levels of growth factors is not clear. In addition, it suggests that targeting cell adhesion molecules, cell-matrix interactions, EC-pericyte interactions, and growth factors involved in angiogenesis may allow both inhibition and eventual regression of the tumor vasculature.

REFERENCES

1. Folkman J. Tumor angiogenesis. Cancer Med 1996; 1:181–204.
2. D'Amore PA. Mechanisms of endothelial growth control. Am J Respir Cell Mol Biol 1992; 6:1–8.
3. Holmgren L, O'Reilly MS, Folkman J. Dormancy of micrometastases: balanced proliferation and apoptosis in the presence of angiogenesis suppression. Nat Med 1995; 1:149–153.
4. Holash J, Maisonpierre PC, Compton D, Boland P, Alexander CR, Zagzag D, et al. Vessel cooption, regression, and growth in tumors mediated by angiopoietins and VEGF. 1999; 284:1994–1998.
5. Folkman J. Fighting cancer by attacking its blood supply. Sci Am 1996; 275:116–119.
6. Hobson B, Denekamp J. Endothelial proliferation in tumours and normal tissues: continuous labelling studies. Br J Cancer 1984; 49:405–413.
7. Dejana E. Endothelial adherens junctions: implications in the control of vascular permeability and angiogenesis. J Clin Invest 1996; 98:1949–1953.
8. Dejana E, Corada M, Lampugnani MG. Endothelial cell-to-cell junctions. FASEB J 1995; 9:910–918.
9. Brooks PC, Montgomery AMP, Rosenfeld M, Reisfeld RA, Hu T, Klier G, et al. Integrin avB3 antagonists promote tumor regression by inducing apoptosis of angiogenic blood vessels. Cell 1994; 79:1157–1164.
10. Eliceiri BP, Cheresh DA. The role of av integrins during angiogenesis. Mol Med 1998; 4:741–750.
11. Ausprunk DH, Falterman K, Folkman J. The sequence of events in the regression of corneal capillaries. Lab Invest 1978; 38:284–94.
12. Dvorak H, Brown L, Detmar M, Dvorak A. Vascular permeability factor/vascular endothelial growth factor, microvascular hyperpermeability, and angiogenesis. Am J Pathol 1995; 146:1029–1039.
13. Benjamin LE, Keshet E. Conditional switching of vascular endothelial growth factor (VEGF) expression in tumors: induction of endothelial cell shedding and regression of hemangioblastoma-like vessels by VEGF withdrawal. Proc Natl Acad Sci U S A 1997; 94:8761–8766.
14. Benjamin LE, Golijanin D, Itin A, Pode E, Keshet E. Selective ablation of immature blood vessels in tumors follows vascular endothelial growth factor withdrawal. J Clin Invest 1999; 103:159–165.
15. Senger DR, Galli SJ, Dvorak AM, Peruzzi CA, Harvey VS, Dvorak HF. Tumor cells

secrete a vascular permeability factor that promotes accumulation of ascites fluid. Science 1983; 219:983–985.
16. Antonetti DA, Barber AJ, Hollinger LA, Wolpert EB, Gardner TW. Vascular endothelial growth factor induces rapid phosphorylation of tight junction proteins occludin and zonula occluden 1. J Biol Chem 1999; 274:23463–23467.
17. Dvorak AM, Kohn S, Morgan ES, Fox P, Nagy JA, Dvorak HF. The vesiculo-vacuolar organelle (VVO)—a distinct endothelial cell structure that provides a transcellular pathway for macromolecular extravasation. J Leuk Biol 1996; 59:100–115.
18. Esser S, Wolburg K, Wolburg H, Breier G, Kurzchalia T, Risau W. Vascular endothelial growth factor induces endothelial cell fenestrations in vitro. J Cell Biol. 1997; 140:947–959.
19. Roberts WG, Palade GE. Increased microvascular permeability and endothelial fenestration induced by vascular endothelial growth factor. J Cell Sci 1995; 108: 2369–2379.
20. Sims DE. The pericyte—a review. Tissue Cell 1986; 18:153–174.
21. Rhodin JAG. The ultrastructure of mammalian arterioles and precapillary sphincters. J Ultrastruct Res 1967; 18:181–223.
22. Rhodin J. Ultrastructure of mammalian venous capillaries, venules, and small collecting veins. J Ultrastruct Res 1968; 25:425–500.
23. Darland DC, D'Amore PA. Blood vessel maturation: vascular development come of age. J Clin Invest 1999; 103:157–158.
24. Eberhard A, Kahlert S, Goede V, Hemmerlein B, Plate KH, Augustin HG. Heterogeneity of angiogenesis and blood vessel maturation in human tumors:implications for antiangiogenic tumor therapies. Cancer, in press.
25. Schlingemann RO, Rietveld FJR, de. Expression of the high molecular weight melanoma-associated antigen by pericytes during angiogenesis in tumors and in healing wounds. Am J Pathol 1990; 136:1393–1405.
26. Sims DE. Recent advances in pericyte biology—implications for health and disease. Can J Cardiol 1991; 7:431–443.
27. Hirschi KK, Rohovsky SA, Beck LH, Smith SR, D'Amore PA. Endothelial cells modulate the proliferation of mural cell precursors via platelet-derived growth factor-BB and heterotypic cell contact. Circ Res, 1999, in press.
28. Dvorak HF, Nagy JA, Feng D, Brown LF, Dvorak AM. Vascular permeability factor/vascular endothelial growth factor and the significance of microvascular permeability in angiogenesis. Curr Top Microbiol Immunol 1999; 237:97–132.

2

The Extracellular Matrix and the Regulation of Angiogenesis

Joseph A. Madri
Yale University School of Medicine, New Haven, Connecticut

I. INTRODUCTION

Angiogenesis, the formation of new blood vessels from preexisting vessels, occurs during development of the vasculature, in selected physiological processes (e.g., ovulation), during the wound healing process, and during the vascularization of tumors. It is a tightly controlled process involving endothelial cell activation, migration, proliferation, multicellular organization and differentiation, stabilization and, in some cases, involution (1–4). As noted in the development and maintenance of all other organ systems, angiogenesis occurs in a complex extracellular matrix environment. The importance of extracellular matrix organization and composition in modulating endothelial and vascular cell behaviors in the process of angiogenesis has been demonstrated in various in vitro and in vivo studies over the past several years (5–13). In this chapter the roles of extracellular matrix composition and organization in modulating vascular cell behavior during in vivo and in vitro vasculogenesis and angiogenesis will be discussed using selected models as examples.

II. EXTRACELLULAR MATRIX COMPONENTS AS MODULATORS OF ENDOTHELIAL CELL BEHAVIOR

The importance of extracellular matrix components in modulating endothelial cell behavior has been recognized since the first successful culture of vascular

---

Supported, in part, by USPHS Grants RO1-HL28373, PO1-DK38979, RO1-HL51018 and PO1-NS35476.

endothelial cells (14). Then, collagenous substrata (gelatin) were shown to confer beneficial growth and culture characteristics to microvascular endothelial cells in culture, including in vitro angiogenesis or ''tube formation'' (14). In the years after these studies, several investigators began using a variety of extracellular matrix components as substrata for the culture microvascular endothelial cells. Such studies documented modulation in a variety of endothelial cell behaviors, including attachment, spreading, proliferation, extracellular matrix synthetic profiles, multicellular organization, and tube formation (7, 8, 15–27). Concurrent and subsequent in vivo angiogenesis studies showed a good correlation between matrix-mediated effects noted in vitro and the presence of matrix components and endothelial cell behavior observed during angiogenesis induced in animal models (26). In vivo, organ culture and tissue culture studies of angiogenesis revealed a complex, spatiotemporal deposition and organization of extracellular matrix components along the angiogenic sprout with eventual formation of a mature basal lamina (28, 29). In vitro, microvascular endothelial cells have interacted with a wide variety of matrix components, including the interstitial collagens, collagenous and noncollagenous components of the basement membrane, and many other noncollagenous extracellular matrix components (4, 6, 26, 27, 30).

Microvascular endothelial cells exhibit varying proliferation rates depending on the underlying extracellular matrix component with which they interact. For example, rat epididymal fat pad-derived microvascular endothelial cells (RFC) exhibit a high proliferative rate when plated on laminin 1, intermediate proliferative rates when plated on collagen types I or V, and low proliferative rates when plated on collagen type IV and fibronectin (26). In addition to effects on proliferation, extracellular matrix components also affect other aspects of endothelial cell behavior. Extracellular matrix composition and concentration modulation of endothelial cell shape and spreading has been appreciated by several investigators and found to affect growth factor responsiveness through integrin engagement-mediated signaling cascades (15–19, 31–33). Culture on different extracellular components has also been observed to modulate the extracellular matrix synthetic profiles of microvascular endothelial cells as well as their ability and propensity to form multicellular complexes, tubelike structures, and fenestrae (3, 7, 20, 34–36). Purified basement membrane components (laminin and type IV collagen) elicit tube formation in cultures of microvascular endothelial cells; Matrigel™, a complex mixture of basement membrane components (laminin 1, type IV collagen, entactin, and heparin sulfate proteoglycan) and growth factors (transforming growth factor beta 1 [TGFβ1], platelet-derived growth factor [PDGF], basic fibroblast growth factor [bFGF], etc.), elicits rapid multicellular organization of endothelial cells leading to meshlike networks of cells in culture (13, 35).

Extracellular matrix-mediated modulation of endothelial cell behavior affects the process of in vivo angiogenesis, as evidenced by the distinct endothelial phenotypes noted among the endothelial cells along an angiogenic sprout that express similar behaviors to endothelial cells cultured on different extracellular matrix components. The migratory cells at the tip of a sprout are invested in cablelike arrays of type V collagen and fibronectin, whereas the proliferating cells distal to these lead cells express and deposit laminin 1 in a diffuse abluminal pattern. Further back along the sprout, the mitotically quiescent differentiating cells rest on a forming basal lamina composed of diffuse fibronectin, laminin, and type IV collagen (5, 26).

III. EXTRACELLULAR MATRIX ORGANIZATION AS A MODULATOR OF ENDOTHELIAL CELL BEHAVIOR

Although useful in clarifying the roles of specific extracellular matrix components in modulating particular aspects of endothelial cell behavior, typical two-dimensional culture systems do not adequately mimic the three-dimensional environment in which most angiogenesis occurs. During the past several years, investigators have used three-dimensional culture systems in their studies of angiogenesis. As noted for a variety of mesenchymal and epithelial cells, endothelial cells cultured in three-dimensional environments (including gels of purified interstitial collagens, basement membrane components, fibrin, and basal lamina and interstitial surfaces of amnion membranes) exhibit significantly different phenotypes compared to their culture in typical two-dimensional culture systems (5–7, 37, 38).

Human umbilical vein endothelial cells (HUVEC) have been shown to form tubelike structures when grown on trypsin-digested fibronectin substrata and deprived of endothelial cell growth factor (12). When HUVEC were cultured on three-dimensional collagen gels and stimulated with phorbol ester (PMA) the cells invaded and migrated into the gels and formed branching, tubelike structures with form lumina and junctional complexes between cells (39–41). In other studies, when HUVEC were dispersed in a type I collagen gel and PMA and angiogenic factors were added, tube formation was observed. Further, the addition of specific β1 integrin antibodies, that is, anti-α2β1, enhanced tube formation, consistent with the concept that matrix-driven, integrin-mediated signaling events are involved in the angiogenic process (38). More recent studies of PMA and angiogenic factor-stimulated HUVEC tube formation in type I collagen gels demonstrated an inhibition of vacuole and lumen formation in the presence of anti-α2β1 (25). This apparent discrepancy is likely due to different culture conditions, passage numbers, and growth factor additions used in these two studies, as well as to differences in the anti-α2β1 reagents used in the two studies. These two studies (25, 38) also described differences in the effects of anti-αvβ3 reagents on tube formation that are not consistent with several recent in vivo angiogenesis studies (42–44). In the study by Gamble et al., anti-αvβ3 was noted to enhance tube formation in fibrin gels but had no appreciable effects in type I collagen

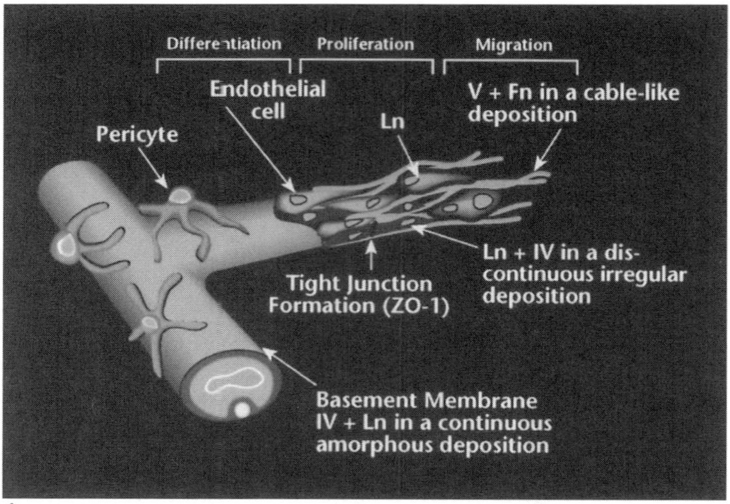

A

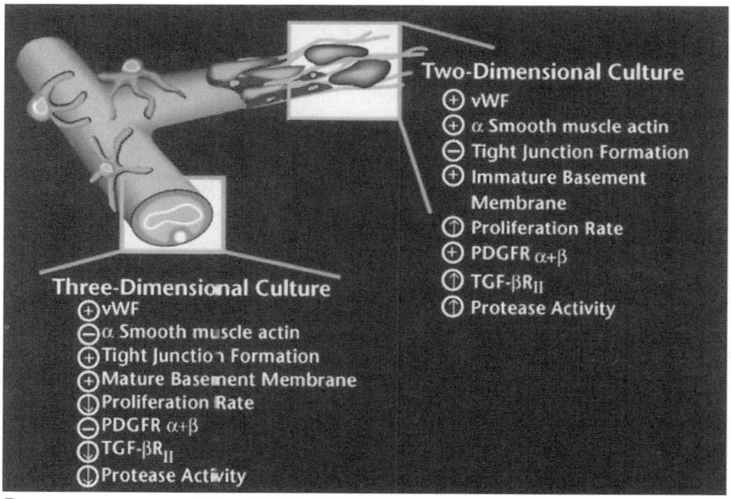

B

Figure 1 Schematic representation of extracellular matrix compositional and organizational changes during angiogenesis. **A**. Cells at the distal tip of the angiogenic sprout deposit and interact with an extracellular matrix having very different composition and organization compared to cells nearer the parent vessel. Cells at the distal tip express several features of undifferentiated EC, having high migratory, proteolytic, and proliferative rates, PDGF receptors, α smooth muscle actin, and a high TGFβ receptor type II to type I ratio. In contrast, cells nearer the parent vessel deposit and interact with a mature basement membrane and express several features of differentiated EC, having low migratory, proteolytic, and proliferative rates, tight junction formation, loss of both PDGFα and

gels. In the Davis and Camarillo study, anti-αvβ3 reagents had no effect on HUVEC lumen formation in type I collagen gels (25). In contrast, Brooks et al. have demonstrated significant inhibition of growth factor-stimulated (vascular endothelial growth factor [VEGF] and bFGF) in vivo angiogenesis by anti-αvβ3 and αvβ5 reagents (44). These apparent discrepancies might reflect differences between in vitro and in vivo models and the use of PMA in the in vitro models described. Thus, in spite of the incompleteness of our understanding of extracellular matrix modulation of angiogenesis, there is accruing evidence that extracellular matrix-mediated integrin engagement that initiates specific signaling pathways is an important modulator of angiogenesis.

The influences of extracellular matrix on the process of angiogenesis have been demonstrated using endothelial cells derived from several vascular beds. When RFC were cultured on the interstitial surface of amnion membranes, the cells invaded and migrated into the interstitial collagen matrix and formed tubelike structures with lumina, junctional complexes between cells, and abluminal deposition of morphologically identifiable basal lamina (45). In later studies these cells, dispersed in three-dimensional type I collagen gels, demonstrated multicellular aggregation followed by tube formation with lumina and tight junction formation at a baseline level in the absence of angiogenic factors, which was enhanced by the addition of angiogenic factors including bFGF, TGFβ1, TGFβ2 and endothelial cell growth factor (ECGF) (8, 46–48).

Bovine aortic endothelial cells (BAEC) have also been shown to form tubes in specific culture conditions. In these studies clonal populations of "sprouting" BAEC were observed to migrate beneath the monolayer of cells and to form tubelike structures, depositing type I collagen and displaying lumina (20, 49).

In both cases, (RFC and BAEC), the presence of cells in the three-dimensional environment has been associated with the morphological end point of tube formation and with dramatic changes in extracellular matrix synthetic profiles, protease/protease inhibitor profiles, and growth factor receptor expression and responsiveness (29, 34, 50, 51). Rat epididymal fat pad cell growth on type I collagen coatings in two-dimensional culture expresses PDGF receptors, exhibits PDGF responsiveness and exhibits an inhibition of proliferation and an extracellular matrix inductive effect in response to TGFβ1. In contrast, RFC cultured in three-dimensional type I collagen gels lose their PDGF receptor expression and

---

β receptors and α smooth muscle actin, and a low TGFβ receptor type II to type I ratio. **B**. Schematic representation of specific culture conditions which mimic the modulation of microvascular EC phenotypes during angiogenesis. Specific culture conditions mimic either EC at the distal tip of an angiogenic sprout (two-dimensional culture) or differentiated EC nearer the parent vessel (three-dimensional culture). *Abbreviations: EC*, endothelial cells; *PDGF*, platelet-derived growth factor; *TGF*, transforming growth factor; *V*, type V collagen; *Fn*, fibronectin; *Ln*, laminin; *IV*, type IV collagen.

responsiveness and exhibit a dramatic reduction in their expression of type II TGFβ receptor. This reduction is associated with a loss of TGFβ1-mediated inhibition of proliferation (34, 50). Placement of RFC in collagen gels also affects protease expression. Culture of RFC on collagen coatings resulted in no changes in expression of urokinase plasminogen activator (uPA) or plasminogen activator inhibitor (PAI)-1 after TGFβ1 treatment, while culture in collagen gels resulted in significant transient uPA and (PAI)-1 induction after TGFβ1 treatment, thought to be required for extracellular matrix remodeling during the early phases of angiogenesis (34). Changes in growth factor responsiveness have been documented in ''sprouting'' BAEC. In contrast to cobblestone BAEC, the tube-forming ''sprouting'' BAEC express PDGF receptors and exhibit both PDGF responsiveness and a proliferative response to TGFβ1 (49, 51). These studies illustrate the importance of extracellular matrix organization in modulating several aspects of the angiogenic response (Fig. 1).

IV. PECAM-1 PHOSPHORYLATION/DEPHOSPHORYLATION: A MODEL FOR EXTRACELLULAR MATRIX-DRIVEN, INTEGRIN-MEDIATED SIGNALING AFFECTING ENDOTHELIAL CELL BEHAVIOR

The roles and control of cell adhesion molecules during angiogenesis are an aspect of endothelial cell behavior that has received attention recently. Two members of this functional family appear early in vasculogenesis: vascular endothelial cadherin (VE cadherin) and platelet endothelial cell adhesion molecule-1 (PECAM-1/CD31) (52–57). These molecules are thought to be involved in the early phases of vessel formation, modulating the adhesive interactions of adjacent endothelial cell processes during tube formation (54, 58–60). Of these two molecules, PECAM-1's tyrosine phosphorylation state, cellular localization, and function are modulated by extracellular matrix-mediated integrin engagement (61). These recent studies have demonstrated that the tyrosine phosphorylation state of PECAM-1 is decreased transiently during in vitro endothelial cell spreading and migration on ECM components and during in vivo vasculogenesis in the murine conceptus (60, 61). In these studies phosphoamino acid analyses and Western blotting using antiphosphotyrosine antibodies showed that endothelial PECAM-1 is tyrosine phosphorylated and that the tyrosine phosphorylation was decreased after endothelial cell spreading and migration on extracellular matrix components but not on plastic. In addition, cell adhesion to anti-integrin antibodies similarly induced PECAM-1 dephosphorylation while concurrently inducing pp125FAK phosphorylation. The tyrosine phosphorylation state of PECAM-1 was found to be mediated by both kinase and phosphatase. The PECAM-1 cytoplasmic sequences flanking tyrosine residues 663 (Y_{663}TEV) and 686 (Y_{686}SEV) are selected for in phosphopeptides that bind to src-homology 2 domains of src family kinases and abl proto-oncogene (62), suggesting that both tyrosine 663 and 686 are potential phosphorylation sites. Furthermore both Y_{663} and Y_{686} were identified as phosphorylation sites by site-directed mutagenesis to phenylalanine. When expressed in 3T3 cells, both mutants (Y to F_{663} and Y to F_{686}) exhibited reduced PECAM-1 phosphorylation compared to 3T3 cells expressing wild-type PECAM. Additionally, F_{686} mutants showed a reversal of PECAM-1 mediated inhibition of 3T3 cell migration and did not localize PECAM-1 to cell borders. These data suggest that β1 integrin engagement signals PECAM-1 dephosphorylation and that this signaling pathway plays a role during endothelial cell migration (Fig. 2) (61, 63).

In our studies we have found that PECAM-1 was more highly phosphorylated in endothelial cells overexpressing c-src and, in in vitro kinase assays, purified c-src phosphorylated a glutathione-s-transferase (GST)-PECAM cytoplasmic tail fusion protein. We also found that the phosphorylated fusion protein did associate with agarose bead-bound c-src. This association appeared to be mediated by c-src-SH2 domain, as tyrosine phosphorylated PECAM-1 could be precipitated by a GST-src-SH2 affinity matrix. The binding to the GST-src-SH2 affinity matrix correlated directly with the level of PECAM-1 phosphorylation. Specifically, more PECAM-1 derived from c-src overexpressing endothelial cells (which is highly tyrosine phosphorylated) was bound to the SH2 affinity matrix than PECAM-1 derived from vector-only transfectants or kinase-negative c-src overexpressing cells (which are less tyrosine phosphorylated) (61, 64). Further, several as yet unidentified phosphoproteins could also be coimmunoprecipitated with wild-type but not with Y to F_{663} or F_{686} mutant PECAM-1 (65).

These data suggest that differential tyrosine phosphorylation of the PECAM-1 cytoplasmic domain could function as a binding site for adaptor proteins, kinases, and phosphatases in signaling cascades. Indeed, further analysis of the PECAM-1 cytoplasmic tail revealed that it resembles an immunoregulatory tyrosine-based activation motif (ITAM) domain, which has been identified in subunits of the T-cell receptor (TCR), B-cell receptor (BCR), Fc receptors, brain immunoglobulin TAM-like molecule (BIT), and natural killer-associated transcripts (NKATs) that function in signal transduction (66–69).

Consensus: **D**XXX-XXXX**D**XX**Y**XX**L**XXXXXXXXXXXXXXXXXXXXX**Y**XX**L**
E **E** **I** **I**
PECAM-1: **D**NKE-PLNS**D**VQ**Y**TE**V**QVSSAEWSHKDLGKKDTETV**Y**SE**V**
663 686

ITAM Consensus and PECAM-1 Sequences

The PECAM-1 ITAM domain may function in a similar manner to the other members of the ITAM family, becoming phosphorylated by a member of

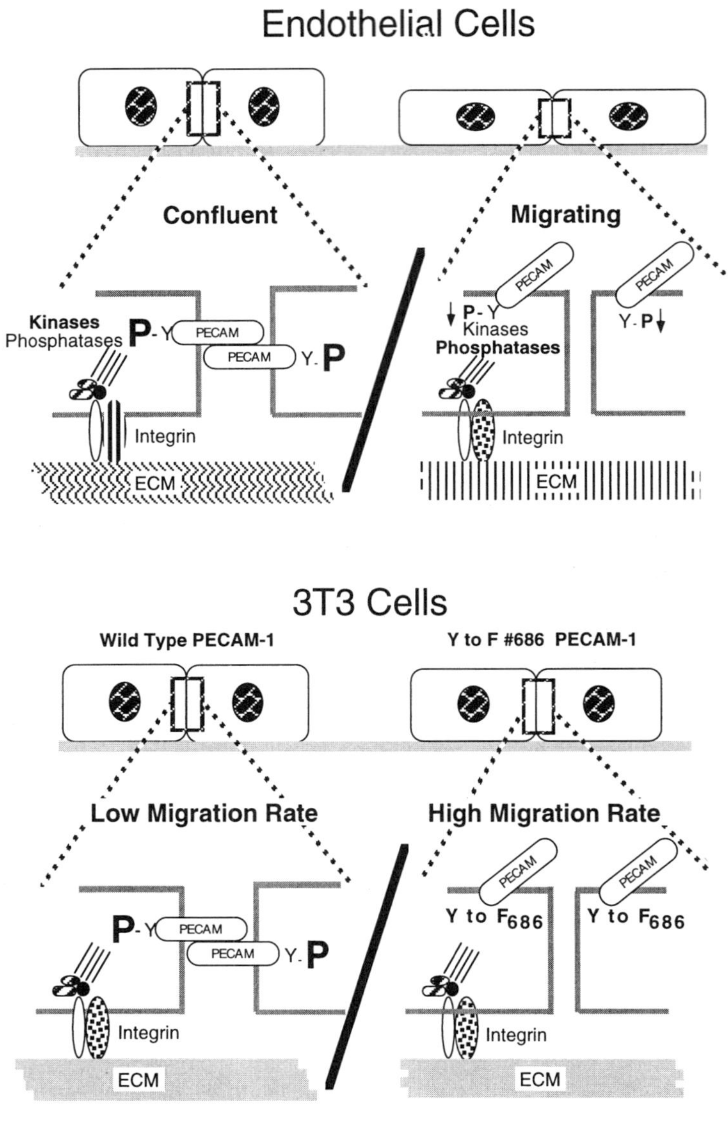

Figure 2 Schematic representation of the dynamic tyrosine phosphorylation/dephosphorylation of PECAM-1 in endothelial cells and 3T3 cells expressing PECAM-1 or a PECAM-1 Y to F_{686} mutation and correlations with migratory state of the cells.

Confluent cultures of endothelial cells exhibit a high level of PECAM-1 tyrosine phosphorylation, with PECAM-1 localized to areas of cell-cell contact along the cell periphery. In contrast, after a stimulus to migrate, endothelial cells exhibit a low level of PECAM-1 tyrosine phosphorylation, with PECAM-1 diffusely localized over the cell surface. Levels of PECAM-1 tyrosine phosphorylation are determined by modulation of kinase and phosphatase activities.

the src kinase family and subsequently bound by a member of the ZAP70/syk family or by other proteins containing single or tandem SH2 domains (61, 65). Thus, the PECAM-1 ITAM domain could serve as a functional branch point of an "outside to inside" signaling cascade, initiated extracellularly by the recognition of a particular extracellular matrix component by an integrin, which would then alter the PECAM-1 tyrosine phosphorylation state by modulating kinase/phosphatase ratios (65, 66, 69, 70). Conversely, the PECAM-1 ITAM domain may also function in an "outside to inside" signaling cascade generated extracellularly by PECAM-1–PECAM-1 engagement, affecting the PECAM-1 ITAM phosphorylation state, initiating a signaling cascade that results in changes in integrin affinity. Experiments using anti-PECAM-1 to ligate PECAM-1 have shown that integrin function can be affected (57, 69, 71, 72). In addition, using migration as a readout, we demonstrated that expression of a Y_{686} to F PECAM-1 construct in BAEC resulted in an increase in migratory rate. This finding is consistent with the notion that the Y_{686} to F PECAM-1 competes with endogenous PECAM-1 in adhesive interactions, thus decreasing "outside-in" signaling by blunting phosphorylation at Y_{686} and subsequent interactions with SH2-containing adaptor and signaling molecules, such as the phosphatase SHP-2 (73).

We have also demonstrated differential tyrosine phosphorylation of PECAM-1 during the formation of blood islands/vessels from clusters of extra-embryonic and embryonic angioblasts in the murine conceptus. We identified differential phosphorylation of tyrosine residue, Y_{686}, in the PECAM-1 cytoplasmic domain (60). In recent studies we demonstrated a correlation between a failure of this transient, dynamic PECAM-1 tyrosine dephosphorylation and arrest of the yolk sac vasculature at the primary capillary plexus stage (74). These findings suggest a pivotal role for PECAM-1 during vasculogenesis that is supported by data demonstrating a role for PECAM-1 in modulating in vitro and in vivo angiogenesis (58). These findings, taken together with knockout mouse studies illustrating critical roles for selected extracellular matrix components (fibronectin), integrin chains ($\alpha5$), and TGFβ1 in embryonic vascular development, suggest the possibility that extracellular matrix-induced integrin-mediated modu-

---

3T3 cells stably expressing wild type PECAM-1 exhibit an inhibition in their migration rate compared to sham-transfected cells. In these cells, PECAM-1 was localized to areas of cell-cell contact along the cell periphery. In contrast, 3T3 cells stably expressing a mutated form of PECAM-1 having a Y to F_{686} mutation that results in a loss of tyrosine phosphorylation, exhibit a high migration rate similar to sham-transfected cells. Furthermore, the mutated PECAM-1 expressed on the surface of these cells is localized diffusely over the cell surface in a pattern similar to that noted for PECAM-1 in migrating endothelial cells. Abbreviation: *PECAM*, platelet endothelial cell adhesion molecule; *ECM*, extracellular matrix.

lation of PECAM-1 tyrosine phosphorylation may be a mechanism by which these embryonic lethal knockouts cause maldevelopment and loss of integrity of the developing vascular system (9–11, 60). Additional studies investigating the cascades and specific proteins involved in extracellular matrix-driven, integrin-mediated PECAM-1 signaling during embryonic vascular development and during large vessel repair and angiogenesis during wound healing will lead to a better understanding of the roles of this molecule in vasculogenesis and angiogenesis.

V. CONTROLLED INVOLUTION AND STABILIZATION OF THE MICROVASCULATURE OF THE GERMINAL MATRIX: THE ROLES OF EXTRACELLULAR MATRIX SYNTHESIS AND ORGANIZATION

The roles of the extracellular matrix in the dynamic regulation of vasculogenesis and angiogenesis are complex. This is well illustrated during brain development (75, 76). Microvascular beds in the brain (as well as other organs and tissues) undergo selective angiogenesis, stabilization, and involution in a tightly regulated fashion (77–79). One particular microvascular bed in which this process is noted is the germinal matrix, a periventricular area from which there is controlled neuronal and glial emigration during development (80–83). During development, the microvascular density is reduced over an extended period, coinciding with the neuronal and glial emigrations and involution of the germinal matrix (84, 85). This controlled vascular involution occurs rapidly after premature delivery and is thought to be a cause of perinatal and early postnatal intraventricular and parenchymal hemorrhage observed in the premature newborn population (81, 86, 87). Animal models of perinatal and early postnatal intraventricular and parenchymal hemorrhage that mimic the human condition have been used to study the roles of extracellular matrix in this process (88–91). Using a beagle pup model, we have found that the period of the highest incidence of intraventricular and parenchymal hemorrhage correlated with a morphologically indistinct and immature vascular basement membrane surrounding the germinal matrix microvessels, few tight junctions, and incomplete astrocytic investiture of the microvessels (81, 86). In the surviving animals, the incidence of intraventricular and parenchymal hemorrhage was noted to decrease over postnatal days 4 to 10. This decrease in hemorrhages correlated with an increased abluminal deposition of basement membrane components, which was followed by increased formation of tight junctions and complete investiture of the surviving vessels by astrocytic endfeet (92) (Fig. 3). These data suggest that the deposition and organization of extracellular matrix components is a prerequisite for, and stimulates the formation of, endothelial cell tight junctions and astrocytic endfeet investiture of the microvessels, forming a competent blood-brain barrier (Fig. 4). The inductive mechanisms and

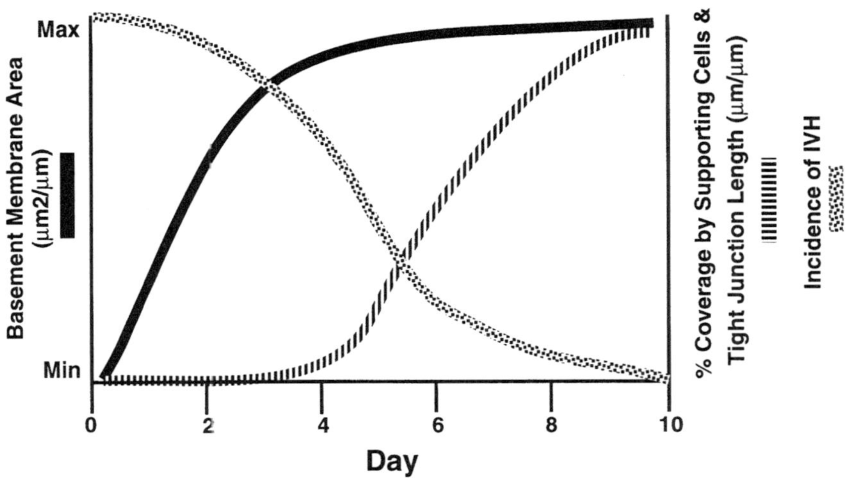

Figure 3 Schematic representation of the temporal relationships of the incidence of intraventricular and parenchymal hemorrhage (*speckled line*), the appearance of basement membrane (*solid line*), and tight junctional complexes and coverage of germinal matrix microvessel abluminal areas by supporting astrocytic cell processes (*hatched line*) from postnatal days 1 to 10.

signal transduction cascades involved in this process are currently unknown; however, treatment of the beagle pups with indomethicin induced a more rapid appearance of basement membrane components that correlated with a reduction in the incidence of intraventricular and parenchymal hemorrhage (87). These data suggest that extracellular matrix deposition and organization elicits endothelial cell tight junction formation and astrocytic endfoot investiture, leading to a stabilized vascular bed resistant to rupture.

Although necessary and useful, animal models are difficult to manipulate and by necessity result in the sacrifice of many animals. Thus, development of in vitro models mimicking the in vivo situation are desirable. To this end we have developed an in vitro culture model using microvascular endothelial cells isolated from beagle pup germinal matrix cultured in three-dimensional type I collagen gels (93, 94). These cells exhibited increased basement membrane component synthesis, decreased proteolytic activity, and robust tube formation compared to standard two-dimensional cultures. Coculture of these microvascular endothelial cells and newborn rat type II astrocytes resulted in endothelial tube formation mimicking in vivo tube formation and stabilization with abluminal basement membrane deposition and astrocytic process investiture of the tubes, mimicking the in vivo process of blood-brain barrier formation (Fig. 5). Further,

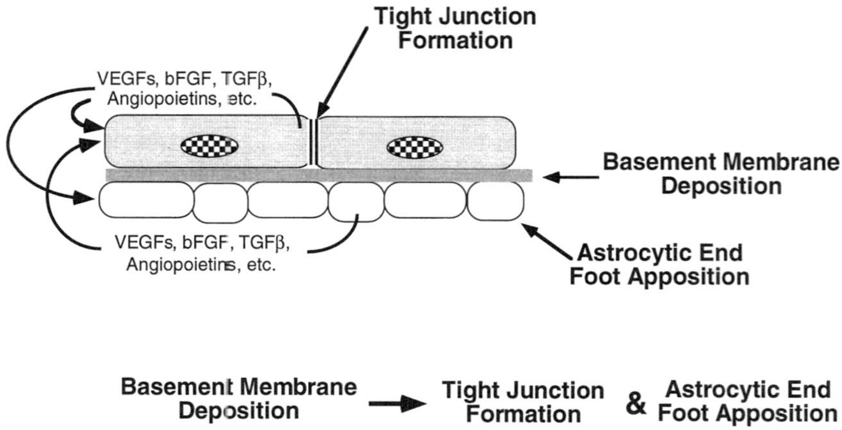

Figure 4 Schematic representation of the development of vascular integrity of the neuronal microvasculature illustrating the initiation of tight junction formation and astrocytic endfoot investiture by deposition and organization of the basement membrane and potential paracrine interactions between the endothelial and supporting astrocytic cells. *Abbreviations*: *VEGF*, vascular endothelial growth factor; *bFGF*, basic fibroblast growth factor; *TGF*, transforming growth factor.

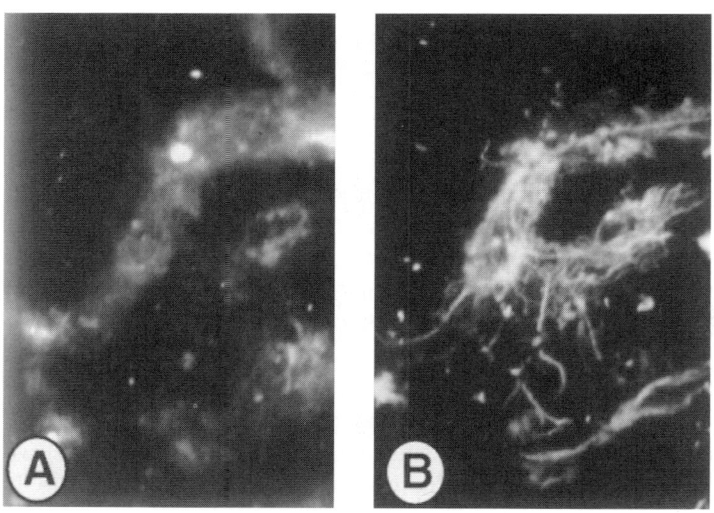

Figure 5 Double-label immunofluorescence micrographs of a three-dimensional coculture of astrocytes with brain microvascular endothelial cells. Scale bar = 50 μm. Original magnification = 400x. **A**. Representative field of the coculture stained with fluorescein conjugated Bandeiraea lectin illustrating diffusely stained branching, tubelike structures. **B**. The same representative field of the coculture stained with antibodies directed against glial fibrillated acid protein and detected with a rhodamine- conjugated secondary antibody illustrating the investiture of segments of the tubelike structures by astrocyte processes. The astrocyte processes are in intimate contact with endothelial cells that have formed tubes.

the endothelial and astrocytic cells comprising these cocultures exhibit mutual paracrine modulation as evidenced by the modulation of both endothelial and astrocytic uPA, mediated by the close presence and interaction of the two cell types in coculture.

VI. EXTRACELLULAR MATRIX AS A MODULATOR OF APOPTOSIS

During brain development the germinal matrix microvascular bed undergoes significant involution (86). There is selective concurrent stabilization and involution of individual vessels in this vascular bed. As discussed above, the synthesis and deposition of vascular basement membrane plays an important role in the stabilization process, driving increased tight junction formation and astrocytic endfoot investiture. Just as important is the process of selective vessel involution. Morphological studies in the beagle pup revealed that the immature germinal matrix vessels (and possibly those vessels destined to undergo involution) exhibit an incomplete investiture by basement membrane and astrocytic endfeet, suggesting a relationship between the presence of astrocytic endfeet, protease levels and basement membrane, and vessel stabilization (81). In vitro studies in which germinal matrix microvascular endothelial cells and astrocytes were cocultured in three-dimensional type I collagen gels are consistent with this notion, as uPA levels were decreased compared to monocultures of endothelial cells (93). These data, and the findings of Cheresh et al. (42–44), suggest that the presence, composition, and physical state of the surrounding extracellular matrix determine endothelial cell adhesive properties, which, in turn, determine apoptotic state of the endothelial cells (Fig. 6).

Data accrued from in vivo and in vitro models showed the importance of soluble factors—VEGF in particular—as modulators of cell survival and the importance of interactions between the extracellular matrix and soluble factors in determining endothelial cell behavior (Fig. 4). Using in vivo models, investigators found that VEGF expression is detectable around stable, quiescent microvessel endothelial cells (93); VEGF expression was found to be decreased during physiological blood vessel regression (95); and VEGF withdrawal resulted in vessel regression (96–98). Using an in vitro model of microvessel formation and stabilization, we have demonstrated that even in the presence of a permissive three-dimensional matrix of native type I collagen and a subendothelial extracellular matrix composed of type IV collagen and laminin, endothelial cells that have been stimulated to form capillary structures require the continued presence of VEGF for survival (99). These studies underscore the importance of the complex interrelationships between the signaling cascades initiated by specific receptors whose engagement is modulated by the composition and organization of the

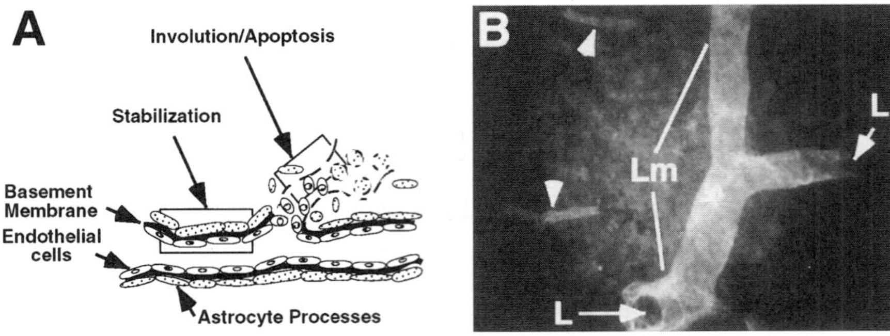

Figure 6 A. Schematic representation of the specific, controlled stabilization and involution/apoptosis of the germinal matrix vasculature during development, resulting in significant reduction in vessel density with the surviving vessels becoming the lenticulostriate vessels. Involution/apoptosis: changes or loss of astrocytic or endothelial cell factors or receptors lead to loss of basement membrane structure and integrity (decreased synthesis/increased proteolysis), which leads to loss of endothelial cell adhesion and apoptosis. Stabilization: formation and stabilization of the basement membrane maintains endothelial cell adhesion, tight junction formation, and astrocytic investiture leading to and maintaining formation of the blood-brain barrier. **B**. Immunofluorescence micrograph (60 μ section) of postnatal day 10 beagle pup germinal matrix illustrating a mature, stabilized vessel segment stained positively for laminin 1 and two smaller, atretic, involuting vessel segments also exhibiting residual laminin staining. *L*, lumen; *Lm*, abluminal laminin staining; *arrows*, involuting vessel segments; *arrowheads*, atretic, involuting vessel segments.

extracellular matrix and the composition and concentrations of soluble factors in blood vessel formation, survival, and involution (99–101) (Fig. 6).

These ongoing studies illustrate the importance, complexity, and interrelationships of cell-matrix, cell-cell, and cell-soluble factor interactions in the regulation of angiogenesis.

VII. CONCLUSIONS

As discussed throughout this chapter, the extracellular matrix has many in vivo and in vitro functions. The use of extracellular matrix preparations has enhanced our ability to culture microvascular endothelial cells from a variety of vascular beds. Extracellular matrix preparations are useful in modulating endothelial cell phenotype and allowing the mimicking of in vivo behavior in defined culture conditions. Extracellular matrix components and mixtures also have aided in the investigation and elucidation of a variety of signaling pathways operational in regulating endothelial cell proliferation, adhesion, spreading, migration, and activation. Further, natural and engineered matrices are playing an increasingly important role in the continued development of artificial blood vessels and endothelial cell-based gene delivery systems. The central importance of the extracellular matrix in the process of angiogenesis also is evident in several of the following chapters in this volume.

REFERENCES

1. Madri JA. The extracellular matrix as a modulator of neovascularization. In: Gallo LL, ed. Cardiovascular Disease: Molecular and Cellular Mechanisms, Prevention, Treatment. New York: Plenum Press, 1987:177–184.
2. Madri JA, Pratt BM. Angiogenesis. In: Clark RF and Henson P, eds. Angiogenesis. New York: Plenum Press, 1988:337–358.
3. Madri JA, Pratt BM, Yannariello-Brown J. Endothelial Cell Extracellular Matrix Interactions: Matrix as a modulator of cell function. In: Simionescu N, Simionescu M, eds. Endothelial Cell Biology in Health and Disease. New York: Plenum Press, 1988:167–188.
4. Madri JA, Sankar S, Romanic AM. Angiogenesis. In: Clark R, ed. Angiogenesis. New York: Plenum Press, 1995:355–371.
5. Nicosia RF, Madri JA. The microvascular extracellular matrix: Developmental changes during angiogenesis in the aortic ring plasma clot model. Am J Pathol 1987;128:78–90.
6. Nicosia RF, Tuszynski GP. Matrix-bound thrombospondin promotes angiogenesis in vitro. J Cell Biol 1994;124:183–193.
7. Madri JA, Williams SK. Capillary endothelial cell cultures: Phenotypic modulation by matrix components. J Cell Biol 1983;97:153–165.
8. Madri JA, Pratt BM, Tucker AM. Phenotypic modulation of endothelial cells by transforming growth factor β depends upon the composition and organization of the extracellular matrix. J Cell Biol 1988;106:1375–1384.
9. Dickson MC, Martin JS, Cousins FM, Kulkarni AB, Karlsson S, Akhurst RJ. Defective haematopoiesis and vasculogenesis in transforming growth factor-1 knock out mice. Development 1995;121:1845–1854.
10. George EL, Georges EN, Patel-King RS, Rayburn H, Hynes RO. Defects in mesodermal migration and vascular development in fibronectin-deficient mice. Development 1993;119:1079–1091.
11. Yang JT, Rayburn H, Hynes RO. Embryonic mesodermal defects in α5 integrin-deficient mice. Development 1993;119:1093–1105.
12. Maciag T, Kadish J, Wilkins L, Stemerman MB, Weinstein R. Organizational behavior of human umbilical vein endothelial cells. J Cell Biol 1982;94:511–520.
13. Vernon RB, Sage EH. Between molecules and morphology: Extracellular matrix and creation of vascular form. Am J Pathol 1995;147:873–883.

14. Folkman J, Haudenschild C. Angiogenesis in vitro. Nature 1980;288:551–556.
15. Ingber DE, Madri JA, Folkman J. Endothelial growth factors and extracellular matrix regulate DNA synthesis through modulation of cell and nuclear shape. In Vitro Cell Dev Biol 1987;23:387–394.
16. Ingber D, Folkman J. How does extracellular matrix control capillary morphogenesis? Cell 1989;58:803–805.
17. Ingber DE, Folkman J. Mechanochemical switching between growth and differentiation during fibroblast growth factor stimulated angiogenesis in vitro: Role of extracellular matrix. J Cell Biol 1989;109:317–330.
18. Ingber DE. Fibronectin controls capillary endothelial cell growth by modulating cell shape. Proc Natl Acad Sci U S A 1990;87:3579–3583.
19. Ingber DE, Prusty D, Frangioni JV, Crague EJ, Lechene C, Schwartz M. Control of intracellular pH and growth by fibronectin in capillary endothelial cells. J Cell Biol 1990;110:1803–1811.
20. Iruela-Arispe ML, Hasselaar P, Sage H. Differential expression of extracellular proteins is correlated with angiogenesis in vitro. Lab Invest 1991;64:174–186.
21. Iruela-Arispe ML, Porter P, Bornstein P, Sage EH. Thrombospondin-1 an inhibitor of angiogenesis is regulated by progesterone in the human endometrium. J Clin Invest 1996;97:403–412.
22. Dejana E, Colella S, Languino LR, Balconi G, Corbascio GC, Marchisio PC. Fibrinogen induces adhesion, spreading, and microfilament organization of human endothelial cells in vitro. J Cell Biol 1987;104:1403–1411.
23. Dejana E, Colella S, Conforti G, Abbadini M, Gaboli M, Marchisio PC. Fibronectin and vitronectin regulate the organization of their respective Arg-Gly-Asp adhesion receptors in cultured human endothelial cells. J Cell Biol 1988;107:1215–1223.
24. Davis GE, Camarillo CW. Regulation of endothelial cell morphogenesis by integrins, mechanical forces and matrix guidance pathways. Exp Cell Res 1995;216: 113–123.
25. Davis GE, Camarillo CW. An alpha2 beta1 integrin dependent pinocytic mechanism involving intracellular vacuole formation and coalescence regulates capillary lumen and tube formation in three-dimensional collagen matrix. Exp Cell Res 1996; 224:39–51.
26. Form DM, Pratt BM, Madri JA. Endothelial cell proliferation during angiogenesis: In vitro modulation by basement membrane components. Lab Invest 1986;55:521–530.
27. Sage EH, Vernon, RB. Regulation of angiogenesis by extracellular matrix: The growth and the glue. J Hypertens 1994;12:S145–S152.
28. Nicosia RF, Madri JA. The extracellular matrix produced during angiogenesis in culture. In: Gallo LL, ed. Cardiovascular Disease: Molecular and Cellular Mechanisms, Prevention, Treatment. New York: Plenum Press, 1987:185–192.
29. Madri JA, Marx M. Matrix composition, organization and soluble factors: Modulators of microvascular cell differentiation in vitro. Kidney Int 1992;41:560–565.
30. Lane TF, Iruela-Arispe ML, Johnson RS, Sage EH. SPARC is a source of copper-binding peptides that stimulate angiogenesis. J Cell Biol 1994;125:929–943.
31. Schwartz MA, Lechene C, Ingber DE. Insoluble fibronectin activates the Na/H antiporter by clustering and immobilizing integrin $\alpha 5\beta 1$, independent of cell shape. Proc Natl Acad Sci U S A 1991;88:7849–7853.

32. Schwartz MA. Spreading of human endothelial cells on fibronectin or vitronectin triggers elevation of intracellular free calcium. J Cell Biol 1993;120:1003–1010.
33. Madri JA, Pratt BM, Yannariello-Brown J. Matrix driven cell size changes modulate aortic endothelial cell proliferation and sheet migration. Am J Pathol 1988; 132:18–27.
34. Sankar S, Mahooti-Brooks N, Bensen L, Centrella M, McCarthy TL, Madri JA. Modulation of transforming growth factor beta receptor expression in microvascular endothelial cells during in vitro angiogenesis. J Clin Invest 1996;97:1436–1446.
35. Grant DS, Iashiro KI, Segui-Real B, Yamada Y, Martin GR, Kleinman HK. Two different laminin domains mediate the differentiation of human endothelial cells into capillary-like structures in vitro. Cell 1989;58:933–943.
36. Carley W, Milici AJ, Madri JA. Extracellular matrix specificity for the differentiation of capillary endothelial cells. Exp Cell Res 1988;178: 426–434.
37. Streuli CH, Bailey N, Bissell MJ. Control of mammary epithelial differentiation: Basement membrane induces tissue-specific gene expression in the absence of cell-cell interaction and morphological polarity. J Cell Biol 1991;115:1383–1395.
38. Gamble JR, Mathias LJ, Meyer G, Kain P, Russ G, Faul R. Regulation of in vitro capillary tube formation by anti-integrin antibodies. J Cell Biol 1993;121:931–943.
39. Montesano R, Orci L. Tumor-promoting phorbol esters induce angiogenesis in vitro. Cell 1985;42:469–477.
40. Montesano R, Vassali JD, Baird A, Guillemin R Orci L. Basic fibroblast growth factor induces angiogenesis in vitro. Proc Natl Acad Sci U S A. 1986;83:7297–7301.
41. Montesano R, Orci L. Phorbol esters induce angiogenesis in vitro from large vessel endothelial cells. J Cell Physiol 1987;130:284–291.
42. Brooks PC, Montgomery AMP, Rosenfeld M, Reisfeld RA, Hu T, Klier G, Cheresh DA. Integrin alpha v beta 3 antagonists promote tumor regression by inducing apoptosis of angiogenic blood vessels. Cell 1994;79:1157–1164.
43. Brooks PC, Clark RAF, Cheresh DA. Requirement of vascular integrin alpha V, beta 3 for angiogenesis. Science 1994;264:569–571.
44. Friedlander M, Brooks PC, Shaffer RW, Kinkaid CM. Definition of two angiogenic pathways by distinct alpha V intergrins. Science 1995;270:1500–1502.
45. Madri JA, Williams SK. Capillary endothelial cell cultures: Phenotypic modulation by matrix components. J Cell Biol 1983;97:153–165.
46. Merwin JR, Anderson J, Kocher O, van Itallie C, Madri JA. Transforming growth factor β1 modulates extracellular matrix organization and cell-cell junctional complex formation during in vitro angiogenesis. J Cell Physiol 1990;142:117–128.
47. Merwin JR, Newman W, Beall D, Tucker A, Madri JA. Vascular cells respond differentially to transforming growth factors-$beta_1$ $beta_2$. Am J Pathol 1991;138: 37–51.
48. Merwin JR, Tucker A, Roberts A, Kondaiah P, Madri JA. Vascular cell responses to transforming growth factor $beta_3$ mimic those of transforming growth factor $beta_1$ in vitro. Growth Factors 1991;5:149–158.
49. Battegay EJ, Rupp J, Iruela-Arispe L, Sage EH, Pech M. PDGF-BB modulates endothelial proliferation and angiogenesis in vitro via PDGF beta-receptors. J Cell Biol 1944;125:917–928.
50. Marx M, Perlmutter R, Madri JA. Modulation of PDGF-receptor expression in mi-

crovascular endothelial cells during in vitro angiogenesis. J Clin Invest 1994;93: 131–139.
51. Iruela-Arispe ML, Sage EH. Endothelial cells exhibiting angiogenesis in vitro proliferate in response to TGF-beta 1. J Cell Biochem 1993;52:414–430.
52. Risau W, Flamme, I. Vasculogenesis. Annu Rev Cell Dev Biol 1995;11:73–91.
53. Navarro P, Caveda L, Breviario F, Mandoteanu I, Lampugnani MG, Dejana E. Catenin-dependent and -independent functions of vascular endothelial cadherin. J Biol Chem 1995,270:30965–30972.
54. Vittet D, Prandini MH, Berthier R, Schweitzer A, Martin-Sisteron A, Uzan G, Dejana E. Embryonic stem cells differentiate in vitro to endothelial cells through successive maturation steps. Blood 1996;88:3424–3431.
55. Albelda SM, Daise M, Levine EM, Buck CA. Identification and characterization of cell-substratum adhesion receptors on cultured human endothelial cells. J Clin Invest 1989;83:1992–2002.
56. Albelda SM, Oliver PD, Romer LH, Buck CA. EndoCAM: A novel endothlial cell-cell adhesion molecule. J Cell Biol 1990;110:1227–1237.
57. Newman PJ. The biology of PECAM-1. J Clin Invest 1997;99:3–8.
58. DeLisser HM, Christofidou-Solomidou M, Strieter RM, Burdick MD, Robinson C, Wexler R, Merwin JR, Madri JA, Albelda SM. Involvement of endothelial PECAM-1/CD31 in angiogenesis. Am J Pathol 1997;151:671–677.
59. Madri JA, Bell L, Merwin JR. Modulation of vascular cell behavior by transforming growth factors beta. Mol Reprod Dev 1992;32:121–126.
60. Pinter E, Barreuther M, Lu T, Madri JA. PECAM-1/CD31 tyrosine phosphorylation state changes during vasculogenesis in the murine conceptus. Am J Pathol 1997; 150:1523–1530.
61. Lu TT, Yan LG. Madri JA. Integrin engagement mediates tyrosine dephosphorylation on platelet-endothelial cell adhesion molecule-1 (PECAM-1). Proc Natl Acad Sci U S A 1996;93:11808–11813.
62. Songyang Z, Shoelson SE, Chaudhuri M, Gish G, Pawson T, Haser WG, King F, Roberts T, Ratnofsky S, Lechleider RJ, Neel BG, Birge RB, Fajardo JE, Chou MM, Hanafusa H, Schaffhausen B, Cantley LC. SH2 domains recognize specific phosphopeptide sequences. Cell 1993;72:767–778.
63. Schimmenti L, Yan HC, Madri JA, Albelda S. Platelet endothelial cell adhesion molecule PECAM-1 modulates cell migration. J Cell Physiol 1992;153:417–428.
64. Bell L, Luthringer DJ, Madri JA, Warren SL. Autocrine angiotensin system regulation of bovine aortic endothelial cell migration and plasminogen activator involves modulation of proto-oncogene pp60c-src expression. J Clin Invest 1992;89:315–320.
65. Lu T, Barreuther M, Davis S, Madri JA. Platelet endothelial cell adhesion molecule-1 (PECAM-1/CD31) is phosphorylatable by c-src, binds src-SH2 domain and exhibits ITAM-like properties. J Biol Chem 1997;272:14442–14446.
66. Cambier J. Antigen and Fc receptor signaling: The awesome power of the immunoreceptor tyrosine-based activation motif (ITAM). J Immunol 1996;155:3282–3285.
67. Colonna M, Samaridis J. Cloning of immunoglobulin-superfamily members associated with HLA-C and HLA-B recognition by human natural killer cells. Science 1995;268:405–408.

68. Ohnishi H, Kubota M, Ohtake A, Sato K, Sano S. Activation of protein-tyrosine phosphatase SH-PTP2 by a tyrosine-based activation motif of a novel brain molecule. J Biol Chem 1996;271:25569–25574.
69. Weiss A. T cell antigen receptor signal transduction: A tale of tails and cytoplasmic protein-tyrosine kinases. Cell 1993;73:209–212.
70. Chan AC, Desai DM, Weiss A. The role of protein tyrosine kinases and protein tyrosine phosphatases in T cell antigen receptor signal transduction. Annu Rev Immunol 1994;12:555–592.
71. Tanaka Y, Albelda SM, Horgan KJ, Seventer GAv, Shimizu Y, Newman W, Hallam J, Newman PJ, Buck CA, Shaw S. CD31 expressed on distinctive T cell subsets is a preferential amplifier of B1 integrin-mediated adhesion. J Exp Med 1992;176: 245–253.
72. Berman ME, Xie Y, Muller W. Roles of platelet/endothelial cell adhesion molecule-1 (PECAM-1, CD31) in natural killer cell transendothelial migration and beta 2 integrin activation. J Immunol 1996;156:1515–1524.
73. Kim CS, Wang T, Madri JA. PECAM-1 expression modulates endothelial cell migration in vitro Lab Invest 1998;78:583–590.
74. Pinter E, Mahooti S, Wang Y, Imhof BA, Madri JA. Hyperglycemia-induced vasculopathy in the murine vitelline vasculature: Correlation with PECAM-1/CD31 tyrosine phosphorylation state. Am J Pathol 1999, in press.
75. DeReuch J. The human periventicular arterial blood supply and the anatomy of cerebral infarctions. Eur Neurol 1971;5:321–324.
76. Risau W. Molecular biology of blood-brain barrier ontogenesis and function. Acta Neurochir 1994;60:109–112.
77. Pepper MS, Belin D, Montesano R, Orci L, Vassali JD. Transforming growth factor β-1 modulates basic fibroblast growth factor-induced proteolytic and angiogenic properties of endothelial cells in vitro. J Cell Biol 1990;111:743–755.
78. Pepper MS, Montesano R. Proteolytic balance and capillary morphogenesis. Cell Differentiation and Development 1990;32:319–328.
79. Pepper MS, Vassali JD, Orci L, Montesano R. Biphasic effect of TGF-beta 1 on in vitro angiogenesis. Exp Cell Res 1993;204:356–363.
80. Ment LR, Stewart WB, Ardito TA, Madri JA. Vascular basement membrane remodeling during germinal matrix maturation in the neonate: Associations with interventricular hemmorhage in the beagle pup model. Stroke 1991;22:390–395.
81. Ment LR, Stewart WB, Ardito TA, Madri MA. Germinal matrix microvascular maturation correlates inversely with the risk period for neonatal intraventicular hemorrhage. Dev Brain Res 1995;84:142–149.
82. Ment LR, Oh W, Ehrenkranz RA, Philip AGS, Schneider K, Katz KH, Taylor KJW, Duncan CC, Makuch RW. Risk period for intraventricular hemorrhage of the preterm neonate is independent of gestational age. Semin Perinatol 1993;17: 338–341.
83. Rorke LB, Pathology of Perinatal Brain Injury. New York: Raven Press, 1982.
84. Grunnet MRL. Morphometry of blood vessels in the cortex and germinal plate of premature neonates. Pediatr Neurol 1989;5:12–16.
85. Povlishock J, Martinez A, Moosy J. The fine structure of blood vessels in the telencephalic germinal matrix in the human fetus. Am J Anat 1977;149:439–452.

86. Ment LR, Stewart WB, Ardito TA, Madri JA. Beagle pup germinal matrix maturation studies. Stroke 1991;22:390–395.
87. Ment LR, Stewart WB, Ardito TA, Huang E, Madri JA. Indomethacin promotes germinal matrix microvessel maturation in the newborn beagle pup. Stroke 1992; 23:1132–1137.
88. Goddard J, Lewis RM, Alcala H, Zeller RS. Intraventicular hemorrhage, an animal model. Biol Neonate 1980;37:39–42.
89. Pasternak JF, Groothuis DR, Fischer JM. Regional cerebral blood flow in the newborn beagle pup: The germinal matrix is a ''low-flow'' structure. Pediatr Res 1982; 7:3–12.
90. Trommer BL, Groothuis DR, Pasternak JF. Quantitative analysis of cerebral vessels in the newborn puppy: The structure of germinal matrix vessels may predispose to hemorrhage. Pediatr Res 1987;22:23–28.
91. Leuschen MP, Shulman RM, Nelson RM. The development of capillaries in the telencephalon of beagle puppies. Anat Rec 1984;208:435–443.
92. Tontsch U, Bauer HC. Glial cells and neurons induce blood-brain barrier related enzymes in cultured cerebral endothelial cells. Brain Res 1990;539:247–253.
93. Ment LR, Stewart WB, Scaramuzzino D, Duncan CC, Madri JA. Germinal matrix microvascular maturation—An in vitro model. In Vitro Cell Dev Biol 1997;33: 684–691.
94. Ment LR, Stewart WB, Fron R, Seashore C, Mahooti S, Scaramuzzino D, Madri JA. Vascular endothelial growth factor mediates reactive angiogenesis in the developing neonatal brain. Dev Brain Res 1997;100:52–61.
95. Takahashi T, Shibuya M. The 230 kDa form of KDR/Flk-1 (VEGF receptor-2) activates the PLC- pathway and partially induces mitotic signals in NIH/3T3 fibroblasts. Oncogene 1997;14:2079–2089.
96. Yuan F, Chen Y, Dellial M, Safabakhsh N, Ferrara N, Jain RK. Time-dependent vascular regression and permeability changes in established human tumor xenografts induced by an anti-vascular endothelial growth factor/vascular permeability factor antibodies. Proc Natl Acad Sci U S A 1996;93:14765–14770.
97. Benjamin LE, Keshet E. Conditional switching of vascular endothelial growth factor (VEGF) expression in tumors: Induction of endothelial cell shedding and regression of hemangioblastoma-like vessels by VEGF withdrawal. Proc Natl Acad Sci U S A 1997;94:8761–8766.
98. Alon T, Hemo I, Itin A, Peer J, Stone J, Keshet E. Vascular endothelial growth factor acts as a survival factor for newly formed retinal vessels and has implications for retinopathy of prematurity. Nat Med 1995;1:1024–1028.
99. Ilan N, Mahooti S, Madri JA. Distinct signal transduction pathways are utilized during the tube formation and survival phases of in vitro angiogenesis. J Cell Sci 1998;111:3621–3631.
100. Haas TL, Davis S, Madri JA. Three dimensional type I collagen lattices induce coordinate expression of matrix metalloproteinases MT1-MMP and MMP-2 in microvascular endothelial cells. J Biol Chem 1998;273:3604–3610.
101. Woodard AS, Garcia-Cardena G, Leong M, Madri JA, Sessa WC, Languino LR. Synergistic activity of the $\alpha v\beta 3$ integrin and the PDGF receptor in microvascular endothelial cells. J Cell Sci 1998;111:469–478.

3

Matrix Metalloproteinases (Matrixins) and Their Inhibitors (TIMPs) in Angiogenesis

Teresa A. Bennett and William G. Stetler-Stevenson
National Cancer Institute, National Institutes of Health, Bethesda, Maryland

I. INTRODUCTION

Angiogenesis is essential for physiological processes such as fetal development and wound healing; however, it also contributes to the evolution of several diseases. The contribution of new vessel formation to the disease may be primary, as in diabetic retinopathy, hemangioma, or Kaposi's sarcoma, or secondary as in rheumatoid arthritis, psoriasis, epithelial malignancies, and cancer metastasis (Folkman and Shing, 1992; Folkman, 1995). Our current view of angiogenesis is that of a balance between positive angiogenic signals and endogenous inhibitors (Folkman, 1997). This stems from the observations that de novo blood vessel formation can be initiated in vivo by the local administration of an exogenous angiogenic factor but is followed by rapid involution after the discontinuation of the angiogenic stimulus. Thus, the sustained angiogenic response associated with many pathological states probably involves both the prolonged release of potent angiogenic stimuli, as well as the removal or down-regulation of antiangiogenic effectors.

Remodeling of the extracellular matrix (ECM) is a prerequisite for the formation of new blood vessels. This involves initial breakdown of the subendothelial basement membrane, as well as turnover of the interstitial matrix during new vessel outgrowth. This proteolytic modification removes the physical barrier (i.e., basement membrane) and prepares a substrate that may stimulate endothelial cell migration. In addition, the action of these proteinases may remove local angiogenesis inhibitors, release angiogenic factors from ECM binding sites, and generate new soluble angiogenesis inhibitors. However, remodeling of the ECM is also a tightly regulated process that is the balance of positive effectors (proteinases) and negative regulators (proteinase inhibitors) (Liotta et al., 1991).

Functional analysis of in vitro and in vivo angiogenesis models has clearly demonstrated the requirement of proteolytic activities in this process. These studies have identified serine proteinases, metalloproteinases, and cysteine proteinases in this process, but what is not clear is the relative contributions of various classes of ECM-degrading proteinases to the overall process. This is certainly due to the interdependence of these different proteinase systems during the complex cellular events involved in cell invasion, migration, and proliferation. In this respect the process of angiogenesis shows several functional similarities to the process of tumor cell invasion. These include demonstration of a specific role for integrin-mediated cell attachment during migration and the requirement of proteolytic remodeling of the ECM. The matrix metalloproteinase (MMP) family has been implicated in both angiogenesis and tumor cell invasion. The contribution of serine proteinases to the process of angiogenesis is reviewed separately.

II. MATRIXIN FAMILY OF PROTEINASES

The MMP, now known as the Matrixins, are a family of zinc atom-dependent, neutral pH optima endopeptidases, active in the extracellular compartment (Birkedal-Hansen, et al., 1993; Ray and Stetler-Stevenson, 1994a). They may be secreted and soluble, cell-surface associated, or membrane type (MT) containing a transmembrane domain. The MMPs were first described in 1967 with the isolation of interstitial collagenase (Jeffrey and Gross, 1967). Shortly thereafter several groups showed that neoplastic transformation was accompanied by a significant increase in the expression of degradative enzymes, including collagenase (Taylor, et al., 1970; Dresden, et al., 1972). A second MMP active in degrading the type IV collagen of basal lamina was isolated from metastatic sarcoma cells (Liotta, et al., 1980; Liotta, et al., 1981). The human Matrixin family is now known to include at least 16 enzymes, which collectively are capable of degrading all components of the ECM (Table 1). Many of these enzymes were originally identified because they were overexpressed in tumor cells or tumor tissue extracts. However, the MMPs are not tumor specific but are expressed at low levels in a number of physiological conditions, such as wound healing, placental development, and embryogenesis.

The MMPs can be subdivided into groups based on their substrate specificities and structural homologies: the collagenases, gelatinases, stromelysins, elastases, and MT. Three collagenases have been identified, interstitial collagenase

Table 1 The Matrix Metalloproteinase Family

Subclass	Enzyme	MMP Number	Substrates (not all proteases in a subgroup will cleave all substrates listed)
Interstitial collagenases	interstitial collagenase	MMP-1	collagens I, II, III,
	neutrophil collagenase	MMP-8	VII and X, gelatins,
	collagenase-3	MMP-13	link protein
Gelatinases	gelatinase A	MMP-2	gelatin, collagens I, IV,
	gelatinase B	MMP-9	V, VII, IX, X, and XI, FBN, LN, VN, link protein, galectin-3, LN-5
Stromelysins	stromelysin-1	MMP-3	proteoglycans, link protein,
	stromelysin-2	MMP-10	FBN, entactin
	matrilysin	MMP-7	pro-MMP-1, -8 and -9, L-selectin
Elastases	metalloelastase	MMP-12	elastin, angiostatin-precursor (FBG), FBN
RXKR secreted type	stromelysin-3	MMP-11	alpha-1-antitrypsin, LN, FBN
RXKR membrane type	MT-1-MMP	MMP-14	pro-MMP-2, collagens
	MT-2-MMP	MMP-15	I, II, III, gelatins,
	MT-3-MMP	MMP-16	FBN, LN, VN
	MT-4-MMP	MMP-17	

Abbreviations: MT-MMP, membrane-type matrix metalloproteinase; *FBN*, fibronectin; *LN*, laminin; *VN*, vitronectin; *FBG*, fibrinogen; link-protein, cross-link regions of collagens.
Matrix metalloproteinase-18 and MMP-19 are not included in this table as they have not yet been fully characterized.

(MMP-1), neutrophil collagenase (MMP-8) and collagenase 3 (MMP-13). These enzymes can degrade the generally proteolytic-resistant fibrillar collagens type I, II, and III (Wilhelm, et al., 1986; Hasty, et al., 1990). There are two type IV collagenases (Collier, et al., 1988; Wilhelm, et al., 1989), termed gelatinase A (MMP-2) and gelatinase B (MMP-9). Both gelatinases cleave collagen types IV, V, VII, X, XI, denatured collagens (gelatins), fibronectin, and laminin. The gelatinases also have been shown to degrade native insoluble elastin (Senior, et al., 1991), and more recently type I collagen and cell surface components such as galectin-3 and basic fibroblast growth factor (bFGF) receptor (Levi, et al., 1996). Three enzymes have been classified as stromelysins, although only stromelysin 1 (MMP-3) and stromelysin 2 (MMP-10) are closely related both by sequence analysis and functionally, degrading various proteoglycan components of the ECM as well as fibronectin and laminin (Wilhelm, et al., 1987; Muller, et al., 1988). Stromelysin 3 (MMP-11) (Bassett, et al., 1990) is in its own subclass. It contains a furin recognition site (RXKR), and its preferred substrate remains a matter of debate. It does not appear to break down known ECM proteins. It is, however, effective in degrading the serine proteinase inhibitor antitrypsin-1 (serpin) and, in doing so, may potentiate the action of serine proteinases such as urokinase-type plasminogen activator (uPA) (Pei, et al., 1994). This serpinase activity also is displayed by other MMPs and supports the hypothesis that the metallo and serine proteinase families act in an interdependent manner.

Two enzymes have been identified that, on the basis of sequence homology, do not belong in the subgroups described above. These are matrilysin (MMP-7) (Quantin, et al., 1989) and metalloelastase (MMP-12) (Shapiro, et al., 1993). Matrilysin is a "truncated" proteinase that can degrade nonfibrillar collagen, fibronectin, and laminin and is thus grouped with the stromelysins. Metalloelastase, as the name suggests, is capable of degrading elastin and is the only member of the elastase subgroup. In 1994, a new subgroup of the Matrixin family was identified. The membrane-type, or MT-MMPs have a C-terminal transmembrane domain that allows them to be anchored in the cell membrane. Currently four members have been identified (MMP-14 to MMP-17) (Sato, et al., 1994; Will and Hinzmann, 1995; Takino, et al., 1995; Puente, et al., 1996). The substrates for most of these enzymes have yet to be established; however, MT1-MMP and MT3-MMP (MMP-14 and MMP-16) appear to be specific activators of latent gelatinase A (Takino, et al., 1995; Strongin, et al., 1995) and new data suggest that all MT-MMPs may have a broad range of substrates that include ECM molecules. More recently MMP-18, an enzyme with some homology to the stromelysins, has been added to the family (Cossins, et al., 1996), and a novel enzyme has been provisionally designated MMP-19, which may represent the first member of a new MMP subgroup (Pendas, et al., 1997).

Additionally, a new gene family has been discovered that encodes membrane proteins with A Distintegrin And Metalloproteinase domain. Called

ADAMs, or adamelysins, these cell surface proteins are composed of an adhesion domain containing a disintegrin sequence, as well as a metalloproteinase domain (Blobel, 1997; Wolfsberg, et al., 1995). Recent reports have implicated MMP involvement in the processing of tumor necrosis factor (TNF) and in the shedding of other cytokines and adhesion molecules. This activity has now been identified and involves ADAMs such as TNF-α-converting enzyme (TACE) (Black, et al., 1997; Moss, et al., 1997).

The synthesis and activation of the MMPs are controlled at several levels, including gene activation and transcription, stability of the mRNA, translation and secretion of proenzymes, binding of proenzymes to cell membranes, activation of enzymes, inhibition by specific inhibitors, and degradation or removal of active enzymes. These enzymes are usually produced as zymogens by a variety of cell types, including fibroblasts, osteoblasts, chondrocytes, and endothelial cells, as well as inflammatory cells such as macrophages, lymphocytes, and neutrophils. The MMP activation is accompanied by proteolytic removal of about 80 amino acid profragments and an approximately 10 kDa decrease in molecular weight. Activation may be accomplished by a plasminogen cascade (Mignatti and Rifkin, 1996), by other members of the MMP family, or by interactions with cell surface components that may trigger an autoactivation mechanism. Until recently, all MMPs were thought to be secreted as proenzymes. However, it now appears that stromelysin-3 (MMP-11) and the MT-MMPs are expressed as active enzymes. These MMPs all contain a RXKR-sequence absent in the other members of this family. The activity of all MMPs is tightly regulated by specific endogenous inhibitors known as the tissue inhibitors of metalloproteinases (TIMPs) and by nonspecific inhibitors such as α_2 macroglobulin. The TIMPs are produced by several cell types and are present in the ECM.

A. Overview of TIMPs

The TIMPs regulate the activation and proteolytic activity of the MMPs (Table 2). The TIMPs were first recognized for their ability to inhibit metalloproteinase activities (Murphy and Docherty, 1992; Birkedal-Hansen, et al., 1993; Denhardt, et al., 1993). Subsequently TIMPs have been shown to be multifunctional proteins demonstrating both erythroid-potentiating ability and cell growth-promoting activities (Docherty, et al., 1985; Stetler-Stevenson, et al., 1992; Hayakawa, 1994; Chesler, et al., 1995). Four different human TIMPs have been identified to date: TIMP-1 (Stricklin and Welgus, 1983; Docherty, et al., 1985; Carmichael, et al., 1986); TIMP-2 (Stetler-Stevenson, et al., 1989; Boone, et al., 1990); TIMP-3 (Pavloff, et al., 1992; Apte, et al., 1994), and TIMP-4 (Greene, et al., 1996). There is a high degree of homology between both proteins and genes in the TIMP family (Douglas, et al., 1997). All have core proteins of approximately 21-22 kDa. Tissue inhibitor of metalloproteinase-1 and TIMP-3 are glycosylated and

Table 2 The TIMP Family

	TIMP-1	TIMP-2	TIMP-3	TIMP-4
Mass of mature protein	28 kDa	21 kDa	24 kDa	22 kDa
Isoelectric point	8.00	6.45	9.04	7.34
Glycosylation	+	−	+	−
Complex	proGel-B	proGel-A	proGel-A, ECM	proGel-A
Gene location	Xq11	17q25	22q12.1–13.2	?
mRNA(s)	0.9 kb	1.1 & 3.5 kb	4.5–5.0 kb	0.97, 1.4, 2.1 and 4.1 kb
Expression	Inducible +TPA −DEX	Constitutive	Inducible +TPA +DEX	?
Major site of expression	ovary, bone	placenta	kidney, brain	heart
MMPs inhibited	ALL	ALL	ALL	?

Abbreviations: TIMP, tissue inhibitors of metalloproteinases; *MMP*, matrix metalloproteinases; *TPA*, 12-0-tetradecanoylphorbal 13-acetate (phorbol 12-myristate 13-acetate); *DEX*, dexamethasone.

run as proteins of 28 and 24 kDa, respectively, on gel electrophoresis (Carmichael, et al., 1986; Apte, et al., 1994); TIMP-2 and TIMP-4 have not been shown to be glycosylated, and are not expected to be, as they do not contain potential glycosylation sites (Stetler-Stevenson, et al., 1989; Liu, et al., 1997).

All of the TIMPs form high affinity, noncovalent, 1:1 stoichiometric complexes with activated MMPs (Murphy and Docherty, 1992; Birkedal-Hansen, et al., 1993; Denhardt, et al., 1993, Murphy, et al., 1994). Although each TIMP is able to interact with all MMPs, some specificity has been demonstrated. Tissue inhibitor of metalloproteinase-1 is a more potent inhibitor for collagenase than TIMP-2; however, TIMP-2 inhibits gelatinase B more effectivily than TIMP-1 (Howard, et al., 1991). Furthermore, TIMP-1 is capable of binding to the latent form of MMP-9, progelatinase B, blocking stromelysin-mediated activation of this enzyme (Goldberg, et al., 1992). Tissue inhibitor of metalloproteinases-2 interacts similarly with MMP-2, binding at a noninhibitory site (Goldberg, et al., 1989). The progelatinase-TIMP-2 complex is believed to be activated at the cell surface by MT1-MMP. Released from the surface, TIMP-2 is presumably in a good position to rebind the activated MMP-2, this time blocking the active site (Strongin, et al., 1995). Tissue inhibitor of metalloproteinases-4 recently has been reported to bind to pro-MMP-2 also (Bigg, et al., 1997). The ability of TIMPs to interact with these proenzymes may add another level of regulation of MMP activity.

As the growing family of TIMPs is characterized, evidence suggests specific, physiological roles for each. As mentioned above, the TIMPs vary in their ability to interact with pro-MMPs. Additionally, TIMP expression and localization varies among members. Although TIMP-1, TIMP-2, and TIMP-4 are soluble proteins, TIMP-3 has poor solubility and is specifically localized in the ECM (Blenis and Hawkes, 1983; Pavloff, et al., 1992). Specific ECM ligands for TIMP-3 have not yet been identified. Tissue inhibitor of metalloproteinases-1 and TIMP-3 are cell cycle-regulated proteins (Leco, et al., 1994; Wick, et al., 1994) and are upregulated by various growth factors, including epidermal growth factor (EGF), transforming growth factor-β (TGF-β), platelet-derived growth factor (PDGF), and interleukin (IL)-1β (Leco, et al., 1994; Fabunmi, et al., 1996; Gatsios, et al., 1996). The TIMP-2 expression is largely constitutive (Denhardt, et al., 1993); TIMP-4 expression has not been fully characterized but appears to be limited, with high expression found only in the normal adult heart (Greene, et al., 1996).

Aside from functioning as inhibitors of MMPs, there is evidence that TIMPs may influence cells directly through receptor-mediated interactions. Tissue inhibitior of metalloproteinases-1 specifically binds to erythroid precursors (Alvalos, et al., 1988; Fraser, et al., 1988) and has erythroid-potentiating activity demonstrated by the ability to stimulate the growth of human and murine erythroid precursors and human erythroleukemia cells (Gasson, et al., 1985; Docherty, et al., 1985). Similarly, TIMP-1 has been shown to stimulate the proliferation of human keratinocytes and specifically binds to these cells with a K_D of 8.7 nM (Bertaux, et al., 1991). Tissue inhibitor of metalloproteinases-1 also promotes the growth of fibroblasts, smooth muscle cells, chondrocytes, breast adenocarcinoma cells, leukemia cells, and lymphoma cells (Hayakawa, et al., 1992). Tissue inhibitor of metalloproteinases-2 also has erythroid-potentiating activity (Stetler-Stevenson, et al., 1992) and recently has demonstrated an ability to bind directly to a number of cells, including HT-1080 fibrosarcoma and MCF-7 breast carcinoma cell lines (Emmert-Buck, et al., 1995). Additionally, TIMP-2 inhibits bFGF-induced human microvascular endothelial cell (MEC) proliferation independent of its ability to inhibit MMP activity (Murphy, et al., 1993).

B. Domain Structure of MMPs and TIMPs

Comparison and alignment of the amino acid sequence for the human MMPs reveal that these proteinases have a minimal domain structure that is conserved between subgroups (Fig. 1). This domain structure has been useful in subgrouping Matrixin family members along these features. The minimal structure comprises a signal peptide, prodomain, and a catalytic domain (Fig. 1a). This minimal struc-

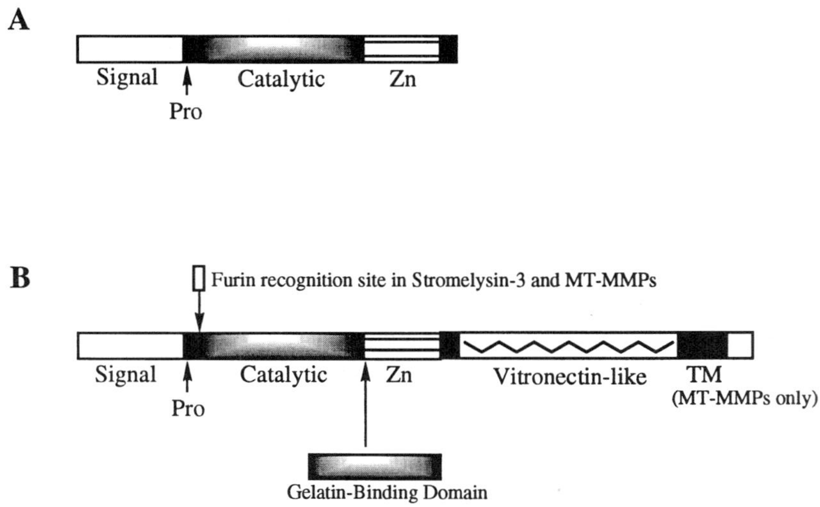

Figure 1 Domain structure of the matrix metalloproteinases. Schematic representation of matrix metalloproteinase (MMP) family. **A**. Minimal structure necessary for MMP activity; figure represents matrilysin (MMP-7). The signal peptide sequence localizes the translation product to the endoplasmic reticulum. The propeptide domain contains a conserved sequence (PRCGXPD) that is the activation locus; cleavage of the prodomain activates the enzyme. The zinc-binding domain contains another conserved sequence (VAAHEXGHXXGXXH) in which the three histidine residues coordinate metal binding. **B**. All MMPs except matrilysin have a C-terminal domain that has homology to hemopexin and vitronectin. The membrane type (MT)-MMPs also have a transmembrane domain and a short cytoplasmic domain. The gelatinases have an additional domain inserted between the catalytic and zinc-binding domains, which shows homology to the type II fibronectin repeats, which binds gelatin. Stromelysin-3 and the MT-MMPs contain a 10-amino acid insertion that has homology to recognition sequences for furin-like enzymes.

ture is observed in matrilysin, the smallest member of the Matrixin family, demonstrating that these are the minimal requirements for proteinase activity. The signal peptide domain is required for trafficking to the endoplasmic reticulum. As shown by X-ray crystallography, the propeptide contains a highly conserved sequence, PRCGVD, in which the cysteine residue coordinates with the zinc atom of the active site to maintain the latency of the proenzyme (Van Wart and Birkdal-Hansen, 1990). Disruption of the sulfhydryl-zinc interaction results in hydration of the zinc and achievement of proteolytic capacity. Detailed analysis of the in vitro activation of several members of the Matrixin family has been completed. These studies suggest that removal of the profragment is a two-step process: the first step produces an obligatory intermediate and is the result of intermolecular proteolytic cleavage, whereas the second step is a rapid intramolecular cleavage (Itoh, et al., 1995; Kleiner and Stetler-Stevenson, unpublished observations).

The catalytic domain contains another highly conserved sequence in which three histidine residues have been identified that coordinate zinc atom binding at the active site. Except for matrilysin, all Matrixin family members contain a C-terminal domain, which shows sequence homology to hemopexin and vitronectin and has a five-bladed propeller-type structure composed of antiparallel β sheets (Libson, et al., 1995) (Fig. 1b). The C-terminal domain of the collagenases, such as MMP-1 and MMP-8, has been implicated in the binding of these proteinases to the fibrillar collagens, types I, II, and III, at a site distinct from the cleavage site that results in positioning of the cleavage site at the enzyme-active site (Murphy, et al., 1992; Bode, 1995). However, the cleavage site specificity does not reside solely in the C-terminal domain, as the catalytic domain also contributes to cleavage specificity as demonstrated using chimeric MMP-1/MMP-3-type recombinant proteinases. For example, stromelysin—MMP-3—does not cleave collagen but does bind through its C-terminal, hemopexin-like domain (Murphy, et al., 1992).

The TIMP family of proteins is classified by the structural similarity among members, as well as by the ability to inhibit MMPs (Fig. 2). There are twelve cysteine residues that are highly conserved in placement and in spacing in all of the TIMPs. Six disulfide bonds divide the mature TIMP into six loop structures

```
       1                                                         50
TIMP-1 CTCVPPHPQT   AFCNSDLVIR   AKFVGTPEVN   QTTLY.....   ..QRYEIKMT
TIMP-2 CSCSPVHPQQ   AFCNADVVIR   AKAVSEKEVD   SGNDIYGNPI   KRIQYEIKQI
TIMP-3 CTCSPSHPQD   AFCNSDIVIR   AKVVGKKLVK   EG......PF   GTLVYTIKQM
TIMP-4 CSCAPAHPQQ   HICHSALVIR   AKISSEKVVP   ASADP.ADTE   KMLRYEIKQI
       * *            *
       51                                                       100
TIMP-1 KMYKGFQALG   DAADIRFVYT   PAMESVCGYF   HRSHNRSEEF   LIAGKLQDGL
TIMP-2 KMFKGPE...   ..KDIEFIYT   APSSAVCGVS   LDVGGKKEYL   IAGKAEGDGK
TIMP-3 KMYRGFTKM.   ..PHVQYIHT   EASESLCGLK   LEVN.KYQYL   LTGRVY.DGK
TIMP-4 KMFKGFEKV.   ..KDVQYIYT   PFDSSLCGVK   LEANSQKQYL   LTGQVLSDGK
                                     *
       101                                                      150
TIMP-1 LHITTCSFVA   PWNSLSLAQR   RGFTKTYTVG   CEECTVFPCL   SIPCKLQSGT
TIMP-2 MHITLCDFIV   PWDTLSTTQK   KSLNHRYQMG   CE.CKITRCP   MIPCYISSPD
TIMP-3 MYTGLCNFVE   RWDQLTLSQR   KGLNYRYHLG   CN.CKIKSCY   YLPCFVTSKN
TIMP-4 VFIHLCNYIE   PWEDLSLVQR   ESLNHHYHLN   CG.CQITTCY   TVPCTISAPN
            *                                 *  *    *        *
       151                                                      200
TIMP-1 HCLWTDQLLQ   GSEKGFQSRH   LACLPREPGL   CTWQSLRSQI   A.........
TIMP-2 ECLWMDWVTE   KNINGHQAKF   FACIKRSDGS   CAWYRGAAPP   KQEFLDIEDP
TIMP-3 ECLWTDMLSN   FGYPGYQSKH   YACIRQKGGY   CSWYRGWAPP   DKSIINATDP
TIMP-4 ECLWTDWLLE   RKLYGYQAQH   YVCMKHVDGT   CSWYRGHLPL   RKEFVDIVQP
        *                         *          *
```

Figure 2 Sequence alignment of the tissue inhibitor of metalloproteinase family (TIMPs). Brackets indicate regions of consensus among the entire family. The asterisks denote conserved cysteine residues.

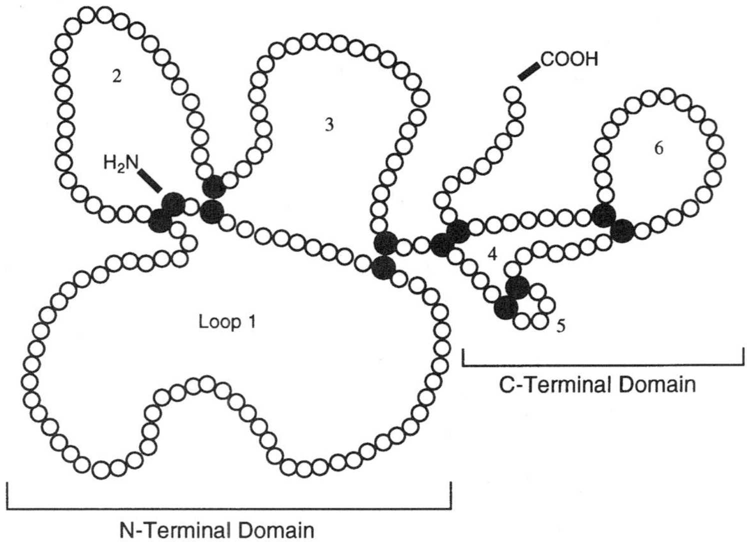

Figure 3 Schematic representation of a tissue inhibitor of metalloproteinase (TIMP). Figure demonstrates loop structure and disulfide bond arrangement of the TIMP molecule. The N-terminal domain is composed of loops 1–3, the C-terminal domain of loops 4–6.

that separate into the N-terminal (loops 1–3) and C-terminal (loops 4–6) domains (Fig. 3) (Douglas, et al., 1997). The MMP inhibitory function of the TIMPs has been localized to the N-terminal regions (Willenbrock and Murphy, 1994; Murphy, et al., 1991). The most highly conserved region in the TIMP family is the first 22 amino acids. This was proposed to be the MMP-inhibitory binding site (Woessner, 1991). However, site-directed mutagenesis studies (O'Shea, et al., 1992), as well as peptide and antibody competition experiments (Bodden, et al., 1994), indicate that TIMP inhibitory activity is distributed throughout the N-terminal domain. X-ray diffraction analysis of MMP-1 (stromelysin) catalytic domain complexes demonstrate that it is the N-terminal amino group of the first cysteine residue that coordinates the active site zinc atom and results in proteinase inhibition (Gomis-Ruth, et al., 1997). The C-terminal regions are more divergent and may be responsible for functions other than MMP inhibition, including TIMP binding to latent MMPs.

The gelatinases are distinguished among the Matrixins by the fact that the proforms of MMP-2 (gelatinase A) and MMP-9 (gelatinase B) are capable of binding the TIMPs. This binding is mediated by the C-terminal domain of the proteinase interacting with the C-terminal region of the TIMP (Goldberg, et al., 1989; Kleiner, et al., 1992; Murphy, et al., 1992; Bigg, et al., 1997). The biological significance of these proproteinase-inhibitor complexes is not clear, but it has been implicated in a cellular mechanism of activation of the MMP, at least for the pro-MMP-2/TIMP-2 complex (Strongin, et al., 1995). The gelatinases are also unique among the Matrixins in that they contain a disruption of the catalytic domain immediately upstream of the zinc atom-binding site. An insertion composed of three fibronectin-type gelatin binding type-II modules is present and has been shown to confer macromolecular substrate-binding ability (Murphy, et al., 1994). The removal of the C-terminal domain does not diminish the substrate-degrading activity of the truncated proteinase. The MT-MMPs have a transmembrane domain inserted in the C-terminal domain such that the catalytic domain is oriented toward the extracellular milieu. Additionally, the MT-MMPs, as well as stromelysin-3, contain a basic amino acid-rich sequence inserted immediately downstream of the prodomain that corresponds to a furin enzyme recognition site, RXKR. This sequence seems to account for the recent demonstration that stromelysin-3 is the first Matrixin family member secreted as an active proteinase and not as a zymogen (Pei and Weiss, 1995). This furin recognition sequence suggests that stromelysin-3 and the MT-MMP can be processed intracellularly in the Golgi vesicles.

Before identification of Matrixin family members with transmembrane domains and furin recognition sequences, it was thought that the MMPs were all secreted, soluble zymogens requiring activation in the extracelluar space. This tended to focus our attention on putative substrates within the ECM and the role of these proteinases in removing and remodeling the physical barrier presented by the ECM. Collectively, the Matrixin family member can degrade all components of the ECM. Many of these studies are done in vitro using purified extracellular macromolecular substrates. What is missing are studies using intact ECM, identification of degradation products from in vitro degradation of the ECM, and in vivo confirmation of the relevance of specific degradation products. However, recent studies have focused on the proteolytic activity of the enzymes at the cell surface and the functional implications of their action on cellular activities, such as adhesion, spreading, and migration. This has led to the identification of new substrates for Matrixin family members, such as laminin-5, and novel activities for these proteolytic degradation fragments, such as stimulation of cell migration (Giannelli, et al., 1997).

C. Activation of MMP

Under some conditions, transcriptional activation of the MMP genes may be a requirement for ECM turnover. Current evidence also suggests that transcriptional activation alone may not be sufficient. Activation of proenzyme forms of these proteinases is required for initiation of matrix degradation and acquisition of the invasive phenotype. The balance of activated proteinases and endogenous inhibitors is crucial for determining the extent of ECM turnover (Stetler-Stevenson, et al., 1993; Mignatti and Rifkin, 1993).

There is very little constitutive expression of MMPs in normal cells. At the level of transcription, many of the MMPs appear to be regulated by similar mechanisms. The MMPs are responsive to cytokines, growth factors, and hormones. In general, most of the MMPs are induced by IL-1β, tumor necrosis factor-α (TNF-α), PDGF, transforming growth factor α (TGF-α), EGF, basic fibroblast growth factor (bFGF), and nerve growth factor (NGF), and are repressed by TGF-β (Birkedal-Hansen, et al., 1993). Interleukin-α appears to be acting as an obligatory intermediate regulator for stimulation of interstitial collagenase expression (Fini, et al., 1994). Sensitivity of individual MMPs to these factors varies from enzyme to enzyme and is tissue specific. Specificity is maintained by induction and repression of distinct MMP family members. Also, many factors must be integrated to elicit a response that is cell specific. Matrix metalloproteinase production is also regulated by the pericellular environment, cell matrix interactions, and components of the ECM (Seftor, et al., 1992; Seftor, et al., 1993; Sweeney, et al., 1991; Werb, et al., 1989; Kato, et al., 1992; Fridman, et al., 1992a; Fridman, et al., 1992b; Bonfil, et al., 1992; Biswas and Dayer, 1979). For example, a number of diverse agents stimulate production of interstitial collagenase by macrophages or epidermal keratinocytes, including calcium influx (Unemori and Werb, 1988), ultraviolet light (Angel, et al., 1985), and cell shape (Werb, et al., 1986). Interleukin-1α and other cytokines also stimulate interstitial collagenase release from fibroblasts in response to interruptions between ECM and cell surface receptors (Uria, et al., 1997). Gelatinase A is unlike most members of the MMP family in that many cell lines in culture demonstrate high levels of constitutive expression of the proteinase. Interestingly, gelatinase A exhibits only a slight response to cytokine and growth factors (Brown, et al., 1990; Overall, et al., 1991; Salo, et al., 1991), and calcium influx suppresses gelatinase A mRNA and protein synthesis (Kohn, et al., 1994). This may indicate a unique role for gelatinase A in matrix homeostasis and suggests that activation of progelatinase A is a critical point in regulation of this enzyme.

The biochemistry of MMP activation has been well characterized through many in vitro studies. The mechanism for mammalian MMP activation is referred to as the ''cysteine switch.'' In this mechanism, an unpaired cysteine residue in the profragment coordinates with the active site zinc atom and maintains the latency of the enzyme (Van Wart and Birkedal-Hansen, 1990). When this cysteine-zinc atom interaction is interrupted by chemical or physical means, a conformational change occurs, and subsequent proteolytic cleavage of the amino-terminal profragment ensues (Birkedal-Hansen, et al, 1993).

Degradation of the ECM is a tightly controlled process. Insufficient degradation would prevent cell migration, whereas excessive degradation would result in loss of substratum for cell attachment to the ECM during migration. Because most MMPs, as well as other degradative proteinases, are secreted as latent enzymes, physiological activation becomes a critical control point. In the case of most of the MMPs evaluated, including collagenases, stromelysins, and gelatinase B, plasmin and uPA have been implicated as the physiological activators (Mignatti and Rifkin, 1993). As uPA binds to a cell-surface receptor, this provides a mechanism for the cell to activate an array of proteinases in close proximity to the cell surface, with the potential to restrict this activation to only a portion of the cell surface, such as the region of cell membrane over invadopodia or adjacent to basement membranes. Interactions occur between the MMPs, which can further enhance activity as illustrated by stromelysin activation of interstitial collagenase and gelatinase B (Ogata, et al., 1992; Azzam and Thompson, 1992). Gelatinase A is not activated by the plasmin/uPA system but can be activated by MT-MMP-1 and -3 (Sato, et al., 1994; Takino, et al., 1995; Shofuda, et al., 1997). The MT-MMPs may prove to be activators of other MMPs as well. Matrix metalloproteinase-2 activation is a key event in endothelial cell invasion, the initial phase of tumor-associated angiogenesis. Inhibition of this enzyme could be an effective treatment for tumor-associated angiogenesis (Benelli, et al., 1994).

III. CELL INVASION

It is now recognized that tumor-induced angiogenesis supports the growth, expansion, and eventual metastasis of many human cancers. Angiogenesis and tumor dissemination are similar to many physiological conditions, such as trophoblast implantation or wound healing, in that all of these processes involve cellular invasion. Studies reveal that cell invasion during the evolution of these processes, both physiological and pathological, share functional similarities. Cell invasion depends on the coordination of cellular adhesion, matrix proteolysis, and migration involving a series of changing and renewing cell-cell and cell-matrix interactions (Stetler-Stevenson, et al., 1993). Liotta and colleagues proposed the original three-step hypothesis to describe tumor cell invasion in 1986 (Liotta, 1986). As an overall scheme for cell invasion, the three steps of attachment, dissolution, and locomotion remain valid today.

We now recognize that the three-step hypothesis can be generalized to all invasive cell types, although the specific molecular events may be different than those originally proposed for tumor cell invasion of the basement membrane (Stetler-Stevenson, et al., 1993). This expanded three-step hypothesis recognizes that directed cellular invasion is the result of a highly coordinated series of cell-matrix interactions that have three distinct phases: (a) modification of cell-cell contacts and establishing new cell-matrix contacts; (b) proteolytic modification of the ECM that removes physical barriers, alters cell-matrix contacts, and prepares matrix to facilitate cell movement; (c) migration of the invasive cell through the proteolysed matrix to establish new matrix contacts. This begins a new cycle and these events are repeated.

These events must be coordinated and integrated so that the leading edge of the invasive cell is forming new contacts with the ECM while the trailing edge is breaking previously formed cell-matrix contacts. Proteolysis of the ECM must be balanced and regulated to preserve the critical cell-matrix contacts that allow traction to occur. Furthermore, these events are not independent of one another. We now know that integrin-mediated cell-matrix interactions can influence proteinase production, and that proteinase activity can alter cell attachment and spreading (Ray and Stetler-Stevenson, 1994a; Seftor, et al., 1992). Understanding how these molecular events of cell invasion during angiogenesis and tumor invasion are coordinated may allow identification of common mechanisms that could be targeted by novel therapeutic interventions.

A. Endothelial Cell Interactions with ECM and MMPs

The invasion of vascular cells is dependent on molecular crosstalk between adhesion receptors (specifically the integrins) and proteinases. Interestingly, stimulators of angiogenesis that mediate MMP expression also seem to induce endothelial cell migration by altering expression of adhesion receptors. Receptors necessary for migration through the interstitial matrix are up-regulated (Defilippi, et al., 1991; Enenstein, et al., 1992), whereas receptors mediating attachment to the basement membrane are down-regulated (Sepp, et al., 1995).

The process of angiogenesis depends on cell-matrix interactions mediated by the vitronectin receptor, integrin $\alpha_v\beta_3$ (Brooks, et al., 1994a; Brooks, et al., 1994b; Brooks, et al., 1995). This receptor is highly expressed on the surface of endothelial cells involved in active angiogenesis in response to bFGF stimulation (Davis, et al., 1993; Brooks, et al., 1994a). The MMP activity in the ECM reveals cryptic sites for $\alpha_v\beta_3$ and $\alpha_v\beta_5$ binding (Davis, 1992; Montgomery, et al., 1994). When this interaction is disrupted through the use of an antagonist of $\alpha_v\beta_3$, the endothelial cells undergo apoptosis and angiogenesis is halted. This can result in tumor regression because of disruption of the angiogenic blood vessels (Brooks, et al., 1994b; Brooks, et al., 1995). The type of angiogenic stimulus may influence the integrin in mediating the endothelial cell invasion and the subsequent autonomy of this process from other growth factors (Friedlander, et al., 1995).

The expression of $\alpha_v\beta_3$ on endothelial cells (or tumor cells) promotes their attachment to partially proteolysed collagen through cryptic RGD-binding sites, which in turn promotes survival of these cells and continuation of the invasive process. Concurrently, ligation of the $\alpha_v\beta_3$ receptor may influence proteinase expression in some tumor cell types (Seftor, et al., 1992). Experimental treatment of human A375M melanoma cells with antibodies against $\alpha_v\beta_3$ results in enhanced in vitro invasive ability of these cells. This was in part caused by enhanced expression of MMP activity, specifically gelatinase A (MMP-2). These findings demonstrate that the first two steps of cell invasion—cell-matrix attachment and ECM proteolysis—are linked with integrin binding, influencing proteinase expression. This may function to coordinate cell attachment with matrix proteolysis.

Of much interest is recent work in which MMP interactions with the ECM have had broader implications than just overcoming barriers to migration. One component of epithelial cell basement membrane, laminin-5, is specifically cleaved by MMP-2, exposing a cryptic site that induces migration of breast epithelial cells (Giannelli, et al., 1997). This site appears to interact with the cells but is not involved in cell adhesion. The cleavage site may either stimulate cell motility or mask a site that suppresses cell motility. Evidence indicating the existence of migratory promoting sites or migratory suppressor sites on other ECM molecules also has been documented (Brooks, 1996; Sato, et al., 1994; Burgeson, et al., 1994; Laurie, et al., 1982). Similarly, vascular smooth muscle cells, which are normally antiproliferative, become mitogenic when the fibrillar collagens around them undergo proteolysis (Koyama, et al., 1996). Fibroblasts from normal and neoplastic human breasts, and two sarcomatous human cancer cell lines, are able to induce the activation of MMP-2 when cultured on type I collagen gels. When these cells were grown on plastic, fibronectin, collagen IV, gelatin, Matrigel, or basement membrane-like HR9 cell matrix, only trace amounts of the activated form of MMP-2 were observed (Azzam and Thompson, 1992). A direct role for type I collagen in MMP-2 processing does not appear to exist; however, this demonstrates a highly dynamic role for ECM molecules in MMP activation.

Additionally, as MMPs degrade ECM, angiogenic factors sequestered there are released. This release of cytokines, together with tumor cell and macrophage production of cytokines, further aid in the growth and infiltration of new blood vessels into the tumor (Lewis, et al., 1995; Cornali, et al., 1996). More recently, there have been reports of MMP involvement with substrates different than ECM molecules or activation of other MMP enzymes. Matrix metalloproteinase-2, but not MMP-9, was shown to release the active soluble ectodomain of FGF receptor-1, which in turn can modulate the angiogenic activity of FGF (Levi, et al., 1996). There also is a role for metalloelastase in angiostatin processing. Angiostatin, a 38 kDa internal fragment of plasminogen, has potent antiangiogenic and antimetastatic activity in its active form (O'Reilly, et al., 1994; Dong, et al., 1996). Several MMPs generate angiostatin-like fragments from plasminogen, including MMP-9 (Patterson and Sang, 1997) and MMP-2 (Stetler-Stevenson, unpublished observation).

Matrix metalloproteinases have been implicated in the shedding of pro-TGF-α, the cell adhesion receptor L-selectin, IL-6 receptor α subunit, β-amyloid precursor protein, and the processing of both TNF-α and its receptor. The cleavage of each of these ectodomains can be inhibited by synthetic proteinase inhibitors specific to MMPs (Arribas, et al., 1996). However, subsequent work has identified a member of the ADAM family of proteins as the proteinase involved in TNF-α processing (Black, et al., 1997). It has not yet been determined if ADAMs are responsible for the shedding of the other ectodomains. However, an important function of ADAM may be to regulate the expression of cell surface proteins.

IV. REQUIREMENT FOR MMPs IN ANGIOGENESIS

That proteolysis is important in angiogenesis was determined in one of the earliest studies of this process. Ausprunk and Folkman (1977) subjected capillary vessels to an angiogenic stimulus and described the sequence of events that occurred around neovascularization. During the new vessel formation, the earliest event was the migration of MEC, preceding proliferation. What is less understood are the relative contributions of various classes of ECM-degrading proteinases. This is almost certainly caused by the interdependence of the different proteinase systems, which must act in concert during the processes of endothelial cell migration, invasion, and vessel formation. Early studies with bovine corneal endothelial cells demonstrated that in vitro invasion through human amniotic membrane can be blocked by both serine proteinase inhibitors, such as aprotinin, and by the MMP inhibitors, TIMP-1, and antigelatinase A antibodies (Mignatti, et al., 1989). In each case, invasion was inhibited by 80% to 90% independently for each inhibitor, supporting the hypothesis that invasion may require the coordinated expression of both classes of proteinase. A role for the cysteine proteinase, cathepsin B, has also been suggested (Mikkelsen, et al., 1995; Sinha, et al., 1995). The following concentrates on evidence of MMP involvement in the angiogenic response.

A positive correlation between the angiogenesis and MMP expression has been demonstrated. Angiogenic factors, including TNF, vascular endothelial growth factor, TGF-α and -β, and prostaglandin can induce MMP production in endothelial cells (Gross, et al., 1982; Moscatelli, et al., 1980, 1985; Montesano and Orci, 1985). The ability of interferons and glucocorticoids to inhibit angiogenic processes correlates with an antagonistic effect in the induction of MMP gene transcription (Shapiro, et al., 1990). In vitro studies with MEC demonstrate that TNF-α induces an endothelial cell-specific up-regulation of collagenase and decreases TIMP production. Matrix metalloproteinase expression and regulation in MEC appears to be unique compared with other cell types, which may be critical for MEC migration in angiogenesis and wound healing (Cornelius, et al., 1995). Endothelial cell-stimulating angiogenesis factor (ESAF) stimulates MEC proliferation in culture (Schor, et al., 1980) and induces angiogenesis on the chick chorioallantoic membrane (Hill, et al., 1983), but has no effect on aortic or large vein endothelial cells (Keegan, et al., 1982). Endothelial cell-stimulating angiogenesis factor also is able to fully activate interstitial collagenase (MMP-1), stromelysin 1 (MMP-3), and gelatinase A (MMP-2). Additionally, the inhibition of these three MMPs by their interaction with TIMPs is reversed by ESAF, yielding fully active MMPs and TIMPs. Endothelial cell-stimulating angiogenesis factor is capable of binding to the active MMPs without interfering with proteinase activity and confers protection against inhibition by TIMPs (McLaughlin and Weiss, 1996).

Additional evidence is based on the ability of proteinase inhibitors, antiproteinase antibodies, and especially the TIMPs to block the angiogenic response (Mignatti and Rifkin, 1996; Pepper, et al., 1996; Johnson, et al., 1994). Endothelial cell migration assayed in modified Boyden chambers in inhibited by TIMP-1 (Johnson, et al., 1994), TIMP-2 (Murphy, et al., 1993), and TIMP-3 (Anand-Apte, et al., 1997). Similarly, Fisher and coworkers (1994) have demonstrated that these TIMPs also inhibit endothelial cell invasion through collagen. Tissue inhibitor of metalloproteinase inhibits angiogenesis in vitro on human amniotic membrane (Mignatti, et al., 1989), and in vivo in a rat corneal angiogenesis assay (Johnson, et al., 1994). Recent experiments with TIMP-3 demonstrated an ability to inhibit angiogenesis in vivo in the chick chorioallentoic membrane assay (Anand-Apte, et al., 1997). The synthetic metalloproteinase inhibitor, batimastat (British Biotech), was shown to reduce the angiogenic response in vivo to heparin-Matrigel implants. In the same study, batimastat inhibited the invasion of human umbilical vein endothelial cells through Matrigel in vitro but did not significantly alter endothelial cell proliferation, haptotaxis, or chemotaxis (Taraboletti, et al., 1995). The endogenous MMP inhibitors may differ in their antiangiogenic activity from synthetic inhibitors because TIMPs also block endothelial cell proliferation and migration.

Interestingly, it seems as though a balance between MMPs and their inhibitors is necessary for angiogenesis. Evidence from in vitro studies indicates that if the level of proteolysis is too high, endothelial cell invasion (and angiogenesis) will be inhibited (Schnaper, et al., 1993). Tube formation by endothelial cells in vitro is increased by addition of recombinant gelatinase A and decreased both by neutralizing antibody and TIMP-2. Although tube network formation was decreased by gelatinase A concentration above a critical level, this decrease was reversed by addition of exogenous TIMP-2. These results suggest that although gelatinase A activity has an important role in angiogenesis, excessive levels of activity will inhibit the process, and regulation by TIMPs may be an important factor (Schnaper, et al., 1993).

An immunohistochemical study of angiogenesis in skin during both fetal development and in adult cutaneous tumors has identified interstitial collagenase as the principle MMP expressed in developing microvessels. Expression of stromelysin, matrilysin, gelatinase A, and gelatinase B was not detected (Karelina, et al., 1995). However, earlier studies showed that antigelatinase A antibodies are able to inhibit endothelial cell invasion in vitro (Mignatti, et al., 1989). Activation of gelatinase A also has been observed in tubule formation in vitro in cocultures of glial cells and central nervous system microvascular endothelial cells (Rao, et al., 1996). As has been suggested by Pepper (1996) and others, the proteinase(s) used in the process of angiogenesis may change according to the type of tissue being vascularized.

The accumulating body of evidence suggests that the remodeling of ECM, whether through normal growth, wound repair, tumor growth, or angiogenesis, is accomplished largely through the action of MMPs, whose activity is the rate-limiting step of ECM degradation (Matrisian, 1990; Woessner, 1994; Birkedal-Hansen, 1995).

V. PROTEINASE-ANTIPROTEINASE BALANCE

Proteolysis and migration through ECM barriers appear to be highly regulated functions in specific physiological circumstances. For invasion to take place, cyclic attachment to, and subsequent release from, matrix components must occur in a directed and controlled manner. This implies that ECM proteolysis, although enhanced in angiogenesis, is still tightly regulated in a temporal and spatial fashion with respect to endothelial cell attachment and migration. Net ECM-degrading proteolytic activity results from the balance between the local concentration of activated enzymes and their endogenous inhibitors. Agents that induce angiogenesis, such as bFGF, will induce endothelial expression of both uPA and plasminogen activator inhibitor (PAI-1), with the balance slightly in favor of uPA (Pepper, et al., 1990). In these assays, a balance in favor of proteinase inhibition resulted in the formation of solid cords of endothelial cells rather than tubes. Montesano and coworkers (1990) have also studied the influence of proteinase-inhibitor balance on the morphology of benign endothelial tumor cell cultures in fibrin gels. Benign endothelial cell lines produced excess proteolytic activity and formed cystic structures in the fibrin gels. The addition of exogenous serine proteinase inhibition resulted in the formation of endothelial cords instead of saccular structures. Thus, proteinase/antiproteinase balance can alter the morphology of the capillary tube, with excessive proteolysis resulting in cystic noninvasive structures. Based on the preliminary studies of Schnaper, et al. (1993), we would predict that a similar balance of MMP and TIMP activity is required to effect a functional angiogenic response.

VI. SUMMARY

Endothelial cell migration appears to be an early event in angiogenesis and vascular remodeling. Matrix metalloproteinase expression and activation are necessary to facilitate this migration. As progress is made in understanding the interactions between MMPs, TIMPs, and ECM components and the cell surface, mechanisms are beginning to appear that suggest complex roles for these molecules other than simply proteinase and substrate. The MMPs remove physical barriers (basement membrane) to cell migration, alter cell adhesion and migration, and unveil cryptic sites in the ECM that can influence cell migration, proliferation, and survival. Additionally, TIMPs appear to be multifunctional molecules participating as inhibitors of MMPs and directly regulating cellular activities, such as proliferation. Although the physiological relevance of much of this work remains to be tested, it provides exciting new possibilities for the interruption of cell invasion in angiogenesis and cancer.

REFERENCES

B.R. Alvalos, S.E. Kaufman, M. Tomonaga, R.W. Williams, D.W. Golde, J.C. Gasson (1988). K562 cells produce and respond to human erythroid-potentiating activity. Blood 71:1720–1725.

P. Angel, J. Rahmsdorf, A. Poting, C. Lucke-Huhle, P. Herrlich (1985). 12-O-tetradecanoylphorbol-13-acetate (TPA) induced gene sequences in human primary diploid fibroblasts and their expression in SV40-transformed fibroblasts. J Cell Biochem 29:351–360.

B. Anand-Apte, M.S. Pepper, E. Voest, K. Iwata, R. Montesano, B.R. Olsen, G. Murphy, S.S. Apte, B. Zetter (1997). Inhibition of angiogenesis by tissue inhibitor of metalloproteinases-3. Invest Ophthalmol Vis Sci 38:817–823.

S.S. Apte, M.G. Mattie, B.R. Olsen (1994). Cloning of the cDNA encoding human tissue inhibitor of metalloproteinase-3 (TIMP-3) and mapping of the TIMP-3 gene to chromosome 22. Genomics 19:86–90.

J. Arribas, L. Coodly, P. Vollmer, T.K. Kishimoto, S. Rose-John, J. Massague (1996). Diverse cell surface protein ectodomains are shed by a system sensitive to metalloprotease inhibitors. J Biol Chem 271:11376–11382.

D.H. Ausprunk, J. Folkman (1977). Migration and proliferation of endothelial cells in preformed and newly formed blood vessels during tumor angiogenesis. Microvasc Res 14:53–65.

H.S. Azzam, E.W. Thompson (1992). Collagen-induced activation of the M_r 72,000 type IV collagenase in normal and malignant human fibroblastoma cells. Cancer Res 52:4540–4544.

P. Basset, J.P. Belloc, C. Wolf, I. Stoll, P. Hutin, J.M. Limacher, O.L. Podhajcer, M.P. Chenard, M.C. Rio, P. Chambon (1990). A novel metalloproteinase gene specifically expressed in stromal cell of breast carcinomas. Nature 348:699–704.

R. Benelli, A. Adatia, B. Ensoli, W.G. Stetler-Stevenson, L. Santi, A. Albini (1994). Inhibition of AID's-Kaposi's sarcoma cell induced endothelial cell invasion by TIMP-2 and a synthetic peptide from the metalloproteinase propeptide: Implications for an anti-angiogenic therapy. Oncol Res 6:251–257.

B. Bertaux, W. Hornebeck, A.Z. Eisen, L. Dubertret (1991). Growth stimulation of human

keratinocytes by tissue inhibitor of metalloproteinases. J Invest Dermatol 97:679–685.
H.F. Bigg, Y.E. Shi, Y.E. Liu, B. Steffensen, C.M. Overall (1997). Specific, high affinity binding of tissue inhibitor of metalloproteinases-4 (TIMP-4) to the COOH-terminal hemopexin-like domain of human gelatinase A. J Biol Chem 272:15496–15500.
H. Birkedal-Hansen, W.G. Moore, M.K. Bodden, L.J. Windsor, B. Birkedal-Hansen, A. DeCarlo, J.A. Engler (1993). Matrix metalloproteinases: A review. Crit Rev Oral Biol Med 4:197–250.
H. Birkedal-Hansen (1995). Proteolytic remodeling of extracellular matrix. Curr Opin Cell Biol 7:728–735.
C. Biswas, J. Dayer (1979). Stimulation of collagenase production by collagen in mammalian cell cultures. Cell 18:1035–1041.
R.A. Black, C.T. Rauch, C.J. Kozlosky, J.J. Peschon, J.L. Slack, M.F. Wolfson, B.J. Castner, K.L. Stocking, R. Reddy, S. Srinivasan, N. Nelson, N. Boiani, K.A. Schooley, M. Gerhart, R. Davis, J.N. Fitzner, R.S. Johnson, R.J. Paxton, C.J. March, D.R. Cerretti (1997). A metalloproteinase disintegrin that releases tumour-necrosis factor-α from cells. Nature 385:729–733.
J. Blenis, S. Hawkes (1983). Transformation sensitive protein associated with the cell substratum of chicken embryo fibroblasts. Proc Natl Acad Sci U S A 80:770–774.
C.P. Blobel (1997). Metalloprotease-disintegrins: Links to cell adhesion and cleavage of TNF alpha and Notch. Cell 90:589–592.
M.K. Bodden, G.J. Harber, B. Birkedal-Hansen, L. Windsor, N.C.M. Caterina, J.A. Engler, H. Birkedal-Hansen (1994). Functional-domains of human TIMP-1 (tissue inhibitor of metalloproteinases). J Biol Chem 269:18943–18952.
W. Bode (1995). A helping hand for collagenases: The haemopexin-like domain. Structure 3:527–530.
R.D. Bonfil, P.A. Medina, D.E. Gomez, E. Farias, A. Lazarowski, M.F. Lucero-Gritti, R.P. Meiss, O.D. Bustuoabed (1992). Expression of gelatinase/type IV collagenase in tumour necrosis correlates with cell detachment and tumor invasion. Clin Exp Metastasis 10:211–220.
T.C. Boone, M.J. Johnson, Y.A. DeClerck, K. Langley (1990). cDNA cloning and expression of a metalloproteinase inhibitor related to tissue inhibitor of metalloproteinases. Proc Natl Acad Sci U S A 87:2800–2804.
P.C. Brooks, R.A. Clark, D.A. Cheresh (1994a). Requirement of vascular integrin alpha v beta 3 for angiogenesis. Science 264:569–571.
P.C. Brooks, A.M. Montgomery, M. Rosenfeld, R.A. Reisfeld, T. Hu, G. Klier, D.A. Cheresh (1994b). Integrin alpha v beta 3 antagonists promote tumor regression by inducing apoptosis of angiogenic blood vessels. Cell 79:1157–1164.
P.C. Brooks, A. Stromblad, R. Klemke, D. Visscher, F.H. Sarkar, D.A. Cheresh (1995). Antiintegrin alpha v beta 3 blocks human breast cancer growth and angiogenesis in human skin [see comments]. J Clin Invest 96:1815–1822.
P.C. Brooks (1996). Role of integrins in angiogenesis. Eur J Cancer 32A:2423–2429.
P.D. Brown, A.T. Levy, I.M. Margulies, L.A. Liotta, W.G. Stetler-Stevenson (1990). Independent expression and cellular processing of Mr 72,000 type IV collagenase and interstitial collagenase in human tumorigenic cell lines. Cancer Res 50:6184–6191.

R.E. Burgeson, M. Chiquet, R. Deutzmann, R. Ekblom, J. Engel, H. Kleinman, G.R. Martin, G. Menequzzi, M. Paulsson, J. Sanes, R. Timpl, K. Tryggvason, Y. Yamada, P.D. Yurchenco (1994). A new nomenclature for the laminins. Matrix Biol 14:209–211.

D.F. Carmichael, A. Sommer, R.C. Thompson, D.C. Anderson, C.G. Smith, H.G. Welgus, G.P. Stricklin (1986). Primary structure and cDNA cloning of human fibroblast collagenase inhibitor. Proc Natl Acad Sci U S A 83:2407–2411.

L. Chesler, D.W. Golde, N. Bersch, M.D. Johnson (1995). Metalloproteinase inhibition and erythroid potentiation are independent activities of tissue inhibitor of metalloproteinases-1. Blood 86:4506–4515.

I.E. Collier, S.M. Wilhelm, A.Z. Eisen, B.L. Marmer, G.A. Grant, J.L. Seltzer, A. Kronberger, C.S. He, E.A. Bauer, G.I. Goldberg (1988). H-*ras* oncogene-transformed human bronchial epithelial (TBE-1) secrete a single metalloproteinase capable of degrading basement membrane collagen. J Biol Chem 263:6579–6587.

E. Cornali, C. Zietz, R. Benelli, W. Weninger, L. Masiello, G. Breier, E. Tschachler, A. Albini, M. Sturzl (1996). Vascular endothelial growth factor regulates angiogenesis and vascular permeability in Kaposi's sarcoma. Am J Pathol 149:1851–1869.

L.A. Cornelius, L.C. Nehring, J.D. Roby, W.C. Parks, H.G. Welgus (1995). Human dermal microvascular endothelial cells produce matrix metalloproteinases in response to angiogenic factors and migration. J Invest Dermatol 105:170–176.

J. Cossins, T.J. Dudgeon, G. Catlin, A.J.H. Bearing, J.M. Clements (1996). Identification of MMP-18, a putative novel human matrix metalloproteinase. Biochem Biophys Res Comm 228:494–498.

G.M. Davis, S.C. Danehower, A. Laurence, J.L. Molony (1993). Identification of a role of the vitronectin receptor and protein kinase C in the induction of endothelial cell vascular formation. J Cell Biol 51:206–218.

G.E. Davis (1992). Affinity of integrins for damaged extracellular matrix: $\alpha v\beta 3$ Binds to denatured collagen type I through RGD sites. Biophys Biochem Res Comm 182: 1025–1031.

P. Defilippi, G. Truffa, G. Stefanuto, F. Altruda, L. Silengo, G. Tarone (1991). Tumor necrosis factor alpha and interferon gamma modulate the expression of the vitronectin receptor (integrin $\beta 3$) in human endothelial cells. J Biol Chem 266:7638–7645.

D.T. Denhardt, B. Feng, D.R. Edwards, E.T. Cocuzzi, U.M. Malyankar (1993). Tissue inhibitor of metalloproteinases (TIMP, aka EPA): Structure, control of expression and biological functions. Pharmacol Ther 59:329–341.

A.J.P. Docherty, A. Lyons, B.J. Smith, E.M. Wright, P.E. Stephens, T.J.R. Harris, G. Murphy, J.J. Reynolds (1985). Sequence of human tissue inhibitor of metalloproteinases and its identity to erythroid-potentiating activity. Nature 318: 66–69.

A. Dong, R. Kumar and I.F. Fidler (1996). Generation of the angiogenesis inhibitor, angiostatin, by Lewis lung carcinoma is mediated by macrophage elastase. Proc Am Assoc Cancer Res 37:403a.

D.A. Douglas, Y.E. Shi, Q.A. Sang (1997). Computational sequence analysis of the tissue inhibitor of metalloproteinase family. J Protein Chem 16:237–255.

M.H. Dresden, S.A. Heilman, J.D. Schmidt (1972). Collagenolytic enzymes in human neoplasms. Cancer Res 32:993–996.

M.R. Emmert-Buck, H.P. Emonard, M.L. Corcoran, H.C. Krutzsch, J-M. Foidart, W.G. Stetler-Stevenson (1995). Cell surface binding of TIMP-2 and pro-MMP-2/TIMP-2 complex. FEBS Lett 364:28–32.

J. Enenstein, N.S. Waleh, R.H. Kramer (1992). Basic FGF and TGFβ differentially modulate integrin expression of human microvascular endothelial cell. Exp Cell Res 203: 499–503.

R.P. Fabunmi, A.H. Baker, E.J. Murray, R.F. Booth, A.C. Newby (1996). Divergent regulation by growth factors and cytokines of 95 kDa and 72 kDa gelatinases and tissue inhibitors of metalloproteinases-1, -2, and -3 in rabbit aortic smooth muscle cells. Biochem J 315:335–342.

M.E. Fini, K.J. Strissel, M.T. Girard, J. West Mays, W.B. Rinehart (1994). Interleukin-1α mediates collagenase synthesis stimulated by phorbal 12-myristate 13-acetate. J Biol Chem 269:11291–11298.

C. Fisher, S. Gilbetson-Beadling, E.A. Powers, G. Petzold, R. Poorman, M.A. Mitchell (1994). Interstitical collagenase is required for angiogenesis in vitro. Dev Biol 162: 499–510.

J. Folkman, Y. Shing (1992). Angiogenesis. J Biol Chem 267:10931–10934.

J. Folkman (1995). Angiogenesis in cancer, vascular, rheumatoid and other disease. Nat Med 1:27–31.

J. Folkman (1997). Angiogenesis and angiogenesis inhibition: An overview. EXS 79:1–8.

J.K. Fraser, F.K. Lin, M.V. Berridge (1988). Expression of high affinity receptors for erythropoietin on human bone marrow cells and on the human erythroleukemic cell line, HEL. Exp Hematol 16:836–842.

M. Friedlander, P.C. Brooks, R.W. Shaffer, C.M. Kincaid, J.A. Varner, D.A. Cheresh (1995). Definition of two angiogenic pathways by distinct alpha v integrins. Science 270:1500–1502.

R. Fridman, T.M. Sweeney, M. Zain, G.R. Martin, H.K. Kleinman (1992a). Malignant transformation of NIH-3T3 cells after subcutaneous co-injection with a reconstituted basement membrane (matrigel). Int J Cancer 51:740–744.

R. Fridman, T.R. Fuerst, R.E. Bird, M. Hayhtya, M. Oelkuct, S. Kraus, D. Kamarek, L.A. Liotta, M.L. Berman, W.G. Stetler-Stevenson (1992b). Domain structure of human 72-kDa gelatinase type IV collagenase. Characterization of proteolytic activity and identification of the tissue inhibitor of metalloproteinase-2 (TIMP-2) binding regions. J Biol Chem 267:15398–15405.

J.C. Gasson, D.W. Golde, S.B. Kaufman, C.A. Westbrook, R.M. Hewick, R.J. Kaufman, G.G. Wong, P.A. Temple, A.C. Leary, E.L. Brown, E.C. Orr, S.C. Clark (1985). Molecular characterization and expression of the gene encoding human erythroid-potentiating activity. Nature 315:768–771.

P. Gatsios, H.D. Haubeck, E.V. De Leur, W. Frisch, S.S. Apte, H. Greiling, P.E. Heinrich, L. Graeve (1996). Oncostatin M differentially regulated tissue inhibitors of metalloproteinases TIMP-1 and TIMP-3 gene expression in human synovial lung cells. Eur J Biochem 241:56–63.

G. Giannelli, J. Falk-Marzillier, O. Schiraldi, W.G. Stetler-Stevenson, V. Quaranta (1997). Induction of cell migration by matrix metalloprotease-2 cleavage of laminin-5. Science 277:225–228.

G.I. Goldberg, B.L. Marmer, G.A. Grant, A.Z. Eisen, S. Wilhelm, C. He (1989). Human 72-kinldalton type IV collagenase forms a complex with a tissue inhibitor of metalloproteases designated TIMP-2. Proc Natl Acad Sci U S A 86:8207–8211.

G.I. Goldberg, A. Strongin, I.E. Collier, L.T. Genrich, B.L. Marmer (1992). Interaction of 92-kDa type IV collagenase with the tissue inhibitor of metalloproteinases prevents dimerization, complex formation with interstitial collagenase, and activation of the proenzyme with stromelysin. J Biol Chem 267:4583–4591.

F.X. Gomis-Ruth, K. Maskos, M. Betz, A. Bergner, R. Huber, K. Suzuki, N. Yoshida, H. Nagase, K. Brew, G.P. Bourenkov, H. Bartunik, W. Bode (1997). Mechanism of inhibition of the human matrix metalloproteinase stromelysin by TIMP-1. Nature 389:77–81.

J. Greene, M. Wang, L.A. Raymond, Y.E. Lui, Y. Shi (1996). Molecular cloning and characterization of human tissue inhibitor of metalloproteinase-4 (TIMP-4). J Biol Chem 271:30375–30380.

J.L. Gross, D. Moscatelli, E.A. Jaffe, D.B. Rifkin (1982). Plasminogen activator and collagenase production by cultured capillary endothelial cells. J Cell Biol 95:974–981.

K.A. Hasty, T.F. Pourmotabbed, G.I. Goldberg, J.P. Thompson, D.G. Spinella, R.M. Stevens, C.L. Mainardi (1990). Human neutrophil collagenase: a distinct gene product with homology to other matrix metalloproteinases. J Biol Chem 265:11421–11424.

T. Hayakawa, K. Yamashita, K. Tanzawa, E. Uchijima and K. Iwata (1992). Tissue inhibitor of metalloproteinases from human bone marrow stromal cell line KM 102 has erythroid-potentiating activity, suggesting its possibly bifunctional role in the hematopoetic microenvironment. FEBS Lett 298:29–32.

T. Hayakawa (1994). Tissue inhibitors of metalloproteinases and their cell growth-promoting activity, mini review. Cell Struct Funct 19:109–114.

C.R. Hill, R.D. Kissun, J.B. Weiss, A. Garner (1983). Angiogenic factor in vitreous from diabetic retinopathy. Experientia 39:583–585.

E.W. Howard, E.C. Bullen, M.J. Banta (1991). Preferential inhibition of 72- and 92-kDa gelatinases by tissue inhibitor of metalloproteinase-2. J Biol Chem 266:13070–13075.

Y. Itoh, S. Briner, H. Nagase (1995). Steps involved in activation of the complex of promatrix metalloprotinase-2 and TIMP-2 by 4-aminophenyl mecuric acetate. Biochem J 308:645–651.

J.J. Jeffrey, J. Gross (1967). Isolation and characterization of a mammalian collagenolytic enzyme. Fed Proc 26:670.

M.D. Johnson, H.R.C. Kim, L. Chesler, G. Tsao-Wu, N. Bouck, P.J. Polverini (1994). Inhibition of angiogenesis by tissue inhibitor of metalloproteinase. J Cell Physiol 160:194–202.

T.V. Karelina, G.I. Goldberg, A.Z. Eisen (1995). Matrix metalloproteinases in blood vessel development in human fetal skin and in cutaneous tumors. J Invest Dermatol 105: 194–202.

Y. Kato, Y. Nakayama, M. Umeda, K. Miyazaki (1992). Induction of 103kDa gelatinase/type IV collagenase by acidic culture conditions in mouse metastatic melanoma cell lines. J Biol Chem 267:11424–11430.

A. Keegan, C.R. Hill, S. Kumar, P. Phillips, A.M. Schor, J.B. Weiss (1982). Purified tumor angiogenesis factor enhances proliferation of capillary, but not aortic, endothelial cells in vitro. J Cell Sci 55:261–276.

D.E. Kleiner, E.J. Unsworth, H.C. Krutzsch, W.G. Stetler Stevenson (1992). Higher order complex formation between the 72-kilodalton type IV collagenase and tissue inhibitor of metalloproteinase-2. Biochemistry 31:1665–1672.

C. Kohn, W. Jacobs, Y.S. Kim, R. Asissandro, W.G. Stetler-Stevenson, L.A. Liotta (1994). Calcium influx modulates MMP-2 expression (72 kDa type IV collagenase, gelatinase A). J Biol Chem 169:21505–21511.

H. Koyama, E.W. Raines, K.E. Bornfeldt, J.M. Roberts, R. Ross (1996). Fibrillar collagen inhibits arterial smooth muscle proliferation through regulation of Cdk2 inhibitors. Cell 87:1069–1078.

G.W. Laurie, C.P. Leblond, G.R. Martin (1982). Localization of type IV collagen, laminin, heparan sulfate proteoglycan, and fibronectin to the basal lamina of basement membranes. J Cell Biol 95:340–344.

K.J. Leco, R. Khokha, N. Pavloff, S.P. Hawkes, D.R. Edwards (1994). Tissue inhibitor of metalloproteinases-3 (TIMP-3) is an extracellular matrix-associated protein with a distinctive pattern of expression in mouse cells and tissues. J Biol Chem 269: 9352–9360.

E. Levi, R. Fridman, H.Q. Miao, Y.S. Ma, A. Yanon, I. Vladavsky (1996). Matrix metalloproteinase 2 releases active soluble ectodomain of fibroblast growth factor receptor 1. Proc Natl Acad Sci U S A 93:7069–7074.

C.E. Lewis, R. Leek, A. Harris, J.O. McGee (1995). Cytokine regulation of angiogenesis in breast cancer: The role of tumor-associated macrophages. J Leukoc Biol 57:747–751.

A.M. Libson, A.G. Gittis, I.E. Collier, B.L. Marmer, G.I. Goldberg, E.E. Lattman (1995). Crystal structure of the haemopexin-like C-terminal domain of gelatinase A [letter]. Nat Struct Biol 2:938–942.

L.A. Liotta, S. Tryggvason, S. Garbisa, I. Hart, C.M. Foltz, S. Shafie (1980). Metastatic potential correlates with enzymatic degradation of basement membrane collagen. Nature 284:67–68.

L.A. Liotta, K. Tryggvason, S. Garbisa, P.G. Robey, A. Abe (1981). Partial purification and characterization of a neutral protease which cleaves type IV collagen. Biochemistry 20:100–104.

L.A. Liotta (1986). Tumor invasion and metastases-role of the extracellular matrix: Rhoads Memorial Award Lecture. Cancer Res 46:1–7.

L.A. Liotta, P.S. Steeg, W.G. Stetler-Stevenson (1991). Cancer metastasis and angiogenesis. An imbalance of positive and negative regulation. Cell 64:327–336.

Y.E. Liu, M. Wang, J. Greene, J. Su, S. Ullrich, H. Li, S. Sheng, R. Alexander, Q.A. Sang, Y.E. Shi (1997). Preparation and characterization of recombinant tissue inhibitor of metalloproteinase 4 (TIMP-4). J Biol Chem 272:20478–20483.

L.M. Matrisian (1990). Metalloproteinases and their inhibitors in matrix remodeling. Trends Genet 6:121–125.

B. McLaughlin, J.B. Weiss (1996). Endothelial-cell-stimulating angiogenesis factor (ESAF) activates progelatinase A (72 kDa type IV collagenase), prostromelysin 1 and procollagenase and reactivates their complexes with tissue inhibitors of metalloproteinases: A role for ESAF in non-inflammatory angiogenesis. Biochem J 317: 739–745.

P. Mignatti, R. Tsuboe, E. Robbins, D.B. Rifkin (1989). In vitro angiogenesis on the human amniotic membrane: Requirement for basic fibroblast growth factor-induced proteinases. J Cell Biol 108:671–682.

P. Mignatti, D.B. Rifkin (1993). Biology and biochemistry of proteinases in tumor invasion. Physiol Rev 73:161–195.

P. Mignatti, D.B. Rifkin (1996). Plasminogen activators and matrix metalloproteinases in angiogenesis. Enz Prot 49:117–137.

T. Mikkelsin, P.S. Yan, K.L. Ho, M. Sameni, B.F. Sloane, M.L. Rosenblum (1995). Immunolocalization of cathepsin B in human glioma—implications for tumor invasion and angiogenesis. J Neurosurg 83:285–290.

R. Montesano, L. Orci (1985). Tumor-promoting phorbol esters induce angiogenesis in vitro. Cell 42:469–477.

R. Montesano, M.S. Petter, U. Mohle-Steinlein, W. Risau, W.F. Wagner, L. Orci (1990). Increased proteolytic activity is responsible for the aberrant morphogenetic behavior of endothelial cells expressing the middle T oncogene. Cell 62:435–445.

A.M. Montgomery, R.A. Reisfeld, S.A. Cheresh (1994). Integrin alpha v beta 3 rescues melanoma cells from apoptosis in three-dimensional dermal collagen. Proc Natl Acad Sci U S A 91:8856–8860.

D. Moscatelli, E. Jaffe, D.B. Rifkin (1980). Tetradecanoly phorbol acetate stimulates latent collagenase production by cultured human endothelial cells. Cell 20:343–351.

D.A. Moscatelli, D.B. Rifkin, E.A. Jaffe (1985). Production of latent collagenase by human umbilical vein endothelial cells in response to angiogenic preparations. Exp Cell Res 156:379–390.

M.L. Moss, S.L. Jin, M.E. Milla, D.M. Bickett, W. Burkhart, H.L. Carter, W.J. Chen, W.C. Clay, J.R. Didsbury, D. Hassler, C.R. Hoffman, T.A. Kost, M.H. Lambert, M.A. Leesnitzer, P. McCauley, G. McGeehan, J. Mitchell, M. Moyer, G. Pahel, W. Rocque, L.K. Overton, F. Schoenen, T. Seaton, J.L. Su, J. Warner, D. Willard, J.D. Becherer (1997). Cloning of a disintegrin metalloproteinase that processes precursor tumor-necrosis factor-alpha. Nature 385:733–736.

D. Muller, B. Quantin, M.C. Gexnel, R. Millon-Collar, J. Abecassis, R. Breathnach (1988). The collagenase gene family in humans consists of at least four members. Biochem J 253:187–192.

A. Murphy, E.J. Unsworth, W.G. Stetler-Stevenson (1993). Tissue inhibitor of metalloproteinases-2 inhibits bFGF-induced human microvascular endothelial cell proliferation. J Cell Physiol 157:351–358.

G. Murphy, A. Houbrechts, M.I. Cockett, R.A. Williamson, M. O'Shea, A.J.P. Docherty (1991). The N-terminal domain of tissue inhibitor of metalloproteinases retains metalloproteinase inhibitory activity. Biochemistry 30:8097–8102.

G. Murphy, J.A. Allan, F. Willenbrock, M.I. Cockett, J. O'Connell, A.J.P. Docherty (1992). The role of the C-terminal domain in collagenase and stromelysin specificity. J Biol Chem 267:9612–9618.

G. Murphy, A.J.P. Docherty (1992). The matrix metalloproteinases and their inhibitors. Am J Respir Cell Mol Biol 7:120–125.

G. Murphy, Q. Nguyen, M.I. Cockett (1994). Assessment of the role of the fibronectin-like domain of gelatinase A by analysis of a deletion mutant. J Biol Chem 269: 6632–6636.

Y. Ogata, M.A. Pratta, H. Nagase, E.C. Arner (1992). Matrix metalloproteinase 9 (92-kDa gelatinase/type IV collagenase) is induced in rabbit articular chondrocytes by cotreatment with interleukin 1 beta and a protein kinase C activator. Exp Cell Res 201:245–249.

M.S. O'Reilly, L. Holmgren, Y. Shing (1994). Angiostatin: A novel angiogenesis inhibitor that mediates the suppression of metastases by a Lewis lung carcinoma. Cell 79: 315–328.

M. O'Shea, F. Willenbrock, R.A. Williamson, M.I. Cockett, R.B. Freedman, J.J. Reynolds, A.J.P. Docherty, G. Murphy (1992). Site-directed mutations that alter the inhibitory activity of the tissue inhibitor of metalloproteinase-1: Importance of the N-terminal region between cysteine 3 and cysteine 13. Biochemistry 31:10146–10152.

C.M. Overall, J.L. Wrana, J. Sodek (1991). Transcriptional and posttranscriptional regulation of 72 kDa gelatinase/type IV collagenase by transforming growth factor-beta-1 in human fibroblasts: Comparisons with collagenase and tissue inhibitor of matrix metalloproteinse gene expression. J Biol Chem 266:14064–14071.

B.C. Patterson, Q-X.A. Sang (1997). Angiostatin-converting enzyme activities of human matrilysin (MMP-7) and gelatinase B/type IV collagenase (MMP-9). J Biol Chem 272:28823–28825.

N. Pavloff, P.W. Staskus, N.S. Kishnani, S.P. Hawkes (1992). A new inhibitor of metalloproteinases from chicken: ChIMP-3. A third member of the TIMP family. J Biol Chem 267:17321–17326.

D. Pei, G. Majmudar and S.J. Weiss (1994). Hydrolytic inactivation of a breast carcinoma cell-derived serpin by human stromelysin-3. J Biol Chem 269:25849–25855.

D. Pei, S.J. Weiss (1995). Furin-dependent intracellular activation of the human stromelysin-3 zymogen. Nature 375:244–247.

A.M. Pendas, V. Knauper, X.S. Puente, E. Llano, M.G. Mattei, S. Apte, G. Murphy, C. Otin-Lopez (1997). Identification and characterization of a novel human matrix metalloproteinase with unique structural characteristics chromosomal location, and tissue distribution. J Biol Chem 272:4281–4286.

M.S. Pepper, D. Belin, R. Montesano, L. Orci, J.D. Vassali (1990). Transforming growth factor-beta 1 modulated basic fibroblast growth factor-induced proteolytic and angiogenic properties of endothelial cells in vitro. J Cell Biol 111:743–755.

M.S. Pepper, R. Montesano, S.J. Mandriota, L. Orci, J.D. Vassalli (1996). Angiogenesis—a paradigm for balanced extracellular proteolysis during cell migration and morphogenesis. Enz Prot 49:138–162.

X.S. Puente, A.M. Pendas, E. Llano, G. Velasco, C. Lopez-Otin (1996). Molecular cloning of a novel membrane-type metalloproteinase from a human breast carcinoma. Cancer Res 56:944–949.

B. Quantin, G. Murphy, R. Breathnach (1989). Pump-1 cDNA codes for a protein with characteristics similar to those of classical collagenase family members. Biochemistry 28:5325–5334.

J.S. Rao, R. Sawaya, Z.L. Gokaslan, W.K.A. Yung, G.W. Goldstein, J. Laterra (1996). Modulation of serine proteinases and metalloproteinases during morphogenic glial-endothelial interactions. J Neurochem 66:1657–1664.

J.M. Ray, W.G. Stetler-Stevenson (1994a). The role of matrix metalloproteases and their inhibitors in tumor invasion, metastasis and angiogenesis. Eur Resp J 7:2062–2072.

J.M. Ray, W.G. Stetler-Stevenson (1994b). Gelatinase A activity directly modulates melanoma cell adhesion and spreading. EMBO J 14:908–917.

T. Salo, J.G. Lyons, R. Rahemtulla, H. Birkedal-Hansen, H. Larjava (1991). Transforming growth factor-β upregulated type IV collagenase expression in cultured human keratinocytes. J Biol Chem 266:11436–11441.

H. Sato, T. Takino, Y. Okada, J. Cao, A. Shinagawa, E. Yamamota, M. Seiki (1994). A matrix metalloproteinase expressed on the surface of invasive tumour cells. Nature 370:61–65.

H.W. Schnaper, D.S. Grant, W.G. Stetler-Stevenson, R. Fritman, G. D'Orazi, A.N. Murphy, R.E. Bird, M. Hoythya, T.R. Fuerst, D.L. French, J.P. Quigley, H.K. Kleinman (1993). Type IV collagenase(s) and TIMPs modulate endothelial cell morphogenesis in vitro. J Cell Physiol 156:235–246.

A.M. Schor, S.L. Schor, J.B. Weiss, R.A. Brown, S. Kumar, P. Phillips (1980). Stimulation by a low-molecular-weight angiogenic factor of capillary endothelial cells in culture. Br J Cancer 41:790–799.

R.E. Seftor, E.A. Seftor, K.R. Gehlsen, W.G. Stetler-Stevenson, P.D. Brown, E. Ruoslahti, M.J. Hendrix (1992). Role of the alpha v beta 3 integrin in human melanoma cell invasion. Proc Natl Acad Sci U S A 89:1557–1561.

R.E.B. Seftor, E.A. Seftor, W.G. Stetler-Stevenson, M.J.C. Hendrix (1993). The 72 kDa type IV collagenase is modulated via differential expression of $\alpha v\beta 3$ and $\alpha 5\beta 1$ integrins during human melanoma cell invasion. Cancer Res 53:3411–3415.

R.M. Senior, G.L. Griffin, C.J. Fliszar, S.D. Shapiro, G.I. Goldberg, H.G. Welgus (1991). Human 92- and 72-kilodalton type IV collagenases are elastases. J Biol Chem 266: 7870–7875.

N.T. Sepp, L.A. Cornelius, N. Romani, L.J. Li, S.W. Caughman, T.J. Lawley, R.A. Swerlick (1995). Polarized expression of basic fibroblast growth factor induced downregulation of the $\alpha 6\beta 4$ integrin complex on human microvascular endothelial cells. J Invest Dermatol 104:266–270.

S.D. Shapiro, E.J. Campbell, D.K. Kobayashi, H.G. Welgus (1990). Immune modulation of metalloproteinase production in human macrophages. J Clin Invest 86:1204–1210.

S.D. Shapiro, D.K. Kobayashi, T.J. Ley (1993). Cloning and characterization of a unique elastolytic metalloproteinase produced by human alveolar macrophages. J Biol Chem 268:23824–23829.

K. Shofuda, H. Yasumitsu, A. Nishihashi, K. Miki, K. Miyazaki (1997). Expression of three membrane-type matrix metalloproteinases (MT-MMPs) in rat vascular smooth muscle cells and characterization of MT3-MMPs with and without transmembrane domain. J Biol Chem 272:9749–9754.

A.A. Sinha, D.F. Gleason, N.A. Staley, M.J. Wilson, M. Sameni, B.F. Sloane (1995). Cathepsin B in angiogenesis of human prostate—an immunohistochemical and immunoelectron microscopic analysis. Anat Rec 241:353–362.

W.G. Stetler-Stevenson, H.C. Krutzsch, L.A. Liotta (1989). Tissue inhibitor of metalloproteinase-2 (TIMP-2). A new member of the metalloproteinase inhibitor family. J Biol Chem 264:17374–17378.

W.G. Stetler-Stevenson, N. Bersch, D.W. Golde (1992). Tissue inhibitor of metalloproteinase-2 (TIMP-2) has erythroid-potentiating activity. FEBS Lett 296:231–234.

W.G. Stetler-Stevenson, S. Aznavoorian, L.A. Liotta (1993). Tumor cell interactions with the extracellular matrix during invasion and metastasis. Annu Rev Cell Biol 9:541–573.

W.G. Stetler-Stevenson, L.A. Liotta, D.E. Kleiner, Jr (1993). Extracellular Matrix 6: Role of matrix metalloproteinases in tumor invasion and metastasis. FASEB J 7:1434–1441.

G.P. Stricklin, H.G. Welgus (1983). Human skin fibroblast collagenase inhibitor. Purification and biochemical characterization. J Biol Chem 258:12252–12258.

A. Strongin, I. Collier, G. Bannikov, B.L. Marmer, G.A. Grant, G.I. Goldberg (1995). Mechanism of cell surface activation of 72kDa type IV collagenase. J Biol Chem 270:5331–5338.

T.M. Sweeney, M.C. Kibbey, M. Zain, R. Fridman, H.K. Kleinman (1991). Basement membrane and the SIKVAV laminin-derived peptide promote tumor growth and metastases. Cancer Metastasis Rev 10:245–254.

T. Takino, H. Sato, A. Shinagawa, M. Seiki (1995). Identification of the second membrane-type matrix metalloproteinase (MT-MMP2) gene from a human placenta cDNA library. MT-MMPs form a unique membrane-type subclass in the MMP family. J Biol Chem 270:23013–23020.

T. Takino, H. Sato, E. Yamamoto, M. Seiki (1995). Cloning of a human gene potentially encoding a novel matrix metalloproteinase having a C-terminal transmembrane domain. Gene 155:293–298.

G. Taraboletti, A. Garofalo, D. Belotti, T. Drudis, P. Borsotti, E. Scanziani, P. Brown, R. Giavazzi (1995). Inhibition of angiogenesis and murine hemangioma growth by batimastat, a synthetic inhibitor of matrix metalloproteinases. J Natl Cancer Inst 87:293–298.

A.C. Taylor, B.M. Levy, J.W. Simpson (1970). Collagenolytic activity of sarcoma tissues in culture. Nature 228:366–367.

E.N. Unemori, A. Werb (1988). Collagenase expression and endogenous activation in rabbit synovial fibroblasts stimulated by calcium ionophore A23187. J Biol Chem 263:16252–16259.

J.A. Uria, M. Stahle-Backdahl, M. Seiki, A. Fueyo, C. Lopez-Otin (1997). Regulation of collagenase-3 expression in human breast carcinomas is mediated by stromal-epithelial cell interactions. Cancer Res 57:4882–4888.

H. Van Wart, H. Birkedal-Hansen (1990). The cysteine switch: A principle of regulation of metalloproteinase activity with potential applicability to the entire matrix metalloproteinase gene family. Proc Natl Acad Sci U S A 87:5578–5582.

A. Werb, R.M. Hembrey, G. Murphy, J. Aggeler (1986). Commitment to expression of the metalloendopeptidases, collagenase and stromelysin: Relationship of inducing events to changes in cytoskeletal architecture. J Cell Biol 102:679–702.

Z. Werb, P.M. Tremble, O. Behrendsten, E. Crowley, C.H. Damsky (1989). Signal transduction through the fibronectin receptor induces collagenase and stromelysin gene expression. J Cell Biol 109:877–889.

M. Wick, C. Burger, S. Brusselbach, E.C. Lucibello, R. Muller (1994). A novel member of human tissue inhibitor of metalloproteinases (TIMP) gene family is regulated during G1 progression, mitogenic stimulation, differentiation, and senescence. J Biol Chem 269:18953–18960.

S.M. Wilhelm, A.Z. Eisen, M. Teter, S.D. Clark, A. Kronberger, G. Goldberg (1986). Human fibroblast collagenase: Glycosylation and tissue-specific levels of enzyme synthesis. Proc Natl Acad Sci U S A 83:3756–3760.

S.M. Wilhelm, I.E. Collier, A. Kronberger, A.Z. Eisen, B.L. Marmer, G.G. Grant, E.A. Bauer, E.I. Goldberg (1987). Human skin fibroblast stromelysin: Structure, glycosylation, substrate specificity, and differential expression in normal and tumourigenic cells. Proc Natl Acad Sci U S A 84:6725–6729.

S.M. Wilhelm, I.E. Collier, B.L. Marmer, A.Z. Eisen, G.A. Grant, G.I. Goldberg (1989). SV40-transformed human lung fibroblasts secrete a 92-kDa Type IV collagenase which is identical to that secreted by normal human macrophages. J Biol Chem 264:17213–17221.

H. Will, B. Hinzmann (1995). cDNA sequence and mRNA tissue distribution of a novel human matrix metalloproteinase with a potential transmembrane segment. Eur J Biochem 231:602–608.

F. Willenbrock, G. Murphy (1994). Structure-function relationships in the tissue inhibitors of metalloproteinases. Am J Respir Crit Care Med 150:S165–S170.

J.F. Woessner, Jr. (1991). Matrix metalloproteinases and their inhibitors in connective tissue remodeling. FASEB J 5:2145–2154.

T.G. Wolfsberg, P. Primakoff, D.G. Myles, J.M. White (1995). ADAM, a novel family of membrane proteins containing A Disintegrin And Metalloproteinase domain: Multipotential functions in cell-cell and cell-matrix interactions. J Cell Biol 131: 275–278.

4

Regulation of Cell Migration in the Process of Angiogenesis

Bela Anand-Apte
Cole Eye Institute, Cleveland Clinic Foundation, Cleveland, Ohio

Bruce R. Zetter
Children's Hospital and Harvard Medical School, Boston, Massachusetts

I. MIGRATION

The morphogenetic events that result in the formation of new capillaries have been well described. Angiogenesis is usually initiated by a localized breakdown of the basement membrane of the parent vessel. A precise spatial and temporal regulation of extracellular proteolytic activity appears be important in this initial process of endothelial cell invasion into the extracellular matrix. After this, endothelial cells migrate into the surrounding ECM within which they form a capillary sprout. Elongation of the sprout occurs by further migration and by endothelial cell proliferation proximal to the migrating front, resulting in the formation of a lumen proximal to the region of proliferation. Anastomoses of contiguous tubular sprouts form a functional capillary loop that is followed by reconstitution of the basement membrane and vessel maturation (1, 2).

Migration of microvascular endothelial cells is a critical component of physiological and pathological angiogenesis. Early studies (1, 3) suggest that endothelial cells first migrate toward an angiogenic stimulus with subsequent mitosis occurring at the more distal aspect of the new capillary. Additional studies by Sholley and colleagues (4) determined that the initial stages of neovascularization, such as capillary budding, could occur in the absence of cell division, mediated primarily by elongation and migration of endothelial cells. It is tantalizing to speculate about the importance of directional endothelium migration to induce directional sprouting of a capillary specifically toward an angiogenic stimulus. This could be important in both tumor and fetal neovascularization, which would require a controlled and directed induction of capillary blood flow. Finally, mathematical and biological models (5, 6) have predicted that the rate of new blood vessel sprouting is primarily determined by endothelial cell migration rate.

A. Directed Versus Random Migration of Endothelial Cells

Before we begin our discussion on endothelial cell motility we need to distinguish between the different types of motile responses of endothelial cells: chemokinesis (random motility), chemotaxis, and haptotaxis.

1. Chemokinesis

Chemokinesis is the induction of random, nondirectional motility in response to a ligand without any orienting cues. Chemokinesis suggests either an increased rate of cellular translocation or an increased distance traveled per unit of time.

2. Chemotaxis

Chemotaxis describes the directional motility response of cells toward a positive gradient of soluble chemoattractant. Angiogenic factors such as vascular endothelial growth factor (VEGF) are chemotactic for endothelial cells. It can be envisioned that the growing tumor secretes angiogenic factors and establishes a chemotactic gradient surrounding it. Endothelial cells in capillaries present in the vicinity of the tumor may sense this gradient and start migrating toward the tumor. Chemotaxis may occur by activating cell surface receptors on endothelial cells in a polarized manner, that is, preferential activation of receptors on the leading edge of the cell. This in turn could stimulate the motile machinery of the cell, including adhesion receptors, actin, myosin, and other cytoskeletal and membrane elements to induce a directional migratory response up to the chemotactic gradient.

3. Haptotaxis

Haptotaxis is the directed migration of cells along a gradient of anchored substrate, such as ECM molecules, which include fibronectin, laminin, collagen, elastin, thrombospondin, and vitronectin. Similar molecular mechanisms as those used during chemotaxis are probably brought into play during the process of haptotaxis. A combination of these different motility responses may be utilized by endothelial cells during angiogenesis in vivo.

B. Positive Regulators of Endothelial Cell Migration and Tumor Angiogenesis

The switch to an angiogenic phenotype in tumors is believed to involve an imbalance in the equilibrium between positive and negative regulators of neovascularization. This might result from either an induction of positive regulatory molecules or an inhibition of negative regulators of angiogenesis.

Morphogenetic events that result in the formation of new capillary blood vessels have been extensively studied. Endothelial cell migration has a crucial role in the formation and maturation of capillary sprouts. After breakdown of the basement membrane of the parent vessel (usually a postcapillary venule), endothelial cells migrate into the surrounding ECM to form a capillary sprout. Further migration and proliferation of endothelial cells result in sprout elongation, which is usually followed by the formation of a lumen. Anastomoses of contiguous sprouts result in a functional capillary loop, and reconstitution of basement membrane leads to vessel maturation. Mathematical models suggest that migration of endothelial cells is the rate limiting step for angiogenesis in vivo (7). The ability of endogenous angiogenic agents to induce migration of endothelial cells has been described in Table 1. Because basic fibroblast growth factor (bFGF) and VEGF are the angiogenic peptides most extensively studied in mouse and human tumors, they will be discussed exclusively in this chapter. Both VEGF and bFGF can induce angiogenesis in an in vivo mouse corneal pocket assay (8). Secretion of these angiogenic factors by tumors may result in the directed migration of endothelial cells toward the tumor, resulting in the directional growth of new capillary sprouts.

1. bFGF

Basic fibroblast growth factor is an 18,000-d heparin-binding protein monomer that can induce migration of endothelial cells and a variety of other effects, such as proliferation, induction of plasminogen activator and collagenase and capillary tube formation (9). Recent evidence suggests that bFGF-stimulated endothelial cell migration is mediated by a pertussis toxin-sensitive GTP-binding protein (10). It has also been reported that phospholipase C gamma activation, phosphotidylinositol hydrolysis, and calcium mobilization are not required for FGF receptor-mediated cell migration (11). The action of bFGF is not restricted to endothelial cells, responses being observed in other cell types in vitro. However, during the process of tumor angiogenesis, bFGF secreted by tumor cells seems to act directly on vascular endothelial cells in vivo.

2. VEGF

Vascular endothelial growth factor is a secreted angiogenic factor with four alternatively spliced isoforms (12). Increased VEGF expression has been associated

Table 1 Positive Regulators of Angiogenesis

Angiogenic Factor	Molecular Weight	Angiogenesis In Vivo Assay	Endothelial Cell Migration	References
Angiogenin	14,100	Rabbit cornea		57
Fibroblast growth factors		Chick CAM	↑	58, 59
Basic	18,000	Rabbit cornea	↑	
Acidic	16,400	Chick CAM	↑	
Granulocyte colony-stimulating factor	17,000	Rabbit cornea	↑	60, 61
Hepatocyte growth factor	92,000	Rat cornea	↑	62–64
Interleukin 8	40,000	Rat cornea	↑	65
Placental growth factor	25,000	Rabbit cornea Chick CAM	↑	66
Platelet-derived endothelial growth factor	45,000	Rat cornea Chick CAM	↑	67
Proliferin	35,000	Rat cornea	↑	68, 69
Transforming growth factor α	5,500	Hamster cheek pouch	↑	70
Transforming growth factor β	25,000	Newborn mouse skin Chick CAM	no	71
Tumor necrosis factor α	17,000	Rat cornea Chick CAM	↑	72–74
Vascular endothelial growth factor	45,000	Rat cornea Chick CAM Transgenic mice	↑	18, 75, 76

Abbreviation: CAM, Chorioallantoic membrane

with a wide variety of tumors, including glioblastoma and colon cancer (13, 14). Vascular endothelial growth factor induces migration of human umbilical vein endothelium and retinal capillary endothelium (15). It has been suggested that the migration of endothelial cells induced by VEGF occurs though stimulation of the KDR receptor (16). Vascular endothelial growth factor homodimers as well as VEGF/placental growth factor heterodimers can induce endothelial cell chemotaxis (17).

Interestingly, checkerboard analysis of migration assays indicate that bFGF acts predominantly as a chemokinetic factor, whereas VEGF was mostly chemotactic for human umbilical vein endothelial cells (18). Also, VEGF and bFGF were not synergistic in endothelial cell migration or proliferation assays in vitro. Synergism between these two factors has been demonstrated in capillary tube morphogenesis assays (19, 20). It is possible that during morphogenesis of capil-

Table 2 Endogenous Angiostatic Inhibitors of Endothelial Cell Migration

Factor	Inhibits Endothelial Cell Migration	Presence in the Circulation	Presence in the ECM	References
Angiostatin	Yes	Yes	NT	77
Interferon alpha	Yes	Yes	NT	78–80
Placental proliferin related protein	Yes	Yes	NT	68
Platelet factor 4	Yes	Yes	No	81, 82
Prolactin (16 kD fragment)	Yes	NT	NT	83, 84
Thrombospondin 1	Yes	Yes	Yes	85–88
TIMP-1	No	Yes	No	38, 39
TIMP-2	No	Yes	No	90
TIMP-3	Yes	NT[a]	Yes	39

[a] NT = not tested.
Abbreviations: ECM, extracellular matrix; *TIMP*, tissue inhibitors of metalloproteinases.

lary tubes, VEGF may act as the primary migration inducer, whereas bFGF may be responsible for induction of proliferation.

C. Negative Regulators of Endothelial Cell Migration and Angiogenesis

The balance of angiogenesis regulation can be altered in favor of new blood vessel growth by inhibition of normally present endogenous negative regulators of angiogenesis. Over the past few years, a number of angiogenesis inhibitors, both endogenous and exogenously derived, have been studied extensively. Table 2 describes some of the endogenous angiogenesis inhibitors that have been identified and their ability to inhibit endothelial cell migration.

II. CLINICAL TRIALS: ANTIANGIOGENIC THERAPY FOR TUMORS

A number of potential angiogenesis inhibitors are now in phase I, II, or III clinical trials (21) for antitumor therapy. These include platelet factor-4 (22), TNP-470 (23), interferon (IFN)-alpha (24–26), carboxy-amidotriazole (CAI[27]), Batimastat (metalloproteinase inhibitor)/marimastat (28–30), and the sulfated peptidoglycan DS4152. Of these PF4, TNP-470, CAI, and IFN-alpha have been tested and shown to inhibit migration of endothelial cells toward both bFGF and VEGF (18, 21, 31–33). These results raise the possibility that some angiogenesis inhibitors may function in vivo by blocking endothelial cell migration.

III. FUTURE DIRECTIONS

Cell migration is a physically integrated complex molecular process involving a multitude of cellular and extracellular components that work together in a dynamic system. Some of these include binding of motility-inducing factor to surface receptors, signal transduction, morphological polarization of the cell, membrane extension, formation of cell-extracellular matrix attachments, contractile force and traction, and release of cell-matrix attachments (34). It can be postulated that endogenous or synthetic inhibitors may act at any one of these levels. A clear understanding of the molecular mechanisms in endothelial migration will aid in the design of molecules with angiostatic capabilities.

Directed endothelial cell migration has a critical role in tumor angiogenesis. This process requires the recognition of guidance cues, probably emanating from tumors in vivo, and their translation by the responding endothelial cells into directional motility before the formation of capillary sprouts. In addition to the initiating cues, the cells need to be able to recognize their ultimate target tissue and stop migrating. These initiating and terminating cues that control endothelial cell motility involved in neovascularization have yet to be determined. It can be hypothesized that under normal physiological conditions, unwarranted endothelial cell migration is kept in check by a tightly regulated balance between

1. Proteolytic molecules and their inhibitors
2. Adhesion stabilizing and destabilizing factors
3. Chemoattractants and chemorepellants

A. Proteolytic Balance During Endothelial Cell Migration and Angiogenesis

Extracellular proteolysis is required for the degradation of the extracellular matrix and migration of endothelial cells during angiogenesis. This process relies on a number of proteases and protease inhibitors secreted by endothelial and nonendothelial cells (35). The plasminogen activator (PA)/plasmin as well as matrix metalloproteinases (MMPs) have been studied and are believed to be regulated during angiogenesis Urokinase plasminogen activator (uPA) and plasminogen activator inhibitor (PAI) activity have been found to be induced in migrating endothelial cells (36, 37). Tissue inhibitor of metalloproteinase-1 (TIMP-1) inhibits migration of endothelial cells in response to adipocyte conditioned medium (38). Recent evidence that TIMP-3 inhibits endothelial cell motility toward VEGF and bFGF suggests that the MMP/TIMP balance might be critical for endothelial cell migration (39). Matrix metalloproteinase-2 colocalized with integrin $\alpha v\beta 3$ on angiogenic blood vessels, which suggests that a single cell surface receptor may regulate both matrix degradation and motility (40). Although it has long been believed that MMPs cause the physical breakdown of the ECM barrier and thereby induce migration, recent studies point to the possibility that MMPs provide a signaling mechanism for cells to begin migration. Laminin-5 is a primary target of MMP-2 cleavage and is critical for cell migration during tissue remodeling and tumor invasion (41). Information on specific MMP/ECM interactions critical for endothelial cell migration will be crucial to understanding the early events in angiogenesis.

B. Balance Between Factors Regulating Adhesion and De-adhesion of Endothelial Cells to Matrix

For a cell to be able to migrate, it should have the preferential ability to form adhesions with the matrix at the leading edge of lamellipodia (42, 43). The mechanisms that initiate and regulate the formation of these adhesive complexes at the leading edge of the cell are unclear. Covalent modifications of certain candidate molecules, such as focal adhesion kinase (FAK), tensin, and paxillin have been implicated in this process (44–52). Recent studies have shown that short-term cell substratum adhesiveness is rate limiting for speed of migration (53). The presence of an optimum adhesiveness for cell migration suggests that this process can be modulated by regulating the amount of ligand (ECM), receptor (integrin) expression, and affinity of binding. A cell bound too tightly to its matrix will not be able to move in any direction. Similarly, a cell with weak matrix interactions will be unable to generate traction at its leading edge to move directionally. It can be hypothesized that tumor cells may release factors that will regulate this process of adhesion/de-adhesion to enable the endothelial cell to move toward it. Further studies to address this hypothesis will be of great interest.

Cell-cell adhesion may also be important for angiogenesis. The soluble form of vascular adhesion molecule 1 (VCAM-1) induces angiogenesis in vivo and migration of human endothelial cells in vitro with no effect on endothelial cell proliferation (54). The angiogenesis-inducing property of VCAM-1 appears to be mediated by its interaction with integrin $\alpha 4\beta 1$ (54). The selectins are another group of transmembrane cell adhesion glycoproteins. The soluble form of E-selectin stimulates endothelial cell migration in vitro, as well as angiogenesis in vivo, in the rat cornea through its interaction with Sialyl-Lewis X (54).

C. Balance Between Chemoattractants and Chemorepellants

Directed endothelial cell migration is similar in principle to the process of axon guidance during development of the nervous system (55). In this system, a combination of attractant and repulsant cues regulate axon pathfinding. UNC-6 and netrin are examples of secreted guidance factors. The same netrin molecule is a chemoattractant for axons but a chemorepellant for trochlear motor neurons (56). This suggests that in addition to chemoattractive cues, chemorepulsive cues may turn out to play an important role in regulating endothelial cell migration during angiogenesis.

A better understanding of the molecular mechanisms involved in directed endothelial cell migration during tumor angiogenesis will enable the creation and use of drugs that inhibit the process in the hope of slowing the progress of rampant tumor growth.

REFERENCES

1. Ausprunk DH, Folkman J. Migration and proliferation of endothelial cells in preformed and newly formed blood vessels during tumor angiogenesis. Microvasc Res 1977;14:53–65.
2. Paku S, Paweletz N. First steps of tumor-related angiogenesis. Lab Invest 1991;65: 334–346.
3. Yamagami I. Electron microscopic study of the cornea I: The mechanism of experimental new vessel formation. Jpn J Ophthalmol 1970;14:41–58.
4. Sholley MM, Ferguson GP, Seibel HR, Montour JL, Wilson JD. Mechanisms of neovascularization. Vascular sprouting can occur without proliferation of endothelial cells. Lab Invest 1984;51:624–634.
5. Stokes CL, Lauffenburger DA. Analysis of the roles of microvessel endothelial cell random motility and chemotaxis in angiogenesis. J Theor Biol 1991;152:377–403.
6. Stokes CL, Rupnick MA, Williams SK, Lauffenburger DA. Chemotaxis of human microvessel endothelial cells in response to acidic fibroblast growth factor. Lab Invest 1990;63:657–668.
7. Stokes CL. Endothelial cell migration and chemotaxis in angiogenesis. EXS 1992; 61:118–124.
8. Kenyon BM, Voest EE, Chen CC, Flynn E, Folkman J, D'Amato RJ. A model of angiogenesis in the mouse cornea. Invest Ophthalmol Vis Sci 1996;37:1625–1632.
9. Rifkin DB, Moscatelli D. Recent developments in the cell biology of basic fibroblast growth factor. J Cell Biol 1989;109:1–6.
10. Sa G, Fox PL. Basic fibroblast growth factor-stimulated endothelial cell movement is mediated by a pertussis toxin-sensitive pathway regulating phospholipase A2 activity. J Biol Chem 1994;269:3219–3225.

11. Clyman RI, Peters KG, Chen YQ, Escobedo J, Williams LT, Ives HE, Wilson E. Phospholipase C gamma activation, phosphotidylinositol hydrolysis, and calcium mobilization are not required for FGF receptor-mediated chemotaxis. Cell Adhes Commun 1994;1:333–342.
12. Park JE, Keller GA, Ferrara N. The vascular endothelial growth factor (VEGF) isoforms: Differential deposition into the subepithelial extracellular matrix and bioactivity of extracellular matrix-bound VEGF. Mol Biol Cell 1993;4:1317–1326.
13. Plate KH, Breier G, Weich HA, Risau W. Vascular endothelial growth factor is a potential tumour angiogenesis factor in human gliomas in vivo. Nature 1992;359: 845–848.
14. Takahashi A, Sasaki H, Kim SJ, Tobisu K, Kakizoe T, Tsukamoto T, Kumamoto Y, Sugimura T, Terada M. Markedly increased amounts of messenger RNAs for vascular endothelial growth factor and placenta growth factor in renal cell carcinoma associated with angiogenesis. Cancer Res 1994;54:4233–4237.
15. Simorre-Pinatel V, Guerrin M, Chollet P, Penary M, Clamens S, Malecaze F, Plouet J. Vasculotropin-VEGF stimulates retinal capillary endothelial cells through an autocrine pathway. Invest Ophthalmol Vis Sci 1994;35:3393–3400.
16. Waltenberger J, Claesson-Welsh L, Siegbahn A, Shibuya M, Heldin CH. Different signal transduction properties of KDR and Fltl, two receptors for vascular endothelial growth factor. J Biol Chem 1994;269:26988–26995.
17. Cao Y, Chen H, Zhou L, Chiang MK, Anand-Apte B, Weatherbee JA, Wang Y, Fang F, Flanagan JG, Tsang ML. Heterodimers of placenta growth factor/vascular endothelial growth factor. Endothelial activity, tumor cell expression, and high affinity binding to Flk-1/KDR. J Biol Chem 1996;271:3154–3162.
18. Yoshida A, Anand-Apte B, Zetter BR. Differential endothelial migration and proliferation to basic fibroblast growth factor and vascular endothelial growth factor. Growth Factors 1996;13:57–64.
19. Pepper MS, Vassalli JD, Montesano R, Orci L. Urokinase-type plasminogen activator is induced in migrating capillary endothelial cells. J Cell Biol 1987;105:2535–2541.
20. Goto F, Goto K, Weindel K, Folkman J. Synergistic effects of vascular endothelial growth factor and basic fibroblast growth factor on the proliferation and cord formation of bovine capillary endothelial cells within collagen gels. Lab Invest 1993;69: 508–517.
21. Folkman J. Seminars in medicine of the Beth Israel hospital, Boston. Clinical applications of research on angiogenesis. N Engl J Med 1995;333:1757–1763.
22. Belman N, Bonnem EM, Harvey HA, Lipton A. Phase I trial of recombinant platelet factor 4 (rPF4) in patients with advanced colorectal carcinoma. Invest New Drugs 1996;14:387–389.
23. Figg WD, Pluda JM, Lush RM, Saville MW, Wyvill K, Reed E, Yarchoan R. The pharmacokinetics of TNP-470, a new angiogenesis inhibitor. Pharmacotherapy 1997;17:91–97.
24. Arnold A, Ayoub J, Douglas L, Hoogendoorn P, Skingley L, Gelmon K, Hirsh V, Eisenhauer E. Phase II trial of 13-cis-retinoic acid plus interferon alpha in non-small-cell lung cancer. The National Cancer Institute of Canada Clinical Trials Group. J Natl Cancer Inst 1994;86:306–309.

25. Cascinu S, Del Ferro E, Ligi M, Graziano F, Castellani A, Catalano G. Phase II trial of 13-cis retinoic acid plus interferon-alpha in advanced squamous cell carcinoma of head and neck, refractory to chemotherapy [letter]. Ann Oncol 1996;7:538.
26. Slabber CF, Falkson G, Burger W, Schoeman L. 13-Cis-retinoic acid and interferon alpha-2a in patients with advanced esophageal cancer: A phase II trial. Invest New Drugs 1996;14:391–394.
27. Kohn EC, Reed E, Sarosy G, Christian M, Link CJ, Cole K, Figg WD, Davis PA, Jacob J, Goldspiel B, Liotta LA. Clinical investigation of a cytostatic calcium influx inhibitor in patients with refractory cancers. Cancer Res 1996;56:569–573.
28. Parsons SL, Watson SA, Steele RJ. Phase I/II trial of batimastat, a matrix metalloproteinase inhibitor, in patients with malignant ascites. Eur J Surg Oncol 1997;23: 526–531.
29. Brown PD. Matrix metalloproteinase inhibitors:A novel class of anticancer agents. Adv Enzyme Regul 1995;35:293–301.
30. Wojtowicz-Praga S, Low J, Marshall J, Ness E, Dickson R, Barter J, Sale M, McCann P, Moore J, Cole A, Hawkins MJ. Phase I trial of a novel matrix metalloproteinase inhibitor batimastat (BB-94) in patients with advanced cancer. Invest New Drugs 1996;14:193–202.
31. Brem H, Gresser I, Grosfeld J, Folkman J. The combination of antiangiogenic agents to inhibit primary tumor growth and metastasis. J Pediatr Surg 1993;28:1253–1257.
32. Brem H, Folkman J. Analysis of experimental antiangiogenic therapy. J Pediatr Surg 1993;28:445–450; discussion 450–451.
33. Sharpe RJ, Byers HR, Scott CF, Bauer SI, Maione TE. Growth inhibition of murine melanoma and human colon carcinoma by recombinant human platelet factor 4. J Natl Cancer Inst 1990;82:848–853.
34. Lauffenburger DA, Horwitz AF. Cell migration: A physically integrated molecular process. Cell 1996;84:359–369.
35. Pepper MS, Montesano R, Mandriota SJ, Orci L, Vassalli JD. Angiogenesis: A paradigm for balanced extracellular proteolysis during cell migration and morphogenesis. Enzyme Protein 1996;49:138–162.
36. Pepper MS, Sappino AP, Montesano R, Orci L, Vassalli JD. Plasminogen activator inhibitor-1 is induced in migrating endothelial cells. J Cell Physiol 1992;153:129–139.
37. Pepper MS, Sappino AP, Stocklin R, Montesano R, Orci L, Vassalli JD. Upregulation of urokinase receptor expression on migrating endothelial cells. J Cell Biol 1993;122:673–684.
38. Johnson MD, Kim HR, Chesler L, Tsao-Wu G, Bouck N, Polverini PJ. Inhibition of angiogenesis by tissue inhibitor of metalloproteinase. J Cell Physiol 1994;160: 194–202.
39. Anand-Apte B, Pepper MS, Voest E, Montesano R, Olsen B, Murphy G, Apte SS, Zetter B. Inhibition of angiogenesis by tissue inhibitor of metalloproteinase-3. Invest Ophthalmol Vis Sci 1997;38:817–823.
40. Brooks PC, Stromblad S, Sanders LC, von Schalscha TL, Aimes RT, Stetler-Stevenson WG, Quigley JP, Cheresh DA. Localization of matrix metalloproteinase MMP-2 to the surface of invasive cells by interaction with integrin alpha v beta 3. Cell 1996;85:683–693.

41. Giannelli G, Falk-Marzillier J, Schiraldi O, Stetler-Stevenson WG, Quaranta V. Induction of cell migration by matrix metalloprotease-2 cleavage of laminin-5. Science 1997;277:225–228.
42. Izzard CS, Lochner LR. Formation of cell-to-substrate contacts during fibroblast motility: An interference-reflexion study. J Cell Sci 1980;42:81–116.
43. Regen CM, Horwitz AF. Dynamics of beta 1 integrin-mediated adhesive contacts in motile fibroblasts. J Cell Biol 1992;119:1347–1359.
44. Wu DY, Goldberg DJ. Regulated tyrosine phosphorylation at the tips of growth cone filopodia. J Cell Biol 1993;123:653–664.
45. Turner CE. Paxillin: A cytoskeletal target for tyrosine kinases. Bioessays 1994;16: 47–52.
46. Schaller MD, Parsons JT. Focal adhesion kinase and associated proteins. Curr Opin Cell Biol 1994;6:705–710.
47. Schaller MD, Parsons JT. FAK-dependent tyrosine phosphorylation of paxillin creates a high-affinity binding site for Crk. Mol Cell Biol 1995;15:2635–2645.
48. Lo SH, Weisberg E, Chen LB. Tensin: A potential link between the cytoskeleton and signal transduction. Bioessays 1994;16:817–823.
49. Davis S, Lu ML, Lo SH, Lin S, Butler JA, Druker BJ, Roberts TM, An Q, Chen LB. Presence of an SH2 domain in the actin-binding protein tensin. Science 1991; 252:712–715.
50. Chen HC, Guan JL. Association of focal adhesion kinase with its potential substrate phosphatidylinositol 3-kinase. Proc Natl Acad Sci U S A 1994;91:10148–10152.
51. Chen HC, Appeddu PA, Parsons JT, Hildebrand JD, Schaller MD, Guan JL. Interaction of focal adhesion kinase with cytoskeletal protein talin. J Biol Chem 1995;270: 16995–16999.
52. Burridge K, Turner CE, Romer LH. Tyrosine phosphorylation of paxillin and pp125FAK accompanies cell adhesion to extracellular matrix: A role in cytoskeletal assembly. J Cell Biol 1992;119:893–903.
53. Palecek SP, Loftus JC, Ginsberg MH, Lauffenburger DA, Horwitz AF. Integrin-ligand binding properties govern cell migration speed through cell-substratum adhesiveness (published erratum appears in Nature 1997 Jul 10;388(6638):210). Nature 1997;385:537–540.
54. Koch AE, Halloran MM, Haskell CJ, Shah MR, Polverini PJ. Angiogenesis mediated by soluble forms of E-selectin and vascular cell adhesion molecule-1. Nature 1995; 376:517–519.
55. Tessier-Lavigne M, Goodman CS. The molecular biology of axon guidance. Science 1996;274:1123–1133.
56. Wadsworth WG, Bhatt H, Hedgecock EM. Neuroglia and pioneer neurons express UNC-6 to provide global and local netrin cues for guiding migrations in *C. elegans*. Neuron 1996;16:35–46.
57. Hu G, Riordan JF, Vallee BL. Angiogenin promotes invasiveness of cultured endothelial cells by stimulation of cell-associated proteolytic activities. Proc Natl Acad Sci U S A 1994;91:12096–12100.
58. Herbert JM, Laplace MC, Maffrand JP. Effect of heparin on the angiogenic potency of basic and acidic fibroblast growth factors in the rabbit cornea assay. Int J Tissue React 1988;10:133–139.

59. Esch F, Baird A, Ling N, Ueno N, Hill F, Denoroy L, Klepper R, Gospodarowicz D, Bohlen P, Guillemin R. Primary structure of bovine pituitary basic fibroblast growth factor (FGF) and comparison with the amino-terminal sequence of bovine brain acidic FGF. Proc Natl Acad Sci U S A 1985;82:6507–6511.
60. Bussolino F, Ziche M, Wang JM, Alessi D, Morbidelli L, Cremona O, Bosia A, Marchisio PC, Mantovani A. In vitro and in vivo activation of endothelial cells by colony-stimulating factors. J Clin Invest 1991;87:986–995.
61. Bussolino F, Colotta F, Bocchietto E, Guglielmetti A, Mantovani A. Recent developments in the cell biology of granulocyte-macrophage colony-stimulating factor and granulocyte colony-stimulating factor: Activities on endothelial cells. Int J Clin Lab Res 1993;23:8–12.
62. Bussolino F, Di Renzo MF, Ziche M, Bocchietto E, Olivero M, Naldini L, Gaudino G, Tamagnone L, Coffer A, Comoglio PM. Hepatocyte growth factor is a potent angiogenic factor which stimulates endothelial cell motility and growth. J Cell Biol 1992;119:629–641.
63. Grant DS, Kleinman HK, Goldberg ID, Bhargava MM, Nickoloff BJ, Kinsella JL, Polverini P, Rosen EM. Scatter factor induces blood vessel formation in vivo. Proc Natl Acad Sci U S A 1993;90:1937–1941.
64. Polverini PJ, Nickoloff BJ. The role of scatter factor and the c-met proto-oncogene in angiogenic responses. EXS 1995;74:51–67.
65. Koch AE, Polverini PJ, Kunkel SL, Harlow LA, Di Pietro LA, Elner VM, Elner SG, Strieter RM. Interleukin-8 as a macrophage-derived mediator of angiogenesis. Science 1992;258:1798–1801.
66. Ziche M, Maglione D, Ribatti D, Morbidelli L, Lago CT, Battisti M, Paoletti I, Barra A, Tucci M, Parise G, Vincenti V, Granger HJ, Viglietto G, Persico MG. Placenta growth factor-1 is chemotactic, mitogenic, and angiogenic. Lab Invest 1997;76:517–531.
67. Ishikawa F, Miyazono K, Hellman U, Drexler H, Wernstedt C, Hagiwara K, Usuki K, Takaku F, Risau W, Heldin CH. Identification of angiogenic activity and the cloning and expression of platelet-derived endothelial cell growth factor. Nature 1989;338:557–552.
68. Jackson D, Volpert OV, Bouck N, Linzer DI. Stimulation and inhibition of angiogenesis by placental proliferin and proliferin-related protein. Science 1994;266:1581–1584.
69. Groskopf JC, Syu LJ, Saltiel AR, Linzer DI. Proliferin induces endothelial cell chemotaxis through a G protein-coupled, mitogen-activated protein kinase-dependent pathway. Endocrinology 1997;138:2835–2840.
70. Grotendorst GR, Soma Y, Takehara K, Charette M. EGF and TGF-alpha are potent chemoattractants for endothelial cells and EGF-like peptides are present at sites of tissue regeneration. J Cell Physiol 1989;139:617–623.
71. Yang EY, Moses HL. Transforming growth factor beta 1-induced changes in cell migration, proliferation, and angiogenesis in the chicken chorioallantoic membrane. J Cell Biol 1990;111:731–741.
72. Leibovich SJ, Polverini PJ, Shepard HM, Wiseman DM, Shively V, Nuseir N. Macrophage-induced angiogenesis is mediated by tumour necrosis factor-alpha. Nature 1987;329:630–632.

73. Frater-Schroder M, Risau W, Hallmann R, Gautschi P, Bohlen P. Tumor necrosis factor type alpha, a potent inhibitor of endothelial cell growth in vitro, is angiogenic in vivo. Proc Natl Acad Sci U S A 1987;84:5277–5281.
74. Olivo M, Bhardwaj R, Schulze-Osthoff K, Sorg C, Jacob HJ, Flamme I. A comparative study on the effects of tumor necrosis factor-alpha (TNF-alpha), human angiogenic factor (h-AF) and basic fibroblast growth factor (bFGF) on the chorioallantoic membrane of the chick embryo. Anat Rec 1992;234:105–115.
75. Koch AE, Harlow LA, Haines GK, Amento EP, Unemori EN, Wong WL, Pope RM, Ferrara N. Vascular endothelial growth factor. A cytokine modulating endothelial function in rheumatoid arthritis. J Immunol 1994;152:4149–4156.
76. Wilting J, Christ B, Bokeloh M, Weich HA. In vivo effects of vascular endothelial growth factor on the chicken chorioallantoic membrane. Cell Tissue Res 1993;274: 163–172.
77. O'Reilly MS, Holmgren L, Chen C, Folkman J. Angiostatin induces and sustains dormancy of human primary tumors in mice. Nat Med 1996;2:689–692.
78. Brouty-Boye D, Zetter BR. Inhibition of cell motility by interferon. Science 1980; 208:516–518.
79. Dvorak HF, Gresser I. Microvascular injury in pathogenesis of interferon-induced necrosis of subcutaneous tumors in mice. J Natl Cancer Inst 1989;81:497–502.
80. Sidky YA, Borden EC. Inhibition of angiogenesis by interferons: Effects on tumor- and lymphocyte-induced vascular responses. Cancer Res 1987;47:5155–5161.
81. Maione TE, Gray GS, Petro J, Hunt AJ, Donner AL, Bauer SI, Carson HF, Sharpe RJ. Inhibition of angiogenesis by recombinant human platelet factor-4 and related peptides. Science 1990;247:77–79.
82. Gengrinovitch S, Greenberg SM, Cohen T, Gitay-Goren H, Rockwell P, Maione TE, Levi BZ, Neufeld G. Platelet factor-4 inhibits the mitogenic activity of VEGF121 and VEGF165 using several concurrent mechanisms. J Biol Chem 1995; 270:15059–15065.
83. D'Angelo G, Struman I, Martial J, Weiner RI. Activation of mitogen-activated protein kinases by vascular endothelial growth factor and basic fibroblast growth factor in capillary endothelial cells is inhibited by the antiangiogenic factor 16-kDa N-terminal fragment of prolactin. Proc Natl Acad Sci U S A 1995;92:6374–6378.
84. Clapp C, Martial JA, Guzman RC, Rentier-Delure F, Weiner RI. The 16-kilodalton N-terminal fragment of human prolactin is a potent inhibitor of angiogenesis. Endocrinology 1993;133:1292–1299.
85. Dameron KM, Volpert OV, Tainsky MA, Bouck N. Control of angiogenesis in fibroblasts by p53 regulation of thrombospondin-1. Science 1994;265:1582–1584.
86. Good DJ, Polverini PJ, Rastinejad F, Le Beau MM, Lemons RS, Frazier WA, Bouck NP. A tumor suppressor-dependent inhibitor of angiogenesis is immunologically and functionally indistinguishable from a fragment of thrombospondin. Proc Natl Acad Sci U S A 1990;87:6624–6628.
87. Rastinejad F, Polverini PJ, Bouck NP. Regulation of the activity of a new inhibitor of angiogenesis by a cancer suppressor gene. Cell 1989;56:345–355.
88. Taraboletti G, Roberts D, Liotta LA, Giavazzi R. Platelet thrombospondin modulates endothelial cell adhesion, motility, and growth: A potential angiogenesis regulatory factor. J Cell Biol 1990;111:765–772.

89. Takigawa M, Nishida Y, Suzuki F, Kishi J, Yamashita K, Hayakawa T. Induction of angiogenesis in chick yolk-sac membrane by polyamines and its inhibition by tissue inhibitors of metalloproteinases (TIMP and TIMP-2). Biochem Biophys Res Commun 1990;171 1264–1271.
90. Murphy AN, Unsworth EJ, Stetler-Stevenson WG. Tissue inhibitor of metalloproteinases-2 inhibits bFGF-induced human microvascular endothelial cell proliferation. J Cell Physiol 1993;157:351–358.

5
Plasmin, Plasmin Inhibitors, and Angiogenesis

Martijn F. B. G. Gebbink
University Medical Center Utrecht, Utrecht, The Netherlands

I. INTRODUCTION

Angiogenesis is a complex process that requires not only proliferation of endothelial cells, but also involves adhesion, migration, and invasion of endothelial cells. In response to angiogenic stimuli, endothelial cells degrade the extracellular matrix (ECM), migrate into the perivascular space, proliferate, and form new blood vessels. Degradation of the ECM is mediated by a large number of proteases, including plasmin and members of the family of matrix metalloproteinases (MMPs). Proteins that regulate the activity of plasmin, such as plasminogen activator (PA) and plasminogen activator inhibitors (PAIs), form complexes with ECM proteins and integrins to regulate adhesion, migration, and invasion. Molecules that interfere with the proteolytic or migratory activity of these complexes may be used to inhibit aberrant angiogenesis in a variety of pathological settings, including neovascularization of tumors. Such molecules promise to be very powerful drugs, and many laboratories and pharmaceutical companies are engaged in finding and developing such angiogenesis inhibitors. The role of plasmin and the cell surface complex of plasmin modulators and integrin $\alpha v\beta 3$ that regulate plasmin activity, cell migration, and invasion are reviewed.

II. PLASMINOGEN

Plasmin is a serine protease formed by the proteolytic cleavage of its zymogen, plasminogen. Human plasminogen is a glycoprotein of 92 kd, synthesized in the liver and maintained in plasma at a concentration of 200 mg/L. The plasminogen molecule consists of 790 amino acids, containing a small preactivation peptide, 5 homologous loop structures called kringles, and a catalytic domain (Fig. 1). Plasminogen is converted to plasmin by cleavage of a single Arg-Val peptide bond. Thus, mature plasmin is composed of two chains: the heavy chain (A chain), containing the N-terminal kringle loops is connected by a disulphide bond to the light chain (B chain), which contains the catalytic domain. Two PA have been identified that cleave plasminogen: tissue plasminogen activator (tPA) and urokinase plasminogen activator (uPA). Like plasminogen, tPA and uPA are single-chain serine proteases that are converted by specific proteolytic cleavage into two-chain polypeptides (1). This step is essential for uPA activation. Proteases that activate uPA include kallikrein, kininogen, and plasmin. Plasmin generates an amplification mechanism. Urokinase plasminogen activator is thought to be primarily involved in cell surface proteolysis, degradation of the extracellular

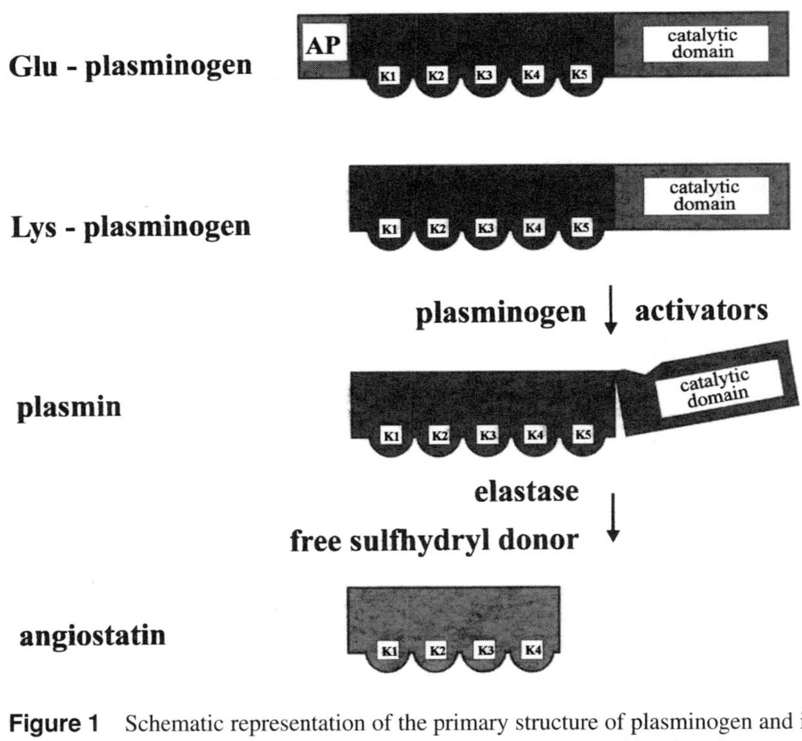

Figure 1 Schematic representation of the primary structure of plasminogen and its proteolytic derivatives. The "activation" of native plasminogen (Glu-plasminogen) to Lys-plasminogen results in a conformational change and binding to fibrinogen with higher affinity. Angiostatin can be generated by elastase (95) or in the presence of free sulfhydryl donors by autoproteolysis (96, 97).

matrix, and cell invasion, whereas tPA plays a primary role in fibrinolysis during blood clot degradation and wound healing. This separation is not absolute and uPA and tPA functions may overlap, especially because a role for tPA in cell invasion and angiogenesis has not been extensively characterized. In contrast to tPA, which is normally only expressed by endothelial cells, uPA is expressed ubiquitously and is known to play a role in migration of cells other than endothelial cells, including epithelial cells, fibroblasts, and tumor cells (2, 3).

The activity of uPA, tPA, and plasmin is tightly controlled by inhibitors, which are members of the serine protease inhibitor superfamily of serpins. Tissue plasminogen activator and uPA are regulated by two PAIs: PAI-1 and PAI-2 (4). The major inhibitor produced by endothelial cells is PAI-1, a 45 kDa protein also expressed by other cell types and present in platelets and plasma. Plasminogen activator inhibitor-2 is mainly expressed by monocytes and macrophages. When complexed with PAI-1 or PAI-2, uPA is rapidly internalized and degraded (5, 6). Plasmin, if not bound to fibrin or the cell surface, is rapidly inhibited by α2-anti-plasmin, its plasma inhibitor (7).

III. PLASMIN SUBSTRATES

As part of the fibrinolytic system, plasmin's major physiological role is to dissolve blood clots. The principal physiological substrate of plasmin is fibrin, the main component of a blood clot. However plasmin has a broad substrate specificity and can degrade a number of other ECM proteins, including fibronectin, laminin, vitronectin, fibrinogen, and proteoglycans. Plasmin does not degrade collagens directly, but it can activate MMPs, including stromelysin, interstitial and type IV collagenases, and latent elastase (8, 9). Other actions of plasmin in the fibrinolytic system include the modification of the coagulation cofactors Va and VIIIa (10, 11) and modulation of platelet membrane receptors, GPIIb-IIIa and GPIb (12;13). Finally plasmin is able to convert latent transforming growth factor beta (TGFβ) to its active form (14, 15). The activation of TGFβ may serve as a feedback mechanism to attenuate further activation of plasminogen by stimulating the production of PAI-1 (16).

IV. THE ROLE OF PLASMIN IN CELL MIGRATION AND INVASION

In addition to its role in the fibrinolytic system, in the past few years much new information concerning the role of plasmin during migration and invasion of cells, including endothelial cells has surfaced. In particular the identification of receptors for uPA and tPA on the surface of endothelial cells that can focus plasmin activity to specific sites and direct migration and invasion has greatly improved our understanding of the role of plasmin and these receptors in the angiogenic process.

V. CELL SURFACE RECEPTORS FOR uPA, tPA AND PLASMINOGEN

Plasminogen, uPA, and tPA are all secreted proteins, but their activity is directed to certain areas on the cell surface by cell surface receptors (17). A specific uPA receptor has been identified and cloned (18). The uPA receptor is bound to the cell surface by a glycosyl phosphatidylinositol (GPI)-anchor, a covalent modification at the c-terminal end of the protein. The uPA receptor is found in focal attachment sites, where it colocalizes and associates with integrins and ECM proteins (19, 20) (see below). Thus this localization limits uPA-generated plasmin action to these focal complexes. Unlike tPA, uPA and the uPA-receptor expression is not limited to endothelial cells. Other cells use the uPA system for plasmin-mediated proteolysis during cell migration and invasion.

Tissue plasminogen activator is the main activator of plasminogen during wound healing, when its primary role is to degrade the fibrin clot. Fibrin binds and activates tPA. However a high affinity cell surface receptor for tPA, annexin II, has recently been identified (21). Annexin-II binds tPA, plasminogen, and plasmin with high affinity and localizes and promotes plasmin generation to the vessel wall (22).

A number of plasminogen binding proteins will directly or indirectly localize plasminogen to the cell surface. In general, plasminogen-binding proteins interact with plasminogen through a carboxy-terminal lysine residue that binds to the lysine-binding sites present in the kringle domains of plasminogen. Direct cell surface receptors include annexin-II, α-enolase, and the platelet integrin glycoprotein GpIIb/IIIa (21, 23–26). Important are the ECM proteins that serve as plasminogen-binding proteins and localize plasminogen indirectly to the cell surface by integrin ECM interactions. Binding sites for plasminogen are present on vitronectin, fibrinogen, fibronectin, collagen, and laminin (27–29).

VI. REGULATION OF PLASMINOGEN ACTIVATORS AND THEIR RECEPTORS BY ANGIOGENIC FACTORS

Quiescent vascular endothelial cells produce but hardly secrete tPA (30). However, the endothelial cells of growing capillaries also express uPA (31), consistent with the suggested role for uPA in the migratory and invasive process.

Basic fibroblast growth factor (bFGF) and vascular endothelial growth factor (VEGF) are two of the most well-characterized angiogenic factors with regard to their effects on endothelial cell proteolytic activity. Both bFGF and VEGF elicit their effects through the binding and subsequent activation of specific cell surface receptor tyrosine kinases. Activation of these receptors induces, among other responses, a proteinase cascade (32, 33). Both bFGF and VEGF increase the activity of tPA and uPA (34, 35). Expression and secretion of these proteases is increased, and the receptor for urokinase (uPAR) is up-regulated (36, 37).

VII. THE ROLE OF INTEGRIN αvβ3

The endothelial cells attach to their underlying basement membrane through integrin receptors that bind ECM proteins, primarily collagen. During angiogenesis, proliferation and migration rely on the ability of endothelial cells temporarily to move along their basement membrane. It has become apparent that vitronectin and its integrin receptors, αvβ3 and αvβ5, play a major role in this process. Endothelial cells under mitogenic stimulation reveal increased levels of the vitronectin receptor, αvβ3. These receptors, which also can bind fibronectin, fibrinogen, and von Willebrand's factor, are required for angiogenesis (38). Antibodies to integrin αvβ3 block angiogenesis induced by bFGF on the chick chorioallantoic membrane. Endothelial cells, as well as some tumor cells, use the αvβ3 to migrate on vitronectin (39, 40). This motility requires the intracellular domain of the integrin receptors and depends on tyrosine kinase-dependent intracellular signaling (40, 41).

VIII. THE LINK BETWEEN PLASMIN, THE ECM INTEGRINS, AND MIGRATION

Both vitronectin and the vitronectin receptors can physically interact with proteins that control the formation of plasmin from plasminogen (Fig. 2). The vitronectin receptor and urokinase plasminogen activator receptor (uPAR) both localize in cell attachment sites (e.g., focal adhesion plaques) (19). Vitronectin in plasma and on cells can associate with PAI-1 (42). Vitronectin can also bind to the urokinase receptor, as well as to PA and plasminogen (20, 27, 43, 44). Thus the uPAR can promote direct adhesion to vitronectin and can serve as an adhesion receptor itself. The binding of vitronectin to uPAR is enhanced by urokinase (20, 43) and can be blocked by a specific peptide (45). Interestingly, it has been shown that transfection of 293 cells with cDNA of the uPAR enhances adhesion of these cells to vitronectin, but decreases integrin β1-mediated adhesion to fibronectin (45). Previously it has been shown that antibodies to αvβ3 abrogate migration of human umbilical cord endothelial cells (46).

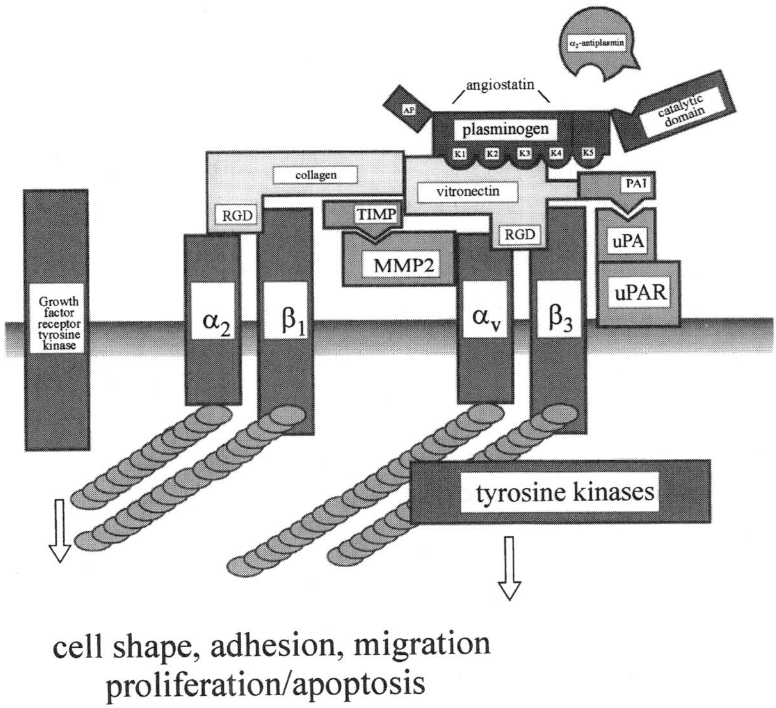

Figure 2 Schematic representation of the cell surface complex that is involved in angiogenesis. In resting state, endothelial cells are tightly bound to the basement membrane, through interaction of extracellular matrix molecules, such as collagen through integrins, mainly of the β1 type. Ligand-bound β1 integrins suppress migration, growth (98) and the synthesis of metalloproteases (99). Angiogenic factors induce expression of plasminogen activators (PAs) and of the β3 integrins, αvβ3 and αvβ5. Angiogenic factors also induce expression of metalloproteases and collagenases, either directly or through ligation of the β3 integrins (100). Ligation of β3 integrins with ligand can subsequently inhibit binding through β1 integrins (101). In other words, binding of vitronectin to αvβ3 can inhibit binding of other integrins to collagen and can facilitate migration. During endothelial migration and proliferation, p53 activity is suppressed by integrin αvβ3. Collagenases can be inhibited by tissue inhibitors of metalloproteases (TIMPs). Plasminogen activator inhibitor (PAI) inhibits PA, thereby regulating plasmin activity and migration. In endothelial cells, both Urokinase plasminogen activator (uPA) and tissue plasminogen activator (tPA) are likely involved in angiogenesis, as well as both vitronectin and fibrinogen (see text). Intracellularly, signaling molecules, including tyrosine kinases such as src (102) and hck (49), regulate cytoskeleton organization, cell migration, secretion, cell proliferation, and apoptosis.

It has become apparent that apart from their role in plasmin formation, uPA and the uPAR directly affect cell adhesion and migration. In fact, migration of endothelial cells can be modulated by uPA and the uPAR even in the absence of proteolytic activity (3, 47, 48). The chemotactic effects of uPA are accompanied by changes in phosphorylation of intracellular proteins (48, 49). The uPAR mediated effects are likely mediated by intracellular signaling mechanism that involves both tyrosine and serine kinases. The uPA-induced signal transduction occurs through activation of hck, a member of the src-family of tyrosine kinases, which associates with the uPAR (49). Such signaling events presumably also underly the uPA- and integrin-mediated effects on the expression of other proteases (50, 51). Taken together, uPA and the uPAR are part of a large complex of proteins (Fig. 2), localized in focal contacts, that coordinate adhesion, migration, and invasion.

IX. PLASMIN AND TUMORIGENESIS

Many studies report elevated levels of uPA in a wide variety of human malignancies, including colon, breast, and prostate cancer (52–55). Abnormal tPA expression is often found in melanoma. In general, high expression levels of uPA, tPA, and PAIs correlate with poor prognosis. Expression of uPA and PAI-1 has been detected in tumor cells, as well as in stromal and endothelial cells. Tumor cell invasion and endothelial cell invasion share many functional similarities, including the uPA system. The actual involvement of uPA in tumor invasion and metastasis has been demonstrated in several models (56–58). For example, human PC3 prostate carcinoma cells transfected with a cDNA-encoding mutant uPA, which lacked protease activity but retained receptor binding, were impaired in the formation of metastasis in vivo. Given the above-mentioned functional similarities between tumor cell invasion and endothelial cell invasion, this soluble uPA mutant may inhibit both angiogenesis and tumor cell invasion. In general, inhibitors of the uPA system (or of metalloproteases) may affect both angiogenesis and tumor cell invasion.

X. INHIBITION OF PLASMIN, ANGIOGENESIS, AND TUMORIGENESIS

As early as 1983, it was demonstrated that antibodies to uPA could inhibit human tumor metastasis in the chorioallantoic membrane assay (59). Furthermore, antibodies to uPA inhibited the number of metastases of Lewis lung carcinoma (60) and local invasion (61). Interestingly a number of other compounds that act through the uPA system also inhibit tumor invasion and metastasis (Table 1).

Table 1 Compounds that Inhibit Angiogenesis and Tumor Growth by the Integrin/uPA/Plasmin Complex[a]

Compound	Mechanism	Effect on endothelial cells and angiogenesis	Effect on metastasis and tumor growth
Plasmin/uPA-related compounds			
Trasylol (aprotinin)	Inhibition of plasmin and other serine proteases	Inhibits invasion of endothelial cells on the human amniotic membrane (103) and tube formation in matrix gels (104–106)	Inhibits metastasis of Lewis lung carcinoma in mice (67)
Cyclocapron (tranexamic acid) and epsilon-amino-caproic acid	Lysine-analogue that inhibits binding of plasminogen to its substrates	Inhibits migration invasion on the human amniotic membrane (103). Antiangiogenic in the cornea assay in rabbits (107)	Inhibits growth of V2 carcinoma in rabbits (69), of Lewis lung carcinoma in mice (108), and of human tumors in nude mice (68, 70). Beneficial effects in humans have been reported (86–88; 109–115)
Amiloride	Inhibition of uPA		Inhibition of human prostate xenografts in SCID mice (116)
p-aminobenzmidine	Inhibition of uPA	Inhibits migration of endothelial cells in matrigels	Inhibition of human prostate cancer in SCID mice (65, 116)
α2-antiplasmin	Inhibition of plasmin		Inhibits in vitro tumor cell invasion through the human amniotic membrane (117)
Anti-uPA antibody	Inhibition of uPA		Inhibition of Lewis lung carcinoma (70) Inhibition of human tumor metastasis and tumor growth in nude mice (59, 60, 118)
PAI-1 (mutants with extended half-life)	Inhibition of uPA		Inhibition of prostate cancer xenografts (116)

ATF-HAS and m1-48Ig (fusions of the N-terminal fragment of uPA)	Inhibition of uPA by blocking uPA binding to uPAR	Changes in cell morphology and remodeling of cytoskeleton (47) Inhibition of neovascularization (81)	Inhibition of in vitro invasion of tumor cells (119) Inhibition of tumor growth (81)
MuPA (proteolytically inactive uPA)	Inhibition of uPA by competition for binding	Inhibition of prostate cancer neovascularization and growth (120)	
Angiostatin and other fragments of plasmin	Unknown, see text	Inhibits proliferation and migration of endothelial cells and neovascularization in the corneal pocket assay (86, 90, 121–123)	Inhibition of metastasis of Lewis lung carcinoma and growth of subcutaneous tumors in mice (86–88, 109)
Integrin αvβ3-related compounds			
LM609 (anti-αvβ3 Ab) and cyclic RGD peptides	Blocks αvβ3 function by blocking ligand binding (antagonists of integrin)	Inhibition of angiogenesis and tumor growth in several assays (38, 85, 124)	
Metalloprotease-related compounds			
TIMP-1 and TIMP-3	Inhibit metalloproteases	Inhibition of endothelial cell proliferation and migration (125, 126)	
Marimastat, Batimastat	Inhibit metalloproteases	Inhibition of endothelial cell invasion (127)	Inhibition of tumor growth in mice (128, 129)
PEX (fragment of MMP-2)	Inhibits MMP-2 activity	Inhibits angiogenesis and tumor growth on the chick CAM (130)	
Other compounds			
MPA, dexamethasone, hydrocortisone, tamoxifen (anticancer steroids)	Up-regulation of PAI-1 (78, 131)	Inhibition of angiogenesis (121)	Preventions of breast cancer growth by tamoxifen (131).

[a] Many other drugs, including tyrosine kinase inhibitors, farnesyl-transferase inhibitors, and inhibitors of eiconasoid synthesis may inhibit angiogenesis and tumor growth in part by directly modulating the function of αvβ3/uPA/plasmin complex.

Abbreviations: *uPA*, Urokinase plasminogen activator; *uPAR*, urokinase plasminogen activator receptor; *PAI*, plasminogen activator inhibitor; *TIMP*, tissue inhibitor of metalloproteinase; *CAM*, chlorioallantoic membrane; *MPA*, medroxyprogesterone acetate.

XI. INHIBITORS OF FIBRINOLYSIS

There is now significant evidence that fibrinolytic enzymes are associated with tumor growth and metastasis. In fact, tumor angiogenesis and processes that occur during wound healing are very similar (62). Angiogenic factors induce hyperpermeability, resulting in the deposition of plasma proteins, including plasminogen, fibrinogen, and vitronectin; hence, the formation of an angiogenic matrix (63). Moreover, similar to what is seen during blood clotting, plasma fibrinogen that extravasates at tumor sites crosslinks to form fibrin (the principal plasmin substrate). Fibrin may then serve as temporary matrix in which new vessels can infiltrate. Fibrinolysis subsequently occurs and can be measured, thereby serving as a prognostic marker (64).

Given the overlap between tumor angiogenesis and wound healing, antifibrinolytic drugs may prevent tumor angiogenesis and tumor growth. These drugs include aprotinin (Trasylol), which inhibits plasmin as well as other serine proteases; tranexamic acid (Cyclocapron) and epsilon amino-caproic acid, which bind to the lysine-binding sites in the kringle domains of plasminogen and inhibit plasmin formation; and p-aminobenzamidine and amiloride, which inhibit uPA. In mouse models, amiloride and p-aminobenzamidine have suppressed the growth of human prostate tumors (65, 66). Aprotinin has been reported to inhibit metastasis of Lewis lung carcinoma in mice (67). Several studies in animals have shown inhibitory effects of tranexamic acid and epsilon amino-caproic acid on tumor growth and metastasis (68–70). Not many promising results in humans have been described thus far, but a few cases have been reported in which antifibrinolytic agents had some inhibitory effects on tumor growth (71–75). However, if used in combination with other angiostatic agents that act through different mechanisms, beneficial effects on treatment of cancer might be obtained.

XII. STEROIDS

A number of anticancer steroids, including medroxyprogesterone and dexamethasone, inhibit angiogenesis (76). Angiostatic steroids inhibit the fibrinolytic activity of endothelial cells (77). In the case of medroxyprogesterone, this inhibition correlated with increased PAI-1 expression (78). Dexamethasone reduces vascular density and PA activity (79) as well as PA activator activity of tumor cells (80). Anticancer steroids may function to inhibit tumor growth, at least in part, by modulating plasmin-mediated invasion of tumor cells and endothelial cells.

XIII. OTHER AGENTS THAT INHIBITED ANGIOGENESIS AND TUMORIGENESIS THROUGH THE uPA SYSTEM

A number of approaches have been taken to design molecules that interfere with uPA-mediated invasion. Most recently, using a very elegant approach, a recombinant uPAR antagonist, containing the epidermal growth factor domain of uPA fused to the Fc portion of human immunoglobulin G (IgG) was used to inhibit primary tumor growth in syngeneic mice (81). This molecule proved to be a potent antagonist of PA and inhibited capillary tube formation, bFGF-induced neovascularization, and B16 melanoma growth in syngeneic mice. Others have used mutated PAI, with an extended half-life to inhibit tumor growth (66).

XIV. ANTAGONISTS OF αvβ3

Angiogenesis can be inhibited by blocking the function of the integrin αvβ3. Recent evidence indicates that integrin αvβ3 antagonists also inhibit tumor growth in mice (82). Intravenous administration of antibodies against αvβ3 prevents tumor growth. The vessel density in areas of neovascularization in the tumor was significantly decreased. The fact that these αvβ3 integrin-negative tumors are inhibited proves that the integrin αvβ3 antagonist effects neovascularization. This is important inasmuch as tumor cells also can use vitronectin and integrin αvβ3 for migration. Much is known about the mechanism by which αvβ3 integrin antagonists inhibit angiogenesis. It has been demonstrated that proper ligation of the vascular integrin αvβ3 is essential for cell survival during angiogenesis and that integrin antagonists trigger apoptosis (83, 84). In the chorioallantoic membrane assay, αvβ3 integrin antagonists induce apoptosis of endothelial cells (85) by suppression of the activity of p53. Suppression of p53 is essential for survival in cells that undergo DNA synthesis. Antagonists of integrin ligation cause activation of p53 and trigger apoptosis. Most importantly, αvβ3 integrin antagonists induce apoptosis of angiogenic blood vessels, whereas pre-existing blood vessels are not affected (85).

XV. ANGIOSTATIN

In 1994 a fragment of plasminogen, named angiostatin, was found that proved to be a potent inhibitor of tumor growth and to regress large tumors. Angiostatin was identified as a circulating factor that mediated the inhibition of metastatic growth in animals carrying a primary Lewis lung carcinoma (86). A number of reports had demonstrated that some tumors, including Lewis lung carcinoma, inhibit the growth, but not the number, of their metastasis. In these cases, the removal of the primary tumor is followed by the rapid growth of distant metastases. It was hypothesized that the primary tumor generates one or more angiogenesis inhibitors. In the distant metastases these inhibitors, by virtue of their longer half-life in the circulation, are in excess to angiogenic simulators and therefore are capable of inhibiting angiogenesis. In the primary tumor, the angiogenic stimulators are theoretically in excess. A threshold size of the primary tumor is necessary for the inhibitory effect. Angiostatin, the first molecule to be discovered to mediate this phenomena, was purified from urine from tumor-bearing mice. Systemic administration of angiostatin blocked neovascularization and growth of metastasis in the absence of the primary tumor. Thereafter, it was shown that angiostatin, when given at a higher dose, can inhibit growth of primary tumors as well (87–89). In vitro, angiostatin inhibits bFGF-induced endothelial cell proliferation and migration (86, 90).

Angiostatin is a proteolytic fragment of plasmin (Fig. 1) and contains the kringles 1 to 4. The mechanism by which angiostatin inhibits endothelial cell proliferation, migration, angiogenesis, and tumor growth is unknown. However it is not unlikely that angiostatin may exert its effect on endothelial cells through integrins, possibly $\alpha v\beta 3$ and $\alpha v\beta 5$, by binding integrin ligands such as fibrin, fibrinogen, and vitronectin. Such a mechanism would result in changes in intracellular signaling similar to those described for uPA (48, 49, 91). The absence of the activation peptide in angiostatin suggests that angiostatin may adopt a conformation that resembles the conformation of the kringles in plasmin. This structure differs from the conformation of native Glu-plasminogen, which explains why angiostatin does not compete with Glu-plasminogen. Thus angiostatin may compete with plasmin for binding sites on endothelial cells and inhibit plasmin-mediated migration and vessel formation in vivo (92). The absence of the protease domain in angiostatin also suggests that it does not bind $\alpha 2$-antiplasmin with high affinity. This may explain why angiostatin is active in the circulation. An attractive, plausible mechanism is that angiostatin binds at focal adhesion sites to vitronectin, fibrinogen, or other $\alpha v\beta 3$ ligands and modulates $\alpha v\beta 3$-mediated integrin function directly, similar to PAI-1 or the N-terminal fragment of uPA.

XVI. PERSPECTIVE

The hypothesis that cancer could be treated by inhibiting angiogenesis was first proposed in 1972 (93). The importance of angiogenesis for the growth of tumors is now well recognized and forms the basis for the concept of antiangiogenic therapy. Major steps have been taken to elucidate this concept further. It has become abundantly clear that cancer and wound healing share striking similarities (94), including the shared role of fibrin and other ECM proteins and plasminogen. At the molecular level, the role of plasminogen and the uPA system, and their connection with integrin-mediated signaling have become obvious. Finally the discovery of angiostatin, a proteolytic fragment of plasminogen as a promising new anticancer drug, has further emphasized the importance of the role for the fibrinolytic system in angiogenesis and tumor growth. The greater understanding of the complex biological processes involved in angiogenesis has provided insight into new therapeutic targets that should lead to successful treatment of cancer in the coming years. A combination of drugs that act on these targets may prove to be most successful.

ACKNOWLEDGMENTS

I would like to thank Dr. Henk M.W. Verheul for helpful discussions. I would like to thank Drs. Patricia D'Amore, Jack Arbiser, and Emile Voest for their comments on the manuscript.

Martijn F.B.G. Gebbink is supported by the Netherlands Cancer Foundation.

REFERENCES

1. Collen D, Lijnen HR, Verstraete M. In: Handin, RI ed. Blood: Principles and Practice of Hematology. Philadelphia: J.B. Lippincott Company, 1995:1261–1288.
2. Del Rosso M, Fibbi G, Dini G, Grappone C, Pucci M, Caldini R, Fimiani M, Lotti T, Panconesi E. J Invest Dermatol 1990; 94:310–316.
3. Odekon LE, Sato Y, Rifkin DB. J Cell Physiol 1992; 150:258–263.
4. Sprengers ED, Kluft C. Blood 1987; 69:381–387.
5. Cubellis MV, Wun TC, Blasi F. EMBO J 1990; 9:1079–1085.
6. Nykjaer A, Conese M, Christensen E, Olson D, Cremona O, Glieman J, Blasi F, Christensen EI, Gliemann J. EMBO J 1997; 16:2610–2620.
7. Holmes WE, Nelles L, Lijnen HR, Collen D. J Biol Chem 1987; 262:1659–1664.
8. Werb Z, Mainardi C, Vater CA, Harris ED. N Engl J Med 1977; 296:1017–1023.
9. Mazzieri B, Masiero L, Zanetta L, Monea S, Onisto M, Garbisa S, Mignatti P. EMBO J 1997; 16:2319–2332.
10. Omar MN, Mann KG. J Biol Chem 1987; 262:9750–9755.
11. Lee CD, Mann KG. Blood 1989; 73:185–190.
12. Stricker RB, Wong D, Shiu DT, Reyes PT, Shuman MA. Blood 1986; 68:275–280.
13. Adelman B, Michelson AD, Greenberg J, Handin RI. Blood 1986; 68:1280–1284.
14. Sato Y, Rifkin DB. J Cell Biol 1989; 109:309–315.
15. Lyons RM, Gentry LE, Purchio AF, Moses HL. J Cell Biol 1990; 110:1361–1367.
16. Saksela O, Moscatelli DA, Rifkin DB. J Cell Biol 1987; 105:957–963.
17. Hajjar KA. Thromb Haemost 1995; 74:294–301.
18. Roldan AL, Cubellis MV, Masucci MT, Behrendt N, Lund LR, Dano K, Blasi F. EMBO J 1990; 9:467–474.
19. Hebert CA, Baker JB. J Cell Biol 1988; 106:1241–1247.
20. Wei Y, Waltz DA, Rao N, Drummond RJ, Rosenberg S, Chapman HA. J Biol Chem 1994; 269:32380–32388.
21. Hajjar KA, Jacovina AT, Chacko J. J Biol Chem 1994; 269:21191–21197.
22. Cesarman GM, Guevara CA, Hajjar KA. J Biol Chem 1994; 269:21198–21203.

23. Miles LA, Dahlberg CM, Plescia J, Felez J, Kato K, Plow EF. Biochemistry 1991; 30:1682–1691.
24. Miles LA, Dahlberg CM, Plow EF. J Biol Chem 1988; 263:11928–11934.
25. Miles LA, Plow EF. Thromb Haemost 1987; 58:936–942.
26. Miles LA, Ginsberg MH, White JG, Plow EF. J Clin Invest 1986; 77:2001–2009.
27. Kost C, Stuber W, Ehrlich HJ, Pannekoek H, Preissner KT. J Biol Chem 1992; 267:12098–12105.
28. Moser TL, Enghild JJ, Pizzo SV, Stack MS. J Biol Chem 1993; 268:18917–18923.
29. Stack MS, Moser TL, Pizzo SV. Biochem J 1992; 284:103–108.
30. Kristensen P, Larsson LI, Nielsen LS, Grondahl-Hansen J, Andreasen PAD. FEBS Lett 1984; 168:33–37.
31. Bacharach E, Itin A, Keshet E. Proc Natl Acad Sci USA 1992; 89:10686–10690.
32. Gross JL, Moscatelli DA, Rifkin DB. Proc Natl Acad Sci USA 1983; 80:2623–2627.
33. Moscatelli DA, Presta M, Mignatti P, Mullins DE, Crowe RM, Rifkin DB. Anticancer Research 1986; 6:861–863.
34. Flaumenhaft R, Abe M, Mignatti P, Rifkin DB. J Cell Biol 1992; 118:901–909.
35. Pepper MS, Ferrara N, Orci L, Montesano R. Biochem Biophys Res Commun 1991; 181:902–906.
36. Mignatti P, Mazzieri RM, Rifkin DB. J Cell Biol 1991; 113:1193–1201.
37. Mandriota SJ, Seghezzi G, Vassalli JD, Ferrara N, Wasi S, Mazzieri RM, Pepper MS. J Biol Chem 1995; 270:9709–9716.
38. Brooks PC, Clark RA, Cheresh DA. Science 1994; 264:569–571.
39. Leavesley DI, Ferguson GD, Wayner EA, Cheresh DA. J Cell Biol 1992; 117: 1101–1107.
40. Filardo EJ, Brooks PC, Deming SL, Damsky C, Cheresh DA. J Cell Biol 1995; 130:441–450.
41. Klemke RL, Yebra M, Bayna EM, Cheresh DA. J Cell Biol 1994; 127:859–866.
42. Declerck PJ, De Mol M, Alessi MC, Baudner S, Paques EP, Preissner KT, Collen D. J Biol Chem 1988; 263:15454–15461.
43. Kanse SM, Kost C, Wilhelm OG, Andreasen PA, Preissner KT. Exp Cell Res 1996; 224:344–353.
44. Moser TL, Enghild JJ, Pizzo SV, Stack MS. Biochem J 1995; 307:867–873.
45. Wei Y, Lukashev M, Simon DI, Bodary SC, Rosenberg S, Doyle MV, Chapman HA. Science 1996; 273:1551–1555.
46. Leavesley DI, Schwartz MA, Rosenfeld M, Cheresh DA. J Cell Biol 1993; 121: 163–170.
47. Lu H, Mabilat C, Yeh P, Guitton JD, Li H, Pouchelet M, Shoevaert D, Soria J, Soria C. FEBS Lett 1996; 380:21–24.
48. Busso N, Masur SK, Lazega D, Waxman S, Ossowski L. J Cell Biol 1994; 126: 259–270.
49. Resnati M, Guttinger M, Valcamonica S, Sidenius N, Blasi F, Fazioli F. EMBO J 1996; 15:1572–1582.
50. Seftor REB, Seftor EA, Stetler-Stevenson WG, Hendrix MJC. Cancer Res 1993; 53:3411–3415.
51. Kim SO, Plow EF, Miles LA. J Biol Chem 1996; 271:23761–23767.

52. Bindal AK, Hammound M, Shi WM, Wu SZ, Sawaya R, Rao JS. J Neurooncol 1994; 22:101–110.
53. de Vries TJ, van Muijen GN, Ruiter DJ. Melanoma Res 1996; 6:79–88.
54. Brunner N, Pyke C, Hansen CH, Romer J, Grondahl-Hansen J, Dano K. Cancer Treat Res 1994; 71:299–309.
55. Duffy MJ, Duggan C, Maguire T, Mulcahy K, Elvin P, McDermott E, O'Higgins N. Enzyme & Protein 1996; 49:85–93.
56. Axelrod JH, Reich R, Miskin R. Mol Cell Biol 1989; 9:2133–2141.
57. Hearing VJ, Law LW, Corti A, Appella E, Blasi F. Cancer Res 1988; 48:1270–1278.
58. Crowley CW, Cohen RL, Lucas BK, Liu G, Shuman MA, Levinson AD. Proc Natl Acad Sci USA 1993; 90:5021–5025.
59. Ossowski LK, Reich E. Cell 1983; 35:611–619.
60. Kobayashi H, Gotoh J, Shinohara H, Moniwa N, Terao T. Thromb Haemost 1994; 71:474–480.
61. Ossowski L. Cancer Res 1992; 52:6754–6760.
62. Dvorak HF, Galli SJ, Dvorak AM. Hum Pathol 1986; 17:122–137.
63. Dvorak HF, Brown LF, Detmar M, Dvorak AM. Am J Pathol 1995; 146:1029–1039.
64. Gandolfo GM, Conti L, Vercillo M. Anticancer Res 1996; 16:2155–2159.
65. Billstrom A, Hartley-Asp B, Lecander I, Batra S, Astedt B. Int J Cancer 1995; 61: 542–547.
66. Jankun J, Keck RW, Skrzypczak E, Swiercz R, Skrzypczak Jankun E. Cancer Res 1997; 57:559–563.
67. Uetsuji S, Yamamura M, Takai S, Hioki K, Yamamoto M. Surg Today 1992; 22: 439–442.
68. Ogawa H, Sekiguchi F, Tanaka N, Ono K, Tanaka K, Kinjo M, Iwakawa AN. Anticancer Res 1982; 2:339–344.
69. Kodama Y, Tanaka K. Gann 1981; 72:411–416.
70. Iwakawa A, Tanaka K. Invasion Metastasis 1982; 2:232–248.
71. Astedt B, Glifberg I, Mattsson W, Trope C. JAMA 1977; 238:154–155.
72. Bramsen T. Acta Ophthalmol 1978; 56:264–269.
73. Astedt B, Mattsson W, Trope C. Acta Medica Scand 1977; 201:491–493.
74. Kikuchi Y, Kizawa I, Oomori K, Matsuda M, Kato K. Acta Obstet Gynecol Scand 1986; 65:453–456.
75. Petrelli NJ, Markus G, Herrera L, Corasanti J, Mittelman A. J Surg Oncol 1986; 33:109–111.
76. Crum R, Szabo S, Folkman J. Science 1985; 230:1375–1378.
77. Ashino-Fuse H, Takano Y, Oikawa T, Shimamura M, Iwaguchi T. Int J Cancer 1989; 44:859–864.
78. Blei F, Wilson EL, Mignatti P, Rifkin DB. J Cell Physiol 1993; 155:568–578.
79. Wolff JE, Guerin C, Laterra J, Bressler J, Indurti RR, Brem H. Brain Res 1993; 604:79–85.
80. Amin W, Karlan BY, Littlefield BA. Cancer Res 1987; 47:6040–6045.
81. Min HY, Doyle LV, Vitt CR, Zandonella CL, Stratton-Thomas JR, Shuman MA, Rosenberg S. Cancer Res 1996; 56:2428–2433.

82. Brooks PC, Stromblad S, Klemke RL, Visscher D, Sarkar FH, Cheresh DA. J Clin Invest 1995; 96:1815–1822.
83. Re F, Zanetti A, Sironi M, Polentarutti N, Lanfrancone L, Dejana E. J Cell Biol 1994; 127:537–546.
84. Stromblad S, Becker JC, Yebra M, Brooks PC, Cheresh DA. J Clin Invest 1996; 98:426–433.
85. Brooks PC, Montgomery AM, Rosenfeld M, Reisfeld RA, Hu T, Klier G. Cell 1994; 79:1157–1164.
86. O'Reilly MS, Holmgren L, Shing Y, Chen C, Rosenthal RA, Moses M, Cao Y, Sage EH, Folkman J. Cell 1994; 79:315–328.
87. O'Reilly MS, Holmgren L, Chen C, Folkman J. Nat Med 1996; 2:689–692.
88. Lee Sim BK, O'Reilly MS, Liang H, Fortier AH, He W, Madsen JW, Lapcevich R, Nacy CA. Cancer Res 1997; 57:1329–1334.
89. Wu YP, van Breugel HH, Lankhof H, Wise RJ, Handin RI, de Groot PG. Arterioscler Thromb Vasc Biol 1996; 16:611–620.
90. Gately S, Twardowski P, Stack MS, Patrick M, Boggio L, Cundiff DL, Madison L, Volpert O, Bouck N, Enghild J, Kwaan HC. Cancer Res 1996; 56:4887–4890.
91. Mirshahi SS, Lounes KC, Lu H, Pujade-Lauraine E, Mishal Z, Benard J, Bernadou A, Soria C, Soria J. FEBS Lett 1997; 411:322–326.
92. Ponting CP, Marshall JM, Cederholm-Williams SA. Blood Coagul Fibrinolysis 1992; 3:605–614.
93. Folkman J. Ann Surg 1972; 175:409–416.
94. Dvorak HF. N Engl J Med 1986; 315:1650–1659.
95. Dong Z, Kumar R, Yang X, Fidler IJ. Cell 1998; 88:801–811.
96. Gately S, Twardowski P, Stack MS, Cundiff DL, Grella D, Castellino FJ, Enghild J, Kwaan HC, Lee F, Kramer RA, Volpert O, Bouck N, Soff GA. Proc Natl Acad Sci USA 1997; 94:10868–10872.
97. Stathakis P, Fitzgerald M, Matthias LJ, Chesterman CN, Hogg PJ. J Biol Chem 1997; 272:20641–20645.
98. Schreiner C, Fisher M, Hussein S, Juliano RL. Cancer Res 1991; 51:1738–1740.
99. Huhtala P, Humphries MJ, McCarthy JB, Tremble PM, Werb Z, Damsky CH. J Cell Biol 1995; 129:867–879.
100. Seftor RE, Seftor EA, Stetler-Stevenson WG, Hendrix MJ. Cancer Res 1993; 53: 3411–3415.
101. Diaz Gonzalez F, Forsyth J, Steiner B, Ginsberg MH. Mol Biol Cell 1996; 7:1939–1951.
102. Hruska KA, Rolnick F, Huskey M, Alvarez U, Cheresh DA. Endocrinology 1995; 136:2984–2992.
103. Mignatti P, Tsuboi R, Robbins E, Rifkin DB. J Cell Biol 1989; 108:671–682.
104. Koolwijk P, van Erck MG, de Vree WJ, Vermeer MA, Weich HA, Hanemaaijer R, van Hinsbergh VW. J Cell Biol 1996; 132:1177–1188.
105. Jimi S, Ito K, Kohno K, Ono M, Kuwano M, Itagaki Y, Ishikawa H. Biochem Biophys Res Commun 1995; 211:476–483.
106. Sato Y, Okamura K, Morimoto A, Hamanaka R, Hamaguchi K, Shimada T, Ono M, Kohno K, Sakata T, Kuwano M. Exp Cell Res 1993; 204:223–229.

107. Ambrus JL, Ambrus CM, Toumbis CA, Forgach P, Karakousis CP, Niswander P, Lane W. J Med 1991; 22:355–369.
108. Tanaka N, Ogawa H, Tanaka K, Kinjo M, Kohga S. Invasion Metastasis 1981; 1: 149–157.
109. Wu Z, O'Reilly MS, Folkman J, Shing Y. Biochem Biophys Res Commun 1997; 236:651–654.
110. Serdengecti S, Buyukunal E, Molinas N, Demirelli FH, Berkarda N, Eyuboglu H, Derman U, Berkarda B. Chemioterapia 1988; 7:122–126.
111. Kikuchi Y, Kizawa I, Oomori K, Matsuda M, Kato K. Acta Obstet Gynecol Scand 1986; 65:453–456.
112. Soma H, Sashida T, Yoshida M, Miyashita T, Nakamura A. Acta Obstet Gynecol Scand 1980; 59:285–287.
113. Bramsen T. Acta Ophthalmol (Copenh) 1978; 56:264–269.
114. Astedt B, Glifberg I, Mattsson W, Trope C. JAMA 1977; 238:154–155.
115. Astedt B, Mattsson W, Trope C. Acta Med Scand 1977; 201:491–493.
116. Jankun J, Keck RW, Skrzypczak JE, Swiercz R. Cancer Res 1997; 57:559–563.
117. Mignatti P, Robbins E, Rifkin DB. Cell 1986; 47:487–498.
118. Ossowski LK, Russo-Payne H, Wilson EL. Cancer Res 1991; 51:274–281.
119. Lu H, Yeh P, Guitton JD, Mabilat C, Desanlis F, Maury I, Legrand Y, Soria C. FEBS Lett 1994; 356:56–59.
120. Evans CP, Elfman F, Parangi S, Conn M, Cunha G, Shuman MA. Cancer Res 1997; 57:3594–3599
121. Yamamoto T, Terada N, Nishizawa Y, Petrow V. Int J Cancer 1994; 56:393–399.
122. Cao Y, Ji RW, Davidson D, Schaller J, Marti D, Sohndel S, McCance SG, O'Reilly MS, Llinas M, Folkman J. J Biol Chem 1996; 271:29461–29467.
123. Cao Y, Chen A, An SSA, Ji R-W, Davidson D, Llinas M, Ji R-W. J Biol Chem 1997; 272:22924–22928.
124. Hammes HP, Brownlee M, Jonczyk A, Sutter A, Preissner KT. Nat Med 1996; 2: 529–533.
125. Anand-Apte B, Pepper MS, Voest EE, Montesano R, Olsen BR, Murphy G, Apte SS, Zetter B. Invest Ophthalmol Vis Sci 1997; 38:817–823.
126. Moses MA, Sudhalter J, Langer R. Science 1990; 248:1408–1410.
127. Taraboletti G, Garofalo A, Belotti D, Drudis T, Borsotti P, Scanziani E, Brown PD, Giavazzi R. J Nat Cancer Inst 1995; 87:293–298.
128. Sledge GWJ, Qulali M, Goulet R, Bone EA, Fife R. J Natl Cancer Inst 1995; 87: 1546–1550.
129. Wang X, Fu X, Brown PD, Crimmin MJ, Hoffman RM. Cancer Res 1994; 54: 4726–4728.
130. Brooks PC, Silletti S, von Schalscha TL, Friedlander M, Cheresh DA. Cell 1998; 92:391–400.
131. Xing RH, Mazar A, Henkin J, Rabbani SA. Cancer Res 1997; 57:3585–3593.

6
Assays to Study Angiogenesis

Robert Auerbach and Wanda Auerbach
University of Wisconsin, Madison, Wisconsin

I. INTRODUCTION

One of the most important technical problems in the study of angiogenesis and antiangiogenesis is the lack of methods that yield meaningful, repeatable, quantitative measurements of the angiogenic process. This is not because there is a dearth of assays or because the assays do not yield quantitative data. Rather, the assays measure a wide range of factors that affect the formation of new blood vessels and one cannot be compared meaningfully with another.

As discussed in previous chapters in this volume, the principal cell involved in angiogenesis is the endothelial cell whose differentiation, migration, proliferation, and structural rearrangement is central to the angiogenic process. Can we not therefore study, singly or collectively, these endothelial cell processes? We can, but one can ask, which kind of endothelial cell? All endothelial cells are not alike. Not only are there structural differences (e.g., fenestrated vs. sinusoidal) but there are significant functional, organ-associated differences. Brain endothelial cells, for example, establish the blood-brain barrier, secrete P-glycoprotein, express brain-specific antigens, and have only a marginal up-regulation of major histocompatibility antigens when stimulated with γ-interferon. Lung endothelial cells secrete large amounts of angiotensin-converting enzyme; lymphatic endothelial cells have an augmented receptor density for vascular endothelial growth factor (VEGF)-C; high endothelial cell venules show structural and cell surface properties specialized to promote rapid transendothelial cell traffic.

Then, too, endothelial cells are not the only cells involved in angiogenesis. The surrounding cells, the extracellular matrix produced in concert by endothelial cells and their apposed mesenchymal cells, and the circulating blood with its cellular and humoral components also are involved. No in vitro assay can be expected to provide a complete correlate for the in vivo process.

Is there only one kind of in vivo angiogenesis? Is angiogenesis a single process? Probably not. There are similarities that reflect the fact that, by definition, angiogenesis always involves the formation of new blood vessels. However, is angiogenesis in the skin like angiogenesis in the retina? Is the process involved in revascularization of grafts the same as the process in neovascularization of tumors? Does blood vessel formation in embryos or in cycling organs such as the ovary have the same properties as angiogenesis that accompanies inflammation?

Part of the solution lies in recognizing the limitations of various assay methods. It is important to recognize what a particular assay can show and, at least as important, what it may fail to show. For example, cultured endothelial cells are extremely delicate and highly sensitive to almost any perturbation of pH or osmolarity, but such perturbations cannot be induced in vivo. Conversely, many compounds are ineffective unless partially broken down or activated. Such breakdown or activation may not occur in vitro, but may be readily attained in vivo. Even within the arena of in vitro tests, endothelial cells may behave differently under different conditions of flow, matrix, medium, or substrate. In vivo tests may also give disparate results, depending on specific microenvironments, organ sites, manner of administration of angiogenic or antiangiogenic agents, hormonal milieu, age of the test animal, or species used.

In the succeeding sections of this volume, we will be describing in vivo and in vitro assay methods. Each may be useful, but each has its limitations. For example, in vitro tests are rapid, readily quantifiable, and consistently reproducible. They can measure specific processes, such as cell motility, cell migration, response to gradients, proliferation, and three-dimensional restructuring. On the other hand, they do not permit the study of the complex physiological interactions that occur in vivo, nor do they generally permit assessment of effects that are indirect (e.g., exerted on nonendothelial cells that in turn produce proteolytic enzymes, growth factors, or cytokines that secondarily act on endothelial cells). In vivo assays are difficult to carry out, frequently requiring tedious surgery or laborious histological preparation and examination. Almost without exception, they are not easily quantifiable and, without exception, they are subject to considerable variability. Species differences may reduce the usefulness of animal models. In vivo tests are almost always more costly, particularly when they involve animals other than rodents.

Several recent reviews have surveyed and compared available angiogenesis assays (1, 2). The purpose of this section is to provide a more detailed description of some of the most frequently used in vivo and in vitro test systems for the measurement of angiogenesis and to evaluate their strengths and weaknesses.

II. PRIMARY CULTURE OF ENDOTHELIAL CELLS

In the early days of tissue culture, explants of embryonic organ rudiments doubtlessly contained endothelial cell precursors, the angioblasts that we know now enter the rudiments during early organ formation (3). Organ explants also contained endothelial cells, for many of the organs had become vascularized before dissection and explantation. Even though endothelial cells were maintained in some of the explants, there was little evidence that endothelial cells flourished under the culture conditions then used, and pure cultures of endothelial cells were not established (4). This was due to two facts: (a) the identification of endothelial cells is difficult in the absence of electron microscopic evidence of junctional complexes and Weibel-Palade bodies; and (b) identification of blood vessels is based on visualization of the vessels by means of the presence of circulating blood, a feature that could not be used in explants. Many morphological attributes of endothelial cells are shared with other cell types. Examples are that sprouting endothelial cells mimic fibroblasts, and that confluent endothelial cells cannot be distinguished from squamous epithelial cells. Therefore, even if endothelial cells had been cultured successfully in the early days, they would not necessarily have been recognized.

Probably the first clear, repeatable cultures of endothelial cells were obtained in 1973, as documented in studies from Eric Jaffe's and Michael Gimbrone's laboratories (5, 6). These cultures, obtained from human umbilical veins, and subsequent cultures obtained from other large vessels such as the bovine aorta, pulmonary vein, and pulmonary artery, were prepared by mild digestion of the internal layer of the vessels by ligation of a segment of the blood vessel, introduction of an enzyme solution into the sealed-off vessel segment, brief incubation, and finally, the elution of the loosened internal lining that was composed of vascular endothelial cells. Culture media used in these studies were standard ones, several passages of the cells were feasible, and the cells retained classic markers of endothelial cells including factor VIII–von Willebrand factor (vWF)-associated antigen and Weibel-Palade bodies. The addition of fibroblast growth factor (bFGF; FGF-2) was recommended by Gospodarowicz and his colleagues (7). Augmentation of the culture medium with bFGF and heparin, which stabilizes FGF, is now the standard protocol for primary endothelial cell cultures. Thilo-Körner et al. have provided a careful comparison of different culture and isolation methods (8). Although their review was prepared 15 years ago, the article is still timely, the principal change since then being the availability of recombinant growth factors that promote endothelial cell survival and proliferation (9).

Microvascular endothelial cells were more refractory to culture, not primarily because their growth properties were different, but because the endothelial cells could not readily be separated from the surrounding pericytes and fibroblasts. In other words, the protocol of introducing collagenase into the lumen of large vessels could not be used for microvascular endothelial cells, because capillaries cannot be cannulated. Collagenase treatment of tissues that included capillaries yielded a mixture of endothelial and nonendothelial cells. The rapid proliferation of the latter (especially in the presence of bFGF) resulted in the endothelial cells present in the initial isolate being overwhelmed and lost by dilution during subsequent passages. The inhibition of endothelial cell proliferation by the accompanying pericytes provided yet another complication (10).

However, in 1979 Folkman, Haudenschild, and Zetter reported successful capillary endothelial cell isolations from the bovine adrenal cortex (11). Their protocols were standard, for example, collagenase treatment and rich culture medium, but they succeeded by dint of patience and perseverance. By plating a dilute suspension of the initial cell isolates, they were able to spot individual small islands of endothelial cells distinct from other islands of fibroblasts and pericytes. By manually removing the nonendothelial cells each day, they ultimately obtained a culture dish enriched for endothelial cells. In such dishes, colonies of endothelial cells could be encircled and plucked for subculture.

Cell-sorting techniques were used by Auerbach et al. (12), who labeled endothelial cells specifically by using monoclonal antibody to angiotensin-converting enzyme, followed by a fluorescent second-step reagent that permitted flow cytometric identification and sorting. The key to successful sorting was to use a protocol that minimized pressure differentials and included a cushion of serum to further reduce the damage that results from rapid pressure changes. Other means for cell sorting using a flow cytometer were developed subsequently, including the use of fluorochrome-tagged acetylated low-density lipoprotein, which identifies the acLDL receptor selective for endothelial cells (13). Fluorochrome-coupled lectins such as Ulex europaeus-I, which is selective for human endothelial cells, or Bandeira simplifolica-I, which identifies murine and porcine endothelial cells, were also shown to be useful (14). Magnetic bead separation is now frequently used, primarily because it is easily available to laboratories that do not have access to the more sophisticated flow cytometers. Magnetic separation generally does not achieve as clean a separation of endothelial cells from nonendothelial cells, but two to three sequential separations can result in reliable purification (15).

Although primary endothelial cell isolations from large vessels use a standard protocol as described above, microvascular endothelial cell isolation requires distinct protocols depending on the source and species used. For example, isolation of microvascular endothelial cells from epididymal fat pads uses differential centrifugation to remove adipocytes. D-valine-containing medium is effective for obtaining kidney endothelial cells because this medium inhibits kidney fibroblast proliferation. Murine brain endothelial cells can be identified by their affinity for peanut agglutinin lectin. Antibodies that identify hematopoietic cells can be used to select against hematopoietic cell contaminants during the isolation of endothelial cells from spleen or lymph node.

The most effective way to improve the yield of microvascular endothelial cells in primary isolation is to increase the proliferation of these cells before isolation. There are several ways to accomplish this. For example, endothelial cells from the retinal vasculature can be more readily obtained from retinas made hypervascular by exposure to oxygen. Similarly, endothelial cells stimulated by implants of tumor cells are more easily established in vitro than are endothelial cells from comparable, normal quiescent blood vessels. Another means of improving the yield of endothelial cells is to use molecular genetic procedures to generate animals carrying transgenes that promote endothelial cell proliferation (16). The advantage of using embryonic sources for endothelial cells is that angiogenesis is an ongoing process during development and, therefore, more of the microvascular endothelial cells are undergoing active cell division.

The yield of endothelial cells is also significantly affected by the addition of growth factors. For example, VEGF, also known as vascular permeability factor (VPF), greatly improves the proliferative rate in vitro. It is important to bear in mind, however, that many growth factors exhibit species specificity. For example, activation of endothelial cells by γ-interferon is species-specific. Tumor necrosis factor (TNF)-α activates both murine and human endothelial cells but is ineffective when added to porcine endothelial cells. Vascular endothelial growth factor-A is stimulatory to vascular endothelial cells, but VEGF-C appears to be selective for lymphatic endothelial cells. Endothelial cells are highly heterogenous with respect to growth factor receptor and, therefore, protocols must be carefully designed to obtain optimal results.

What emerges clearly from the foregoing examples is that successful primary endothelial cell isolation is unlikely to be achieved by following standard "cookbook" protocols. Rather, each cell source, varying either in organ source or species, has distinct, although often subtle differences, attention to which may make the difference between success and failure.

In using microvascular endothelial cell cultures for angiogenesis assays, the following points should be kept in mind:

1. Many organ-specific markers are lost on long-term culture, but primary cultures such as those described here generally do not give enough cell numbers. Several passages in vitro are required. This is particularly true for endothelial cell isolations from small animals such as mice and rats.
2. Growth factors act as selective agents, promoting growth of only those microvascular endothelial cells that express the receptors for those factors. By adding basic fibroblast growth factor, for example, those endothelial cells that express the receptor(s) for FGF-2 will proliferate dif-

ferentially. Because the endothelial cells that finally proliferate in primary isolates rarely exceed 0.1% of the initially plated suspension, the cells established in vitro may not be characteristic of the endothelial cell population encountered in patent capillaries, and therefore may not represent the in vivo reality.

3. For many studies, it will be important that microvascular endothelial cells be used. It is always tempting to use large, vessel-derived endothelial cells for in vitro study of angiogenesis, because these cells can be obtained in adequate numbers in primary culture. They can be used directly or in early passage and they also tend to be more stable in vitro. However, angiogenesis, such as that seen during neovascularization of tumors, during wound healing, or in the estrus cycle, involves microvascular endothelial cells, and for this reason endothelial cells from umbilical vein, aorta, or pulmonary artery and vein may not be an adequate substitute for organ-specific microvascular endothelial cells.

In the long run, we may need to return to the early studies of organ explants, studies that date back to the pioneering experiments of Alexis Carrel, Warren Lewis, and Alexander Maximow (see [4] for bibliography). In their studies and others carried out in the 1920s, endothelial cells survived in explants that retained three-dimensional organotypic organization. It is in such cultures that the endothelium is most representative of in vivo conditions. Three-dimensional culture systems such as the aortic ring explant method developed by Nicosia (17) is a valuable modern extension of these classic studies. The next step in the development of endothelial cell culture technology may not be to improve methods of isolation, but rather to improve methods of coculture and organ explantation, using contemporary advances in growth factor, cell surface receptor and cell signaling technologies to optimize organ survival and cell-cell interactions in vitro.

III. ASSAYS FOR ENDOTHELIAL CELL PROLIFERATION AND MIGRATION

As has been already discussed in earlier chapters in this volume, angiogenesis involves both endothelial cell migration and endothelial cell proliferation, and both of these attributes of the angiogenic process have been used as in vitro correlates for angiogenesis. Whenever endothelial cells leave an existing blood vessel to migrate toward an angiogenic stimulus, they do so while maintaining continuity with the original endothelium. Hence, proliferation must always take place to allow the continued extension of the leading endothelial cell away from the parent vessel. In the absence of migration, angiogenesis cannot occur; in the absence of proliferation, angiogenesis cannot continue (1, 2, 18).

A. Cell Migration Assays

1. Directed Cell Migration

Because endothelial cells move in oriented fashion toward an angiogenic stimulus, they must be able to detect a gradient of the angiogenesis-inducing factor(s). For this reason the method of choice has been to use a Boyden chamber-type (transwell) assay (19, 20). In such chambers, endothelial cells are plated on top of a filter and permitted to migrate across the filter in response to a differential concentration of the test angiogenic factor. By varying the concentration of test substance above and below the filter of the transwell culture dish or Boyden chamber, a ''checkerboard'' type of analysis can be carried out. When the concentration of test factor is higher above than below the filter, cells will move less than when the concentration of test factor is higher below the filter. When the concentration of test factor is identical in both chambers, the number of cells migrating across the filter represents the baseline of nonspecific motility.

A major advantage of the transwell assay system is its extreme sensitivity to small differences in concentration of test substances. Its major disadvantages are the relative difficulty of setting up the assay, problems in maintaining transfilter gradients for prolonged periods, and the difficulty in obtaining accurate cell counts when relatively small numbers of cells traverse the filter.

2. Cell Motility Assays

Because angiogenic factors tend to increase overall motility, an increase in cell movement itself can be a measure of angiogenic response. This increase in motility is, of course, seen in the transwell assays just described, in which the number of cells migrating across the filter is determined both in the absence of test factor and in the presence of equal amounts of test factor above and below the filter. However, there are easier and more readily quantifiable assays for cell motility.

A frequently used cell motility test has been derived from the phagokinetic track assay methods originally developed by Albrecht Buehler. In the original assay, colloidal gold-plated coverslips were used to serve as a substrate for the movement of cells. As cells move they displace the colloidal gold, leaving a track that can be measured both for directional properties and total area. Zetter et al. (21) demonstrated that this assay could be used to quantitate cell motility of endothelial cells. Obeso and Auerbach (22) subsequently modified the assay to permit large-scale screening. In the modified assay, 1 μM-diameter beads are affixed to the bottom of 96-well microtiter plates. When endothelial cells are added, they settle on the bead monolayer and generate tracks similar to those produced by the colloidal gold. Image analysis software can then be used to measure the size and directionality of the tracks (23, 24).

3. Monolayer Migration Assays

In what has been described as a ''wound healing assay,'' endothelial cell monolayers are prepared and permitted to reach confluence. Either manually or by use of a scraping tool, a portion of the monolayer is cleared of endothelial cells, thereby providing a margin from which endothelial cells can migrate to fill the denuded region. The rate of cell migration is then monitored microscopically (25).

Quantitation here is somewhat more arbitrary than in either the transwell or bead migration assays. Use of a grid to produce reproducible, replicate areas of denudation improves quantitation. However, it is imperative to run control and experimental groups under identical conditions of confluence, and the denuded areas must be precise. A major advantage of this assay is that the cells can be observed microscopically and the migration can be recorded by time lapse photography.

4. Cell Migration in Three-Dimensional Organ Culture

A closer approximation to in vivo endothelial cell migration may be achieved by combining organ culture techniques with cell migration analysis. The prototype for this assay is the aortic ring assay developed by Roberto Nicosia and his colleagues (17, 26). In this assay, segments of aorta are explanted in collagen or fibrin gels to achieve a culture environment that permits three-dimensional growth and cell migration. Quantitation is achieved by measuring the number and length of microvessel outgrowths from the primary explant. Inducers or inhibitors of angiogenesis can be added at various time points, and quantitation can be obtained sequentially by making measurements at different time points during a culture period that may extend to 14 days (27, 28).

B. Cell Proliferation Assays

Cell proliferation of endothelial cells has long been a favorite means for measuring angiogenic and antiangiogenic activity of test substances. The procedures are easy and reproducible, the assay lends itself to precise quantitation, large numbers of cultures can be set up—thus providing the means to obtain dose/response data—and there is little day-to-day variation (9).

Unfortunately these assays are probably the least informative for assessment of angiogenesis-inducing factors. This is because, although cell proliferation is essential for angiogenesis, only a few proliferation-inducing factors are endothelial cell–specific, the one major exception being VEGF. On the other hand, factors that influence the ability of endothelial cells to proliferate secondarily, that is, where factors affect endothelial cells in some specific manner that is subsequently manifested by an inhibition of endothelial cell proliferation, the assay can prove useful, at least as a primary screen.

There appear to be no proliferation assays that are unique for endothelial cells. Endothelial cells that have been established are capable of cell division. Thus any marker of cell division can be used for assessment of proliferation. There are two major classes of proliferation assays: those that determine net cell number and those that evaluate cell cycle kinetics.

1. Assessment of Effects on Cell Number

DNA synthesis is generally determined by use of radioisotopically labeled thymidine incorporation. By determining the total incorporation at some specific time point, the amount of DNA synthesized, reflected in an increase in isotope incorporation, is a measure of the number of cells in S-phase during the period of exposure to the isotope. Assuming that the relative number of dividing cells is constant, the amount of thymidine incorporation correlates with the number of cells present during the labeling period. An alternate method is to stain cells with a DNA-binding dye and then evaluate the amount of bound dye using a colorimeter or enzyme-linked immunosorbent assay (ELISA) reader (9).

Another option is to determine net cell number. This can readily be achieved by use of a hemocytometer, or more accurately by use of an electronic counter such as the Coulter Counter.

2. Cell Cycle Analysis

Although there are many means of determining cell cycle, the most readily available assay uses flow cytometric analysis of cells labeled with various DNA-binding molecules. Perhaps the most frequently used method involves the exposure of cells to bromodeoxyuridine (BrDU) for a short period, followed by staining with propidium iodide (PI) and a fluorochrome-tagged antibody to BrDU. Propidium iodide staining to saturation provides a measure of total DNA/cell, whereas the BrDU/anti-BrDU staining identifies and quantitates the cells that have incorporated BrDU. Standard cell cycle information can be obtained by analysis of correlated displays of BrDU content with PI content. Pulse/chase protocols can get precise information on the rate of cell division.

3. Apoptosis

Both the standard TUNEL assay and flow cytometric determination of DNA content of individual cells permits estimates of the number of cells undergoing apoptosis. By combining data from apoptosis assays with either cell cycle or total cell number data, it is possible to gain a reasonable picture of proliferation/survival of endothelial cells exposed to angiogenic or antiangiogenic agents.

C. In Vivo/In Vitro Assays

The following chapters will describe in vivo assays for angiogenesis, and, as has already been pointed out in the introduction to this chapter, it is important to recognize both the advantages and the limitations of assay methods. Sometimes, it may be best to combine the best features of each, and two examples illustrate this point.

1. The In Vitro Chick Embryo Chorioallantoic Membrane Assay

Although the chick embryo chorioallantoic membrane (CAM) assay is considered an in vivo (actually in ovo) assay, it has been possible to use culture techniques to achieve in vivo conditions. The in vitro assay is carried out by placing the entire chick egg contents on the third to fourth day of incubation into a petri dish, where the embryo can continue to grow and develop (29). Grafts or test materials can be placed on the CAM after 4 to 5 days of further incubation, and vascular changes can be monitored repeatedly during a subsequent 3 to 5 day incubation period (30). In addition to providing the opportunity for periodic monitoring and photographic documentation, the method permits multiple grafts to be placed on the same embryonic membrane. The method also has been used to study grafts and test materials placed on the yolk sac membrane immediately after initiation of the embryo culture.

2. In Vitro Assessment of In Vivo Angiogenesis

Because in vivo quantitation is difficult to achieve, in vitro methods can be used to obtain such information. For example, when sponge implants or Matrigel plugs containing angiogenesis-inducing factors become impregnated with endothelial cells, they can be removed from test animals and incubated in vitro. Under appropriate conditions, endothelial cells will then migrate out of the sponge or Matrigel, and their behavior in vitro, their expression of inducible cell surface antigens, their proliferative rate, and their migratory behavior can be determined (31).

IV. CONCLUDING REMARKS

New methods and significant modifications or adaptations of established methods will continue to appear, especially with the exponential increase of angiogenesis and antiangiogenesis research that we have experienced in the past several years. We must be constantly aware that improvements in methodology may be of critical importance for the specific research questions under investigation in various laboratories. No hard-cover text will be able to replace the need for alertness to new literature and for communication among investigators in the field.

REFERENCES

1. Auerbach R, Auerbach W, Polakowski I. Assays for angiogenesis: a review. 1991; Pharmacol Therap 51:1–11.
2. Jain RK. Quantitative angiogenesis assays: progress and problems. 1997; Nature Med 3:1203–1208.
3. Noden DM. Embryonic origins and assembly of blood vessels. 1989; Am Rev Resp Dis 140:1097–1103.
4. Murray MR, Kopech G. A Bibliography of the Research in Tissue Culture. 1884–1950. An Index to the Literature of the Living Cell Cultivated In Vitro. New York: Academic Press, 1953.
5. Jaffe EA, Nachmann RL, Becker CG. Culture of human endothelial cells derived from umbilical cord veins. J Clin Invest 1973; 52:2745–2756.
6. Gimbrone MA, Cotran RS, Folkman J. Human vascular endothelial cells in culture. Growth and DNA synthesis. J Cell Biol 1974; 60:673–684.
7. Gospodarowicz D, Brown KD, Birdwell CR, Zetter BR. Control of proliferation of human vascular endothelial cells. Characterization of the response of human umbilical vein endothelial cells to fibroblast growth factor, epidermal growth factor and thrombin. J Cell Biol 1978; 77:774–788.
8. Thilo-Körner DGS, Heinrich D, Temme H. Endothelial cells in culture. A literature survey on isolation, harvesting, cultivation, medium and serum composition, cell counting, gas atmosphere, and confluency rates. In: Thilo-Körner DGFS, Freshney IR, eds. The Endothelial Cell—A Pluripotent Control Cell of the Vessel Wall. Basel: S. Karger 1983:158–202.
9. Freshney RI. Culture of Animal Cells. 3rd ed. New York: Wiley-Lisds, 1994.
10. Orlidge A, D'Amore PA. Inhibition of capillary endothelial cell growth by pericytes and smooth muscle cells. J Cell Biol 1987; 105:1455–1462.
11. Folkman J, Haudenschild CC, Zetter BR. Long-term culture of capillary endothelial cells. Proc Natl Acad Sci U S A 1979; 76:5217–5221.
12. Auerbach R, Alby L, Grieves J, Joseph J, Lindgren C, Morrissey LW, Sidky YA, Tu M, Watt SL. A monoclonal antibody against angiotensin-converting enzyme: Its use as a marker for murine, bovine, and human endothelial cells. Proc Natl Acad Sci U S A 1982; 79:7891–7895.
13. Voyta JC, Via DP, Butterfield CE, Zetter BR. Identification and isolation of endothelial cells based on their increased uptake of acetylated-low density lipoprotein. J Cell Biol 1984; 99:2034–2040.
14. Wang SJ, Greer P, Auerbach R. Isolation and propagation of yolk sac-derived endothelial cells from a hypervascular transgenic mouse expressing a Gain-of-Function *fps/fes* proto-oncogene. In Vitro Cell Dev Biol 1996; 32:292–299.
15. Plendl J, Hartwell L, Auerbach R. Organ-specific change in Dolichos biflorus lectin

binding by myocardial endothelial cells during in vitro cultivation. In Vitro Cell Dev Biol 1993; 29A:25–31.
16. Martin M, Schoecklmann H, Foster G, Barley-Maloney L, McKanna J, Daniel TO. Identification of a subpopulation of human renal microvascular endothelial cells with capacity to form capillary-like cord and tube structures. In Vitro Cell Dev Biol Anim 1997; 33:161–269.
17. Nicosia RF, Ottinetti A. Growth of microvessels in serum-free matrix culture of rat aorta: a quantitative assay of angiogenesis in vitro. Lab Invest 1990; 63:115–122.
18. Auerbach W, Auerbach R. Angiogenesis inhibition: a review. Pharmacol Therap 1994; 63:265–311.
19. Glaser BM, D'Amore PA, Seppa H, Seppa S, Schiffomann E. Adult tissues contain chemoattractants for vascular endothelial cells. Nature 1980; 288:483–484.
20. Alessandri G, Raju K, Gullino PM. Mobilization of capillary endothelium in vitro induced by effectors of angiogenesis in vivo. Cancer Res 1983; 43:1790–1797.
21. Zetter BR. Assay of capillary endothelial cell migration. Methods Enzymol 1987; 147:135–144.
22. Obeso JL, Auerbach R. A new microtechnique for quantitating cell movement in vitro using polystyrene bead monolayers. J Immunol Methods 1984; 70:141–152.
23. Weber J, Meyer KC, Banda P, Calhoun W, Auerbach R. Studies of bronchoalveolar lavage (BAL) cells and fluids in pulmonary sarcoidosis. II. Enhanced capacity of BAL fluids from patients with pulmonary sarcoidosis to induce cell movement in vitro. Am Rev Resp Dis 1989; 140:1450–1454.
24. Obeso J, Weber J, Auerbach R. A hemangioendothelioma-derived cell line: its use as a model for the study of endothelial cell biology. Lab Invest 1990; 63:259–269.
25. Pepper MS, Belin D, Montesano R, Orci L, Vassali JD. Transforming growth factor-beta 1 modulates basic fibroblast growth factor-induced proteolytic and angiogenic properties of endothelial cells in vitro. J Cell Biol 1990; 111:743–775.
26. Nicosia RF, Bonanno E, Smith N. Fibronectin promotes the elongation of microvessels during angiogenesis in vitro. J Cell Physiol 1993; 154:654–661.
27. Nicosia RF, Lin YJ, Hazelton D, Qian X-H. Endogenous regulation of angiogenesis in the rat aorta model. Role of vascular endothelial growth factor. Am J Pathol 1997; 151:1379–1386.
28. Nicosia RF, Bonanno E. Inhibition of angiogenesis in vitro by Arg-Gly-Asp-containing synthetic peptide. Am J Pathol 1991; 138:829–833.
29. Auerbach R, Kubai L, Knighton D, Folkman J. A simple procedure for the long term cultivation of chicken embryos. Dev Biol 1974; 41:391–394.
30. Form DM, Auerbach R. PGE_2 and angiogenesis. Proc Soc Exp Biol Med 1983; 172: 214–218.
31. Polakowski IJ, Lewis MK, Muthukkaruppan VR, Erdman B, Kubai L, Auerbach R. A ribonuclease inhibitor expresses anti-angiogenic properties and leads to reduced tumor growth in mice. Am J Pathol 1993; 143:1–11.

7

Screening for Angiogenesis Inhibitors with the Chick Chorioallantoic Membrane and the Mouse Corneal Micropocket Assays

Robert J. D'Amato
Harvard Medical School, Boston, Massachusetts

I. INTRODUCTION

The identification of compounds that can inhibit blood vessel growth has relied on the development of specific models of angiogenesis. Both in vitro and in vivo models have contributed to the screening of specific angiogenesis inhibitors. Although in vitro models are rapid and inexpensive, they focus on only a single component of the overall angiogenic process. In vivo angiogenesis models may model more closely the angiogenesis in biologically relevant settings. Results obtained from studies of putative inhibitors of angiogenesis using in vivo models most accurately extrapolate to mechanisms of angiogenesis observed clinically.

The selection of an appropriate angiogenic model requires the consideration of several important questions. First, how will angiogenesis be induced? Ischemia or inflammation can cause the production of angiogenic growth factors (1, 2). These same growth factors can be exogenously implanted into biological tissue to stimulate new blood vessel growth. The selection of the induction method will likely depend on the particular biological question to be addressed. Second, how will the potential inhibitory compound be delivered once new blood vessel growth has been initiated? Third, how will the effect of a compound on angiogenesis be assessed? The induction of new blood vessels can be measured readily in some systems, such as the corneal micropocket assay. In other systems, such as the retinal models, the quantification of new blood vessel growth can be technically difficult. Fourth, issues concerning spontaneous regression of induced blood vessels also need to be addressed for each model under consideration. For example, in the corneal micropocket assay, spontaneous regression is typically seen after 6 days, whereas in the tumor models, spontaneous regression of angiogenesis rarely occurs. The following discussion will focus on two important in vivo models of angiogenesis, the chick chorioallantoic membrane (CAM) assay and the corneal micropocket assay.

II. CHICK CHORIOALLANTOIC MEMBRANE

The CAM is a critical component of the oxygen exchange system of the developing chick embryo. The membrane originates from the embryo and gradually grows to cover the surface of the egg. The membrane is normally highly vascular and transparent, allowing any alteration in blood vessel growth to be easily seen.

To investigate the effects of a particular compound, a pellet containing the compound is placed on the surface of the membrane on day 6 of embryogenesis (3, 4). After 48 hours, the membrane surrounding the pellet is examined for alterations of growing vascularity. An inhibitory effect appears as an avascular zone surrounding the pellet containing the test compound (Fig. 1). In general, the results of these experiments are scored qualitatively. A range of inhibitor concentrations can be tested. However, a "larger" avascular zone does not necessarily correlate with the potency of a potential inhibitor. The size of the avascular zone depends on many factors, including the solubility and stability of the test chemical under the conditions of the assay.

The CAM assay system is relatively inexpensive and rapid. Like other in vivo models, the CAM assay has the advantage of assessing all of the steps important in new blood vessel growth. Consequently, it is useful for testing the inhibitory capabilities of compounds with a wide range of biological activities including inhibitors of endothelial cell migration, proliferation, or basement membrane degradation.

Unfortunately, a number of disadvantages are also associated with the CAM assay. False negative responses can result from compounds that are either highly soluble or highly insoluble. Highly soluble drugs may be released from the pellet too rapidly to allow the inhibitory effect to be observed. Highly insoluble drugs often are not released from the pellet at all. False negative responses also can result from compounds that are not stable during the 48-hour incubation at 37°. Some proteins that function as inhibitors of angiogenesis will not demonstrate an effect with the CAM assay because their activity is species specific. This problem can be addressed in other systems, such as cell culture assays, by

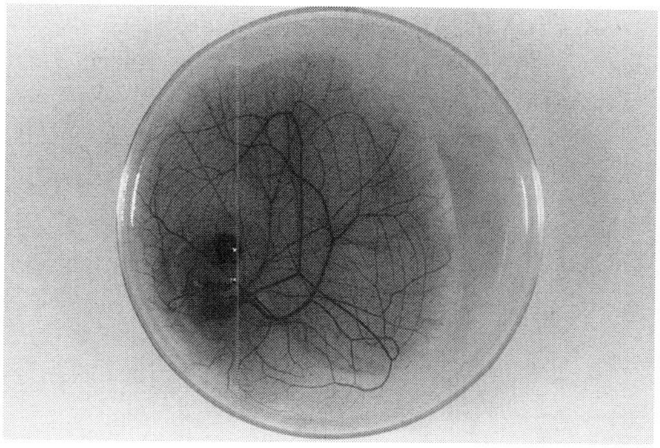

A

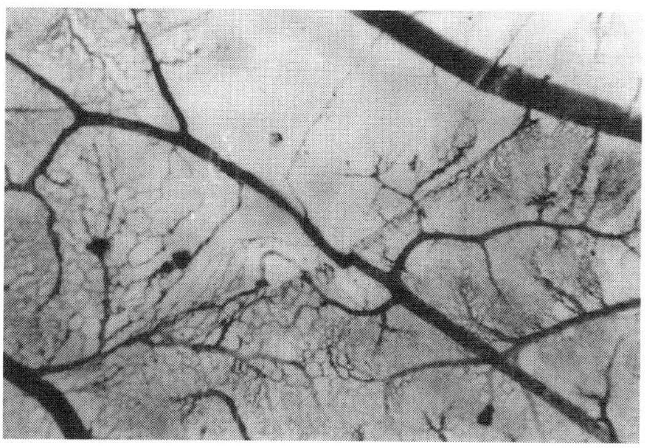

B

Figure 1 A. Six-day-old chick embryo incubated in a petri dish. **B**. Higher magnification view of an inhibitory zone on the chick chorioallantoic membrane. The pellet with test compound has been removed to fully expose the area of capillary drop-out at the top of the photo.

using endothelial cells derived from the same species as the putative inhibitor. Other instances of false negative results on the CAM may be seen if a compound requires metabolic activation to be antiangiogenic. Because hepatic activation does not occur on the surface of the CAM, compounds requiring hepatic metabolism will not appear to be active inhibitors.

In some instances the CAM assay also can produce false positive results. Some compounds may produce a distinct avascular zone, yet they are not specific inhibitors of angiogenesis. Compounds that fall into this category are antimitotic compounds that inhibit the growth of all cell types, including the proliferation of endothelial cells required for blood vessel growth. Other technical problems with the assay also may produce misleading results. Many compounds are locally irritating and form scars that can mask the inhibitory effects. Also pellets may sometimes float in the amniotic fluid surrounding the yolk, preventing the release of drug in a specific area.

In general, the CAM assay is useful as an initial rapid qualitative screen to test the activity of a potential inhibitor. Those compounds that give positive results can be further investigated using other systems to define the specific activity and potency of the test compound.

III. CORNEAL MICROPOCKET ASSAY

The cornea is the most external structure of the eye. Normally, it is transparent and avascular. The accessibility and transparency of the cornea make it an ideal site for the study of experimental neovascularization. A number of different methods to induce neovascularization in the cornea have been developed. These methods fall into four groups. First, immune-related angiogenesis can be incited by infectious agents, immune rejection (graft rejection), or wounds produced by thermal, mechanical, or chemical injury to the cornea (5–11). Second, tumors that induce neovascularization can be grown in the cornea (12–14). Third, with the advent of slow-release polymers including Elvax and Hydron, pellets can be implanted with specific growth factors or other angiogenic factors to stimulate angiogenesis (15–22). Fourth, some systemic nutritional deficiencies (for example vitamin A deficiency) and genetic abnormalities are associated with corneal neovascularization (23–25).

Early experimental corneal models used rabbits because the relatively large eye facilitated the required surgical manipulation. Recently, rodents have been used for these procedures. The advantages of rodents include availability of rodent-specific reagents, the ability to modify genetic conditions (i.e., use of skid mice), and their relative low cost. Our laboratory has found the mouse corneal micropocket model to be reliable as a screening assay (Fig. 2). In this model, pellets consisting of a Hydron base impregnated with 80 ng of basic fibroblast growth factor (bFGF) and 40 μg of sucralfate are implanted into the cornea. To investigate other growth factors besides bFGF, pellets can be made with vascular endothelial growth factor (VEGF), IL-8 or others (26). Sucralfate is used in the pellets to stabilize the bFGF and protect it from degradation by the alcohol used in forming the Hydron. Also, sucralfate binds to the bFGF and releases it slowly from the pellet over many days. It is important that the pellets be highly uniform and contain the same amount of bFGF. We standardize the formation of pellets by using a mold to form them. A paste of sucralfate, bFGF, and Hydron is spread on a mesh and then the fibers of the mesh are pulled apart, releasing square pellets. These pellets are visualized with a microscope and sorted for size and

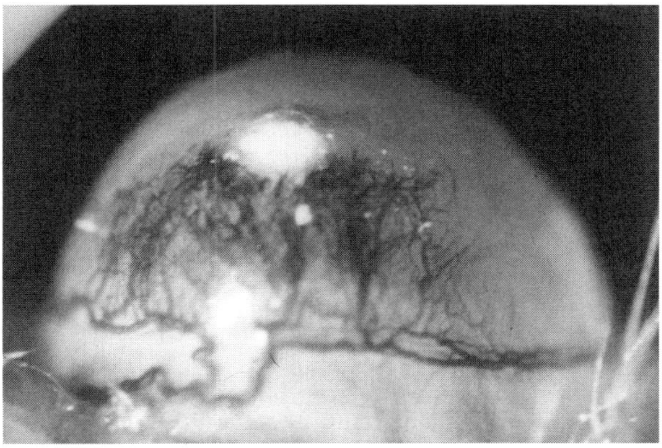

Figure 2 Mouse corneal micropocket assay. A white pellet containing basic fibroblast growth factor and sucralfate has been implanted into the cornea. After 5 days, the blood vessels clearly can be seen growing up to the pellet through the normally avascular cornea.

uniformity. Micropockets are surgically constructed by making a half-thickness corneal incision followed by a dissection through the middle of the cornea using a blunt spatula to create a potential space.

After implanting bFGF pellets in corneal micropockets of mice, neovascularization is induced on day 2 and continues through day 8. There is very little edema or inflammation, as the vessels are stimulated directly by an angiogenic factor. The maximum neovascular response is present on day 5, and this time point is used for grading and comparing angiogenesis inhibitors that are generally systemically administered daily after pellet implantation. Measurements of corneal neovascularization are easily obtained noninvasively with a slit lamp biomicroscope. Quantification can be performed by computerized image analysis. For initial screening, the length and width of the sector of new vessels can be measured. The approximate area of neovascularization can then be calculated using a simple formula.

Histology of corneal neovascularization induced by bFGF pellets typically reveals the presence of vessels throughout the corneal stroma. The response is primarily angiogenic; generally only an occasional inflammatory cell is observed. The importance of the inflammation associated with angiogenesis has been discussed frequently. I feel that the most important distinction is whether the inflammation is the primary source of the angiogenic stimulus or whether it is a minor component associated with the angiogenesis. Any time blood vessels grow into an area, these vessels will leak some fluid and allow some inflammatory cells to egress. Induction of neovascularization by specific growth factors such as VEGF produces a minimal number of inflammatory cells. In contrast, burn or endotoxin models produce hundreds of inflammatory cells that serve to produce the primary angiogenic stimulus. All of the in vivo models will have some component of inflammation; however, in some models it can be only a minimal component.

It has been speculated that certain growth factors may predominate in different types of physiologic angiogenesis. For instance, VEGF may be more important in tumors and bFGF may be more important in wound healing or restenosis. Therefore, certain compounds that have preferential inhibitory activity toward one cytokine might give an advantage in targeting a specific disease. By implanting a variety of growth factors into the cornea, the relative potency of each inhibitor can be tested. Additionally, the specific interaction of a growth factor with a particular inhibitor can be evaluated. Each inhibitor has its own profile of inhibitory activity. Some inhibitors have a specific interaction with only one growth factor. Other agents, such as thalidomide, inhibit bFGF-induced and VEGF-induced neovascularization equally. Determining the profile of actions of an angiogenesis inhibitor with different growth factors may help direct the development of the agent as treatment for appropriate disease states.

The route of administration of putative angiogenesis inhibitors used in in vivo models can be important, because differences are often seen when comparing local to systemic administration. For example, minocyclin inhibits blood vessel growth when incorporated into pellets placed directly into the cornea; however, we have not been able to detect inhibition when it is given orally. Results from experiments using local administration of inhibitors cannot be generalized to other routes of administration inasmuch as the high millimolar concentrations of drugs incorporated into pellets are rarely able to be achieved in the bloodstream by systemic administration.

A last factor for consideration relates to regression of vessels in animal models. In the mouse corneal micropocket model, vessels begin to regress after about day 6. This is thought to be caused by the depletion of growth factor in the pellet and the effect of endogenous inhibitors normally present in the cornea. Very few models of angiogenesis have no spontaneous regression. Thus most angiogenesis models are only useful for screening inhibitors during a short period when neovascularization is actively induced before spontaneous regression occurs. However, in tumors, new blood vessels do not regress. Because the persistent and aggressive neovascular response of tumors cannot be modeled well with slow release pellets, putative angiogenesis inhibitors must be tested separately in animal tumor models.

Tumor angiogenesis can be evaluated in situ by staining and quantifying the tumor's vascular density. The decrease in the vascular density of tumors corresponds with the degree of angiogenesis inhibition. Tumor-induced vessels also can be seen growing toward the tumor (prior to invasion into the tumor mass) when tumors are implanted into the cornea. Some compounds may inhibit angiogenesis in tumor systems by causing direct toxicity to the tumor, which could cause a reduction in growth factor production by the tumor. Decreased tumor angiogenesis may be secondary to effects of a drug on the tumor or it may be due to direct effects of the drug on the tumor vasculature. Models of isolated angiogenesis that use sustained release of growth factors, such as the corneal micropocket model, can help to differentiate these actions.

To conclude, I have attempted to outline how our laboratory performs screening assays to identify inhibitors of angiogenesis. Every model has strengths and weaknesses. Results from studies using models that closely mimic a specific disease are not readily generalized to other disorders. However, general models used to quantify angiogenesis are often not broadly applicable to individual disease states because of the requirements for specific growth factors and other unique aspects of a particular disease processes. Ultimately, several different models must be used to predict reliably the efficacy of any putative inhibitor. The abundance of these models allows reliable pharmacological development of new inhibitors of angiogenesis.

REFERENCES

1. Knighton DR, Hunt TK, Scheuenstuhl H, Halliday BJ, Werb Z, Banda MJ. Oxygen tension regulates the expression of angiogenesis factor by macrophages. Science 1983; 221:1283–1285.
2. Shweiki D, Itin A, Soffer D, Keshet E. Vascular endothelial growth factor induced by hypoxia may mediate hypoxia-initiated angiogenesis. Nature 1992; 359:843–845.
3. Auerbach R, Kubai L, Knighton D, Folkman J. A simple procedure for the long-term cultivation of chicken embryos. Dev Biol 1974; 41(2):391–394.
4. Crum R, Szabo S, Folkman J. A new class of steroids inhibits angiogenesis in the presence of heparin or a heparin fragment. Science 1985; 230:1375–1378.
5. McCracken JS, Burger PC, Klintworth GK. Morphologic observations on experimental corneal vascularization in the rat. Lab Invest 1979; 41(6):519–530.
6. Karasek E, Heder G. The rabbit cornea model for detecting neovascularization effects. Z Versuchstierkunde 1981; 23(1):59–66.
7. Fournier GA, Lutty GA, Watt S, Fenselau A, Patz A. A corneal micropocket assay for angiogenesis in the rat eye. Invest Ophthalmol Vis Sci 1981; 21:351–354.
8. Mahoney JM, Waterbury LD. Drug effects on the neovascularization response to silver nitrate cauterization of the rat cornea. Curr Eye Res 1985; 4(5):531–535.
9. Epstein RJ, Stulting RD. Corneal neovascularization induced by stimulated lymphocytes in inbred mice. Invest Ophthalmol Visual Sci 1987; 28(9):1505–1513.
10. Li WW, Grayson G, Folkman J, D'Amore PA. Sustained-release endotoxin. A model for inducing corneal neovascularization. Invest Ophthalmol Visual Sci 1991; 32(11): 2906–2911.
11. Amano S, Sawa M, Ishii Y. Keratoepithelioplasty in rat: Development of a model and histological study. Japan J Ophthalmol 1992; 36:407–416.
12. Gimbrone MA Jr, Cotran RS, Leapman SB, Folkman J. Tumor growth and neovas-

cularization: An experimental model using the rabbit cornea. J Natl Cancer Inst 1974; 52(2):413–427.
13. Ryu S, Albert DM. Evaluation of tumor angiogenesis factor with the rabbit cornea model. Invest Ophthalmol Visual Sci 1979; 18(8):831–841.
14. Muthukkaruppan VR, Kubai L, Auerbach R. Tumor-induced neovascularization in the mouse eye. J Natl Cancer Inst 1982; 69(3):699–708.
15. Langer R, Folkman J. Polymers for sustained release of proteins and other macromolecules. Nature 1976; 263:797–800.
16. BenEzra D. Neovasculogenic ability of prostaglandins, growth factors, and synthetic chemoattractants. Am J Ophthalmol 1978; 88:455–461.
17. Muthukkaruppan VR, Auerbach R. Angiogenesis in the mouse cornea. Science 1979; 205:1416–1418.
18. Gospodarowicz D, Bialecki H, Thakral TK. The angiogenic activity of fibroblast and epidermal growth factor. Exp Eye Res 1979; 28:501–514.
19. Gaudric A, N'guyen T, Moenner M, Glacet-Bernard A, Barritault D. Quantification of angiogenesis due to basic fibroblast growth factor in a modified rabbit corneal model. Ophthalmic Res 1992; 24(3):181–188.
20. Rieck P, Assouline M, Savoldelli M, Hartmann C, Jacob C, Pouliquen Y, Courtois Y. Recombinant human basic fibroblast growth factor (Rh-bFGF) in three different wound models in rabbits: Corneal wound healing effect and pharmacology. Exp Eye Res 1992; 54(6):987–998.
21. Kenyon BM, Voest EE, Chen CC, Flynn E, Folkman J, D'Amato RJ. A model of angiogenesis in the mouse cornea. Invest Ophthalmol Visual Sci 1996; 37(8):1625–1632.
22. Loughnan M, Chatziftefanou K, Flynn E, Adamis T, Shing Y, D'Amato R, Folkman J. Experimental corneal neovascularization using sucralfate and bFGF. Aust N Z J Ophthalmol 1996; 24(3):289–295.
23. Fromer CH, Klintworth GK. An evaluation of the role of leukocytes in the pathogenesis of experimentally induced corneal vascularization. Am J Pathol 1975; 79:531–554.
24. Leure-Dupree AE. Vascularization of the rat cornea after prolonged zinc deficiency. Anat Rec 1986; 216(1):27–32.
25. Smith RS, Hawes NL, Kuhlmann SD, Heckenlively JR, Chang B, Roderick TH, Sundberg JP. Cornl: A mouse model for corneal surface disease and neovascularization. Invest Ophthalmol Visual Sci 1996; 37(2):397–404.
26. Strieter RM, Kunkel SL, Elner VM, Martonyi CL, Koch AE, Polverini PJ, Elner SG. Interleukin-8: A corneal factor that induces neovascularization. Am J Pathol 1992; 141(6):1279–1284.

8

Capillary Morphogenesis In Vitro

Cytokine Interactions and Balanced Proteolysis

Roberto Montesano and Michael S. Pepper
University of Geneva Medical Center, Geneva, Switzerland

I. INTRODUCTION

The series of morphogenetic events that result in the formation of new capillary blood vessels has been well described. Angiogenesis begins with localized breakdown of the basement membrane of the parent vessel (usually a postcapillary venule). Endothelial cells then migrate into the surrounding extracellular matrix (ECM) within which they form a capillary sprout. As the sprout elongates by migration and proliferation of endothelial cells, a lumen is gradually formed proximal to the migrating front. Contiguous tubular sprouts subsequently anastomose to form functional capillary loops, and vessel maturation is accomplished by reconstitution of the basement membrane (1–4). Angiogenesis is thus characterized by alterations in at least three endothelial cell functions: (a) modulation of interactions with the ECM, which requires alterations of cell-ECM contacts and the production of matrix-degrading proteolytic enzymes; (b) an initial increase and subsequent decrease in locomotion (migration), which allows the cells to translocate toward the angiogenic stimulus and to stop once they reach their destination; and (c) an increase in proliferation, which provides new cells for the growing and elongating vessel, and a subsequent return to the quiescent state once the vessel is formed. Together these cellular functions contribute to the process of capillary morphogenesis, that is, the formation of patent tubelike structures.

Despite our detailed knowledge of the sequential steps of the neovascularization process from descriptive in vivo studies and the identification of a host of angiogenesis-modulating cytokines, the molecular mechanisms of angiogenesis are incompletely understood. The two most widely used assays for studying angiogenesis in vivo are the chick chorioallantoic membrane (5) and the rabbit corneal micropocket (6). More recently described quantitative in vivo assays involve subcutaneous implantation of various three-dimensional substrates to which angiogenesis-regulating factors can be added. These include polyester sponges (7), polyvinylalcohol foam discs covered on both sides with Millipore filters (the disc angiogenesis system) (8), and Matrigel, a basement membrane-rich ECM (9). These assays have been used for many years to describe the morphologically identifiable events that occur during angiogenesis. They have been important in the identification of positive and negative regulators. The in vivo assays described above are essential to establish whether a given molecule stimulates blood vessel formation in the intact organism. However, their interpretation is frequently complicated by the fact that the experimental conditions may inadvertently favor inflammation, and that under these conditions the angiogenic response is elicited indirectly, at least in part, through the activation of inflammatory or other nonendothelial cells. Although this may be relevant to some settings in which angiogenesis occurs in vivo, it does not allow study of the consequences of the direct interaction of angiogenesis regulators with endothelial cells. To circumvent this drawback, in vitro assays using populations of cultured endothelial cells have been developed for several of the cellular components of the angiogenic process. Based on the geometry of the assay, these can be classified as either two-dimensional or three-dimensional. Conventional two-dimensional assays include measurement of endothelial cell proliferation, migration, and production of proteolytic enzymes such as matrix metalloproteinases (MMPs) and plasminogen activators (PAs) (10). Three-dimensional assays have as their end point the formation of capillarylike cords or tubes by endothelial cells cultured either on the surface of (planar models) or within simplified ECMs. These assays include: (a) long-term culture of endothelial cells in dishes coated with a thin layer of ECM proteins (11–17); (b) short-term culture of endothelial cells on a thick gel of basement membranelike matrix (18–21); (c) suspension of endothelial cells within a three-dimensional collagen gel (22); (d) radial growth of branching tubules from rings of rat aorta (23) or from fragments of either rat adipose tissue microvessels (24) or human placental blood vessels (25) embedded in collagen or fibrin gels; (e) radial growth of tubular sprouts from endothelial cells grown on microcarrier beads embedded in a fibrin gel (26).

Because in the living organism angiogenesis occurs in a three-dimensional ECM microenvironment, we have designed culture systems that allow the reestablishment of three-dimensional interactions between microvascular endothelial cells and the surrounding ECM. In this review, we summarize work from our laboratory on the use of these in vitro assays that accurately recapitulate the invasive nature of the angiogenic process and allow for histotypic morphogenesis, that is, for the formation of patent capillarylike tubes whose abluminal surface is in direct contact with the ECM.

II. THREE-DIMENSIONAL INTERACTION WITH COLLAGEN FIBRILS PROMOTES THE ORGANIZATION OF ENDOTHELIAL CELLS INTO TUBE-LIKE STRUCTURES

In vivo, microvascular endothelial cells experience a different ECM environment, depending on whether they are in a resting state or are undergoing sprouting and migration during angiogenesis. In the normal quiescent state, endothelial cells rest on a specialized ECM, the basement membrane, which contains predominantly type IV collagen and laminin. During angiogenesis, however, these cells focally degrade their investing basement membrane, and subsequently migrate into the interstitial matrix of the surrounding connective tissue, which consists mainly of type I collagen (1, 27). In an attempt to understand the role of the ECM in the process of angiogenesis, we have studied the interactions of endothelial cells with three-dimensional gels of reconstituted type I collagen fibrils. We found that when a monolayer of microvascular endothelial cells on the surface of a collagen gel is covered with a second layer of collagen, it reorganizes within a few days into a network of branching and anastomosing tubules (Fig. 1). These findings demonstrate that a three-dimensional interaction with collagen fibrils plays an important role in driving capillary morphogenesis (28).

III. THREE-DIMENSIONAL ASSAY OF ENDOTHELIAL CELL INVASION AND TUBE MORPHOGENESIS

In the studies described above (28), formation of capillarylike tubules was experimentally induced by embedding endothelial cells within a three-dimensional collagen matrix. During angiogenesis in vivo, however, the morphogenetic events that culminate in the formation of new capillary blood vessels are intimately associated with the activation of an invasive process, that is, the local breakdown of the microvascular basement membrane and the penetration of endothelial sprouts into the interstitial ECM. The question of how normally quiescent endothelial cells acquire invasive properties that endow them with the ability to breach the mechanical barriers of the ECM is central to the understanding of the mechanisms of angiogenesis. Cell invasiveness in angiogenesis and in

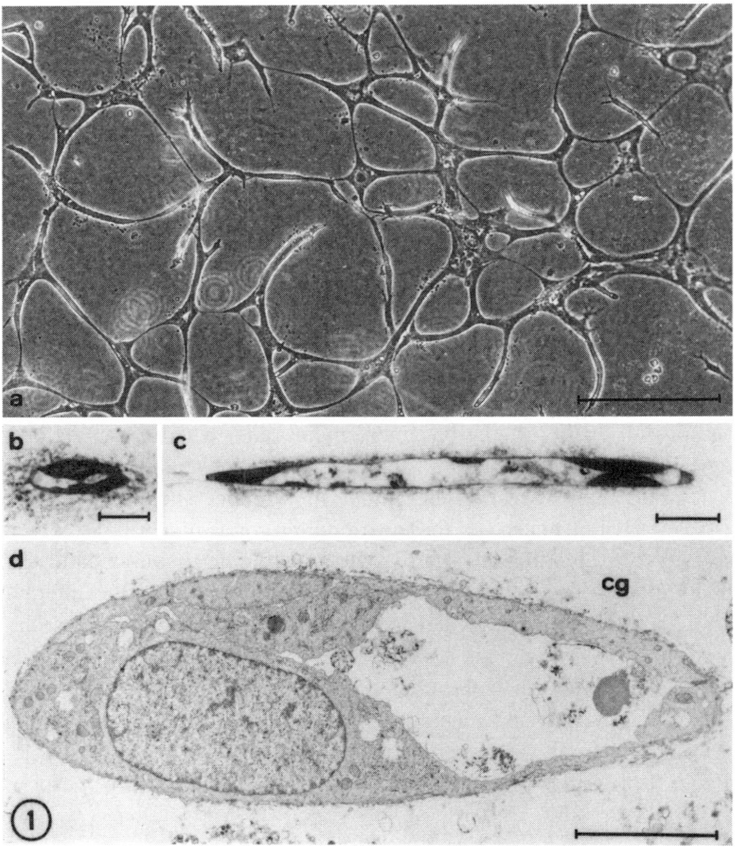

Figure 1 **a**. Collagen matrix promotes the organization of endothelial cells into capillarylike tubules. Phase contrast microscopy of a culture of microvascular endothelial cells grown initially on top of a collagen gel and subsequently covered with a second layer of collagen. Four days after being overlaid, the existing monolayer has reorganized into a network of branching and anastomosing cords of endothelial cells. **b–d**. Sections for light **(b, c)** and electron **(d)** microscopy perpendicular to a culture of capillary endothelial cells sandwiched between two collagen layers as in **(a)**. The endothelial cells surround a central lumen to form capillarylike tubular structures. *Abbreviations: cg*, collagen gel. **(a)**: bar = 200 μm; **(b)**: bar = 10 μm; **(c)**: bar = 20 μm; **(d)**: bar = 5 μm.
(a) From News in Physiological Sciences 1990; 5:75–95, by copyright permission of The American Physiological Society. **(b–d)** From The Journal of Cell Biology 1983; 97:1648–1652, by copyright permission of The Rockefeller University Press.

other biological processes is believed to require the elaboration of proteolytic enzymes that act in the extracellular environment and that include essentially MMPs (e.g., interstitial collagenases, gelatinases, and stromelysins) and serine proteases, in particular PA/plasmin system (29–32). The central component of the PA/plasmin system is plasmin, whose principal physiological role is fibrinolysis, and which has been suggested to activate latent MMPs and growth factors. Plasmin is generated from its inactive precursor plasminogen by the activity of two PAs: urokinase-type PA (uPA) and tissue-type PA (tPA). Urokinase PA activity can be localized to the cell surface through binding to a specific high affinity receptor (uPAR), and uPA and tPA are subject to inhibition by specific physiological PA inhibitors (PAI-1 and PAI-2) (33).

Our earlier studies, described above (28), had shown that endothelial cells grown on a collagen gel form a monolayer on the surface of the gel and do not invade the underlying matrix. We next asked whether induction of matrix-degrading protease synthesis might allow endothelial cells to penetrate into the collagen matrix, as they do during angiogenesis in vivo. To investigate this possibility, confluent monolayers of either microvascular or large vessel endothelial cells on collagen gels were treated with phorbol myristate acetate (PMA), a tumor promoter that significantly stimulates the production of collagenase and PAs (34) (Table 1). Whereas control endothelial cells were confined to the surface of the gels, PMA-treated endothelial cells invaded the underlying collagen matrix, within which they formed capillarylike tubular structures (Fig. 2a,b) (35, 36).

Table 1 Inducers of Angiogenesis in Collagen Gel Model

Cytokines:	References:
bFGF	52
aFGF + heparin	unpublished
$VEGF_{165}$	55
$VEGF_{121}$	unpublished
Activators of protein kinase C:	
PMA	35
Bryostatin I (200ng/ml)	unpublished
Mezerein (100ng/ml)	unpublished
Others:	
Sodium orthovanadate	65
Hyaluronan oligosaccharides	131

Abbreviations: bFGF, basic fibroblast growth factor; *aFGF*, acidic fibroblast growth factor; *VEGF*, vascular endothelial growth factor.

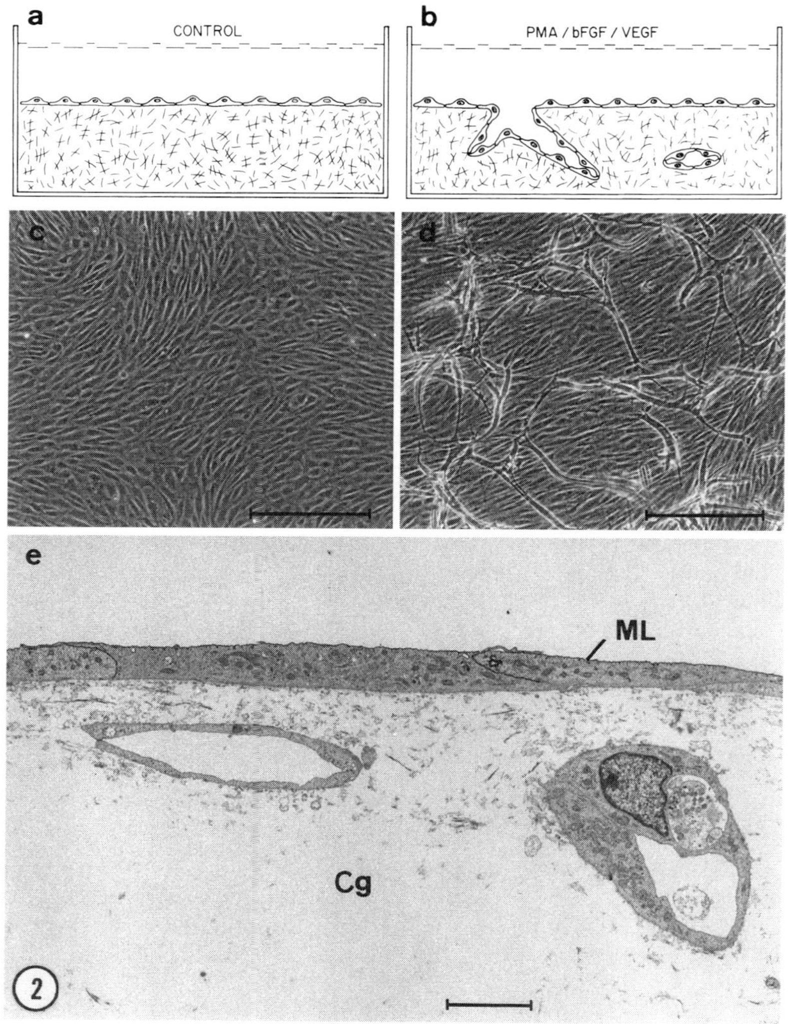

Figure 2 Collagen gel invasion model for the study of angiogenesis in vitro. **a**. Endothelial cells grown on the surface of a three-dimensional collagen gel form a confluent monolayer without invading the underlying matrix (control). **b**. Addition of either the protein kinase C activator phorbol myristate acetate (PMA) or the physiological angiogenic cytokines basic fibroblast growth factor (bFGF) and vascular endothelial growth factor (VEGF) induces the cells to invade the underlying gel and to form capillarylike tubular structures. Invasion and tube formation are also induced by sodium orthovanadate, an inhibitor of phosphotyrosine phosphatases (65). **c**. When viewed from above by phase contrast microscopy, the endothelial cells are seen to form a monolayer on the surface of the gel. **d**. Three days after addition of bFGF, the cells have formed a network of branching cords. **e**. When the invading cell cords are viewed in cross section by electron microscopy, their tubular nature, morphologically similar to capillaries seen in vivo, can be appreciated. *Abbreviations: ML*, endothelial monolayer; *Cg*, collagen gel. **(c, d)**: bar = 200 μm; **(e)**: bar = 10 μm.

Table 2 Inhibitors of Angiogenesis in Collagen Gel Model

Cytokines:	References:
TGF-β[a]	67, 69
TNF-α[a]	unpublished
IFN-α2a	153
Oncostatin M, LIF, IL-6, IL-11	51, 97, and unpublished
Steroids and metabolites:	
2-methoxyestradiol	150
Synthetic angiostatic steroids (U-24067, U-42129)	153
Dexamethasone (1 nm-1μm)	unpublished
Hydrocortisone (100 ng/ml-10 μg/ml)	unpublished
Protease inhibitors:	
TIMP-2, TIMP-3	38
Synthetic MMP inhibitors	unpublished
α2-antiplasmin	unpublished
Others:	
Genistein and isoflavonoid analogues	149 and unpublished
Retinoic acid	153
Heparin	153
Suramin[a]	153
Protamine (100μg/ml)	unpublished
dbcAMP (1 mM)	unpublished
IBMX (1.5 mM); Theophylline (1.5 mM)	unpublished
LiCl (10–30 mM)	unpublished

[a] Biphasic effect
Abbreviations: TGF, transforming growth factor; *TNF*, tumor necrosis factor; *IFN*, interferon; *LIF*, leukemia inhibitory factor; IFN, interferon; *TIMP*, tissue inhibitor of metalloproteinase; *MMP*, matrix metalloproteinase; *dbcAMP*, dibutyryl cyclic AMP; *IBMX*, isobutylmethylxanthine.

The finding that invasion and tube formation are associated with degradation of collagen fibrils and are prevented either by the metal chelator 1,10-phenanthroline (35), by synthetic low molecular weight MMP inhibitors (37; R. Montesano and M.S. Pepper, unpublished data), or by recombinant tissue inhibitors of metalloproteinases (TIMPs) (37, 38) (Table 2) suggests an important role for interstitial collagenases or other metalloproteinases in angiogenesis.

The collagen gel invasion assay described above has been used by several

---

(a, b, e) From Curr Top Microbiol Immunol 1996; 213/II:31–67, by copyright permission of Springer-Verlag. **(c, d)** From Front Endocrinol 1994; 6:43–66, by copyright permission of Ares-Serono Symposia (152).

groups to investigate the effect of various cytokines or tumor cell-conditioned media, as well as the role of proteolytic enzymes in angiogenesis in vitro (37, 39–46). In addition, a modified version of this assay using Millipore chambers has been described by Okamura et al. (47) and by Sakuda et al. (48).

IV. BASIC FIBROBLAST GROWTH FACTOR AND VASCULAR ENDOTHELIAL GROWTH FACTOR INDUCE ANGIOGENESIS IN VITRO

The experiments described above indicated that endothelial cells, even after repeated passage in culture, retain the potential to express a latent ''angiogenic program'' that may be switched on by appropriate signals. To establish whether physiological messengers could elicit an angiogenic response similar to that induced by PMA, microvascular endothelial cells grown on collagen gels were treated with basic fibroblast growth factor (bFGF), a well-characterized angiogenic polypeptide (49–51). As previously observed in response to PMA, bFGF induced endothelial cells to invade the underlying collagen matrix and to form capillarylike tubules (Fig. 2). Concomitantly, bFGF stimulated endothelial cells to produce PAs (52). These results demonstrate that, in vitro, bFGF can induce two essential components of angiogenesis, namely invasion of a three-dimensional ECM and morphogenesis of endothelial tubules. In addition, because bFGF is unable to induce tubule formation in conventional culture systems, these studies highlight the importance of three-dimensional cell-ECM interactions in promoting an appropriate angiogenic response in endothelial cells after exposure to angiogenic factors.

After studying the response of endothelial cells to bFGF, we examined the potential effect in our system of a number of other cytokines that have been reported to be angiogenic in vivo. Among these agents, only vascular endothelial growth factor (VEGF), which is currently considered to be one of the most important physiological regulators of angiogenesis (51, 53, 54), was able to induce endothelial cell invasion and tube formation (see Fig. 4c) (55, 56). Like bFGF, VEGF also increased the expression of uPA by endothelial cells (57).

V. PROTEOLYTIC BALANCE AND CAPILLARY MORPHOGENESIS

The coordinate modulation of invasive behavior and PA production by PMA, bFGF, and VEGF (see above), together with our demonstration of an increase in uPA and uPAR expression in endothelial cells migrating from the edge of an experimental wound in vitro (58, 59), supported the proposed role for the PA/plasmin system (34) in angiogenesis. The expression of proteolytic activity by endothelial cells must, however, be tightly controlled to prevent inappropriate matrix degradation. That the balance between proteases and protease inhibitors might be important for normal capillary morphogenesis was first demonstrated in experiments in which fibrin gels were substituted for collagen gels in our in vitro angiogenesis assay. The reasoning was that angiogenesis often occurs in a fibrin-rich matrix, for example during wound healing or as a consequence of vascular hyperpermeability in inflammation and tumors. In striking contrast to what we had observed with collagen gels, we noted that upon addition of the angiogenic stimulus to endothelial cells cultured on a fibrin gel, the underlying gel was rapidly lysed. The absence of a three-dimensional substrate, therefore, precluded invasion and the formation of capillarylike tubules. However, inhibition of excessive fibrinolysis by addition of serine protease inhibitors allowed for preservation of a three-dimensional matrix into which endothelial cells migrated to form tubelike structures (60). This study highlights the notion that although increased protease activity is clearly associated with the invasive phenotype, protease inhibitors play an equally important, albeit permissive, role in angiogenesis by preventing excessive and unnecessary matrix destruction and ensuring the integrity of the ECM scaffold (60).

Additional support for the role of protease inhibitors in normal capillary morphogenesis has come from our observations on the behavior of endothelial cells expressing the polyoma virus middle-T (mT) oncogene. It had been shown previously that mT induces cystlike endothelial tumors when expressed in chimeric or transgenic mice (61, 62). Furthermore, when endothelial cells expressing mT (End. cells) were isolated from these tumors and injected into mice, hemorrhagic cystlike tumors (endotheliomas) were also induced (63). We have developed an in vitro correlate of endothelioma formation by embedding End. cells into three-dimensional fibrin gels. In contrast to normal endothelial cells, which formed a network of capillarylike tubules in fibrin gels, End. cells formed large cystlike structures that bear striking resemblance to endotheliomas observed in vivo (Figure 3a,b). When studying the proteolytic properties of these cells, we found that they displayed increased PA activity when compared to endothelial cells that do not express mT, and that this could be accounted for by an increase in uPA and a decrease in PAI-1 activity. With these observations in mind, we asked what would happen if we attempted to reduce the excess proteolysis by adding protease inhibitors to the culture system. We found that when serine protease inhibitors were added to the cultures, the End. cells, instead of forming cysts, now formed branching capillarylike tubules (Figure 3c, d) (64). These results demonstrated that excessive proteolytic activity is not compatible with normal capillary morphogenesis, but that by reducing this activity through the addition of serine protease inhibitors, normal morphogenetic properties could be restored to the cells. A more detailed discussion of the properties of mT-expressing endothelial cells and their relevance to vascular tumors in humans can be found in ref. 63.

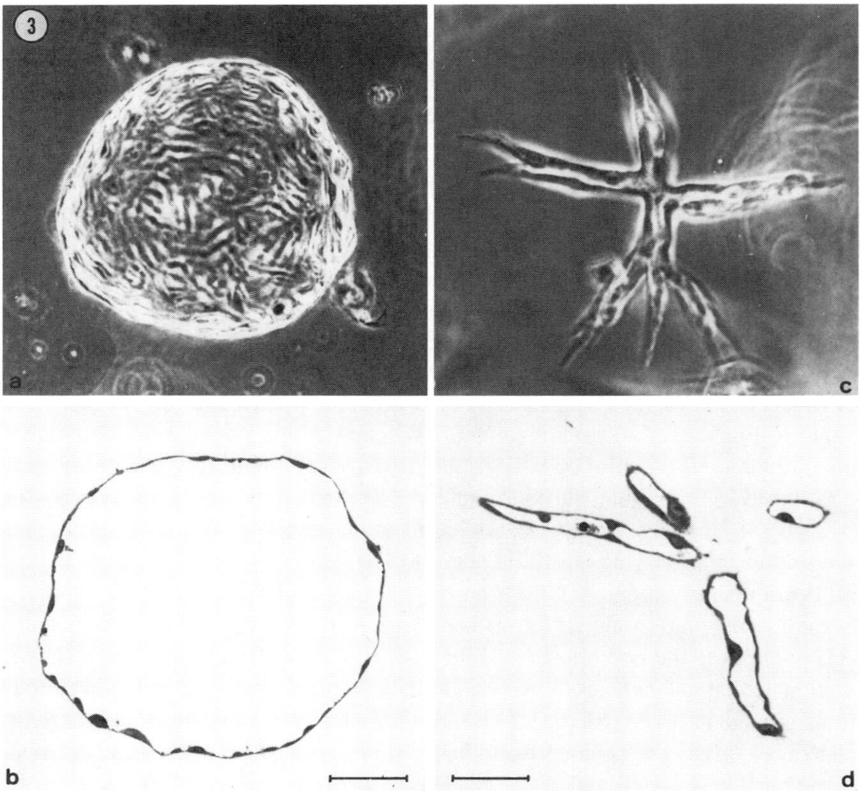

Figure 3 Morphogenetic behavior of mT-expressing endothelial cells grown within fibrin gels under control conditions or in the presence of exogenously added serine protease inhibitors. **a**. Spherical cyst formed by mT-expressing endothelial cells grown within a fibrin gel (phase-contrast microscopy). In this picture, the focus is approximately on the equatorial plane of the cyst. The endothelial cells lining the floor and the roof of the cavity appear blurred in the center of the cyst. **b**. Semithin section of an endothelial cyst. The large cavity is lined by a continuous monolayer of flattened endothelial cells. **c, d**. Branching capillarylike tubules formed by mT-expressing endothelial cells grown within a fibrin gel in the presence of the serine protease inhibitors ϵ-aminocaproic acid (**c**) or Trasylol (**d**). (**a, b**): bar = 100 μm; (**c, d**): bar = 50 μm.
(**a–c**) From Cell 1990; 62 435–445, by copyright permission of Cell Press. (**d**) From *Endothelial and Mucus Secreting Cells,* Pozzi E, ed., 1991: p. 1–17, by copyright permission of Masson S.p.A.

A protective role for protease inhibitors was also suggested by the finding that PMA, bFGF, sodium orthovanadate and VEGF, four agents that induce invasion and tube formation in the three-dimensional in vitro model described above (35, 36, 52, 55, 65), increase not only uPA in microvascular endothelial cells (10, 34, 52, 57, 65), but also PAI-1 (57, 66, 67). Similarly, wound-induced two-dimensional migration is characterized by a concomitant increase in uPA as well as PAI-1 (58, 59, 68). In an attempt to understand better the respective roles of proteases and protease inhibitors in angiogenesis, we studied the modulation of uPA and PAI-1 by bFGF and transforming growth factor (TGF)-β1, a cytokine that greatly increases PAI-1 production by endothelial cells (66, 67). In addition to increasing PAI-1, we observed that TGF-β1 also increased uPA expression in microvascular endothelial cells. However, when using the ratio of uPA/PAI-1 mRNA as a reflection of the potential proteolytic activity of the cells, the net response to TGF-β1 was always antiproteolytic, in contrast to the large increase in potential proteolysis observed in response to bFGF. When cells were exposed to both bFGF and TFG-β1, levels of potential proteolysis as represented by the uPA/PAI-1 mRNA ratio mimicked those seen in controls (67).

Knowing that TGF-β1 was capable of modulating bFGF-induced proteolysis, we next assessed its effect on bFGF-induced capillarylike tube formation in vitro. Experiments aimed at addressing this problem were performed in fibrin rather than collagen gels to assay more specifically for the PA system. In response to bFGF, the cells invaded the underlying gel, resulting in the formation of branching tubelike structures with large, ectatic lumina. When added alone, TGF-β1 had no effect. However, when coadded with bFGF, lumen diameter of capillarylike tubes was significantly reduced. Although this was true at both 500 pg/ml and 5 ng/ml TGF-β1, doses that increased and decreased bFGF-induced invasion respectively (see next section), the presence of a lumen was less frequently observed at 5 ng/ml than at 500 pg/ml. Furthermore, lumen size at 500 pg/ml TGF-β1 was reduced to a size that was physiologically more relevant (67, 69). Because the creation of a hollow space (i.e., the lumen) within the fibrin gel is dependent on fibrinolysis, these findings suggest that the antiproteolytic effect of TGF-β1, which results from a large increase in PAI-1, is likely to be responsible, at least in part, for the reduction in lumen size.

In addition to the model described above, in which tubule formation is induced by exogenous stimuli, a three-dimensional model of spontaneous angiogenesis has been developed for the purpose of identifying potential physiological inhibitors. Endothelial cells are seeded onto a nonadhesive agarose substrate, which results in the formation of solid-cell aggregates floating in the culture medium. These aggregates are then embedded into three-dimensional collagen or fibrin gels. After a few hours, endothelial sprouts begin to grow out spontaneously from the original aggregate, resulting after a few days in the formation of radially disposed hollow endothelial tubes. The observation that the capillary lumen is devoid of ECM suggests that lumen formation is proteolysis-dependent. When the serine protease inhibitor Trasylol was added to fibrin gel cultures, the cells migrated out as solid endothelial cords, that is, lumen formation was completely inhibited. These findings demonstrate that lumen formation in fibrin gels requires extracellular serine protease activity (70). Inasmuch as cartilage is one of the few avascular tissues in the body, we also determined whether chondrocytes might produce a factor that inhibits endothelial sprout formation in vitro using the model just described. When chondrocytes were coincorporated in collagen or fibrin gels with endothelial cell aggregates or added to the culture medium above the gel, sprout formation normally seen in controls was greatly inhibited. On the basis of antibody inhibition studies, we demonstrated that a chondrocyte-derived TGF-β1 was partially responsible for inhibition of sprout formation in this experimental system (70).

VI. INTERACTIONS BETWEEN ANGIOGENESIS-MODULATING CYTOKINES

Very little is known about interactions between angiogenesis-modulating cytokines. It is highly likely, however, that endothelial cells are rarely (if ever) exposed to a single cytokine during physiological and pathological processes. To explore potential interactions between cytokines, we have used the collagen gel invasion assay described above, in which the extent of endothelial tube formation in response to angiogenic factors can be quantitated by measuring the total additive length of all cellular structures that have penetrated from the surface monolayer into the underlying gel.

A. Synergism Between bFGF and VEGF

Using our three-dimensional model, we first assessed the effect of simultaneous addition of bFGF and VEGF on the in vitro angiogenic response. We found that, when added simultaneously, VEGF and bFGF induced an in vitro angiogenic response that was far greater than the sum of the effects elicited by either agent separately and that occurred with greater rapidity than the response to either cytokine alone (Figs. 4 and 5a). These results demonstrate that, by acting in concert, these two cytokines have a potent synergistic effect on the induction of angiogenesis in vitro (55). In attempting to understand the mechanisms responsible for this synergistic effect, we initially assessed the effect of coaddition of bFGF and VEGF in conventional two-dimensional in vitro assays of endothelial cell proliferation, migration, and PA-mediated extracellular proteolysis. In none of these situations was the effect of simultaneous addition of bFGF and VEGF greater than additive (71–73). However, we, and others, have detected a syner-

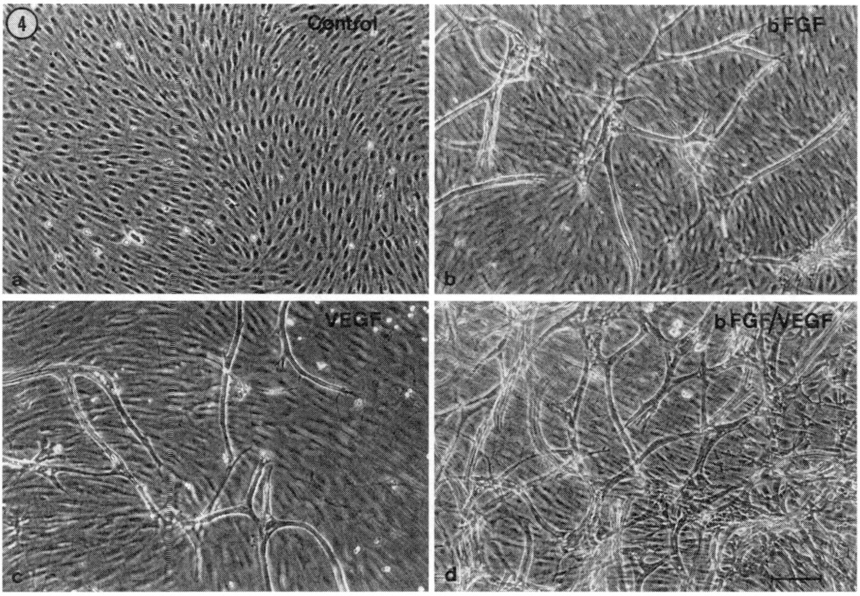

Figure 4 Synergistic effect of coadded bFGF and VEGF on angiogenesis in vitro. **a**. Endothelial cells are grown on the surface of a three-dimensional collagen gel as described in Figure 2. Under these conditions, the cells do not invade the underlying matrix (control). When treated with bFGF (10 ng/ml) **(b)** or VEGF (30 ng/ml) **(c)** for 4 days, the cells invade the underlying matrix and form branching cell cords within the gel. When coadded **(d)**, bFGF and VEGF induce an invasive response that is greater than additive. Bar = 100 μm. *Abbreviations: bFGF*, basic fibroblast growth factor; *VEGF*, vascular endothelial growth factor.

gistic effect of bFGF and VEGF on endothelial proliferation when the cells are grown in a three-dimensional ECM (74; M.S. Pepper et al., unpublished data). Our subsequent approach has been to determine whether bFGF and VEGF might modulate expression of receptors for FGF and VEGF in monolayer culture. We have found that although neither cytokine, either alone or in combination, is capable of modulating expression of FGF receptor-1, bFGF increases expression of VEGF receptor-2 (VEGFR-2 or Flk-1) in bovine endothelial cells (75).

What are the implications of these findings? Modulation of new capillary blood vessel formation may serve as an alternative/adjunct to current therapeutic modalities in several angiogenesis-associated diseases (76). At first sight, the redundancy of angiogenesis-regulating cytokines might suggest that therapeutic strategies based on neutralization of single angiogenic factors might be unrealis-

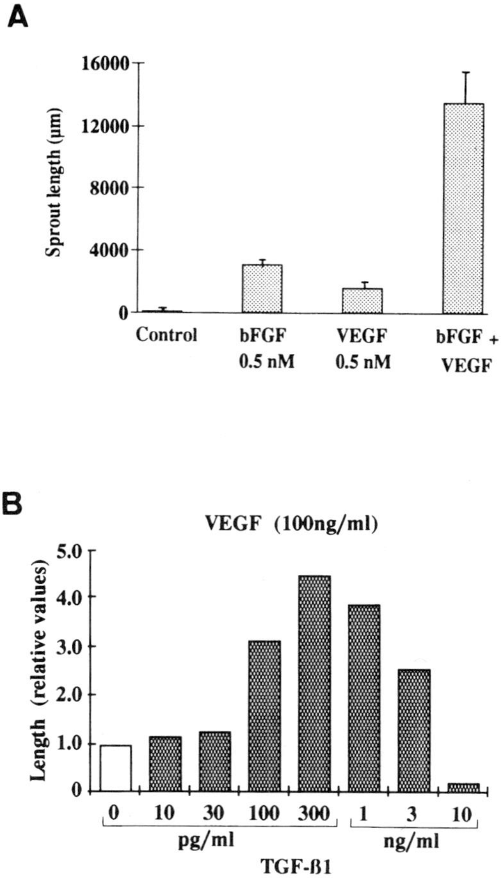

Figure 5 Interactions between angiogenesis-modulating cytokines. **A**. Quantification of the synergistic effect of bFGF and VEGF on in vitro angiogenesis. Endothelial cell invasion was quantitated by measuring the length of all cell cords that had penetrated beneath the surface monolayer. At equimolar concentrations (0.5 nM), bFGF was about twice as potent as VEGF. Coaddition of the two cytokines induced an invasive response that was greater that additive. **B**. Quantitative analysis of the effect of TGF-β1 on VEGF-induced collagen gel invasion. Confluent monolayers of microvascular endothelial cells were treated for 4 days with both VEGF (100 ng/ml) and TGF-β1, or with VEGF alone, and the length of invading cell cords determined. **(A)** From Biochem Biophys Res Commun 1992; 189:824–831. **(B)** From Exp Cell Res 1993; 204:356–363, by copyright permission of Academic Press. *Abbreviations: bFGF*, basic fibroblast growth factor; *VEGF*, vascular endothelial growth factor; *TGF*, transforming growth factor.

tic. If, however, the synergism we have observed in vitro is relevant to the endogenous regulation of angiogenesis in vitro, angiogenesis would be more prominent in tumors or other pathological settings in which more than one angiogenic factor is produced. This may justify antiangiogenesis strategies based on the neutralization of a single angiogenic factor, as this would reduce the synergistic effect. On the other hand, recent work has demonstrated that administration of angiogenic factors can enhance the growth of collateral vessels in animal models of coronary, peripheral, and cerebral arterial occlusion (77–79). We have suggested that the effect of coaddition of two cytokines whose interaction is synergistic would be greater than that derived from the addition of one of these cytokines alone (55). Support for this hypothesis has recently been provided by an in vivo study in which coadministered bFGF and VEGF synergized in the induction of collateral blood vessel formation in a rabbit model of hind limb ischemia (80). In summary, our findings on the synergism between bFGF and VEGF may have relevance both to understanding the biology of angiogenesis (51) as well as to positive and negative therapeutic modulation of this process. Our observations also highlight the importance of a three-dimensional environment for the study of angiogenesis in vitro: had we relied exclusively on traditional two-dimensional assays of proliferation, migration, or proteolysis, the synergism between bFGF and VEGF would not have been detected.

B. Biphasic Effect of TGF-β1 on In Vitro Angiogenesis

Transforming growth factor-β is an angiogenesis-modulating cytokine that has been described as being pro- or antiangiogenic, depending on the nature of the assay (81). In vivo, TGF-β is a potent inducer of angiogenesis (82, 83), and this effect is believed to be mediated by secretory products of TGF-β-recruited connective tissue and inflammatory cells (83–86). In vitro, however, TGF-β inhibits a number of essential components of the angiogenic process. These include endothelial cell proliferation (87–89), migration (89, 91), and extracellular proteolytic activity (66, 67, 92). Results from three-dimensional in vitro assays demonstrate that the response to TGF-β also varies depending on the assay used. Thus, TGF-β inhibits endothelial cell invasion of three-dimensional collagen gels (89), as well as the invasion of the explanted amnion (93). In addition, as described above, TGF-β at 500 pg/ml reduces lumen size, and at 5 ng/ml completely inhibits lumen formation within three-dimensional fibrin gels (67, 69). These results support the notion that TGF-β is a direct-acting inhibitor of ECM invasion and tube formation. However, it also has been reported that TGF-β promotes organization of endothelial cells into tubelike structures (22, 94). These apparently conflicting results may be reconciled by considering that TGF-β might have different functions on vessel formation at different stages of the angiogenic process (81). When acting directly on endothelial cells, it may inhibit invasion and vessel formation. Once sprout formation has occurred, TGF-β may be necessary for the inhibition of further endothelial cell replication and migration and to induce vessel organization and functional maturation. An additional possibility is that the direct effect of TGF-β on endothelial cell function is concentration dependent, particularly because this cytokine has been described as a bifunctional regulator in a variety of other biological processes (95).

The effect of a wide range of concentrations of TGF-β1 on bFGF- or VEGF-induced angiogenesis was assessed in our three-dimensional in vitro model. We found that in the presence of TGF-β1, bFGF- or VEGF-induced invasion was increased at 200 to 500 pg/ml of TGF-β1 and decreased at 5 to 10 ng/ml of TGF-β1 (Fig. 5B). The inhibitory effect at relatively high concentrations is in accord with previous studies in which endothelial cell invasion of three-dimensional collagen gels (89) or the explanted amnion (93) were inhibited by TGF-β1 at 1 to 10 ng/ml. These results clearly demonstrate that the effect of TGF-β1 on bFGF- or VEGF-induced in vitro angiogenesis is concentration dependent (69).

The mechanisms responsible for the biphasic effect of TGF-β1 are not known. One hypothesis is based on alterations in the net balance of extracellular proteolysis (96). Thus, at the dose of TGF-β1 that potentiates bFGF- or VEGF-induced invasion, an optimal balance between proteases and protease inhibitors may be achieved at the cell surface. This allows for focal pericellular matrix degradation, while at the same time protecting the matrix against excessive degradation and inappropriate destruction (71). However, we also have evidence to suggest that integrin expression is differentially affected at these various concentrations of TGF-β1 (96a). The relative contribution of these parameters, namely proteases and integrins, to the modulation of capillary morphogenesis by TGF-β1 is currently under investigation. To summarize the effects of TGF-β on the angiogenic response, the direct effect of TGF-β on endothelial cells not only varies at different stages of the angiogenic process, but is also concentration dependent. Thus, in addition to its indirect angiogenic effect, TGF-β could either promote or inhibit angiogenesis when acting directly on endothelial cells (81).

To summarize: Using a three-dimensional model of in vitro angiogenesis, we have demonstrated that important interactions exist between different cytokines in the in vitro angiogenic response. Synergism was observed between bFGF and VEGF, and TGF-β1 had a biphasic effect on bFGF- or VEGF-induced invasion. We have also found that leukemia inhibitory factor, oncostatin M, interleukin-6, and interleukin-11, all of which signal through the gp130 signal converter, inhibit bFGF- or VEGF-induced angiogenesis in vitro (97, 51; Pepper et al., unpublished data). These interactions appear to be limited to the cytokines indicated, as a large number of other cytokines we tested in our collagen gel model had no effect on invasion or tube formation, either on their own or in combination with bFGF or VEGF (98). We suggest that the temporally coordinated and concentration-dependent activity of a limited number of cytokines is necessary for the control of different elements of the angiogenic process in specific and appropriate settings in vitro.

VII. SYNERGISTIC EFFECT OF HYALURONAN OLIGOSACCHARIDES AND VEGF ON ANGIOGENESIS IN VITRO

In addition to diffusible cytokines, ECM components including collagens (13, 28), laminin (19, 99) and other glycoproteins (14, 100, 101) have been shown to be important in angiogenesis. Hyaluronan (hyaluronic acid, HA), a glycosaminoglycan composed of repeating disaccharide units of D-glucuronate and N-acetylglucosamine, is one of the most abundant constituents of the ECM. Originally considered primarily as a structural moiety, HA has now emerged as an important signaling molecule (102–104). Hyaluronic acid is involved in a number of developmental processes (105, 106) and has been shown to promote cell proliferation (107), differentiation (108, 109), and motility (110–113). The diverse biological activities of HA are believed to be mediated, at least in part, through interaction with specific cell-surface receptors such as CD44 and RHAMM (114–120) resulting in activation of intracellular signalling events (121, 122). Hyaluronic acid obtained from different tissue sources exhibits considerable variation in size, and its biological activity has been shown to be critically dependent on molecular mass in a number of experimental systems, including angiogenesis (123, 124). Native high-molecular-weight HA is antiangiogenic (125), whereas HA degradation products of specific size (3 to 10 disaccharide units) stimulate endothelial cell proliferation (122, 126, 127) and migration (110, 122, 128), and induce angiogenesis in the chick chorioallantoic membrane assay (129), in rat skin (128), and in a cryoinjured skin graft model (130).

We wished to determine whether HA or its degradation products influence endothelial cell invasion of a three-dimensional ECM. Using our collagen gel assay we found that, like bFGF and VEGF (see above), oligosaccharides of HA (OHA) induce endothelial cells to invade the underlying gel within which they form capillarylike tubes, with an optimal effect at approximately 0.5 to 2 μg/ml OHA (Fig 6a). Strikingly, coaddition of OHA (0.5 to 2 μg/ml) and VEGF (30 ng/ml), but not coaddition of OHA and bFGF (10 ng/ml), induced an in vitro angiogenic response that was greater than the sum of the effects elicited by either agent separately (Fig. 6b, c). In contrast to OHA, native high-molecular-weight HA (nHA) was consistently inactive, either when added alone or in combination with VEGF or bFGF (Fig. 6) (131). Because, as discussed earlier, endothelial

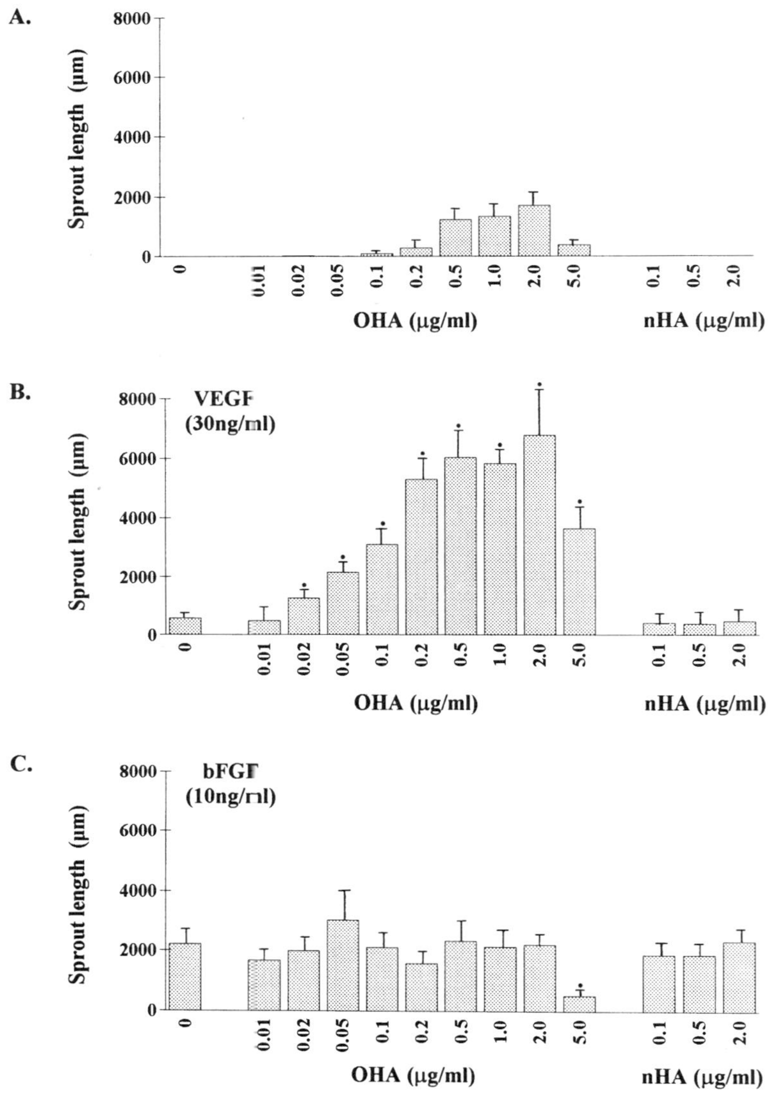

Figure 6 Synergistic effect of OHA and VEGF on angiogenesis in vitro. Confluent monolayers of endothelial cells on collagen gels were treated with OHA or nHA at the indicated concentrations (**A**), cotreated with OHA or nHA and VEGF (**B**), or cotreated with OHA or nHA and bFGF (**C**). Invasion was quantified after 4 days and results are expressed as mean total additive length (in µm) ± s.e.m. of all sprouts that had penetrated beneath the surface monolayer in three randomly selected photographic fields from each of at least three separate experiments per experimental condition. *$P < 0.001$. Oligosaccharides of HA stimulate angiogenesis in vitro in a dose-dependent manner (**A**) and synergize with VEGF (**B**), but not with bFGF (**c**). Native high-molecular-weight hyaluronic acid has no significant effect on invasion, either when added alone (**A**) or in combination

cell invasion is believed to require extracellular proteolytic activity, we also investigated the effect of OHA on the PA/plasmin system. Oligosaccharides of HA (0.01 to 1 μg/ml), but not nHA, induced a dose-dependent increase in mRNA levels of uPA, uPAR and PAI-1 and a parallel increase in the functional activity of uPA and PAI-1, as determined by zymography and reverse zymography, respectively. The effects of OHA on proteolytic activity were additive with those of VEGF but not with those of bFGF, which on its own induced a near-maximal response (131).

The mechanisms by which OHA stimulates endothelial cell invasion of collagen gels and modulate their PA-mediated extracellular proteolytic activity are not known. However, in bovine endothelial cells, OHA recently has been found to induce phosphorylation and activation of mitogen-activated protein (MAP) kinase (122), as well as up-regulation of early response genes such as c-fos, c-jun and jun-B (123), which are known to control the expression of a number of other genes including those of matrix-degrading proteases. Because HA receptors, including a CD44-like transmembrane protein, have been identified in bovine endothelial cells (127, 132–134), it is conceivable that OHA promotes endothelial cell invasion and tube formation by activating intracellular signaling pathways that ultimately result in modulation of pericellular proteolysis. The molecular mechanisms responsible for the specific synergistic interaction between OHA and VEGF in the induction of angiogenesis in vitro are also unknown. Oligosaccharides of HA and VEGF might activate independent but converging intracellular signaling pathways, resulting in a synergistic effect, or OHA might up-regulate expression of high-affinity VEGF receptors such as Flk-1. Alternatively, as has been shown for heparinlike glycosaminoglycans (135–138), OHA may complex with VEGF molecules, thereby increasing ligand half-life or facilitating multivalent VEGF binding and receptor oligomerization.

Although exogenously added OHA promotes angiogenesis in in vitro and in vivo assays, it has not yet been clearly established whether endogenous OHA can act as a physiological regulator of angiogenesis. Several observations suggest the potential involvement of OHA in angiogenesis associated with reparative and pathological processes. In a number of clinical settings, including wound healing, rheumatoid arthritis, vasoproliferative retinopathy, and cancer, angiogenesis occurs in close proximity to HA-rich tissues or fluids (139–145). Hyaluromic acid catabolism has been shown to be very rapid: in skin for instance, up to 25% of injected HA is degraded locally in 24 hours (103). Although most vertebrate hyaluronidases characterized so far are lysosomal, HA-degrading activities with

---

with VEGF or bFGF (**B, C**). From Lab Invest 1996; 75:249–262, by copyright permission of Williams and Wilkins. *Abbreviations: OHA*, oligosaccharides of hyaluronic acid; *VEGF*, vascular endothelial growth factor; *nHA*, native high-molecular-weight hyaluronic acid; *bFGF*, basic fibroblast growth factor.

near-neutral pH optima recently have been shown to be expressed by tumor cells and to induce angiogenesis in vivo (146, 147). It is conceivable that breakdown of high-molecular-weight HA occurs in the extracellular space during pathological processes. This would result in the production of OHA, which in addition to being angiogenic on their own, could synergize with VEGF, which has been shown to be overexpressed in all the clinical settings mentioned above (53, 54). Based on our in vitro studies, we propose that the potential therapeutic effect of coadministration of VEGF and OHA deserves to be investigated in situations that would benefit from stimulation of angiogenesis, particularly in animal models of coronary or peripheral arterial insufficiency.

VIII. THE COLLAGEN GEL INVASION SYSTEM AS A BIOASSAY FOR THE IDENTIFICATION OF ADDITIONAL REGULATORS OF ANGIOGENESIS

In addition to its use as an experimental system for investigating the mechanisms of angiogenesis, the collagen gel invasion model provides a convenient alternative to widely used endothelial cell proliferation assays for the identification of positive and negative regulators of angiogenesis (98). Endothelial cell proliferation represents only one component of the angiogenic process. In contrast, collagen gel invasion assays rely on the detection of biological activities that induce both endothelial cell proliferation and migration into a three-dimensional ECM substratum, as well as morphogenesis of capillary tubes, all of which are essential components of the angiogenic process. The use of the collagen gel invasion system as a bioassay is exemplified by the coculture experiments described below.

In an attempt to identify additional regulators of angiogenesis, we have developed a coculture system that allows the study of paracrine interactions between microvascular endothelial cells and other types of normal or tumoral cells. In this assay, cells that potentially may produce angiogenic factors are suspended within a collagen gel and overlaid with an additional collagen gel devoid of cells, onto which endothelial cells are subsequently seeded and grown to confluence. Among the cell types we have cocultured with endothelial cells in this experimental system, Swiss mouse embryo 3T3 fibroblasts induced a robust in vitro angiogenic response. When microvascular or large vessel endothelial cells grown on the upper cell-free collagen gel layer attained confluence, numerous cell cords began to extend from the surface monolayer into the underlying collagen matrix. Over the next few days of coculture, these cords elongated, branched progressively, and developed patent lumina (148). Extensive radial outgrowth of endothelial sprouts was also observed in a second coculture model in which a collagen disc containing a suspension of endothelial cells was surrounded by an annular collagen gel containing Swiss 3T3 cells. Conditioned medium from Swiss 3T3 cells mimicked the effect of coculture by inducing endothelial cell invasion and tube formation and increased endothelial cell uPA activity (148). The nature of the factor(s) produced by Swiss 3T3 cells that induces angiogenesis in vitro has not yet been determined, but available evidence suggests that it is likely to be different from a number of well-characterized angiogenic cytokines.

In addition to representing a convenient assay for the detection of positive regulators of angiogenesis in conditioned media, the collagen gel invasion model also can be exploited in the search of new agents, either pharmacological or physiological, which inhibit angiogenesis. Thus, Fotsis et al. (149) have demonstrated that genistein, an isoflavonoid present in high concentrations in the urine of subjects consuming a diet rich in soya, is a potent inhibitor of bFGF-induced angiogenesis in our three-dimensional in vitro model (Table 2). The same investigators have also identified an endogenous estrogen metabolite in human urine, namely 2-methoxyestradiol, which is a potent inhibitor of bFGF-induced tubule formation in collagen gels (Table 2) and of tumor neovascularization in vivo (150).

IX. POTENTIAL CLINICAL IMPLICATIONS OF IN VITRO STUDIES OF ANGIOGENESIS

Because angiogenesis plays an important role in a wide range of physiological and pathological processes, its modulation provides a useful alternative/adjunct to current therapeutic modalities in several diseases characterized by local hyper- or hypovascularity (76, 79).

Inhibition of angiogenesis has long been recognized as a potential strategy for cancer treatment (151). Although angiogenesis is required for the growth of solid tumors beyond 1 to 2 mm^3, under physiological conditions it is only required for wound healing and reproductive functions. Complete inhibition of angiogenesis should be well tolerated by most adults. Inhibition of angiogenesis also is of potential benefit in the treatment of ocular neovascularization (e.g., diabetic proliferative retinopathy) and of life-threatening hemangiomas. The redundancy of angiogenesis-stimulating cytokines may hinder therapeutic strategies based on neutralization of angiogenic factors. Because sprouting endothelial cells must invade and translocate across the ECM regardless of the nature of the angiogenic stimulus, targeting cellular processes such as extracellular proteolysis may overcome the problems of growth factor redundancy. We believe that a better understanding of the factors that regulate the invasive and proteolytic properties of endothelial cells may facilitate the design of angiostatic agents capable of inhibiting inappropriate blood vessel growth in a variety of clinical settings. Identification of additional inhibitors of angiogenesis is potentially of great importance, because different antiangiogenic agents may act through diverse mechanisms and may achieve a maximum therapeutic effect when administered in appropriate combinations.

Stimulation of angiogenesis, on the other hand, has been shown to accelerate the healing of wounds and peptic ulcers and to promote growth of collateral vessels in ischemic diseases. Recent work has demonstrated that administration of angiogenic factors can enhance the growth of collateral vessels in animal models of myocardial, peripheral, and cerebral arterial insufficiency (77, 78). We are confident that the use of in vitro systems will contribute to the development of appropriate therapeutic strategies by allowing for the identification of additional physiological stimulators of angiogenesis and of other examples of synergistic interactions, such as those we have previously shown for the combination of bFGF and VEGF (55) and of OHA and VEGF (131). Evidence from recent in vivo studies (80) suggests that in situations in which stimulation of angiogenesis is desired, the benefit derived from coaddition of two agents whose interaction is synergistic would be greater than that derived from the addition of only one of these agents.

ACKNOWLEDGMENTS

We would like to thank Dr. J.-D. Vassalli for his important contributions to our work, and Dr. L. Orci for continued support, advice, and constructive criticism. We are also grateful to J. Rial-Robert, C. Di Sanza, and M. Quayzin for excellent technical assistance and to F. Hellal for preparing the manuscript. We apologize for not having cited our many colleagues who have provided the cytokines and other potential regulators listed in Tables 1 and 2 and wish to acknowledge their invaluable contributions. Work performed in the authors' laboratory has been supported by the Swiss National Science Foundation, the Juvenile Diabetes Foundation International, and the Sir Jules Thorn Charitable Overseas Trust.

REFERENCES

1. Ausprunk DH, Folkman J. Migration and proliferation of endothelial cells in preformed and newly formed blood vessels during angiogenesis. Microvasc Res 1977; 14:53–65.
2. Folkman J, Klagsbrun M. Angiogenic factors. Science 1987; 235:442–447.
3. Paku S, Paweletz N. First steps of tumor-related angiogenesis. Lab Invest 1991; 65:334–346.
4. Folkman J, Shing Y. Angiogenesis. J Biol Chem 1992; 267:10931–10934.
5. Klagsbrun M, Knighton D, Folkman J. Tumor angiogenesis activity in cells grown in tissue culture. Cancer Res 1976; 36:110–114.
6. Gimbrone MA Jr, Cotran RS, Leapman SB, Folkman J. Tumor growth and neovas-

cularization: An experimental model using the rabbit cornea. J Natl Cancer Inst 1974; 52:413–427.
7. Andrade SP, Fan T-PD, Lewis GP. Quantitative in-vivo studies on angiogenesis in a rat sponge model. Br J Exp Pathol 1987; 68:755–766.
8. Fajardo LF, Kowalski J, Kwan HH, Prionas SD, Allison AC. The disc angiogenesis system. Lab Invest 1988; 58:718–724.
9. Passaniti A, Taylor RM, Pili R, Guo Y, Long PV, Haney JA, Pauly RR, Grant DS, Martin GR. A simple, quantitative method for assessing angiogenesis and antiangiogenic agents using reconstituted basement membrane, heparin, and fibroblast growth factor. Lab Invest 1992; 67:519–528.
10. Moscatelli D, Presta M, Rifkin DB. Purification of a factor from human placenta that stimulates capillary endothelial cell protease production, DNA synthesis and migration. Proc Natl Acad Sci U S A 1986; 83:2091–2095.
11. Folkman J, Haudenschild C. Angiogenesis in vitro. Nature 1980; 288:551–555.
12. Maciag T, Kadish J, Wilkins L, Stemerman MB, Weinstein R. Organizational behavior of human umbilical vein endothelial cells. J Cell Biol 1982; 94:511–520.
13. Madri JA, Williams SK. Capillary endothelial cell cultures: Phenotypic modulation by matrix components. J Cell Biol 1983; 97:153–165.
14. Ingber DE, Folkman J. Mechano-chemical switching between growth and differentiation during growth factor-stimulated angiogenesis in vitro: Role of the extracellular matrix. J Cell Biol 1989; 109:317–330.
15. Iruela-Arispe M, Hasselaar P, Sage H. Differential expression of extracellular proteins is correlated with angiogenesis in vitro. Lab Invest 1991; 64:174–186.
16. Iruela-Arispe ML, Sage EH. Endothelial cells exhibiting angiogenesis in vitro proliferate in response to TGF-β1. J Cell Biochem 1993; 52:414–430.
17. Battegay EJ, Rupp J, Iruela-Arispe L, Sage EH, Pech M. PDGF-BB modulates endothelial proliferation and angiogenesis in vitro via PDGFβ-receptors. J Cell Biol 1994; 125:917–928.
18. Kubota Y, Kleinman HK, Martin GR, Lawley TJ. Role of laminin and basement membrane in the morphological differentiation of human endothelial cells into capillary-like structures. J Cell Biol 1988; 107:1589–1598.
19. Grant DS, Tashiro KI, Segui-Real B, Yamada Y, Martin GR, Kleinman HK. Two different laminin domains mediate the differentiation of human endothelial cells into capillary-like structures in vitro. Cell 1989; 58:933–943.
20. Vernon RB, Sage EH. Between molecules and morphology: Extracellular matrix and creation of vascular form. Am J Pathol 1995; 147:873–883.
21. Vernon RB, Lara SL, Drake CJ, Iruela-Arispe ML, Angello JC, Little CD, Wight TN, Sage EH. Organized type I collagen influences endothelial patterns during "spontaneous angiogenesis in vitro": Planar cultures as models of vascular development. In Vitro Cell Dev Biol 1995; 31:120–131.
22. Madri JA, Pratt BM, Tucker AM. Phenotypic modulation of endothelial cells by transforming growth factor-β depends on the composition and organization of the extracellular matrix. J Cell Biol 1988; 106:1357–1384.
23. Nicosia RF, Ottinetti A. Growth of microvessels in serum-free matrix culture of rat aorta. Lab Invest 1990; 63:115–122.
24. Hoying JB, Boswell CA, Williams SK. Angiogenic potential of microvessel frag-

ments established in three-dimensional collagen gels. In Vitro Cell Dev Biol 1996; 32:409–419.

25. Brown KJ, Maynes SF, Bezos A, Maguire DJ, Ford MD, Parish CR. A novel in vitro assay for human angiogenesis. Lab Invest 1996; 75:539–555.
26. Nehls V, Drenckhahn D. A novel, microcarrier-based in vitro assay for rapid and reliable quantification of three-dimensional cell migration and angiogenesis. Microvasc Res 1995; 50:311–322.
27. Madri JA, Pratt BM. Angiogenesis. In: Clark RAF, Henson PM, eds. The Molecular and Cellular Biology of Wound Repair. New York: Plenum Press, 1988:337–358.
28. Montesano R, Orci L, Vassalli P. In vitro rapid organization of endothelial cells into capillary-like networks is promoted by collagen matrices. J Cell Biol 1983; 97:1648–1652.
29. Alexander CA, Werb Z. Extracellular matrix degradation. In: Hay ED, ed. Cell Biology of Extracellular Matrix. 2d ed. New York: Plenum Press, 1991:255–302.
30. Liotta LA, Steeg PS, Stetler-Stevenson WG. Cancer metastasis and angiogenesis: An imbalance of positive and negative regulation. Cell 1991; 64:327–366.
31. Mignatti P, Rifkin DB. Plasminogen activators and angiogenesis. In: Günthert U, Birchmeier W, eds. Current Topics in Microbiology and Immunology. Vol. 213-I: Attempts to Understand Metastasis Formation. Berlin and Heidelberg: Springer Verlag, 1996:31–49.
32. Pepper MS, Montesano R, Mandriota SJ, Orci L, Vassalli J-D. Angiogenesis: A paradigm for balanced extracellular proteolysis during cell migration and morphogenesis. Enzyme Protein 1996; 49:138–162.
33. Vassalli J-D, Sappino A-P, Belin D. The plasminogen activator/plasmin system. J Clin Invest 1991; 88:1067–1072.
34. Gross JL, Moscatelli D, Jaffe EA, Rifkin DB. Plasminogen activator and collagenase production by cultured capillary endothelial cells. J Cell Biol 1982; 95:974–981.
35. Montesano R, Orci L. Tumor-promoting phorbol esters induce angiogenesis in vitro. Cell 1985; 42:469–477.
36. Montesano R, Orci L. Phorbol esters induce angiogenesis in vitro from large vessel endothelial cells. J Cell Physiol 1987; 130:284–291.
37. Fisher C, Gilberston-Beadling S, Powers EA, Petzold G, Poorman R, Mitchell MA. Interstitial collagenase is required for angiogenesis in vitro. Dev Biol 1994; 162: 499–510.
38. Anand-Apte B, Pepper MS, Voest E, Montesano R, Olsen B, Murphy G, Apte SS, Zetter B. Inhibition of angiogenesis by tissue inhibitor of metalloproteinase-3 (TIMP-3). Invest Ophtalmol Vis Sci 1997; 38:817–823.
39. Leibovich SJ, Polverini J, Shepard HM, Wiseman DM, Shively V, Nuseir N. Macrophage-induced angiogenesis is mediated by tumour necrosis factor-α. Nature 1987; 329:630–632.
40. Yasunaga C, Nakashima Y, Sueishi K. A role of fibrinolytic activity in angiogenesis. Quantitative assay using in vitro method. Lab Invest 1989; 61:698–704.
41. Mawatari M, Okamura K, Matsuda T, Hamanaka R, Mizoguchi H, Higashio K, Kohno K, Kuwano M. Tumor necrosis factor and epidermal growth factor modulate

migration of human microvascular endothelial cells and production of tissue-type plasminogen activator and its inhibitor. Exp Cell Res 1991; 192:574–580.
42. Gajdusek CM, Luo Z, Mayberg MR. Basic fibroblast growth factor and transforming growth factor beta-1: Synergistic mediators of angiogenesis in vitro. J Cell Physiol 1993; 157:133–144.
43. Sato Y, Okamura K, Morimoto A, Hamanaka R, Hamaguchi K, Shimada T, Ono M, Kohno K, Sakata T, Kuwano M. Indispensable role of tissue-type plasminogen activator in growth factor-dependent tube formation of human microvascular endothelial cells in vitro. Exp Cell Res 1993; 204:223–229.
44. Laaroubi K, Delbé J, Vacherot P, Desgranges P, Tardieu M, Jaye M, Barritault D, Courty J. Mitogenic and in vitro angiogenic activity of human recombinant heparin affin regulatory peptide. Growth Factors 1994; 10:89–98.
45. Wang D-Y, Kao C-H, Yang VC, Chen J-K. Glycosaminoglycans enhance phorbol ester-induced proteolytic activity and angiogenesis in vitro. In Vitro Cell Dev Biol 1994; 30A:777–782.
46. Deroanne CF, Colige AC, Nusgens BV, Lapiere CM. Modulation of expression and assembly of vinculin during in vitro fibrillar collagen-induced angiogenesis and its reversal. Exp Cell Res 1996; 224:215–223.
47. Okamura K, Morimoto A, Hamanaka R, Ono M, Kohno K, Uchida Y, Kuwano M. A model system for tumor angiogenesis: Involvement of transforming growth factor-α in tube formation of human microvascular endothelial cells induced by esophageal cancer cells. Biochem Biophys Res Commun 1992; 186:1471–1479.
48. Sakuda H, Nakashima Y, Kuriyama S, Sueishi K. Media conditioned by smooth muscle cells cultured in a variety of hypoxic environments stimulates in vitro angiogenesis. A relationship to transforming growth factor-β1. Am J Pathol 1992; 141: 1507–1516.
49. Baird A, Klagsbrun M. The fibroblast growth factor family. Cancer Cells 1991; 3: 239–243.
50. Basilico C, Moscatelli D. The FGF family of growth factors and oncogenes. Adv Cancer Res 1992; 59:115–165.
51. Pepper MS, Mandriota SJ, Vassalli J-D, Orci L, Montesano R. Angiogenesis-regulating cytokines: Activities and interactions. In: Günthert U, Birchmeier W, eds. Current Topics in Microbiology and Immunology. Vol. 213-II: Attempts to Understand Metastasis Formation. Berlin and Heidelberg: Springer-Verlag, 1996:31–67.
52. Montesano R, Vassalli J-D, Baird A, Guillemin R, Orci L. Basic fibroblast growth factor induces angiogenesis in vitro. Proc Natl Acad Sci U S A 1986; 83:7297–7301.
53. Ferrara N. The role of vascular endothelial growth factor in pathological angiogenesis. Breast Cancer Res Treat 1995; 36:127–137.
54. Dvorak HF, Brown LF, Detmar M, Dvorak AM. Vascular permeability factor/vascular endothelial growth factor, microvascular hyperpermeability and angiogenesis. Am J Pathol 1995; 146:1029–1039.
55. Pepper MS, Ferrara N, Orci L, Montesano R. Potent synergism between vascular endothelial growth factor and basic fibroblast growth factor in the induction of angiogenesis in vitro. Biochem Biophys Res Commun 1992; 189:824–831.
56. Bikfalvi A, Sauzeau C, Moukadiri H, Maclouf J, Busso N, Bryckaert M, Plouet J,

Tobelem G. Interaction of vasculotropin/vascular endothelial growth factor with human umbilical vein endothelial cells: Binding, internalization, and biological effects. J Cell Physiol 1991; 149:50–59.

57. Pepper MS, Ferrara N, Orci L, Montesano R. Vascular endothelial growth factor (VEGF) induces plasminogen activators and plasminogen activator inhibitor-1 in microvascular endothelial cells. Biochem Biophys Res Commun 1991; 181:902–906.
58. Pepper MS, Vassalli J-D, Montesano R, Orci L. Urokinase-type plasminogen activator is induced in migrating capillary endothelial cells. J Cell Biol 1987; 105: 2535–2541.
59. Pepper MS, Sappino A-P, Stocklin R, Montesano R, Orci L, Vassalli J-D. Upregulation of urokinase receptor expression on migrating endothelial cells. J Cell Biol 1993; 122:673–684.
60. Montesano R, Pepper MS, Vassalli J-D, Orci L. Phorbol ester induces cultured endothelial cells to invade a fibrin matrix in the presence of fibrinolytic inhibitors. J Cell Physiol 1987; 132:509–516.
61. Bautch VL, Toda S, Hassell JA, Hanahan D. Endothelial cell tumors develop in transgenic mice carrying polyoma virus middle T oncogene. Cell 1987; 51:529–538.
62. Williams RL, Risau W, Zerwes HG, Drexler H, Aguzzi A, Wagner EF. Endothelioma cells expressing the polyoma middle T oncogene induce hemangiomas by host cell recruitment. Cell 1989; 57:1053–1063.
63. Pepper MS, Tacchini-Cottier F, Sabapathy TK, Montesano R, Wagner EF. Endothelial cells transformed by polyoma virus middle-T oncogene: A model for hemangiomas and other vascular tumors. In: Lewis CE, Bicknell R, Ferrara N, eds. Tumor Angiogenesis. Oxford: Oxford University Press, 1997:310–331.
64. Montesano R, Pepper MS, Möhle-Steinlein U, Risau W, Wagner EF, Orci L. Increased proteolytic activity is responsible for the aberrant morphogenetic behavior of endothelial cells expressing the middle T oncogene. Cell 1990; 62:435–445.
65. Montesano R, Pepper MS, Belin D, Vassalli J-D, Orci L. Induction of angiogenesis in vitro by vanadate, an inhibitor of phosphotyrosine phosphatases. J Cell Physiol 1988; 134:460–466.
66. Saksela O, Moscatelli D, Rifkin DB. The opposing effects of basic fibroblast growth factor and transforming growth factor beta on the regulation of plasminogen activator activity in capillary endothelial cells. J Cell Biol 1987; 105:957–963.
67. Pepper MS, Belin D, Montesano R, Orci L, Vassalli J-D. Transforming growth factor-beta 1 modulates basic fibroblast growth factor-induced proteolytic and angiogenic properties of endothelial cells in vitro. J Cell Biol 1990; 111:743–755.
68. Pepper MS, Sappino A-P, Montesano R, Orci L, Vassalli J-D. Plasminogen activator inhibitor-1 is induced in migrating endothelial cells. J Cell Physiol 1992; 153: 129–139.
69. Pepper MS, Vassalli J-D, Orci L, Montesano R. Biphasic effect of transforming growth factor-beta-1 on in vitro angiogenesis. Exp Cell Res 1993; 204:356–363.
70. Pepper MS, Montesano R, Vassalli J-D, Orci L. Chondrocytes inhibit endothelial sprout formation in vitro: Evidence for the involvement of a transforming growth factor-beta. J Cell Physiol 1991; 146:170–179.

71. Pepper MS, Vassalli J-D, Orci L, Montesano R. Angiogenesis in vitro: Cytokine interactions and balanced extracellular proteolysis. In: Maragoudakis ME, Gullino PM, Lelkes PI, eds. Angiogenesis. Molecular Biology, Clinical Aspects. New York: Plenum Press, 1994:149–170.
72. Mandriota SJ, Seghezzi G, Vassalli J-D, Ferrara N, Wasi S, Mazzieri R, Mignatti P, Pepper MS. Vascular endothelial growth factor increases urokinase receptor expression in vascular endothelial cells. J Biol Chem 1995; 270:9709–9716.
73. Yoshida A, Anand-Apte B, Zetter BR. Differential endothelial migration and proliferation to basic fibroblast growth factor and vascular endothelial growth factor. Growth Factors 1996; 13:57–64.
74. Goto M, Goto K, Weindel K, Folkman J. Synergistic effects of vascular endothelial growth factor and basic fibroblast growth factor on the proliferation and cord formation of bovine capillary endothelial cells within collagen gels. Lab Invest 1993; 69:508–517.
75. Pepper MS, Mandriota SJ. Regulation of vascular endothelial growth factor receptor-2 (Flk-1) expression in vascular endothelial cells. Exp Cell Res 1998; 241:414–425.
76. Pepper MS. Positive and negative regulation of angiogenesis: From cell biology to the clinic. Vasc Med, 1996:259–266.
77. Höckel M, Schlenger K, Doctrow S, Kissel T, Vaupel P. Therapeutic angiogenesis. Arch Surg 1993; 128:423–429.
78. Symes JF, Sniderman AD. Angiogenesis: Potential therapy for ischaemic disease. Curr Opin Lipidol 1994; 5:305–312.
79. Folkman J. Clinical applications of research on angiogenesis. N Engl J Med 1995; 333:1757–1763.
80. Asahara T, Bauters C, Zheng LP, Takeshita S, Bunting S, Ferrara N, Symes JF, Isner J-M. Synergistic effects of vascular endothelial growth factor and basic fibroblast growth factor on angiogenesis in vivo. Circulation 1995; 92 (suppl II):II-365–II-371.
81. Pepper MS. Transforming growth factor-beta: Vasculogenesis, angiogenesis and vessel wall integrity. Cytokine Growth Factor Rev, 1997:21–43.
82. Roberts AB, Sporn MB, Assoian RK, Smith JM, Roche NS, Wakefield LM, Heine UI, Liotta LA, Falanga V, Kehrl JH, Fauci AS. Transforming growth factor type β: Rapid induction of fibrosis and angiogenesis in vivo and stimulation of collagen formation in vitro. Proc Natl Acad Sci U S A 1986; 83:4167–4171.
83. Yang EY, Moses HL. Transforming growth factor β1-induced changes in cell migration, proliferation, and angiogenesis in the chicken chorioallantoic membrane. J Cell Biol 1990; 111:731–741.
84. Wahl SM, Hunt DA, Wakefield LA, McCartney-Francis N, Wahl LM, Roberts AB, Sporn MB. Transforming growth factor type β induces monocyte chemotaxis and growth factor production. Proc Natl Acad Sci U S A 1987; 84:5788–5792.
85. Wiseman DM, Polverini PJ, Kamp DW, Leibovich SJ. Transforming growth factor beta (TGFβ) is chemotactic for human monocytes and induces their expression of angiogenic activity. Biochem Biophys Res Commun 1988; 157:793–800.
86. Phillips GD, Whitehead RA, Knighton DR. Inhibition by methylprednisolone acetate suggests an indirect mechanism for TGF-β induced angiogenesis. Growth Factors 1992; 6:77–84.

87. Baird A, Durkin T. Inhibition of endothelial cell proliferation by type β-transforming growth factor: Interactions with acidic and basic fibroblast growth factors. Biochem Biophys Res Commun 1986; 138:476–482.
88. Fràter-Schröder M, Müller G, Birchmeier W, Böhlen P. Transforming growth factor-beta inhibits endothelial cell proliferation. Biochem Biophys Res Commun 1986; 137:295–302.
89. Müller G, Behrens J, Nussbaumer U, Böhlen P, Birchmeier W. Inhibitory action of transforming growth factor-β on endothelial cells. Proc Natl Acad Sci U S A 1987; 84:5600–5604.
90. Heimark RL, Twardzik DR, Schwartz SM. Inhibition of endothelial regeneration by type-beta transforming growth factor from platelets. Science 1986; 233:1078–1080.
91. Sato Y, Rifkin DB. Autocrine activities of basic fibroblast growth factor: Regulation of endothelial cell movement, plasminogen activator synthesis, and DNA synthesis. J Cell Biol 1988; 107:119–1205.
92. Pepper MS, Montesano R, Orci L, Vassalli J-D. Plasminogen activator-inhibitor-1 is induced in microvascular endothelial cells by a chondrocyte-derived transforming growth factor-beta. Biochem Biophys Res Commun 1991; 176:633–638.
93. Mignatti P, Tsuboi R, Robbins E, Rifkin DB. In vitro angiogenesis on the human amniotic membrane: Requirements for basic fibroblast growth factor-induced proteases. J Cell Biol 1989; 108:671–682.
94. Merwin JR, Anderson JM, Kocher O, van Itallie CM, Madri JA. Transforming growth factor-β1 modulates extracellular matrix organization and cell-cell junctional complex formation during in vitro angiogenesis. J Cell Physiol 1990; 142: 117–128.
95. Nathan C, Sporn M. Cytokines in context. J Cell Biol 1991; 113:981–986.
96. Pepper MS, Montesano R. Proteolytic balance and capillary morphogenesis. Cell Diff Dev 1990; 32:319–328.
96a. Collo G, Pepper MS. Endothelial cell integrin α5β1 expression is modulated by cytokines and during migration in vitro. J Cell Sci 1999; 112:569–578.
97. Pepper MS, Ferrara N, Orci L, Montesano R. Leukemia inhibitory factor (LIF) is a potent inhibitor of in vitro angiogenesis. J Cell Sci 1995; 108:73–83.
98. Montesano R, Pepper MS. Three-dimensional in vitro assay of endothelial cell invasion and capillary tube morphogenesis. In: Little CD, Mironov V, Sage EH, eds. Vascular Morphogenesis. Boston: Birkaüser Verlag, 1998:79–110.
99. Nicosia RF, Bonanno E, Smith M, Yurchenco P. Modulation of angiogenesis in vitro by laminin-entactin complex. Dev Biol 1994; 164:197–206.
100. Lane TF, Iruela-Arispe ML, Johnson RS, Sage EH. SPARC is a source of copper-binding peptides that stimulate angiogenesis. J Cell Biol 1994; 125:929–943.
101. Canfield AE, Schor AM. Evidence that tenascin and thrombospondin-1 modulate sprouting of endothelial cells. J Cell Sci 1995; 108:797–809.
102. Toole BP. Hyaluronan and its binding proteins, the hyaladherins. Curr Opin Cell Biol 1990; 2:839–844.
103. Laurent TC, Fraser JRE. Hyaluronan. FASEB J 1992; 6:2397–2404.
104. Knudson CB, Knudson W. Hyaluronan-binding proteins in development, tissue homeostasis, and disease. FASEB J 1993; 7:1233–1241.

105. Toole BP. Proteoglycans and hyaluronan in morphogenesis and differentiation. In: Hay ED, ed. Cell Biology of Extracellular Matrix. 2d ed. New York: Plenum Press, 1991:305–341.
106. Fenderson BA, Stamenkovic I, Aruffo A. Localization of hyaluronan in mouse embryos during implantation, gastrulation and organogenesis. Differentiation 1993; 54:85–98.
107. Yoneda M, Yamagata M, Sakaru S, Kimata K. Hyaluronic acid modulates proliferation of mouse dermal fibroblasts in culture. J Cell Sci 1988; 90:265–273.
108. Kujawa MJ, Carrino DA, Caplan AI. Substrate-bonded hyaluronic acid exhibits a size-dependent stimulation of chondrogenic differentiation of stage 24 limb mesenchymal cells in culture. Dev Biol 1986; 144:519–528.
109. Kujawa M, Pechak DG, Fiszman MY, Caplan AI. Hyaluronic acid bonded to cell culture surfaces inhibits the program of myogenesis. Dev Biol 1986; 113:10–16.
110. West DC, Kumar S. Endothelial cell proliferation and diabetic retinopathy. Lancet 1988; 1:715–716.
111. Boudreau N, Turley EA, Rabinovitch M. Fibronectin, hyaluronan and hyaluronan binding protein contribute to increased ductus arteriosus smooth muscle cell migration. Dev Biol 1991; 143:235–247.
112. Turley EA, Austen L, Vandeligt K, Clary C. Hyaluronan and a cell-associated hyaluronan binding protein regulate the locomotion of Ras-transformed cells. J Cell Biol 1991; 112:1041–1047.
113. Savani RC, Wang C, Yang B, Zhang S, Kinsella MG, Wight TN, Stern R, Nance DM, Turley EA. Migration of bovine aortic smooth muscle cells after wounding injury. The role of hyaluronan and RHAMM. J Clin Invest 1995; 95:1158–1168.
114. Aruffo A, Stamenkovic I, Mulnick M, Underhill CB, Seed B. CD44 is the principal cell surface receptor for hyaluronate. Cell 1990; 61:1303–1313.
115. Culty M, Miyake K, Kincaide PW, Silorski E, Butcher E, Underhill AM. The hyaluronate receptor is a member of the CD44 (H-CAM) family of cell surface glycoproteins. J Cell Biol 1990; 111:2765–2774.
116. Miyake K, Underhill CB, Lesley J, Kincaide PW. Hyaluronate can function as a cell adhesion molecule and CD44 participates in hyaluronate recognition. J Exp Med 1990; 172:69–75.
117. Stamenkovic I, Aruffo A, Amiot M, Seed B. The hematopoietic and epithelial forms of CD44 are distinct polypeptides with different adhesion potentials for hyaluronate-bearing cells. EMBO J 1991; 10:343–348.
118. Banerjee SD, Toole BP. Monoclonal antibody to chick embryo hyaluronan-binding protein: Changes in distribution of binding during early brain development. Dev Biol 1991; 146:186–197.
119. Hardwick C, Hoare K, Owens R, Hohn HP, Hook M, Moore D, Cripps V, Austen L, Nance DM, Turley EA. Molecular cloning of a novel hyaluronan receptor that mediates tumor cell motility. J Cell Biol 1992; 117:1343–1350.
120. Sherman L, Sleeman J, Herrlich P, Ponta H. Hyaluronate receptors: Key players in growth, differentiation, migration and tumor progression. Curr Opin Cell Biol 1994; 6:726–733.
121. Hall CL, Wang C, Lange LA, Turley EA. Hyaluronan and the hyaluronan receptor

RHAMM promote focal adhesion turnover and transient tyrosine kinase activity. J Cell Biol 1994; 126:575–588.
122. Slevin M, Krupinski J, Kumar S, Gaffney J. Angiogenic oligosaccharides of hyaluronan induce protein tyrosine kinase activity in endothelial cells and activate a cytoplasmic signal transduction pathway resulting in proliferation. Lab Invest 1988; 78:987–1003.
123. Rooney P, Kumar S, Ponting J, Wang M. The role of hyaluronan in tumor neovascularization. Int J Cancer 1995; 60:632–636.
124. Rooney P, Kumar P, Ponting J, Kumar S. The role of collagens and proteoglycans in tumor angiogenesis. In: Bicknell R, Lewis CE, Ferrara N, eds. Tumor Angiogenesis. Oxford: Oxford University Press, 1997. In press.
125. Feinberg RN, Beebe DL. Hyaluronate in vasculogenesis. Science 1983; 220:1177–1179.
126. West DC, Kumar S. The effects of hyaluronate and its oligosaccharides on endothelial cell proliferation and monolayer integrity. Exp Cell Res 1989; 183:179–196.
127. Sattar A, Kumar S, West DC. Does hyaluronan have a role in endothelial cell proliferation of the synovium? Semin Arthritis Rheum 1992; 22:37–43.
128. Sattar A, Rooney P, Kumar S, Pye D, West DC, Scott I, Ledger P. Application of angiogenic oligosaccharides of hyaluronan increase blood vessel numbers in skin. J Invest Dermatol 1994; 103:573–579.
129. West DC, Hampson IN, Arnold F, Kumar S. Angiogenesis induced by degradation products of hyaluronic acid. Science 1985; 228:1324–1326.
130. Lees VC, Fan T-PD, West DC. Angiogenesis in a delayed revascularization model is accelerated by angiogenic oligosaccharides of hyaluronan. Lab Invest 1995; 73: 259–266.
131. Montesano R, Kumar S, Orci L, Pepper MS. Synergistic effect of hyaluronan oligosaccharides and vascular endothelial growth factor on angiogenesis in vitro. Lab Invest 1996; 75:249–262.
132. Bourguignon LYW, Lokeshwar VB, He J, Chen X, Bourguignon GJ. A CD44-like endothelial cell transmembrane glycoprotein (GP 116) interacts with extracellular matrix and ankyrin. Mol Cell Biol 1992; 12:4464–4471.
133. Banerjee SD, Toole BP. Hyaluronan-binding protein in endothelial cell morphogenesis. J Cell Biol 1992; 119:643–652.
134. Lokeshwar VB, Iida N, Bourguignon LYW. The cell adhesion molecule, GP 116, is a new CD44 variant (ex14/v10) involved in hyaluronic acid binding and endothelial proliferation. J Biol Chem 1996; 271:23853–23864.
135. Tessler S, Rockwell P, Hicklin D, Cohen T, Levi B-Z, Witte L, Lemischka IR, Neufeld G. Heparin modulates the interaction of $VEGF_{165}$ with soluble and cell associated Flk-1 receptors. J Biol Chem 1994; 269:12456–12461.
136. Schlessinger J, Lax I, Lemmon M. Regulation of growth factor activation by proteoglycans: What is the role of the low affinity receptors? Cell 1995; 83:357–360.
137. Faham S, Hileman RE, Fromm JR, Lindhart RJ, Rees DC. Heparin structure and interactions with basic fibroblast growth factor. Science 1996; 271:1116–1120.
138. Ornitz DM, Herr AB, Nilsson M, Westman J, Svahn C-M, Waksman G. FGF binding and FGF receptor activation by synthetic heparan-derived di- and trisaccharides. Science 1995; 268:432–436.

139. Toole BP, Biswas C, Gross J. Hyaluronate and invasiveness of the rabbit V2 carcinoma. Proc Natl Acad Sci U S A 1979; 76:6199–6203.
140. Turley EA, Tretiak M. Glycosaminoglycans produced by murine melanoma variants in vivo and in vitro. Cancer Res 1985; 45:5098–5105.
141. Iozzo R. Proteoglycans: Structure, function, and role in neoplasia. Lab Invest 1985; 53:373–396.
142. Weigel PH, Fuller GM, LeBoeuf RD. A model for the role of hyaluronic acid and fibrin in the early events during the inflammatory response and wound healing. J Theor Biol 1986; 119:219–234.
143. Knudson W, Biswas C, Li XQ, Nemee RE, Toole BP. The role and regulation of tumor-associated hyaluronan. In: Evered D, Whelau J, eds. The Biology of Hyaluronan. Ciba Foundation Symposium Vol. 143. Chichester: John Wiley and Sons, 1989:150–169.
144. Bertrand P, Girard N, Delpech B, Duval C, D'Anjour J, Dance JP. Hyaluronan (hyaluronic acid) and hyaluronectin in the extracellular matrix of human breast carcinomas. Int J Cancer 1992; 52:1–6.
145. Ponting J, Kumar S, Pye D. Localization of hyaluronan and hyaluronectin in normal and tumour breast tissues. Int J Oncology 1993; 2:889–893.
146. Lokeshwar VB, Lokeshwar BL, Pham HT, Block NL. Association of elevated levels of hyaluronidase, a matrix-degrading enzyme, with prostate cancer progression. Cancer Res 1996; 56:651–657.
147. Liu D, Pearlman E, Diaconu E, Guo K, Mori H, Haqqi T, Markowitz S, Willson G, Sy M-S. Expression of hyaluronidase by tumor cells induces angiogenesis in vivo. Proc Natl Acad Sci U S A 1996; 93:7832–7837.
148. Montesano R, Pepper MS, Orci L. Paracrine induction of angiogenesis in vitro by Swiss 3T3 fibroblasts. J Cell Sci 1993; 105:1013–1024.
149. Fotsis T, Pepper M, Adlercreutz H, Fleischmann G, Hase T, Montesano R, Schweigerer L. Genistein, a dietary-derived inhibitor of in vitro angiogenesis. Proc Natl Acad Sci U S A 1993; 90:2690–2694.
150. Fotsis T, Zhang Y, Pepper MS, Adlercreutz H, Montesano R, Nawroth PP, Schweigerer L. The endogenous oestrogen metabolite 2-methoxyoestradiol inhibits angiogenesis and suppresses tumor growth. Nature 1994; 368:237–239.
151. Folkman J. Tumor angiogenesis: Therapeutic implications. N Engl J Med 1971; 285:1182–1186.
152. Montesano R, Vassalli J-D, Orci L, Pepper MS. The role of growth factors and extracellular matrix in angiogenesis and epithelial morphogenesis. In: Sizonenko PC, Aubert ML, Vassalli J-D, eds. Frontiers in Endocrinology. Vol. 6: Developmental Endocrinology. Rome: Ares-Serono Symposia Publications, 1994:43–66.
153. Pepper MS, Vassalli J-D, Wilks JW, Schweigerer L, Orci L, Montesano R. Modulation of microvascular endothelial cell proteolytic properties by inhibitors of angiogenesis. J Cell Biochem 1994; 55:419–434.

9
Skin Fold Chamber Models

Michael Leunig
University of Berne, Berne, Switzerland

Konrad Messmer
Institute for Surgical Research, Ludwig-Maximilians-University of Munich, Munich, Germany

I. INTRODUCTION

To date, most research on biological principles of angiogenesis has been conducted in vitro, with only a little information provided from in vivo research. This despite the fact that the concept of the angiogenesis dependence of tumors was initiated and promoted by Folkman and coworkers (1) using in vivo assays such as the chicken chorioallantoic membrane and the rabbit cornea.

Although findings obtained by molecular and cell biology are fundamental for uncovering mechanisms of angiogenesis, they often fail to be reproducible in vivo. Thus, for the evaluation of concepts of angiogenesis identified in vitro, experimental models that closely reflect the complex environment present in the in vivo situation are required (2–4). Ongoing advances in biotechnology, such as genetically engineered molecules, cells, or animals as well as refined techniques in intravital microscopy provide an increasing array of options for the quantitative breakdown of the in vivo situation. In this chapter we will describe the technical aspects and experimental applications of skin fold chamber preparations as an experimental in vivo assay for the study of angiogenesis in mice.

II. TECHNICAL ASPECTS

For chronic monitoring of angiogenesis, microcirculation, and transport, the instrumented skin has frequently been used. Sandison was the first to implant chambers into animals for microscopy in living tissues (5). Since then, various chambers have been developed and implanted into various sites such as the cheek pouch, the ear, or the dorsal skin to investigate angiogenesis and microcirculation in both animals (3, 4, 6) and humans (7). The tissue under microscopic observation in skin fold chambers was either newly formed granulation tissue (8–20) or preformed tissue, such as striated skin muscle and subcutaneous tissue (21–61). In granulation tissue chambers, the thin two-dimensional granulation tissue layer sandwiched between two cover glasses provides a high optical quality that cannot be met by preformed tissue preparations, and that is used in rats (5, 8–13, 15–19), but rarely in mice (14). However, granulation tissue resembles a healing wound and undesired signals and stimuli of inflammation might be present (35). In addition, the confined space between both cover glasses restricts implantation of tissues and might change pathophysiological parameters such as hydrostatic tissue pressure.

In this chapter, preformed tissue skin fold chambers will be described in more detail. The material currently used in the fabrication of chambers is titanium (Workshop, Institute for Surgical Research, University of Munich, Germany), which is biocompatible and more resistant to mechanical stress than the formerly used coated aluminum. Mice suitable for this preparation should be 2 to 3 months old (25 to 30 g), healthy (virus free) without nutritional deficiencies (vitamins, etc.) and not distressed (bite wounds). To implant skin fold chambers (Fig. 1), mice are anesthetized (ketamine chloride 7.5 mg and xylacine 2.5 mg per 100 g b.w.), skin is shaved at the site of chamber implantation, and two symmetrical frames, which are mirror images of each other, are fixed so as to sandwich the

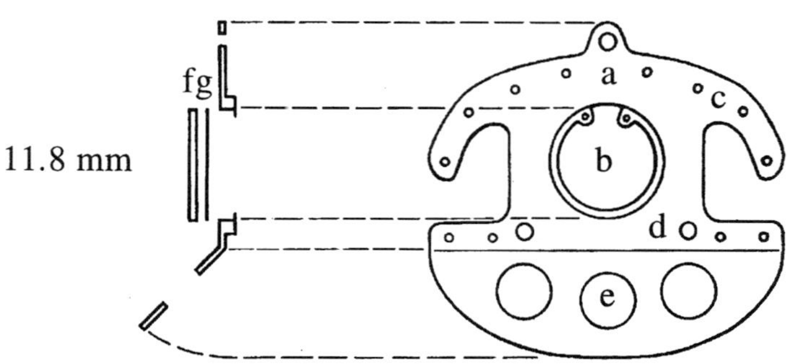

Figure 1 Titanium skin fold chambers **(a)** are inserted into the extended double layer of the dorsal skin of small rodents. The central area **(b)** is the field of interest for intravital microscopy. Drill holes of varying sizes are used for suture **(c)** or screw fixation **(d)** of the chamber on the skin fold, or for weight reduction **(e)**. A retaining ring **(f)** keeps the removable cover slip **(g)** in place. (Modified from Ref. 6).

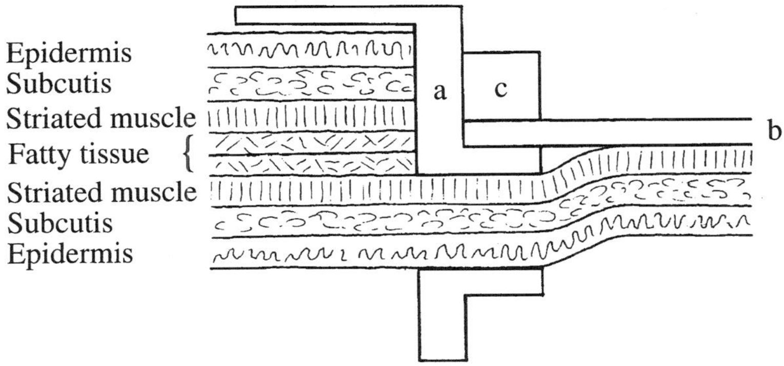

Figure 2 High magnification cross-sectional view of a mounted skin fold chamber (**a**). For implantation of the skin fold chamber, one part of the double layer of the skin is removed entirely including the subcutaneous fat tissue of the remaining skin, which at the end of surgery is sealed by the removable cover glass (**b**) kept in place by the retaining ring (**c**). (Modified from Ref. 33).

extended double layer of the skin (Fig. 1). One layer of the skin is resected in a circular area of approximately 15 mm in diameter, and the remaining layer, consisting of epidermis, subcutaneous tissue, and the striated muscle, is protected by a removable transparent cover slip incorporated into one of the frames (Fig. 2). All microsurgical procedures are performed aseptically under a microscope. Mice endure skin fold chambers (Fig. 3) well, as reflected by maintenance of

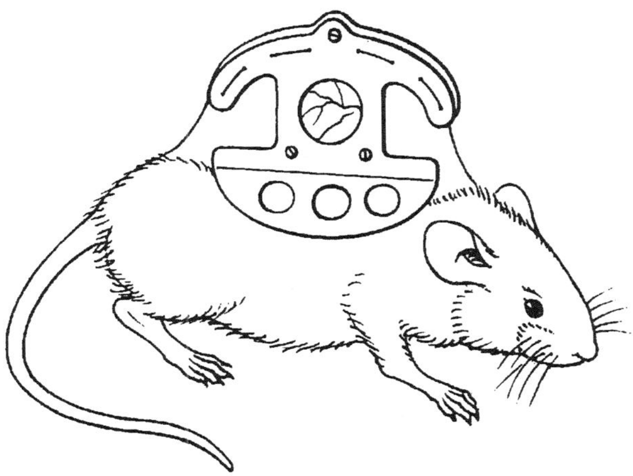

Figure 3 Schematic of a mouse fitted with a dorsal skin fold chamber.

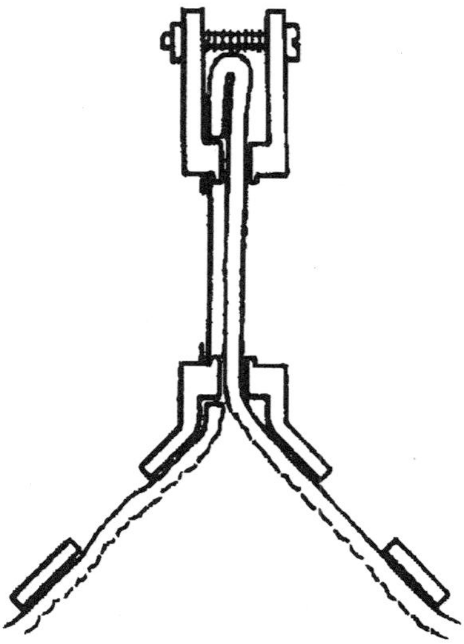

Figure 4 Cross-sectional view of a mounted skin fold chamber. The skin is sealed by only one removable cover glass, enabling implantation of various tissues.

regular sleeping and feeding habits. After a recovery period of 24 to 48 hours, chambers meeting the criteria of intact microcirculation (62) are used as sites for implantation of several tissues (Fig. 4). The recent adaptation of skin fold chambers to immunodeficient mice widened the spectrum of transplantation from syngeneic rodent to human xenografts (Fig. 5).

For intravital microscopy, the chamber preparation containing the transplanted tissue is placed under a microscope and high resolution visualization of the tissue of interest is performed by transillumination or epi-illumination techniques. Excitation of fluorescent dyes labeling blood cells/compartments or fluorescence indicators reflecting the biochemical status of the local microenvironment by light possessing appropriate physical qualities (wavelength, pulsed light, etc.) can be used for the identification and exact quantification of a broad variety

---

Figure 5 Intravital microscopy of **(a)** LS174T human adenocarcinoma xenograft (Bar: 2 cm) and **(b)** an isografted neonatal femur (Bar: 1 mm) 16 days after implantation into dorsal skin fold chamber in immunodeficient mice. **c**. FITC-dextran and fluorescence microscopy facilitate the contrast enhancement of the intravascular space of newly formed blood vessels induced various tissues such as neonatal bone (Bar: 100 μm). (Photographs taken by Michael Leunig at the Steele Lab for Tumor Biology, MGH, Harvard Medical School, Boston, MA).

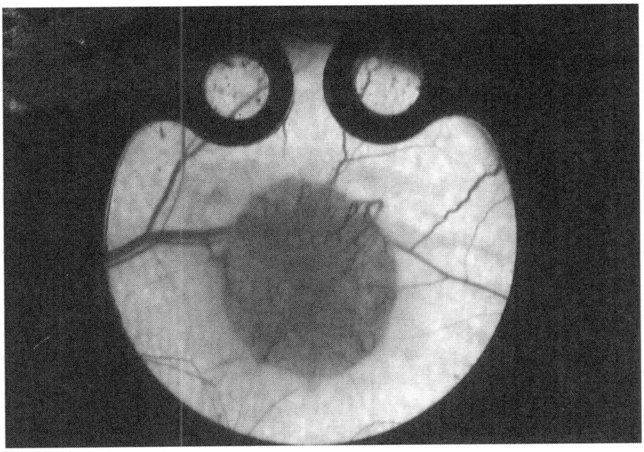

(a)

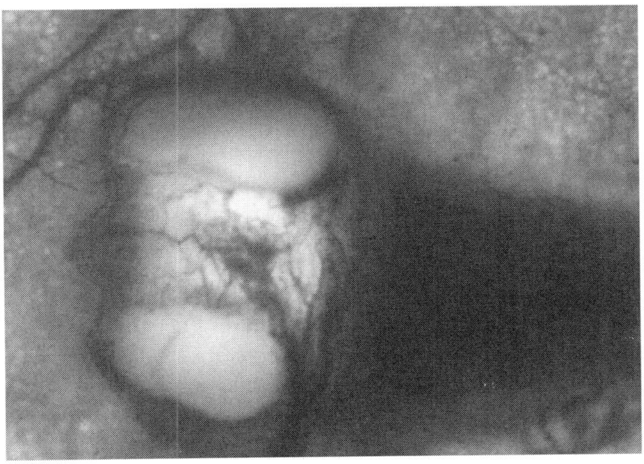

(b)

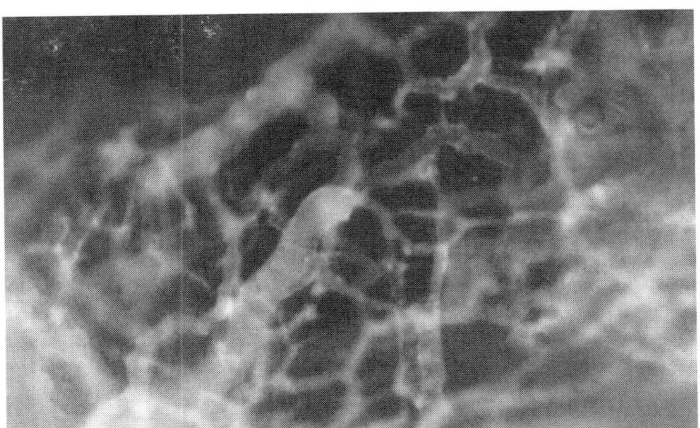

(c)

of in vivo processes (e.g., reactive oxygen species, pH, pO_2, Ca^{2+}, etc.) (63–65). Microscopic images are recorded by means of low-light-level cameras on videotapes or directly digitized and stored on the hard disc of an image analysis system. Even extremely weak fluorescence yield can be successfully detected by photomultipliers.

Angiogenesis can be assessed by qualitative and quantitative measures. Morphological phenomena (dilation of capillaries, sprout formation, sinusoidal vessels, etc.) occurring during the initial phase of angiogenesis are qualitatively described and frequently difficult to image because of local tissue impairment (hemorrhage, inflammatory response, edema, etc.). The functional integrity of the more mature vascular network is quantitatively assessed by computerized image analysis of capillary density, microcirculatory (red blood cell [RBC]-velocity, leukocyte-endothelium interaction, etc.) and transport parameters (vascular permeability to macromolecules, etc.). Recently, mathematical modeling using fractal analysis has been used to identify common mechanisms underlying the process of angiogenesis (percolation or diffusion-limited aggregation).

III. EXPERIMENTAL APPLICATIONS

Since the pioneering work of Algire and colleagues (21), skin fold chambers have been used for the quantitative characterization of rodent, and more recently, human tumor xenografts (Table 1). These studies commonly revealed that the tumor microcirculation does not conform to the standard microvascular organization (46). Although intravital microscopy has been used for the analysis of the angioarchitecture of implanted tissues, its strength definitely rests on the ability to provide a dynamic portrayal of rapid processes associated with angiogenesis, microvascular perfusion and the functional analysis of intravascular, transvascular, interstitial, and cellular processes. Specifically, the visualization of dynamic events occurring in the microcirculation and microenvironment uncovered a wide variety of characteristics of nonneoplastic and tumor tissue and their implications for health and disease that were not identifiable by in vitro techniques alone. Intravital microscopy using skin fold chambers served as a research tool to characterize the distribution of macromolecules throughout the vascular space, across the microvascular wall, through the interstitium, and across cell membranes. Enhanced permeability of tumor microvasculature (20, 33, 36, 41, 51) has been identified as a central factor contributing to the interstitial hypertension in tumors (31, 53), which increases during successive stages of angiogenesis (53). To analyze the interstitial movement of macromolecules, fluorescence recovery after photobleaching has been applied successfully in vivo (33, 56) and promises novel information on the composition of the interstitial matrix.

Table 1 Skin Fold Chambers in Rodents and In Vivo Microscopy Have Been Used for the Chronic Visualization and Quantitative Assessment of Angiogenesis, Microcirculation, and Transport Characteristics of Various Tissues.

Tissue	Species	Substrate	References
Neoplastic tissues:			
Cells:	Hamsters	Tumors	(26, 28, 36, 44)
	Mice	Tumors	(32, 37, 40, 41, 43, 45, 46, 54, 56, 57, 59)
Fragments:	Hamsters	Tumor	(25)
	Mice	Tumor	(15)
	Rats	Tumors	(8–14, 16–20)
Spheroids:	Mice	Tumors	(42, 51, 55, 56)
Nonneoplastic tissues:			
Cells:	Hamsters	Pancreatic islets	(31, 33, 47, 48)
	Mice	Pancreatic islets	(35, 38, 52)
Tissues/Organs:	Hamsters	Bone	(27)
		Spleen	(29)
	Mice	Bone	(22, 39, 46, 50, 58, 61)
Synthetics:			
Prosthesis:	Hamsters	Vascular graft	(30)
Release device:	Mice	Gels (bFGF/VPF)	(57)

Abbreviations: bFGF, basic fibroblast growth factor; *VPF*, vascular permeability factor.

Besides these mainly physiological studies, skin fold chamber preparations have been applied to study the effect of tumoricidal agents acting by direct cell-mediated or indirect vascular mechanisms. In skin fold chamber preparations in mice, tumor angiogenesis was successfully inhibited by linomide (43) and, more recently, by antivascular endothelial growth factor neutralizing antibody (55). Intravascular processes such as leukocyte-endothelium interaction were analyzed subsequent to tumor necrosis factor (TNF)-α (45) or photodynamic treatment (44), showing a more pronounced up-regulation in normal tissue compared to tumor tissue. Intravital microscopic studies revealed that angiotensin II increased the vascular area by increasing blood flow selectively in tumors (16), thus potentially improving chemotherapeutic and diagnostic effects in patients. The analysis of the microvasculature subsequent to hyperthermia (28) or photodynamic therapy (17) yielded information on the susceptibility of tumor vessels to these physical treatment procedures. Hyperthermic and photodynamic therapy significantly impair microvascular perfusion, eliciting a cessation of tumor blood flow, thus greatly contributing to the tumoricidal action of these treatments. The transport characteristics of photosensitizers within tumors (36) suggested that tumor selectivity of these molecules results, in part, from the enhanced leakiness of the tumor microvasculature.

These are examples of in vivo information obtained by means of skin fold chamber, and although tumors have been used frequently as tissue of interest in these preparations, nonneoplastic implants were also studied by some investigators. Angiogenesis and microcirculation of tissues such as bone (2, 22, 27, 39, 46, 49, 50, 58, 60, 61), pancreatic islets (31, 33, 38, 52), spleen (29), growth factor-containing gels (57), and artificial vascular grafts (30) have been quantified, revealing the strong angiogenic potential of biologically intact nonneoplastic tissues. Although the angiogenic response to pancreatic islets of Langerhans was inhibited by linomide, indomethacin (50) or anti-basic fibroblast growth factor (bFGF) antibodies (61) failed to suppress angiogenesis in transplanted femora. Reducing the biologic potency of bone by heating or freezing, as is done for banking bone, significantly reduced angiogenic response toward the implanted tissue (58).

Angiogenesis, microcirculation, and transport represent events of major significance during normal development and as a cause of, or accompaniment to disease. Recognizing this, biomedical research has to focus on the in vivo aspects to advance the current understanding of health and disease. The use of intravital microscopy for the in vivo analysis of transfected cells expressing certain angiogenic, immunological, and other signals will reveal new clues on the regulation of in vivo processes such as wound repair, tumor development, etc. The successful transfer of the skin fold chamber technique to mice with certain immunodeficiencies opened the door to the use of transgenic animals (66), developing spontaneous tumors at sites such as the skin, in addition to studying the microvasculature of transplanted tumors. Skin fold models have certain limitations and cannot replace other assays; however, they create an experimental situation that facilitates the in vivo assessment of angiogenesis and mediated phenomena—important events that are far from being understood. Specifically, with the discovery of concepts that are proposed to modulate angiogenesis (67, 68), sensitive assays providing a high spatial and temporal resolution are required to characterize the in vivo activity of these mediators.

REFERENCES

1. Folkman J. How is blood vessel growth regulated in normal and neoplastic tissue? G.H.A. Clowes memorial award lecture. Cancer Res 1986; 46:467–473.
2. Messmer K, Funk W, Endrich B, Zeintl H. The perspectives of new methods in microcirculation research. Prog Appl Microcirc 1984; 6:77–90.
3. Menger MD, Lehr HA. Scope and perspectives of intravital microscopy—bridge over from in vitro to in vivo. Immunol Today 1993; 14:519–522.

4. Leunig M, Messmer K. Intravital microscopy in tumor biology: Current status and future perspectives (review). Int J Oncol 1995; 6:413–417.
5. Sandison JC. The transparent chamber of the rabbit's ear giving a complete description of improved techniques of construction and introduction and general account of growth and behavior of living cells and tissues seen with the microscope. Am J Anat 1928; 41:447–472.
6. Nolte D, Menger MD, Messmer K. Microcirculatory models of ischemia-reperfusion in skin and striated muscle. Int J Microcirc 1995; 15:9–16.
7. Brånemark PL, Aspegren K, Breine U. Microcirculatory studies in man by high resolution vital microscopy. Angiology 1964; 15:329–332.
8. Reinhold HS. Improved microcirculation in irradiated tumors. Eur J Cancer 1971; 7:273–280.
9. Eddy HA, Casarett HW. Development of the vascular system in the hamster malignant neurilemmoma. Microvasc Res 1972; 6:63–82.
10. Yamaura H, Sato H. Studies on the developing vascular system of rat hepatoma. J Natl Cancer Inst 1974; 53:1229–1240.
11. Reinhold HS, Blachiewicz B, Block A. Oxygenation and reoxygenation in ''sandwich'' tumors. Bibl Anat 1977; 15:270–272.
12. Endrich B, Intaglietta M, Reinhold HS, Gross JF. Hemodynamic characteristics in microcirculatory blood channels during early tumor growth. Cancer Res 1979; 39: 17–23.
13. Endrich B, Reinhold HS, Gross JF, Intaglietta M. Tissue perfusion inhomogeneity during early tumor growth in rats. J Natl Cancer Inst 1979; 62:387–395.
14. Peters W, Teixeira M, Intaglietta M, Gross JF. Microcirculatory studies in rat mammary carcinoma. I. Transparent chamber method, development of microvasculature, and pressures in tumor vessels. J Natl Cancer Inst 1980; 65:631–642.
15. Falkvoll K, Rofstad EK, Brustad T, Marton P. A transparent chamber for the dorsal skin fold of athymic mice. Exp Cell Biol 1984; 52:260–268.
16. Hori K, Suzuki M, Abe I, Sato S, Sato H. Increase in tumor vascular is due to increased blood flow by angiotensin II in rats. J Natl Cancer Inst 1984; 74:453–459.
17. Star W, Marijnissen HPA, van-den-Berg-Block AE, Versteeg JAC, Franken KAP, Reinhold HS. Destruction of rat mammary tumor and normal tissue microcirculation by hematoporphyrin derivative photoradiation observed in vivo in sandwich observation chambers. Cancer Res 1986; 46:2532–2540.
18. Dewhirst MW, Tso CY, Oliver R, Gustafson CS, Secomb TW, Gross JF. Morphologic and hemodynamic comparison of tumor and healing normal tissue microvasculature. Int J Radiat Oncol Biol Phys 1989; 17:91–99.
19. Wu NZ, Klitzman B, Dodge R, Dewhirst MW. Diminished leukocyte-endothelium interaction in tumor microvessels. Cancer Res 1992; 52:4265–4268.
20. Wu NZ, Da D, Rudoll TL, Needham D, Whorton AR, Dewhirst MW. Increased microvascular permeability contributes to the preferential accumulation of stealth liposomes in tumor tissue. Cancer Res 1993; 53:3765–3770.
21. Algire GH, Chalkley HW, Legallais FY, Park HD. Vascular reactions of normal and malignant tissues in vivo. I. Vascular reaction of mice to wounds and to normal and neoplastic transplants. J Natl Cancer Inst 1945; 6:73–85.

22. Sabet TY, Hidvegi EB, Ray RD. Bone immunology. J Bone Joint Surg 1961; 43-A:1007–1021.
23. Brånemark PL, Aspegren K, Breine U. Microcirculatory studies in man by high resolution vital microscopy. Angiology 1964; 15:329–332.
24. Endrich B, Asaishi K, Goetz AE, Messmer K. Technical report. A new chamber technique for microvascular studies in unanesthetized hamsters. Res Exp Med 1980; 177:125–134.
25. Asaishi K, Endrich B, Götz AE, Messmer K. Quantitative analysis of microvascular structure and function in the amelanotic melanoma A-Mel-3. Cancer Res 1981; 41: 1898–1904.
26. Oda T, Lehmann A, Endrich B. Capillary blood flow in the amelanotic melanoma of the hamster after isovolemic hemodilution. Biorheology 1984; 21:509–520.
27. Funk W, Endrich B, Messmer K. A novel method for follow-up studies of the microcirculation in non-malignant tissue implants. Res Exp Med 1986; 186:259–270.
28. Endrich B, Hammersen F, Messmer K. Hyperthermia-induced changes in tumor microcirculation. Recent Results Cancer Res 1988; 107:44–59.
29. Foitzik T, Funk W, Roth H, Messmer K. Splenic implants: Influence of particle size and fibrin fixation on vascularization and angioarchitecture. Pediatr Surg Int 1988; 4:263–268.
30. Menger MD, Hammersen F, Walter P, Messmer K. Neovascularization of prosthetic vascular graft. Quantitative analysis of angiogenesis and microhemodynamics by means of intravital microscopy. Thorac Cardiovasc Surg 1990; 38:139–145.
31. Menger MD, Jäger S, Walter P, Hammersen F, Messmer K. A novel technique for studies of the microvasculature of transplanted pancreatic islets of Langerhans in vivo. Int J Microcirc Clin Exp 1990; 9:103–117.
32. Leunig M, Yuan F, Menger MD, Boucher Y, Goetz AE, Messmer K, Jain RK. Angiogenesis, microvascular architecture, microhemodynamics, and interstitial fluid pressure during early growth of human adenocarcinoma LS174T in SCID mice. Cancer Res 1992; 52:6553–6560.
33. Menger MD, Vajkoczy P, Leiderer R, Jäger S, Messmer K. Influence of experimental hyperglycemia on microvascular blood perfusion of pancreatic islet isografts. J Clin Invest 1992; 90:1361–1369.
34. Berk DA, Yuan F, Leunig M, Jain RK. Fluorescence photobleaching with Fourier spatial analysis: A new method for measurement of interstitial diffusion in thick tissues. Biophys J 1993; 65:2428–2436.
35. Lehr HA, Leunig M, Menger MD, Nolte D, Messmer K. Dorsal skinfold chamber technique for intravital microscopy on striated muscle in nude mice. Am J Pathol 1993; 143:1055–1062.
36. Leunig M, Richert C, Gamarra F, Lumper M, Vogel E, Jocham D, Goetz AE. Tumor localization kinetics of photofrin and three synthetic porphyrinoids in an amelanotic melanoma of the hamster. Br J Cancer 1993; 67:225–234.
37. Yuan F, Leunig M, Berk D, Jain RK. Microvascular permeability of albumin, vascular surface area and vascular volume measured in human adenocarcinoma LS174T using dorsal chamber in SCID mice. Microvasc Res 1993; 45:269–289.
38. Borgström P, Torres Filho IP, Vajkoczy P, Strandgarden K, Polacek J, Hartley-Asp

B. The quinoline-3-carboxamide linomide inhibits angiogenesis in vivo. Cancer Chemother Pharmacol 1994; 34:280–286.

39. Leunig M, Yuan F, Berk DA, Gerweck LE, Jain RK. Angiogenesis and growth of isografted bone: Quantitative in vivo assay in nude mice. Lab Invest 1994; 71:300–307.
40. Torres Filho IP, Leunig M, Yuan F, Intaglietta M, Jain RK. Microvascular and interstitial pO2 profiles in a human tumor in SCID mice. Proc Natl Acad Sci 1994; 91: 2091–2085.
41. Yuan F, Leunig M, Huang SK, Berk DA, Papahadjopoulos D, Jain RK. Microvascular permeability and interstitial penetration of sterically stabilized (stealth) liposomes in a human tumor xenograft. Cancer Res 1994; 54:3352–3356.
42. Vajkoczy P, Goldbrunner R, Farhadi M, Vince G, Schilling L, Tonn JC, Schmideck P, Menger MD. Glioma cell migration is associated with glioma-induced angiogenesis in vivo. Int J Dev Neurosci 1999; 17:557–563.
43. Borgström P, Torres Filho IP, Hartley-Asp B. Inhibition of angiogenesis and metastases of the Lewis-lung cell carcinoma by the quinoline-3-carboxamide, Linomide. Anticancer Res 1995; 15:719–728.
44. Dellian M, Abels C, Kuhnle GHE, Goetz AE. Effects of photodynamic therapy on leucocyte-endothelium interaction differences between normal and tumour tissue. Br J Cancer 1995; 72:1125–1130.
45. Fukumura D, Salehi HA, Witwer B, Tuma R, Melder RJ, Jain RK. TNF-α-induced leukocyte adhesion in normal and tumor vessels: Effect of tumor type, transplantation site, and host strain. Cancer Res 1995; 55:4824–4829.
46. Gazit Y, Berk DA, Leunig M, Baxter LT, Jain RK. Scale-invariant behavior and vascular network formation in normal and tumor tissue. Phys Rev Lett 1995; 75: 2428–2431.
47. Hansell P, Maione TE, Borgström P. Selective binding of platelet factor 4 to regions of active angiogenesis in vivo. Am J Physiol 1995; 269:H829–836.
48. Hansell P, Olofsson M, Maione TE, Arfors KE, Borgström P. Differences in binding of platelet factor 4 to vascular endothelium in vivo and endothelial cells in vitro. Acta Physiol Scand 1995; 154:449–459.
49. Leunig M, Yuan F, Berk DA, Jain RK. An experimental in vivo model to quantitatively analyze vascularization and growth of grafted bone: Technical report. Osteologie 1995; 4:201–206.
50. Leunig M, Yuan F, Gerweck LE, Berk DA, Jain RK: Quantitative analysis of angiogenesis and growth of bone: Effect of indomethacin exposure in a combined in vitro-in vivo approach. Res Exp Med 1995; 195:275–288.
51. Torres Filho IP, Hartley-Asp B, Borgström P. Quantitative angiogenesis in a syngeneic tumor spheroid model. Microvasc Res 1995; 49:212–226.
52. Vajkoczy P, Menger MD, Simpson E, Messmer K. Angiogenesis and vascularization of murine pancreatic islet isografts. Transplantation 1995; 60:123–127.
53. Yamada S, Melder R, Leunig M, Ohkubo C, Jain RK. Leukocyte rolling increases with age. Blood 1995; 86:4707–4708.
54. Yuan F, Dellian M, Fukumura H, Leunig M, Berk DA, Jain RK. Vascular permeability in a human tumor xenograft: Molecular size dependence and cut-off size. Cancer Res 1995; 55:3752–3756.

55. Borgström P, Hillan KJ, Sriramarao P, Ferrara N. Complete inhibition of angiogenesis and growth of microtumors by anti-vascular endothelial growth factor neutralizing antibody: Novel concepts of angiostatic therapy from intravital microscopy. Cancer Res 1996; 56:4032–4039.
56. Boucher Y, Leunig M, Jain RK. Interstitial fluid pressure increases during the successive stages of tumor angiogenesis. Cancer Res 1996; 56:4264–4266.
57. Dellian M, Witwer BP, Salehi HA, Yuan F, Jain RK. Quantification and physiological characterization of angiogenic vessels in mice: Effect of basic fibroblast growth factor, vascular growth factor/vascular permeability factor, and host microenvironment. Am J Pathol 1996; 149:59–71.
58. Leunig M, Yuan F, Berk DA, Gerweck LE, Jain RK. Heating or freezing of bone: Effect on angiogenesis induction and growth potential in mice. Acta Orthop Scand 1996; 67:383–388.
59. Berk DA, Yuan F, Leunig M, Jain RK. Direct in vivo measurement of targeted binding in a human tumor xenograft. Proc Natl Acad Sci U S A 1997; 94:1785–1790.
60. Harris AG, Schropp A, Schütze E, Kromback F, Messmer K. Implementation of the microdialysis method in the hamster dorsal skinfold chamber. Res Exp Med 1999; 199:141–152.
61. Leunig M, Yuan F, Gerweck LE, Jain RK. Effect of bFGF and angiogenesis and growth of isografted bone: Quantitative in vitro and in vivo analysis in mice. Int J Mic Clin Exp 1997; 17:1–9.
62. Sewell IA. Studies of the microcirculation using transparent tissue observation chambers inserted in the hamster cheek pouch. J Anat 1966; 100:839–856.
63. Rumsey WL, Vanderkooi JM, Wilson DF. Imaging of phosphorescence: A novel method for measuring oxygen distribution in perfused tissue. Science 1988; 241: 1649–1651.
64. Suematsu M, Schmid-Schoenbein GW, Chavez-Chavez RH, Yee TT, Tamatani T, Miyasaka M, Delano FA, Zweifach BW. In vivo visualization of oxidative changes in microvessels during neutrophil activation. Am J Physiol 1993; 264:H881–H891.
65. Them A. Intracellular ion concentrations in the brain: Approaches towards in situ confocal imaging. Adv Exp Med Biol 1993; 333:145–175.
66. Adams JM, Cory S. Transgenic models of tumor development. Science 1991; 254: 1161–1177.
67. Folkman J, Klagsbrun M. Angiogenic factors. Science 1987; 235:442–447.
68. Klagsbrun M, D'Amore PA. Regulators of angiogenesis. Annu Rev Physiol 1991; 53:217–239.

10

Protease Assays and Their Use in the Discovery of Novel Regulators of Angiogenesis

Li Yan, Inmin Wu, and Marsha A. Moses
Children's Hospital and Harvard Medical School, Boston, Massachusetts

I. INTRODUCTION

The role of extracellular proteolysis in the process of neovascularization should not be underestimated. Among the most well-studied, angiogenesis-relevant enzyme systems are the plasminogen activator (PA)-plasmin family and the matrix metalloproteinase (MMP) family of enzymes. A series of recent reviews has documented, in detail, the involvement of these two enzyme systems in the regulation of angiogenesis (1–3). Mignatti and Rifkin have recently highlighted the critical involvement of proteolysis in the process of angiogenesis by writing, "Thus, from a biochemical point of view, capillary formation can be thought of as resulting from alternate cycles of activation and inhibition of extracellular proteolysis." (2)

Indeed, the profound importance of extracellular proteolysis in the formation of a new capillary from a pre-existing vessel was apparent in the earliest studies of the events required for successful neovascularization. In the first electron microscopic analysis of capillary formation, Ausprunk and Folkman (4) described the sequence of events by which a new, tumor-induced capillary forms. In the earliest stages, the basal lamina of the parent venule is proteolytically degraded and the endothelial cells (EC) begin to migrate away from the parent vessel toward the angiogenic stimulus. Shortly thereafter, the nascent capillary structure begins to establish a new lamina propria, an event that requires the cells to synthesize and accumulate matrix components. This event must occur against a backdrop of reduced proteolysis in that immediate microenvironment. Eventually, the extension of the new capillary sprout also involves the degradation of the new basement membrane as endothelial cells invade the surrounding matrix.

Since the importance of local proteolysis was first appreciated in this early study, an accumulating body of evidence has demonstrated that the activity of the PA and MMP enzyme systems is a key requirement for successful neovascularization. The angiogenesis-related consequences of these proteolytic activities include the breaching of the pericapillary membrane of the parent venule by the ECs as they begin to form the new microvessel (capillary sprouting), EC migration and invasion through the extracellular matrix (ECM) in response to an angiogenic stimulus, formation of a patent lumen, release of angiogenic factors stored in the ECM, cytokine regulation, and the processing of matrix components into angiogenesis-relevant fragments (1–3).

Many of the studies that have provided the evidence supporting these important roles of local proteolysis in capillary morphogenesis have used a series of specific functional enzymatic assays to determine enzyme and endogenous inhibitor activity within the context of studying a particular component of the angiogenic process, such as migration, proliferation, and others. In this chapter, we will briefly review the most commonly used enzyme assay systems and provide the reader with an example of the use of this strategy to discover inhibitors of angiogenesis.

II. PROTEASE ASSAYS

A. Immunochemical Assays

Over the past two decades, a variety of monoclonal and polyclonal antibodies have been developed that are useful in the detection and identification of different MMPs, tissue inhibitors of matrix metalloproteinases (TIMPs), and components of other proteinase systems, such as urokinase-type plasminogen activator (uPA), tissue-specific PA, uPA receptor (uPAR), and PA inhibitors (PAIs). Immunochemical assays using these antibodies include standard Western blot, enzyme-linked immunosorbent assay (ELISA), radioimmunoassay (RIA) and immunoprecipitation. Because of their sensitivity and convenience, these methods are routinely used in the detection and quantification of enzymes in cell culture media, body fluids, and tissue extracts. Use of monoclonal antibodies raised against specific polypeptide regions of these proteins also enables investigators to distinguish, for example, between highly homologous MMP family members. However, an important limitation of many of these immunochemical methods is their inability to distinguish between the active and latent forms of some of these proteases (e.g., MMPs) or to detect proteases present as enzyme: inhibitor complexes. Therefore, because these assays reflect only the total levels of proteases, they are not necessarily the assays of choice for identifying the operative proteolytic activities in vivo.

B. Functional Protease Assays

As mentioned above, many ECM-degrading enzymes are produced as latent proenzymes or zymogens. As an important step in controlling the activities of these proteases, the proenzymes are secreted into the extracellular environment, where they are subsequently activated. In addition, the active enzymes can be rapidly neutralized by their endogenous inhibitors. As a direct consequence of these regulatory mechanisms, active proteases usually account for only a small percentage of total enzyme produced. Therefore, in many circumstances, determination of the actual enzymatic activities and their activity state (i.e., latent vs. active) is essential to realistically assessing the true proteolytic profile of a particular sample. Three commonly used functional assays are described below.

1. Substrate Gel Electrophoresis (Zymography)

Substrate gel electrophoresis, or zymography, has long been used as a convenient assay for MMPs and PAs (5–7). Substrate gel electrophoresis essentially uses a modified SDS-polyacrylamide gel copolymerized with substrates of proteases. Routinely used substrates include gelatin/denatured collagen for MMP-2 (72 kDa type IV collagenase, gelatinase A) and MMP-9 (92 kDa type IV collagenase, gelatinase B), casein and proteoglycan for MMP-3 (stromelysin-1), and MMP-1 (interstitial collagenase), and plasminogen for PA. This method has been successful in assessing the levels of these proteases in tissues, cell culture media, and various biological fluids. Substrate is added to the standard Laemmli acrylamide polymerization mixture at a final concentration of 0.2 to 1.0 mg/ml. Experimental samples are mixed with nonreducing sample buffer (0.25 M Tris-HCl, pH 6.8, 10% SDS, 50% glycerol, and 0.1% bromophenol blue). After electrophoresis, the gel is incubated in 2.5% Triton X-100 with gentle shaking for 30 minutes with one change of detergent solution. This step slowly removes SDS from the gel, and a small percentage of proteases are refolded and activated. Gels are then rinsed and incubated overnight at 37°C in substrate buffer (50 mM Tris-HCl buffer, pH 8.0, 5 mM $CaCl_2$, and 0.02% NaN_3). After incubation, the gels are stained for 30 minutes in 0.5% Coomassie Blue R-250 in acetic acid:isopropyl alcohol:water (1:3:6), followed by destaining in water. Proteolytic activities appear as clear zones, demonstrating lysis of the substrate in the gels, against a background of the dark-stained gel. Quantitative densitometry is often performed on the gels to provide quantitative information about the enzyme species detected.

Zymography is a system sensitive enough to detect and reliably quantitate picogram amounts of MMPs and levels of PAs in the range of 0.05 U/ml when carefully performed (7, 8). In addition to being a relatively sensitive assay, zymography permits the user to distinguish between different species of enzymes (e.g., MMP-2, Mr 72 kDa vs. MMP-9, Mr 92 kDa) on the basis of their different mobilities through the gels. This same principle also enables the use of zymography to discriminate between zymogens (latent) and active forms of enzymes that may be simultaneously present in a sample. For example, with respect to MMP latency, one might use zymography to study the sequential activation steps of these enzymes, which might be occurring naturally or as a result of treatment with mercurial agents, by screening for the characteristic decrease in molecular size that is indicative of the removal of a segment of the N-terminus of the enzyme. This assay does not necessary reflect actual physiological proteolytic activities, because endogenous inhibitors can be separated from their cognate proteases upon electrophoresis, whereas their activities are counterbalanced by these inhibitors in vivo.

A modification of standard zymography—reverse zymography—can be used to detect and quantitate the activity of proteases inhibitors in biological samples (9). Active proteases are incorporated into the gel, and after electrophoresis, the substrate in the gel is digested by the incorporated proteases except at the locations where the inhibitors are present, appearing as dark bands on a relatively bright background.

2. Solid-Phase Substrate Assay

For detection of total proteolytic activity present in biological samples, radiolabeled substrates have been used in a number of quantitative assay systems. Solid-phase substrate assays use radiolabeled substrates (e.g., ^{14}C-type I collagen) that are either dried as thin films on culture plates (10) or covalently bound to microcarriers (11) The degradation of substrates by proteolytic activities in the test samples is accompanied by the release of soluble radioactive fragments, which is measured by liquid scintillation counting. These solid-phase substrate assays are capable of detecting proteolytic activities in the nanomolar range. For convenience, these assays easily can be adapted to be performed in microtiter plates for quick processing of larger numbers of samples in the form of either purified preparations or crude cell culture media and tissue extracts. A similar assay system using ^{125}I-labeled fibrin can be used for quantitating PA activity (12). These methods can also be modified to detect inhibitor activities (13).

3. Soluble Substrate Assay

As an alternative to the use of solid-phase substrates, radiolabeled substrates can be used in a water-soluble form. One of the most frequently used soluble substrate assays is a classic collagenase assay (14). Simply put, purified collagen is radiolabeled with ^{3}H or ^{14}C by acetylation and used as a substrate for collagenases. Samples containing collagenase activity are then incubated with radiolabeled collagen. Proteolytic fragments released by collagenase cleavage remain in the supernatants after trichloroacetic acid (TCA) precipitation. The radioactivity of the supernatants represents the amount of proteolytic fragments generated by collagenase cleavage and is proportional to the enzymatic activity contained in the sample. This is a relatively accurate assay for enzymatic activity and can be adapted easily for assays of different proteases by using specific substrates, such as casein, proteoglycans (PGs), or synthetic substrates. These assays, however, are critically dependent on the final concentration of the acid used to precipitate undigested molecules. They are also not particularly sensitive in detecting proteolytic activities in unactivated biological samples and usually require an additional activation step using organic mercuric compounds (15).

In the case of PA a coupled photometric system has been developed by Coleman and Green (16). The system consists of a two-step reaction. In the first step, plasminogens are converted into plasmin by PA activities in the samples. In the second step, the resulting plasmin reacts with thiobenzyl-benzyloxycarbonyl-L-lysinate (Z-Lys-SBzl), a general substrate for trypsin-like enzymes, to form Z-lysine and benzyl mercaptan, which in turn reacts with 5,5′-dithiobis (2-nitrobenzoic acid) (DTNB) to form the colored thiophenolate anion. This method has been adapted for use in a 96-well format using an automatic microplate spectrophotometer for handling large numbers of biological samples simultaneously. The modified method also permits discrimination between tPA and uPA in cell culture-conditioned media (17).

In recent years, the use of fluorogenic peptides for measuring activity of MMPs has been developed by several laboratories (18–21). This method uses peptides consisting of amino acid sequences specifically recognized by different MMPs as synthetic substrates. A fluorophore and a light-absorbing group (quencher) are chemically attached to these substrates. In the intact molecules, the fluorogenic group is repressed by the quencher. Once the substrate is proteolytically cleaved by enzyme, the effect of the quencher is eliminated, and the fluorogenic group is activated. Thus, fluorescence emission is specifically correlated with the cleavage of substrate and reflects the specific proteolytic activities in the sample.

The first generation of these substrates contain the lipophilic fluorophores or quenchers that are not soluble in water, thereby limiting their use in the assay of biological samples. Recently, a water-soluble fluorogenic MMP substrate containing the charged EDANS/Dabcyl group was developed and successfully used in the study of relatively complex samples such as human umbilical vein endothelial cells (HUVEC) cell culture media and synovial fluid (22). Its convenience and specificity will make this new method a very useful tool in studying proteases in more complex biological fluids.

C. In Situ Detection of Proteases

Matrix degradation by extracellular proteases is a tightly regulated event, both temporally and spatially. Expression of enzymatic activities is controlled at the level of tissue, cell type and even subcellular specificity. The restriction of certain enzymatic activities to discrete tissue or cellular compartments ensures the successful local remodeling of ECM. All of the methods mentioned above are designed to assess the enzymatic levels or activities in an entire biological sample. For example, extraction of tissues is required for the biochemical assays and precludes the possibility of detecting the cell types expressing proteolytic activities. Here, we describe three methods to detect localized expression of mRNA, protein, and enzymatic activities in tissue samples or cultured cells.

1. In Situ Hybridization

In situ hybridization using antisense RNA or cDNA probes to determine the cell types that express proteolytic enzymes has become a powerful tool in understanding the fundamental mechanisms underlying biological events such as embryonic implantation, tumor metastasis, and angiogenesis (23). Using recombinant DNA techniques, researchers can generate a probe corresponding to a specific region of proteases of interest: Tissue sections of interest can be incubated with these probes under stringent conditions allowing only specific binding of probes with mRNA containing complementary sequences. The specific probes that bind can then be detected by different colorimetric, fluorescent, or autoradiographic methods to reveal the distribution of protease gene products in situ (24). The specificity of this assay permits the user to discriminate between cells that express proteases of interest from their closely surrounding neighbors that may not. This assay also enables investigators to follow expression patterns of molecules of interest during a dynamic process (such as wound healing, for example) by analyzing tissue samples at different stages in the process being studied. In the case of MMPs, the detection of gene products often has been impeded by low copy numbers. However, a new method, *I*S-RT-PCR, which combines reverse transcription reaction (RT), polymerase chain reaction (PCR), and in situ hybridization has greatly improved the sensitivity of the system and has recently been shown to detect transiently expressed MMP genes (25).

2. Histochemical Localization of Proteases

Matrix-degrading enzymes are usually synthesized upon demand and secreted extracellularly where they are activated. Although in situ hybridization can specifically determine which cells express these proteases, the actual distribution of the final gene products, such as the protein, does not necessary correlate with its cellular origins (26). For example, as a function of the invasive, metastatic nature of tumor cells, it had been assumed that the tumor cells were exclusively responsible for producing the various MMPs used to invade and to metastasize. However, in colorectal cancers for example, MMP-9 and TIMP-1 mRNA were observed in the peritumor stroma cells rather than in tumor cells themselves (27). Based on the use of traditional immunohistochemical techniques, it was suggested that this stromal protease, which was immunodetected at the ''leading edge'' of the invading tumor, could be facilitating the migration and invasion of the tumor cells in that immediate microenvironment (27). Therefore, it continues to be important to attempt to localize the site of proteolytic activity, and standard immunocytochemical methods using commercially available antibodies can be a useful approach to doing so.

3. In Situ Zymography

As discussed above, local matrix-degrading activities, in particular those of the MMPs, are controlled not only by the expression and secretion of these enzymes, but also by their extracellular activation and their temporal and spatial relationship with corresponding inhibitors. These local proteolytic activities can be studied using a method known as in situ zymography (28–30). In this system, quickly frozen tissue sections are overlaid by a thin layer of substrates of proteases of interest, such as gelatin, casein, or fibrin. The slides are then incubated at 37°C in a humidified chamber that facilitates substrate degradation. Proteolytic activities present in the analyzed samples are revealed by lytic zones in the substrate layer, which in turn leads to changes in the light-reflecting index, or fluorogenic property, if the substrate is fluorescently labeled. These changes can then be examined under a dark-field or fluorescent microscope. In situ zymography is a method of detecting proteolytic activities that preserves the tissue integrity and that at least spatially, closely resembles the in vivo situation. Combined with in situ hybridization and immunocytochemistry, in situ zymography can be a valuable tool to dissect the functions of proteases in various complex biological processes, such as tumor cell invasion and angiogenesis.

III. PROTEASE ASSAYS AS TOOLS IN ANGIOGENESIS INHIBITOR DISCOVERY

In addition to being used as experimental endpoints in and of themselves, protease assays of the types outlined above have been used successfully to understand the mechanisms of action of various angiogenic factors as well as to monitor the purification of angiogenesis inhibitors. In fact, the use of a radiometric enzyme assay for collagenase inhibition (^{14}C-solid collagen fibril assay), coupled with an assay that measures the inhibition of growth-factor stimulated capillary EC proliferation, was successfully used to purify, identify, and characterize the first TIMP shown to inhibit angiogenesis in vivo and in vitro (13).

This work had at its foundation a series of studies that demonstrated that cartilage, a relatively avascular and tumor-resistant tissue, contained inhibitors of neovascularization. The earliest reports documenting the presence of antiangiogenesis inhibitors in cartilage used the rabbit corneal pocket assay and demonstrated that angiogenesis could be suppressed by implants of native rabbit cartilage tissue (31). The next series of studies showed that cartilage extracts could indeed inhibit EC proliferation in culture (32) and implicated the inhibition of extracellular proteolysis as a potential mechanism of action of these extracts (33). Shortly thereafter, partially purified preparations of bovine cartilage extracts were shown to contain collagenase inhibitory activity as well as inhibitors of neovascularization in vivo (34, 35).

The macromolecule responsible for this cartilage-derived inhibition of angiogenesis was identified in 1990, when our laboratory first reported the purification of a cartilage-derived TIMP (13). To purify this antiangiogenic agent from such an intractable tissue as cartilage, a series of four different chromatography steps that followed multiple extraction and precipitation steps were required. These chromatography steps included gel filtration on A-1.5m Sepharose in the presence of 4M guanidine-HCl, ion exchange chromatography on a Bio-Rex 70 cation exchange column, a second size-exclusion step on a Sephadex G-75 column, and finally reverse-phase high-performance liquid chromatography (HPLC) on a C4 column. These data are presented in detail elsewhere (13). Importantly, we chose to monitor fractions eluted from each of these purification columns for two different bioactivities: MMP inhibition using a radiometric enzyme assay for collagenase inhibition (^{14}C-collagen fibril assay) and fibroblast growth factor (FGF)-stimulated EC growth inhibition using a colorimetric assay that measures the number of EC in culture. Each of these assays was conducted using a 96-well tissue culture plate format that allowed the screening of large numbers of column fractions. From the earliest screening experiments, we detected a copurification of the two inhibitory bioactivities throughout the entire purification protocol. The single protein ultimately purified was identified as a cartilage-derived inhibitor (CDI) of MMPs. This purified protein possessed the two distinct bioactivities that had comigrated during purification. In addition to its ability to inhibit collagenase activity, CDI also inhibited FGF-driven capillary EC proliferation (IC_{50} = 67 nM), and growth factor-stimulated EC migration (IC_{50} = 16 nM). Finally, we were able to demonstrate that CDI was a potent inhibitor of embryonic angiogenesis in the chick chorioallantoic assay (13) and of tumor-induced angiogenesis in the corneal pocket assay (36). Subsequently, other MMP inhibitors also have been shown to inhibit angiogenesis (37–41). Through the use of an experimental strategy similar to that described above, the single cell type in cartilage, the chondrocyte, was eventually shown to be the source of this antiangiogenic TIMP (42).

ACKNOWLEDGMENTS

The authors gratefully acknowledge support from The American Cancer Society (RGP97013) and the National Heart, Lung and Blood Institute, National Institutes of Health (HL57669).

REFERENCES

1. Pepper MS, Montesano R, Mandriota SJ, Orci L and Dominique JD. Angiogenesis: A paradigm for balanced extracellular proteolysis during cell migration and morphogenesis. Enz Prot 1996; 49:138–162.
2. Mignatti P, Rifkin DB. Plasminogen activators and matrix metalloproteinases in angiogenesis. Enz Prot 1996; 49:117–137.
3. Moses, MA. The regulation of neovascularization by matrix metalloproteinases and their inhibitors. Stem Cells 1997; 15:180–189.
4. Ausprunk DH, Folkman J. Migration and proliferation of endothelial cells in preformed and newly formed blood vessels during tumor angiogenesis. Microvasc Res 1977; 14:53–65.
5. Herron GS, Werb Z, Dwyer K, Banda MJ. Secretion of metalloproteinases by stimulated capillary endothelial cells. I. Production of procollagenase and prostromelysin exceeds expression of proteolytic activity. J Biol Chem 1986; 261:2810–2813.
6. Heussen C, Dowdle EB. Electrophoretic analysis of plasminogen activators in polyacrylamide gels containing sodium dodecyl sulfate and copolymerized substrates. Anal Biochem 1980; 102:196–202.
7. Mussoni L, Lawrence D, Loskutoff DJ. A direct, plasmin-independent assay for plasminogen activator. Thromb Res 1984; 34:241–254.
8. Kleiner DE, Stetler-Stevenson WG. Quantitative zymography: Detection of picogram quantities of gelatinases. Anal Biochem 1994; 218:325–329.
9. Oliver GW, Leferson JD, Stetler-Stevenson WG, Kleiner DE. Quantitative reverse zymography: Analysis of picogram amounts of metalloproteinase inhibitors using gelatinase A and B reverse zymograms. Anal Biochem 1997; 244:161–166.
10. Johnson-Wint B. A quantitative collagen film collagenase assay for large numbers of samples. Anal Biochem 1980; 104:174–181.
11. Manicourt DH, Lefebvre V. An assay for matrix metalloproteinases and other proteases acting on proteoglycans, casein, or gelatin. Anal Biochem 1993; 215:171–179.
12. Levin EG. Quantitation and properties of the active and latent plasminogen activator inhibitors in cultures of human endothelial cells. Blood 1986; 67:1309–1313.
13. Moses MA, Sudhalter J, Langer R. Identification of an inhibitor of neovascularization from cartilage. Science 1990; 248:1408–1410.
14. Cawston TE, Barrett AJ. A rapid and reproducible assay for collagenase using [1-^{14}C] acetylated collagen. Anal Biochem 1979; 99:340–345.
15. Nagase H, Enghild JJ, Suzuki K, Salvesen G. Stepwise activation mechanisms of the precursor of matrix metalloproteinase 3 (stromelysin) by proteinases and (4-aminophenyl) mercuric acetate. Biochemistry 1990; 29:5783–5789.

16. Coleman PL, Green GD. A coupled photometric assay for plasminogen activator. In: Lorand L, ed. Methods in Enzymology. San Diego; Academic Press, 1980; 80: 408–414.
17. Leprince P, Rogister B, Moonen G. A colorimetric assay for the simultaneous measurement of plasminogen activators and plasminogen activator inhibitors in serum-free conditioned media from cultured cells. Anal Biochem 1989; 177:341–346.
18. Stack MS, Gray RD Comparison of vertebrate collagenase and gelatinase using a new fluorogenic substrate peptide. J Biol Chem 1989; 264:4277–4281.
19. Knight CB, Willenbrock F, Murphy G. A novel coumarin-labelled peptide for sensitive continuous assays of the matrix metalloproteinases. FEBS Lett 1992; 296:263–266.
20. Nagase H, Fields CG, Fields GB. Design and characterization of a fluorogenic substrate selectively hydrolyzed by stromelysin 1 (matrix metalloproteinase-3). J Biol Chem 1994; 269:20952–20957.
21. Bicket DM, Green MD, Berman J, Dezube M, Howe AS, Brown PJ, Roth JT, McGeehan GM. A high throughput fluorogenic substrate for interstitial collagenase (MMP-1) and gelatinase (MMP-9). Anal Biochem 1993; 212:58–64.
22. Beekman B, Drijfhout JW, Bloemhoff W, Ronday HK, Tak PP, Koppele JM. Convenient fluorometric assay for matrix metalloproteinase activity and its application in biological media. FEBS Lett 1996; 390:221–225.
23. Birkedal-Hansen H. Proteolytic remodeling of extracellular matrix. Curr Opin Cell Biol 1995; 7:728–735.
24. Tessarollo L, Parada LF. In situ hybridization. Methods Enzymol 1995; 254:419–430.
25. Haupt LM, Thompson EW, Griffiths LR, Irving MG. *I*S-RT-PCR assay detection of MT-MMP in a human breast cancer cell line. Biochem Mol Biol Int 1996;39: 553–561.
26. Crawford HC, Matrisian LM. Tumor and stromal expression of matrix metalloproteinases and their role in tumor progression. Invasion Metastasis 1994; 14:234–245.
27. Zeng ZS, Guillem JG Distinct pattern of matrix metalloproteinase 9 and tissue inhibitor of metalloproteinase 1 mRNA expression in human colorectal cancer and liver metastases. Br J Cancer 1995; 72:575–582.
28. Gross J, Lapiere CM. Collagenolytic activity in amphibian tissues: A tissue culture assay. Proc Natl Acad Sci U S A 1962; 48:1014–1022.
29. Sappino AP, Huarte J, Vassalli JD, Belin D. Sites of synthesis of urokinase and tissue-type plasminogen activators in the murine kidney. J Clin Invest 1990; 87: 962–970.
30. Galis ZS, Sukhova GK, Libby P. Microscopic localization of active proteases by in situ zymography: Detection of matrix metalloproteinase activity in vascular tissue. FASEB 1995; 9:974–980.
31. Brem H, Folkman J. Inhibition of tumor angiogenesis mediated by cartilage. J Exp Med 1975; 41:427–439.
32. Eisenstein R, Kuettner KE, Neopolitan C, Soble LW, Sorgente N. The resistance of certain tissues to invasion. III. Cartilage extracts inhibit the growth of fibroblasts and endothelial cells in culture. Am J Pathol 1975; 81:337–347.
33. Sorgente N, Kuettner KE, Soble L, Eisenstein R. The resistance of certain tissues

to invasion. II. Evidence for extractable factors in cartilage which inhibit invasion by vascularized mesenchyme. Lab Invest 1975; 32:217–222.

34. Langer R, Brem H, Falterman R, Klein K, Folkman J. Isolation of a cartilage factor that inhibits tumor neovascularization. Science 1976; 193:70–72.
35. Langer R, Conn H, Vacanti J, Haudenschild C, Folkman J. Control of tumor growth by infusion of an angiogenesis inhibitor. Proc Natl Acad Sci U S A 1980; 77:4331–4335.
36. Moses MA, Langer R. Inhibitors of angiogenesis. Biotechnology (NY) 1991; 9:630–634.
37. Takigawa M, Nishida Y, Suzuki F, Kishi J, Yamashita K, Hakawaya T. Induction of angiogenesis in chick yolk-sac membrane by polyamines and its inhibition by tissue inhibitors of metalloproteinases (TIMP-1 and TIMP-2). Biochem Biophys Res Commun 1990; 171:1264–1271.
38. Tamargo RJ, Bok RA, Brem H. Angiogenesis inhibition by minocycline. Cancer Res 1991; 51:672–675.
39. Murphy AN, Unsworth EJ, Stetler-Stevenson WG. Tissue inhibitor of metalloproteinases-2 inhibits bFGF-induced human microvascular endothelial cell proliferation. J Cell Physiol 1993; 157:351–358.
40. Johnson MD, Kim HC, Chesler L, Tsao-Wu G, Bouck N, Polverini PJ. Inhibition of angiogenesis by tissue inhibitor of metalloproteinase. J Cell Physiol 1994; 160: 194–202.
41. Taraboletti G, Garafola A, Belotti D, Drudis T, Borsotti P, Scanziani E, Brown PD, Giavazzi R. Inhibition of angiogenesis and murine hemangioma growth by batimastat, a synthetic inhibitor of matrix metalloproteinases. J Natl Cancer Inst 1995; 87: 293–298.
42. Moses MA, Sudhalter J, Langer R. Isolation and characterization of an inhibitor of neovascularization from scapular chondrocytes. J Cell Biol 1992; 119:474–481.

11

Vascular Endothelial Growth Factor/Vascular Permeability Factor

Multiple Biological Activities for Promoting Angiogenesis

Donald R. Senger
Beth Israel Deaconess Medical Center, Boston, Massachusetts

I. BACKGROUND: VEGF ISOFORMS, RELATED PROTEINS, AND VEGF RECEPTORS

Vascular endothelial growth factor (VEGF), also known as vascular permeability factor (VPF), is a potent cytokine that is critically important, both for normal developmental angiogenesis and for the neovascularization associated with numerous pathologies, including cancer. Vascular endothelial growth factor/VPF was identified independently as an acute inducer of microvascular hyperpermeability in vivo (1–3) and as a selective endothelial cell mitogen in vitro (4). Subsequently, it was established that both the vascular permeability and mitogenic activities were represented by the same 43,000 M_r disulfide-bonded dimeric protein that exhibits low but significant sequence homology to the A and B chains of platelet-derived growth factor (5–7).

Three principal, naturally occurring isoforms of human VEGF have been identified through sequence analyses of isolated cDNA clones. These variants encode polypeptides that, upon cleavage of the signal peptide, are predicted to contain 189, 165, and 121 amino acids (4). Analysis of the human VEGF gene

Supported by National Institutes of Health Grant No. CA77357.

indicated that the coding sequences are split among eight exons and that the various isoforms arise from alternative splicing of mRNA (8). Similarly, the mouse VEGF gene consists of eight exons, although the predicted sequence of each of the mouse VEGF isoforms contains one fewer amino acid than the corresponding human VEGF polypeptides (9, 10).

Thus far, the principal functional differences between the different VEGF isoforms appear to relate primarily to the respective affinities of these variants for heparin (11). Vascular endothelial growth $factor_{121}$ has little or no affinity for heparin; $VEGF_{165}$ binds heparin moderately; and $VEGF_{189}$, which contains an additional cluster of basic amino acids encoded by exon 6, binds heparin with greatest affinity. Unlike $VEGF_{121}$ and $VEGF_{165}$, $VEGF_{189}$ is largely retained at the cell surface, presumably through interactions with heparan sulfate proteoglycans (12). Thus, alternative splicing of VEGF mRNA appears to generate isoforms of this cytokine, which effectively differ in solubility within the extracellular matrix and therefore in the rate of diffusion from sites of synthesis.

Vascular endothelial growth factor stimulates endothelial cells through two receptor tyrosine kinases: Flt-1 (fms-like tyrosine kinase-1, also known as VEGFR-1) and KDR/Flk-1 (kinase insert domain-containing receptor/fetal liver kinase-1, also known as VEGFR-2) (13). Vascular endothelial growth $factor_{165}$ also binds neuropilin-1, a receptor for members of the semaphorin/collapsin protein family that regulate the guidance of neuronal cell axons (14). This interaction appears to be isoform specific because $VEGF_{121}$ is not bound by neuropilin. Through binding to neuropilin, $VEGF_{165}$ binding to KDR/Flk-1 is enhanced, and therefore neuropilin may serve to regulate $VEGF_{165}$/KDR interactions, rather than serve as a receptor for direct cytokine signaling (14).

Scanning mutagenesis of $VEGF_{165}$ has provided identification of different regions of this molecule that are involved in binding Flt-1 and KDR/Flk-1; and, in particular, these studies determined that structural elements of $VEGF_{165}$ that mediate binding to KDR/Flk-1 are essential for $VEGF_{165}$-stimulation of microvascular endothelial cell growth (15). By contrast, $VEGF_{165}$ mutants that were deficient in Flt-1 binding but exhibited normal binding to KDR/Flk-1 were fully active in promoting endothelial cell proliferation. Consistent with these findings, previous studies with transfected aortic endothelial cells, which normally lacked endogenous VEGF receptors, had demonstrated that KDR/Flk-1 is important for the mitogenic response of these cells to $VEGF_{165}$, and that cells transfected for Flt-1 expression failed to proliferate upon VEGF stimulation (16). Thus, these experiments collectively have implicated KDR/Flk-1 as important for VEGF stimulation of endothelial cell proliferation and have suggested that ligation of the Flt-1 receptor by VEGF serves a distinctly different function. Further support for these conclusions has come from analyses of mutant mouse embryos that are homozygous for targeted mutations of either the KDR/Flk-1 or Flt-1 genes. Both of these null mutations are lethal in utero; however, Flt-1 mutants formed endothelial cells, yet failed to assemble them into normal vascular channels (17). In contrast, KDR/Flk-1 mutants failed to generate mature endothelial cells (18), consistent with a role for this receptor in endothelial cell differentiation and proliferation.

Placenta growth factor (PlGF), a dimeric protein that displays 53% identity with the platelet-derived growth factor region of VEGF (19), also binds Flt-1, but it does not bind KDR/Flk-1 (20, 21). Consistent with this receptor specificity, PlGF displays little or no mitogenic activity for endothelial cells (20). Naturally occurring VEGF/PlGF heterodimers, formed through disulfide linkage of conserved cysteine residues, are active as endothelial cell mitogens (22), most probably because they are able to bind and activate KDR/Flk-1 (23). Vascular endothelial growth factor-B, a recently described cytokine that, like PlGF, shares considerable sequence homology with VEGF, also heterodimerizes with VEGF (24). Although the functional consequences of VEGF-B heterodimerization with VEGF have yet to be elucidated, the VEGF-B homodimer, which like VEGF is encoded by eight exons (25), has been shown to be mitogenic for endothelial cells (24). Vascular endothelial growth factor-C, another recently described member of the VEGF family, stimulates growth of endothelial cells through interactions with both KDR/Flk-1 and Flt-4 (26, 27). Flt-4 expression becomes restricted to lymphatic endothelium during development (28), suggesting a dual function for VEGF-C in promoting the development of both venous and lymphatic vessels (23, 26, 29, 30).

Two additional members of the VEGF family, VEGF-D (31) and VEGF-E (32), also have been identified recently, and so it is apparent that this group of cytokines is complex and that this complexity provides the potential for considerable diversity in endothelial cell signaling. Additional diversity is likely provided through heterodimerization of the various individual polypeptides through disulfide linkage of conserved cysteine residues. For VEGF, disulfide-linked dimerization of polypeptide chains is essential for biological activity (33, 34). Presumably such dimerization allows VEGF to ligate two receptor tyrosine kinase molecules simultaneously, leading to noncovalent receptor dimerization, receptor phosphorylation, and signal transduction (35, 36). Thus, if heterodimerization of VEGF with a related polypeptide occurs naturally, as predicted from studies in vitro (22), such heterodimerization may provide for ligand-mediated pairing of different receptors. Finally, additional complexity in the VEGF protein family is predicted by findings that mRNAs encoding VEGF and VEGF-related proteins are alternatively spliced (11, 20, 25). As demonstrated for VEGF, alternative splicing of these mRNAs is likely important for providing cytokine populations that are differentially retained by extracellular matrix (11, 12).

II. CENTRAL IMPORTANCE OF VEGF FOR ANGIOGENESIS

Notwithstanding the complexity of the VEGF family of proteins, much has been learned specifically about the biology of VEGF, including the regulation of VEGF expression and its relationship to angiogenesis and the mechanisms by which this cytokine promotes neovascularization. In particular, and although there are potentially numerous angiogenesis factors (37), considerable evidence has accumulated indicating that VEGF is an angiogenic cytokine of central importance. Vascular endothelial growth factor angiogenic activity has been demonstrated in numerous experimental models, including the chick chorioallantoic membrane (38–40), rabbit ischemic hind limb (41), tumor xenografts and subcutaneous implants in mice (42–44), and a primate model of iris neovascularization (45). Additionally, both infusion of exogenous VEGF and overexpression of VEGF endogenously were found to induce hypervascularization of avian embryos (46, 47).

Conversely, antagonists of VEGF function and specific inhibition of VEGF expression inhibit angiogenesis. For example, blocking monoclonal VEGF antibody inhibited tumor vascularization and growth in nude mice (48–50) and promoted vascular regression in established tumor xenografts (51). Furthermore, a dominant-negative mutant of the VEGF receptor KDR/Flk-1 inhibited tumor growth by preventing vascularization (52, 53). In the eye, antisense oligonucleotide inhibition of VEGF expression inhibited the neovascularization associated with retinopathy of prematurity (54). A soluble VEGF receptor (KDR/Flk-1) chimera also inhibited proliferative retinopathy (55), and blocking VEGF antibody inhibited retinal ischemia-associated iris neovascularization (56). By contrast, intraocular injection of exogenous VEGF prevented the retinal vaso-obliteration that occurs in animals exposed to hyperoxia (57, 58), suggesting that VEGF, in addition to its function as an angiogenesis factor, also serves to promote endothelial cell survival. In vitro experiments have indicated that VEGF promotes endothelial cell survival through KDR/Flk-1-mediated activation of phosphatidylinositol 3′-kinase (59). Finally, targeted inactivation of the VEGF gene in mice has led to the fundamentally important observation that the deletion of only a single VEGF allele results in disruption of normal blood vessel development and embryonic death in utero (60). Thus, it has been firmly established that proper development of the embryonic vasculature strictly requires a level of VEGF expression greater than that provided by a single functional VEGF allele.

Considerable additional support for the central importance of VEGF for angiogenesis has come from many studies on the expression of VEGF and its receptors. These investigations, which are only partially summarized here, have established that elevated expression of VEGF and its receptors correlate both temporally and spatially with vascularization during embryogenesis (61–63) and with the angiogenesis associated with wound healing (64), cancer (65–67), rheumatoid arthritis (68), psoriasis (69), delayed hypersensitivity reactions (70), and proliferative retinopathies (71–73). Thus, VEGF has been demonstrated to promote angiogenesis in a variety of experimental systems and to be overexpressed in a diversity of settings in which angiogenesis is prominent. Vascular endothelial growth factor overexpression can be induced by cytokines (69, 74), and tumor cells overexpress VEGF as a consequence of malignant transformation (75). However, it appears that induction of VEGF overexpression by hypoxia, through mechanisms involving transcriptional induction, increased mRNA stability and c-Src activation (76–80), is most generally important to a variety of pathologies and wound healing and possibly to normal development (57, 58, 81, 82). Moreover, hypoxic induction of VEGF expression is important in cancer, particularly in regions of tumor necrosis (81, 83).

III. MECHANISMS BY WHICH VEGF PROMOTES ANGIOGENESIS

A. Regulation of Plasma Protein Extravasation and Functional Interactions Between Plasma Proteins and Endothelial Cell Proteins Induced by VEGF

Stimulation of endothelial cell growth is undoubtedly an important mechanism by which VEGF promotes angiogenesis. However, the association of other biological activities with VEGF suggests that the mechanisms by which this cytokine promotes angiogenesis are likely to be complex and to involve far more than stimulation of endothelial cell growth. Specifically, and as indicated by its alternative designation as vascular permeability factor, VEGF is a potent inducer of increased microvascular permeability (2, 3, 84, 85). Vascular endothelial growth factor increases extravasation of blood plasma proteins from the dermal microvasculature of guinea pigs within minutes, with a molar potency 50,000 times greater than that of histamine (3). Moreover, in vitro VEGF potently and rapidly increases the hydraulic conductivity of isolated microvessels (85). The VEGF-mediated increase in microvessel permeability involves functional activation of vesicular-vacuolar organelles present in the cytoplasm of endothelial cells (86, 87). Vascular endothelial growth factor also has been implicated in the induction of interendothelial cell gaps and endothelial fenestrations (88).

Given that VEGF potently increases microvascular permeability resulting in plasma protein extravasation from the blood, an important question arises as to the significance of plasma protein extravasation for VEGF-driven angiogenesis. Investigations on VEGF regulation of gene expression in microvascular endothelial cells have yielded several independent findings that offer insights into an answer to this question. In particular, the available data suggest that stimulation of angiogenesis by VEGF involves multiple functionally important interactions between specific endothelial cell proteins induced by VEGF and specific plasma proteins that extravasate as a consequence of VEGF-induced microvascular hyperpermeability (89).

Figure 1 summarizes much of the supporting data for the foregoing hypothesis. As indicated on the left side of the diagram, VEGF stimulation of endothelial cells in vitro induces expression of osteopontin (OPN) (90), urokinase-type plasminogen activator (uPA) (91), tissue-type plasminogen activator (tPA) (91), plasminogen activator inhibitor-1 (PAI-1) (91), tissue factor (TF) (92), $\alpha_v\beta_3$ integrin (90), and the uPA receptor (uPAR) (93). The right side of Figure 1 shows that VEGF induces extravasation of plasma proteins, including coagulation factors and fibrinogen (Fg) (94), fibronectin (Fn), vitronectin (Vn), and plasminogen (A.P. Sergiou and D.R. Senger, unpublished data). Thus, the functional relationships between the proteins induced in endothelial cells by VEGF and the plasma proteins that extravasate as a consequence of VEGF-induced microvascular hyperpermeability can be assigned to three general categories: 1) activation of the extrinsic coagulation pathway and generation of active thrombin from prothrombin; 2) adhesive interactions between endothelial cell surface integrins and extracellular matrix; and 3) regulation of extracellular proteolysis. However, as illustrated in Figure 1, many of the proteins serve functions that relate to multiple categories. For example, VEGF induction of tissue factor and activation of extravasated coagulation factors of the extrinsic coagulation pathway lead to the generation of active thrombin, which converts soluble fibrinogen to insoluble fibrin (94), thus modifying the composition of the extracellular matrix. In contrast to soluble fibrinogen, insoluble fibrin significantly enhances tPA activity (95); consequently, induction of tissue factor by VEGF may indirectly facilitate the generation of active plasmin from extravasated plasminogen. Plasmin is an important protease capable of degrading matrix proteins both directly and indirectly through activation of locally expressed matrix metalloproteinases (MMPs) (96). Interestingly, plasminogen is not only a precursor to plasmin but also the precursor to angiostatin, which inhibits angiogenesis (97).

Another consequence of activation of extravasated coagulation factors involves cleavage of induced osteopontin by thrombin, thus enhancing both the adhesive and cell migration-promoting activity of this extracellular matrix protein (90, 98, 99). Both intact osteopontin and its thrombin-cleaved form are ligands for the $\alpha_v\beta_3$ integrin (98, 99), and this integrin is induced on dermal microvascular endothelial cells by VEGF (90). The $\alpha_v\beta_3$ integrin also is induced on newly formed blood vessels of wound granulation tissue (100), and antibodies to $\alpha_v\beta_3$ have been demonstrated to block angiogenesis (101, 102). In addition to osteopontin, the three major adhesive proteins present in blood plasma—fibrinogen, fibronectin, and vitronectin—are ligands for the $\alpha_v\beta_3$ integrin and, as noted above, extravasate as a consequence of VEGF-induced microvascular hyperpermeability. Thus, osteopontin, Fg, Fn, and Vn all likely participate in the regulation

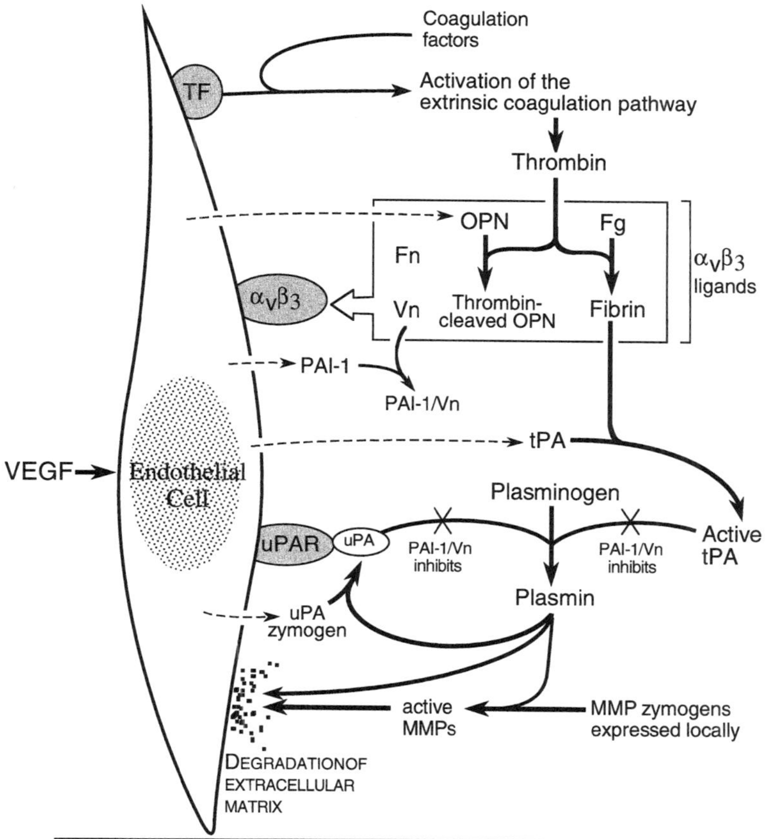

I) Endothelial cell proteins induced by VEGF

Secreted	*Cell Surface*
OPN uPA tPA PAI-1	TF $\alpha_V\beta_3$ uPAR

II) Functionally related plasma proteins which extravasate due to VEGF - induced microvascular hyperpermeability

Coagulation factors
Fg
Fn
Vn
Plasminogen

Figure 1 Functional relationships between specific proteins induced in endothelial cells by VEGF and specific proteins that extravasate from blood plasma as a consequence of VEGF-induced microvascular hyperpermeability suggest that interactions between these two protein populations are fundamental to the mechanism by which VEGF promotes angiogenesis. *Abbreviations: VEGF*, vascular endothelial growth factor; *OPN*, osteopontin; *uPA*, urokinase-type plasminogen activator; *tPA*, tissue-type plasminogen activator; *PAI-1*, plasminogen activator inhibitor-1; $\alpha_v\beta_3$, $\alpha_v\beta_3$ integrin; *TF*, tissue factor; *uPAR*, uPA receptor (uPAR is also a receptor for Vn—not shown); *Fg*, fibrinogen; *Fn*, fibronectin; *Vn*, vitronectin; *MMP*, matrix metalloproteinase. PAI-1/Vn is a stable complex that inhibits both uPA and tPA. (From Ref. 89. With permission).

of endothelial cell adhesion and migration during VEGF-driven angiogenesis. Moreover, the availability and utility of these four ligands for regulation of these processes is coordinated by VEGF induction of $\alpha_v\beta_3$ together with VEGF induction of microvascular hyperpermeability.

In contrast to fibrin, which indirectly promotes plasminogen activation by enhancing tPA activity (95), Vn antagonizes plasminogen activation through binding and stabilization of PAI-1 (103, 104). Plasminogen activator inhibitor-1 inhibits both tPA and uPA (105), and it is likely that Vn/PAI-1 complexes bound to Vn receptors serve to inhibit plasminogen activation at the cell surface (106). Conversely, vascular uPA and uPAR, which as indicated above are both induced by VEGF, serve to promote pericellular activation of plasminogen. Urokinase-type plasminogen activator is expressed as a zymogen but is readily converted to its active form by plasmin (107). Although not illustrated in Figure 1, Vn also has been reported to bind to uPAR (108). Thus, extravasation of Vn may inhibit proteolysis at the endothelial cell surface through binding and stabilization of PAI-1 and through binding to uPAR. Vitronectin also may influence endothelial cell adhesion directly through such interactions. Additional consequences for Vn/PAI-1 association (not illustrated) include inhibition of thrombin (109) and inhibition of Vn binding to $\alpha_v\beta_3$ (110).

Because investigations on the regulation of endothelial cell gene expression by VEGF are at an early stage, it is highly probable that the functional relationships illustrated in Figure 1 represent only a fraction of the total complexity, and that more relationships between extravasated plasma proteins and endothelial cell proteins induced by VEGF will be identified. Moreover, given the potential for considerable functional overlap, some of these interactions may not be essential for angiogenesis. Examples of the latter may include interactions involving either Vn or PAI-1 because homozygous null mice lacking expression of these proteins develop with an apparently normal vasculature (111–113). However, it remains a possibility that angiogenesis associated with wound healing or various pathologies is affected in these Vn or PAI-1-deficient animals, particularly because the composition of extracellular matrix associated with vascular development in the embryo is very probably distinct from the matrix present in, for example, wounds and tumors (114, 115). Regardless, the many important functional relationships between specific proteins induced in endothelial cells by VEGF and specific plasma proteins that extravasate as a consequence of VEGF-induced vascular hyperpermeability predict that the sum of interactions between these two protein populations are crucial for VEGF-driven angiogenesis.

B. VEGF Induction of Collagen Receptor Expression by Endothelial Cells

Vascular endothelial growth factor induces expression of the $\alpha v\beta 3$ integrin in dermal microvascular endothelial cells (90). As previously noted, this integrin serves as a receptor for several ligands, including osteopontin, Fg, Fn, and Vn—all of which are present in the provisional extracellular matrix during VEGF-driven angiogenesis (Figure 1). Nonetheless, angiogenesis very often proceeds in a microenvironment that is also very rich in interstitial collagens; and, for example, collagens normally account for about 75% of the dry weight of skin. Therefore, it is reasonable to expect that in addition to $\alpha v\beta 3$, VEGF might also regulate collagen receptor expression by endothelial cells. Indeed, VEGF potently induces dermal microvascular endothelial cells to express the $\alpha 1\beta 1$ and $\alpha 2\beta 1$ integrins, both of which bind interstitial collagens (116). Moreover, a combination of $\alpha 1$-blocking and $\alpha 2$-blocking antibodies significantly inhibited VEGF-driven angiogenesis in mouse skin without detectable effects on the pre-existing vasculature (116), thereby implicating the $\alpha 1\beta 1$ and $\alpha 2\beta 1$ integrins as functionally important for VEGF-driven angiogenesis. Thus, VEGF induces dermal microvascular endothelial cells to express at least three cell surface integrins—$\alpha 1\beta 1$, $\alpha 2\beta 1$, and $\alpha v\beta 3$—and thereby indirectly regulates endothelial cell interactions with most of the major components of extracellular matrix. Also, as noted previously, VEGF regulates the matrix protein composition of the extravascular compartment by promoting either extravasation or induction of specific matrix components. Therefore, VEGF potently regulates endothelial cell adhesion during angiogenesis through multiple mechanisms, as summarized in Figure 2. Through these mechanisms for regulating endothelial cell adhesion, VEGF also very probably regulates endothelial cell migration.

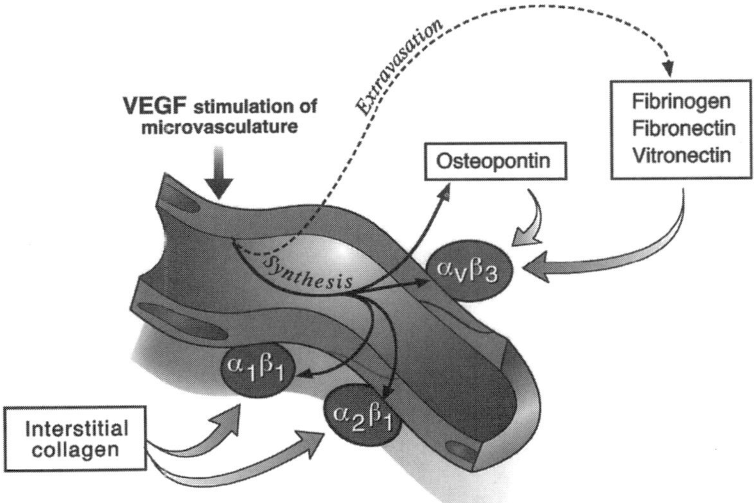

Figure 2 Vascular endothelial growth factor regulates the composition of extracellular matrix and endothelial cell expression of cell surface integrins that serve as receptors for matrix proteins.

In conclusion, the collective evidence suggests that VEGF promotes angiogenesis not only by stimulating endothelial cell growth but also through induction of microvascular hyperpermeability and induction of endothelial cell gene expression. Numerous important functional relationships between specific endothelial cell proteins induced by VEGF and specific plasma proteins that extravasate as a consequence of VEGF-induced microvascular permeability suggest that interactions between the endothelial cell and plasma protein compartments are crucial for VEGF-driven angiogenesis. Many of these interactions between endothelial cell and plasma proteins serve in the remodeling of the provisional extracellular matrix together with the regulation of endothelial cell adhesion and migration. Finally, VEGF induction of collagen receptor expression serves to augment endothelial cell interactions with the pre-existing, collagen-rich microenvironment during the process of neovascularization.

REFERENCES

1. Dvorak HF, Orenstein NS, Carvalho AC, Churchill WH, Dvorak AM, Galli SJ, Feder J, Bitzer AM, Rypysc J, Giovinco P. Induction of a fibrin-gel investment: An early event in line 10 hepatocarcinoma growth mediated by tumor-secreted products. J Immunol 1979; 122(1):166–174.
2. Senger DR, Galli SJ, Dvorak AM, Perruzzi CA, Harvey VS, Dvorak HF. Tumor cells secrete a vascular permeability factor that promotes accumulation of ascites fluid. Science 1983; 219:983–985.
3. Senger DR, Connolly DT, Van De Water L, Feder J, Dvorak HF. Purification and NH2-terminal amino acid sequence of guinea pig tumor-secreted vascular permeability factor. Cancer Res 1990; 50:1774–1778.
4. Ferrara N, Henzel WJ. Pituitary follicular cells secrete a novel heparin-binding growth factor specific for vascular endothelial cells. Biochem Biophys Res Commun 1989; 161:851–858.
5. Keck PJ, Hauser SD, Krivi G, Sanzo K, Warren T, Feder J, Connolly DT. Vascular permeability factor. An endothelial cell mitogen related to PDGF. Science 1989; 246:1309–1312.
6. Leung DW, Cachianes G, Kuang W-J, Goeddel DV, Ferrara N. Vascular endothelial growth factor is a secreted angiogenic mitogen. Science 1989; 246:1306–1309.
7. Conn G, Bayne ML, Soderman DD, Kwok PW, Sullivan KA, Palisi TM, Hope DA, Thomas KA. Amino acid and cDNA sequences of a vascular endothelial cell mitogen that is homologous to platelet-derived growth factor. Proc Natl Acad Sci U S A 1990; 87:2628–2632.
8. Tischer E, Mitchell R, Hartman T, Silva M, Gospodarowicz D, Fiddes JC, Abraham JA. The human gene for vascular endothelial growth factor. Multiple protein forms are encoded through alternative exon splicing. J Biol Chem 1991; 266(18):11947–11954.

9. Shima DT, Kuroki M, Deutsch U, Ng Y-S, Adamis AP, D'Amore PA. The mouse gene for vascular endothelial growth factor. Genomic structure, definition of the transcriptional unit, and characterization of transcriptional and post-transcriptional regulatory sequences. J Biol Chem 1996; 271(7):3877–3883.
10. Claffey KP, Wilkison WO, Spiegelman BM. Vascular endothelial growth factor: Regulation by cell differentiation and activated second messenger pathways. J Biol Chem 1992; 267:16317–16322.
11. Neufeld G, Cohen T, Gitay-Goren H, Poltorak Z, Tessler S, Sharon R, Gengrinovitch S, Levi B-Z. Similarities and differences between the vascular endothelial growth factor (VEGF) splice variants. Cancer Metastasis Rev 1996; 15:153–158.
12. Park JE, Keller G-A, Ferrara N. The vascular endothelial growth factor (VEGF) isoforms: Differential deposition into the subepithelial extracellular matrix and bioactivity of extracellular matrix-bound VEGF. Mol Biol Cell 1993; 4:1317–1326.
13. Mustonen T, Alitalo K. Endothelial receptor tyrosine kinases involved in angiogenesis. J Cell Biol 1995; 129:895–898.
14. Soker S, Takashima S, Miao HQ, Neufeld G, Klagsbrun M. Neuropilin-1 is expressed by endothelial and tumor cells as an isoform-specific receptor for vascular endothelial growth factor. Cell 1998; 92(6):735–745.
15. Keyt BA, Nguyen HV, Berleau LT, Duarte CM, Park J, Chen H, Ferrara N. Identification of vascular endothelial growth factor determinants for binding KDR and FLT-1 receptors. J Biol Chem 1996; 271(10):5638–5646.
16. Waltenberger J, Claesson-Welsh L, Siegbahn A, Shibuya M, Heldin C-H. Different-signal transduction properties of KDR and Flt1, two receptors for vascular endothelial growth factor. J Biol Chem 1994; 269(43):26988–26995.
17. Fong G-H, Rossant J, Gertsenstein M, Breltman ML. Role of the Flt-1 receptor tyrosine kinase in regulating the assembly of vascular endothelium. Nature 1995; 376:66–70.
18. Shalaby F, Rossant J, Yamaguchi TP, Gertsenstein M, Wu X-F, Breltman ML, Schuh AC. Failure of blood-island formation and vasculogenesis in Flk-1-deficient mice. Nature 1995; 376:62–66.
19. Maglione D, Guerriero V, Viglietto G, Delli-Bovi P, Persico MG. Isolation of a human placenta cDNA coding for a protein related to the vascular permeability factor. Proc Natl Acad Sci U S A 1991; 88:9267–9271.
20. Park JE, Chen HH, Winer J, Houck KA, Ferrara N. Placenta growth factor. Potentiation of vascular endothelial growth factor bioactivity, in vitro and in vivo, and high affinity binding to Flt-1 but not to Flk-1/KDR. J Biol Chem 1994; 269(41): 25646–25654.
21. Terman BI, Khandke L, Dougher-Vermazan M, Maglione D, Lassam NJ, Gospodarowicz D, Persico MG, Bohlen P, Eisinger M. VEGF receptor subtypes KDR and FLT1 show different sensitivities to heparin and placenta growth factor. Growth Factors 1994; 11:187–195.
22. DiSalvo J, Bayne ML, Conn G, Kwok PW, Trivedi PG, Soderman DD, Palisi TM, Sullivan KA, Thomas KA. Purification and characterization of a naturally occurring vascular endothelial growth factor/placenta growth factor heterodimer. J Biol Chem 1995; 270(13):7717–7723.

23. Cao Y, Chen H, Zhou L, Chiang M-K, Anand-Apte B, Weatherbee JA, Wang Y, Fang F, Flanagan JG, Tsang ML-S. Heterodimers of placenta growth factor/vascular endothelial growth factor. Endothelial activity, tumor cell expression, and high affinity binding to Flk-1/KDR. J Biol Chem 1996; 271(6):3154–3162.
24. Olofsson B, Pajusola K, Kaipainen A, von Euler G, Joukov V, Saksela O, Orpana A, Pettersson RF, Alitalo K, Eriksson U. Vascular endothelial growth factor B, a novel growth factor for endothelial cells. Proc Natl Acad Sci U S A 1996; 93: 2576–2581.
25. Townson S, Lagercrantz J, Grimmond S, Silins G, Nordenskjold M, Weber G, Hayward N. Characterization of the murine VEGF-related factor gene. Biochem Biophys Res Commun 1996; 220:922–928.
26. Joukov V, Pajusola K, Kaipainen A, Chilov D, Lahtinen I, Kukk E, Saksela O, Kalkkinen N, Alitalo K. A novel vascular endothelial growth factor, VEGF-C, is a ligand for the Flt4 (VEGFR-3) and KDR (VEGFR-2) receptor tyrosine kinases. EMBO J 1996; 15(2):290–298.
27. Lee J, Gray A, Yuan J, Louh S-M, Avraham H, Wood WI. Vascular endothelial growth factor-related protein: A ligand and specific activator of the tyrosine kinase receptor Flt4. Proc Natl Acad Sci U S A 1996; 93:1988–1992.
28. Kaipainen A, Korhonen J, Mustonen T, van Hinsbergh VWM, Fang G-H, Dumont D, Breitman M, Alitalo K. Expression of the fms-like tyrosine kinase 4 gene becomes restricted to lymphatic endothelium during development. Proc Natl Acad Sci U S A 1995; 92:3566–3570.
29. Oh SJ, Jeltsch MM, Birkenhager R, McCarthy JE, Weich HA, Christ B, Alitalo K, Wilting J. VEGF and VEGF-C: Specific induction of angiogenesis and lymphangiogenesis in the differentiated avian chorioallantoic membrane. Dev Biol 1997; 188(1):96–109.
30. Jeltsch M, Kaipainen A, Joukov V, Meng X, Lakso M, Rauvala H, Swartz M, Fukumura D, Jain RK, Alitalo K. Hyperplasia of lymphatic vessels in VEGF-C transgenic mice [published erratum appears in Science 1997; 277(5325):463]. Science 1997; 276(5317):1423–1425.
31. Achen MG, Jeltsch M, Kukk E, Makinen T, Vitali A, Wilks AF, Alitalo K, Stacker SA. Vascular endothelial growth factor D (VEGF-D) is a ligand for the tyrosine kinases VEGF receptor 2 (Flk1) and VEGF receptor 3 (Flt4). Proc Natl Acad Sci U S A 1998; 95(2):548–553.
32. Ogawa S, Oku A, Sawano A, Yamaguchi S, Yazaki Y, Shibuya M. A novel type of vascular endothelial growth factor, VEGF-E (NZ-7 VEGF), preferentially utilizes KDR/Flk-1 receptor and carries a potent mitotic activity without heparin-binding domain. J Biol Chem 1998; 273(47):31273–31282.
33. Potgens AJG, Lubsen NH, van Altena MC, Vermeulen R, Bakker A, Schoenmakers JGG, Ruiter DJ, de Waal RMW. Covalent dimerization of vascular permeability factor/vascular endothelial growth factor is essential for its biological activity. J Biol Chem 1994; 269(52):32879–32885.
34. Claffey KP, Senger DR, Spiegelman BM. Structural requirements for dimerization, glycosylation, secretion, and biological function of VPF/VEGF. Biochim Biophys Acta 1995; 1246:1–9.
35. Dougher-Vermazen M, Hulmes JD, Bohlen P, Terman BI. Biological activity and

phosphorylation sites of the bacterially expressed cytosolic domain of the KDR VEGF-receptor. Biochem Biophys Res Commun 1994; 205(1):728–738.

36. Heldin C-H. Dimerization of cell surface receptors in signal transduction. Cell 1995; 80:213–223.
37. Folkman J, Shing Y. Minireview: Angiogenesis. J Biol Chem 1992; 267(16): 10931–10934.
38. Wilting J, Christ B, Weich HA. The effects of growth factors on the day 13 chorioallantoic membrane (CAM): A study of $VEGF_{165}$ and PDGF-BB. Anat Embryol 1992; 186:251–257.
39. Wilting J, Christ B, Bokeloh M, Weich HA. In vivo effects of vascular endothelial growth factor on the chicken chorioallantoic membrane. Cell Tissue Res 1993; 274: 163–172.
40. Wilting J, Birkenhager R, Eichmann A, Kurz H, Martiny-Baron G, Marme D, McCarthy JEG, Christ B, Weich HA. $VEGF_{121}$ induces proliferation of vascular endothelial cells and expression of flk-1 without affecting lymphatic vessels of the chorioallantoic membrane. Dev Biol 1996; 176:76–85.
41. Takeshita S, Zheng LP, Brogi E, Kearney M, Pu L-Q, Bunting S, Ferrara N, Symes JF, Isner JM. Therapeutic angiogenesis: A single intraarterial bolus of vascular endothelial growth factor augments revascularization in a rabbit ischemic hind limb model. J Clin Invest 1994; 93:662–670.
42. Potgens AJG, Lubsen NH, van Altena MC, Schoenmakers JGG, Ruiter DJ, de Waal RMW. Vascular permeability factor expression influences tumor angiogenesis in human melanoma lines xenografted to nude mice. Am J Pathol 1995; 146(1):197–209.
43. Claffey KP, Brown LF, del Aguila LF, Tognazzi K, Yeo K-T, Manseau EJ, Dvorak HF. Expression of vascular permeability factor/vascular endothelial growth factor by melanoma cells increases tumor growth, angiogenesis, and experimental metastasis. Cancer Res 1996; 56:172–181.
44. Kondo S, Matsumoto T, Yokoyama Y, Ohmori I, Suzuki H. The shortest isoform of human vascular endothelial growth factor/vascular permeability factor (VEGF/VPF_{121}) produced by *Saccharomyces cerevisiae* promotes both angiogenesis and vascular permeability. Biochim Biophys Acta 1995; 1243:195–202.
45. Tolentino MJ, Miller JW, Gragoudas ES, Chatzistefanou K, Ferrara N, Adamis AP. Vascular endothelial growth factor is sufficient to produce iris neovascularization and neovascular glaucoma in a nonhuman primate. Arch Ophthalmol 1996; 114:964–970.
46. Drake CJ, Little CD. Exogenous vascular endothelial growth factor induces malformed and hyperfused vessels during embryonic neovascularization. Proc Natl Acad Sci U S A 1995; 92:7657–7661.
47. Flamme I, von Reutern M, Drexler HCA, Syed-Ali S, Risau W. Overexpression of vascular endothelial growth factor in the avian embryo induces hypervascularization and increased vascular permeability without alterations of embryonic pattern formation. Dev Biol 1995; 171:399–414.
48. Kim KJ, Li B, Winer J, Armanini M, Gillett N, Phillips HS, Ferrara N. Inhibition of vascular endothelial growth factor-induced angiogenesis suppresses tumor growth in vivo. Nature 1993; 362:841–844.

49. Warren RS, Yuan H, Matli MR, Gillett NA, Ferrara N. Regulation by vascular endothelial growth factor of human colon cancer tumorigenesis in a mouse model of experimental liver metastasis. J Clin Invest 1995; 95:1789–1797.
50. Asano M, Yukita A Matsumoto T, Kondo S, Suzuki H. Inhibition of tumor growth and metastasis by an immunoneutralizing monoclonal antibody to human vascular endothelial growth factor/vascular permeability $factor_{121}$. Cancer Res 1995; 55: 5296–5301.
51. Yuan F, Chen Y, Dellian M, Safabakhsh N, Ferrara N, Jain RK. Time-dependent vascular regression and permeability changes in established human tumor xenografts induced by an anti-vascular endothelial growth factor/vascular permeability factor antibody. Proc Natl Acad Sci U S A 1996; 93:14765–14770.
52. Millauer B, Shawver LK, Plate KH, Risau W, Ullrich A. Glioblastoma growth inhibited in vivo by a dominant-negative Flk-1 mutant. Nature 1994; 367(6463): 576–579.
53. Millauer B, Longhi MP, Plate KH, Shawver LK, Risau W, Ullrich A, Strawn LM. Dominant-negative inhibition of Flk-1 suppresses the growth of many tumor types in vivo. Cancer Res 1996; 56:1615–1620.
54. Robinson GS, Pierce EA, Rook SL, Foley E, Webb R, Smith LEH. Oligodeoxynucleotides inhibit retinal neovascularization in a murine model of proliferative retinopathy. Proc Natl Acad Sci U S A 1996; 93:4851–4856.
55. Aiello LP, Pierce EA, Foley ED, Takagi H, Chen H, Riddle L, Ferrara N, King GL, Smith LEH. Suppression of retinal neovascularization in vivo by inhibition of vascular endothelial growth factor (VEGF) using soluble VEGF- receptor chimeric proteins. Proc Natl Acad Sci U S A 1995; 92:10457–10461.
56. Adamis AP, Shima DT, Tolentino MJ, Gragoudas ES, Ferrara N, Folkman J, D'Amore PA, Miller JW. Inhibition of vascular endothelial growth factor prevents retinal ischemia-associated iris neovascularization in a nonhuman primate. Arch Ophthalmol 1996; 114:66–71.
57. Alon T, Hemo I, Itin A, Pe'er J, Stone J, Keshet E. Vascular endothelial growth factor acts as a survival factor for newly formed retinal vessels and has implications for retinopathy of prematurity. Nature Med 1995; 1(10):1024–1028.
58. Pierce EA, Foley ED, Smith LEH. Regulation of vascular endothelial growth factor by oxygen in a model of retinopathy of prematurity. Arch Ophthalmol 1996; 114: 1219–1228.
59. Gerber HP, McMurtrey A, Kowalski J, Yan M, Keyt BA, Dixit V, Ferrara N. Vascular endothelial growth factor regulates endothelial cell survival through the phosphatidylinositol 3′-kinase/Akt signal transduction pathway. Requirement for Flk-1/KDR activation. J Biol Chem 1998; 273(46):30336–30343.
60. Carmeliet P, Ferreira V, Breier G, Pollefeyt S, Kieckens L, Gertsenstein M, Fahrig M, Vandenhoeck A, Harpal K, Eberhardt C. Abnormal blood vessel development and lethality in embryos lacking a single VEGF allele. Nature 1996; 380:435–442.
61. Millauer B, Wizigmann-Voos S, Schnurch H, Martinez R, Moller NPH, Risau W, Ullrich A. High affinity VEGF binding and development expression suggest Flk-1 as a major regulator of vasculogenesis and angiogenesis. Cell 1993; 72:835–846.
62. Quinn TP, Peters KG, De Vries C, Ferrara N, Williams LT. Fetal liver kinase 1

is a receptor for vascular endothelial growth factor and is selectively expressed in vascular endothelium. Proc Natl Acad Sci U S A 1993; 90:7533–7537.

63. Peters KG, De Vries C, Williams LT. Vascular endothelial growth factor receptor expression during embryogenesis and tissue repair suggests a role in endothelial differentiation and blood vessel growth. Proc Natl Acad Sci U S A 1993; 90:8915–8919.
64. Brown LF, Yeo K-T, Berse B, Yeo T-K, Senger DR, Dvorak HF, Van De Water L. Expression of vascular permeability factor (vascular endothelial growth factor) by epidermal keratinocytes during wound healing. J Exp Med 1992; 176:1375–1379.
65. Brown LF, Berse B, Jackman RW, Tognazzi K, Manseau EJ, Senger DR, Dvorak HF. Expression of vascular permeability factor (vascular endothelial growth factor) and its receptors in adenocarcinomas of the gastrointestinal tract. Cancer Res 1993; 53:4727–4735.
66. Brown LF, Berse B, Jackman RW, Tognazzi K, Manseau EJ, Dvorak HG, Senger DR. Increased expression of vascular permeability factor (vascular endothelial growth factor) and its receptors in kidney and bladder carcinomas. Am J Pathol 1993; 143:1255–1262.
67. Berkman RA, Merrill MJ, Reinhold WC, Monacci WT, Saxena A, Clark WC, Robertson JT, Ali IU, Oldfield EH. Expression of the vascular permeability factor/vascular endothelial growth factor gene in central nervous system neoplasms. J Clin Invest 1993; 91:153–159.
68. Fava RA, Olsen NJ, Spencer-Green G, Yeo K-T, Yeo T-K, Berse B, Jackman RW, Senger DR, Dvorak HF, Brown LF. Vascular permeability factor/endothelial growth factor (VPF/VEGF): Accumulation and expression in human synovial fluids and rheumatoid synovial tissue. J Exp Med 1994; 180:341–346.
69. Detmar M, Brown LF, Claffey KP, Yeo K-T, Kocher O, Jackman RW, Berse B, Dvorak HF. Overexpression of vascular permeability factor/vascular endothelial growth factor and its receptors in psoriasis. J Exp Med 1994; 180:1141–1146.
70. Brown LF, Olbricht SM, Berse B, Jackman RW, Matsueda G, Tognazzi KA, Manseau EJ, Dvorak HF, Van De Water L. Overexpression of vascular permeability factor (VPF/VEGF) and its endothelial cell receptors in delayed hypersensitivity skin reactions. J Immunol 1995; 154:2801–2807.
71. Aiello LP, Avery RL, Arrigg PG, Keyt BA, Jampel HD, Shah ST, Pasquale LR, Thieme H, Iwamoto MA, Park JE. Vascular endothelial growth factor in ocular fluid of patients with diabetic retinopathy and other retinal disorders. N Engl J Med 1994; 331:1480–1487.
72. Adamis AP, Miller JW, Bernal M-T, D'Amico DJ, Folkman J, Yeo T-K, Yeo K-T. Increased vascular endothelial growth factor levels in the vitreous of eyes with proliferative diabetic retinopathy. Am J Opthalmol 1994; 118:445–450.
73. Pierce EA, Avery RL, Foley ED, Aiello LP, Smith LEH. Vascular endothelial growth factor/vascular permeability factor expression in a mouse model of retinal neovascularization. Proc Natl Acad Sci U S A 1995; 92:905–909.
74. Brogi E, Wu T, Namiki A, Isner JM. Indirect angiogenic cytokines upregulate VEGF and bFGF gene expression in vascular smooth muscle cells, whereas hypoxia upregulates VEGF expression only. Circulation 1994; 90(2):649–652.

75. Senger DR, Perruzzi CA, Feder J, Dvorak HF. A highly conserved vascular permeability factor secreted by a variety of human and rodent tumor cell lines. Cancer Res 1986; 46:5629–5632.
76. Levy AP, Levy NS, Wegner S, Goldberg MA. Transcriptional regulation of the rat vascular endothelial growth factor gene by hypoxia. J Biol Chem 1995; 270(22): 13333–13340.
77. Shima DT, Deutsch U, D'Amore PA. Hypoxic induction of vascular endothelial growth factor (VEGF) in human epithelial cells is mediated by increases in mRNA stability. FEBS Lett 1995; 370:203–208.
78. Ikeda E, Achen MG, Breier G, Risau W. Hypoxia-induced transcriptional activation and increased mRNA stability of vascular endothelial growth factor and C6 glioma cells. J Biol Chem 1995; 270(34):19761–19766.
79. Levy AP, Levy NS, Goldberg MA. Post-transcriptional regulation of vascular endothelial growth factor by hypoxia. J Biol Chem 1996; 271(5):2746–2753.
80. Mukhopadhyay D, Tsiokas L, Zhou XM, Foster D, Brugge JS, Sukhatme VP. Hypoxic induction of human vascular endothelial growth factor expression through c-Src activation. Nature 1995; 375:577–581.
81. Shweiki D, Itin A, Soffer D, Keshet E. Vascular endothelial growth factor induced by hypoxia may mediate hypoxia-initiated angiogenesis. Nature 1992; 359:843–845.
82. Detmar M, Brown LF, Berse B, Jackman RW, Elicker BM, Dvorak HF, Claffey KP. Hypoxia regulates the expression of vascular permeability factor/vascular endothelial growth factor (VPF/VEGF) and its receptors in human skin. J Invest Dermatol 1997; 108:263–268.
83. Shweiki D, Neeman M, Itin A, Keshet E. Induction of vascular endothelial growth factor expression by hypoxia and by glucose deficiency in multicell spheroids: Implications for tumor angiogenesis. Proc Natl Acad Sci U S A 1995; 92:768–772.
84. Collins PD, Connolly DT, Williams TJ. Characterization of the increase in vascular permeability induced by vascular permeability factor in vivo. Br J Pharmacol 1993; 109:195–199.
85. Bates DO, Curry FE. Vascular endothelial growth factor increases hydraulic conductivity of isolated perfused microvessels. Am J Physiol 1996; 271:H2520–2528.
86. Dvorak HF, Brown LF, Detmar M, Dvorak AM. Vascular permeability factor/vascular endothelial growth factor, microvascular hyperpermeability, and angiogenesis. Am J Pathol 1995; 146(5):1029–1039.
87. Feng D, Nagy JA, Hipp J, Dvorak HF, Dvorak AM. Vesiculo-vacuolar organelles (VVOs) and the regulation of venule permeability to macromolecules by vascular permeability factor, histamine and serotonin. J Exp Med 1996; 183(5):1981–1986.
88. Roberts WG, Palade GE. Increased microvascular permeability and endothelial fenestration induced by vascular endothelial growth factor. J Cell Sci 1995; 108:2369–2379.
89. Senger DR. Molecular-framework for angiogenesis. A complex web of interactions between extravasated plasma proteins and endothelial cell proteins induced by angiogenic cytokines. Am J Pathol 1996; 149(1):1–7.
90. Senger DR, Ledbetter SR, Claffey KP, Papadopoulos-Sergiou A, Perruzzi CA, Detmar M. Stimulation of endothelial cell migration by vascular permeability fac-

tor/vascular endothelial growth factor through cooperative mechanisms involving the $\alpha_v\beta_3$ integrin, osteopontin, and thrombin. Am J Pathol 1996; 149(1):293–305.
91. Pepper MS, Ferrara N, Orci L, Montesano R. Vascular endothelial growth factor (VEGF) induces plasminogen activators and plasminogen activator inhibitor-1 in microvascular endothelial cells. Biochem Biophys Res Comm 1991; 181(2):902–906.
92. Clauss M, Gerlach M, Gerlach H, Brett J, Wang F, Familletti PC, Pan Y-CE, Olander JV, Connolly DT, Stern D. Vascular permeability factor: A tumor-derived polypeptide that induces endothelial cell and monocyte procoagulant activity, and promotes monocyte migration. J Exp Med 1990; 172:1535–1545.
93. Mandriota SJ, Seghezzi G, Vassalli J-D, Ferrara N, Wasi S, Mazzieri R, Mignatti P, Pepper MS. Vascular endothelial growth factor increases urokinase receptor expression in vascular endothelial cells. J Biol Chem 1995; 270(17):9709–9716.
94. Dvorak HF, Senger DR, Harvey VS, McDonagh J. Regulation of extravascular coagulation by microvascular permeability. Science 1985; 227:1059–1061.
95. Hoylaerts M, Rijken DC, Lijnen HR, Collen D. Kinetics of the activation of plasminogen by human tissue plasminogen activator. J Biol Chem 1982; 257(6):2912–2919.
96. Matrisian LM. The matrix-degrading metalloproteinases. BioEssays, 1992; 14(7): 455–463.
97. O'Reilly MS, Holmgren L, Shing Y, Chen C, Rosenthal RA, Moses M, Lane WS, Cao Y, Sage EH, Folkman J. Angiostatin: A novel angiogenesis inhibitor that mediates the suppression of metastases by a Lewis lung carcinoma. Cell 1994; 79:315–328.
98. Senger DR, Perruzzi CA, Papadopoulos-Sergiou A, Van De Water L. Adhesive properties of osteopontin: Regulation by a naturally occurring thrombin-cleavage in close proximity to the GRGDS cell-binding domain. Mol Biol Cell 1994; 5:565–574.
99. Senger DR, Perruzzi CA. Cell migration promoted by a potent GRGDS-containing thrombin-cleavage fragment of osteopontin. Biochim Biophys Acta 1996; 1314: 13–24.
100. Brooks PC, Clark RAF, Cheresh DA. Requirement of vascular integrin $\alpha_v\beta_3$ for angiogenesis. Science 1994; 264:569–571.
101. Brooks PC, Montgomery AMP, Rosenfeld M, Reisfeld RA, Hu T, Klier G, Cheresh DA. Integrin $\alpha_v\beta_3$ antagonists promote tumor regression by inducing apoptosis of angiogenic blood vessels. Cell 1994; 79:1157–1164.
102. Drake CJ, Cheresh DA, Little CD. An antagonist of integrin $\alpha_v\beta_3$ prevents maturation of blood vessels during embryonic neovascularization. J Cell Sci 1995; 108: 2655–2661.
103. Preissner KT, Grulich-Henn J, Ehrlich HJ, Declerck P, Justus C, Collen D, Pannekoek H, Muller-Berghaus G. Structural requirements for the extracellular interaction of plasminogen activator inhibitor 1 with endothelial cell matrix-associated vitronectin. J Biol Chem 1990; 265(30):18490–18498.
104. Seiffert D, Ciambrone G, Wagner NV, Binder BR, Loskutoff DJ. The somatomedin B domain of vitronectin. J Biol Chem 1994; 269(4):2659–2666.
105. Keijer J, Linders M, Wegman JJ, Ehrlich HJ, Mertens K, Pannekoek H. On the

target specificity of plasminogen activator inhibitor 1: The role of heparin, vitronectin, and the reactive site. Blood 1991; 78(5):1254–1261.
106. Ciambrone GJ, McKeown-Longo PJ. Plasminogen activator inhibitor type I stabilizes vitronectin-dependent adhesions in HT-1080 cells. J Cell Biol 1990; 111: 2183–2195.
107. Wun T-C, Ossowski L, Reich E. A proenzyme form of human urokinase. J Biol Chem 1982; 257(12):7262–7268.
108. Wei Y, Waltz DA, Rao N, Drummond RJ, Rosenberg S, Chapman HA. Identification of the urokinase receptor as an adhesion receptor for vitronectin. J Biol Chem 1994; 269(51):32380–32388.
109. Preissner KT, De Boer H, Pannekoek H, De Groot PG. Thrombin regulation by physiological inhibitors: The role of vitronectin. Semin Thromb Hemost 1996; 22(2):165–172.
110. Stefansson S, Lawrence DA. The serpin PAI-1 inhibits cell migration by blocking integrin $\alpha v\beta 3$ binding to vitronectin. Nature 1996; 383:441–443.
111. Zheng X, Saunders TL, Camper SA, Samuelson LC, Ginsburg D. Vitronectin is not essential for normal mammalian development and fertility. Proc Natl Acad Sci U S A 1995; 92:12426–12430.
112. Carmeliet P, Kieckens L, Schoonjans L, Ream B, Van Nuffelen A, Prendergast G, Cole M, Bronson R, Collen D, Mulligan RC. Plasminogen activator inhibitor-1 gene-deficient mice. I. Generation by homologous recombination and characterization. J Clin Invest 1993; 92:2746–2755.
113. Carmeliet P, Stassen JM, Schoonjans L, Ream B, van den Oord JJ, De Mol M, Mulligan RC, Collen D. Plasminogen activator inhibitor-1 gene-deficient mice. II. Effects on hemostasis, thrombosis, and thrombolysis. J Clin Invest 1993; 92(6): 2756–2760.
114. Dvorak HF. Tumors: Wounds that do not heal. Similarities between tumor stroma generation and wound healing. N Engl J Med 1986; 315(26):1650–1659.
115. Brown LF, Papadopoulos-Sergiou A, Berse B, Manseau EJ, Tognazzi K, Perruzzi CA, Dvorak HF, Senger DR. Osteopontin expression and distribution in human carcinomas. Am J Pathol 1994; 145:610–623.
116. Senger DR, Claffey KP, Benes JE, Perruzzi CA, Sergiou AP, Detman M. Angiogenesis promoted by vascular endothelial growth factor: Regulation through alpha1beta1 and alpha2beta1 integrins. Proc Natl Acad Sci U S A 1997; 94(25):13612–13617.

12
Tie Receptors, Ang Ligands

Yuji Gunji, Arja Kaipainen, Kristiina Iljin, Eola Kukk-Valdre, Berndt Enholm, and Kari Alitalo
Haartman Institute, University of Helsinki, Helsinki, Finland

I. INTRODUCTION

The Tie-receptor family consists of two known endothelial tyrosine kinases: Tie-1 and Tie-2/Tek. These have two immunoglobulin homology domains, three fibronectin type III homology domains, and three epidermal growth factor (EGF) homology domains in their extracellular region, followed by a hydrophobic transmembrane domain and an intracellular tyrosine kinase domain split by a kinase insert (Fig. 1). Tie-1 was originally cloned from a human erythroleukemia cell cDNA library (1). In addition, mouse, rat, and bovine homologues have been isolated (2–4). The main Tie-1 mRNA transcript of 4.4 kb encodes a 135 kDa glycosylated protein. However, a differentially spliced alternative form of Tie-1 lacking the EGF homology domain 1 has also been described (1). Tie-2 shares a 46% amino acid sequence identity with Tie-1. It was cloned from several sources and has also been designated as *tek* and *hyk* (3, 5–9). The 4.6 kb Tie-2 mRNA encodes a 140 kDa glycoprotein (10). Although Tie-1 is still an orphan receptor, four ligands for Tie-2 (angiopoietins 1–4) have been reported (11–13).

II. POINT MUTATION OF THE Tie-2 GENE IS IMPLICATED IN VENOUS MALFORMATIONS

The Tie-2 gene has been mapped to chromosome 9p21 (14) and rare familial venous malformations (VMs) have been linked to the locus (15). Venous malfor-

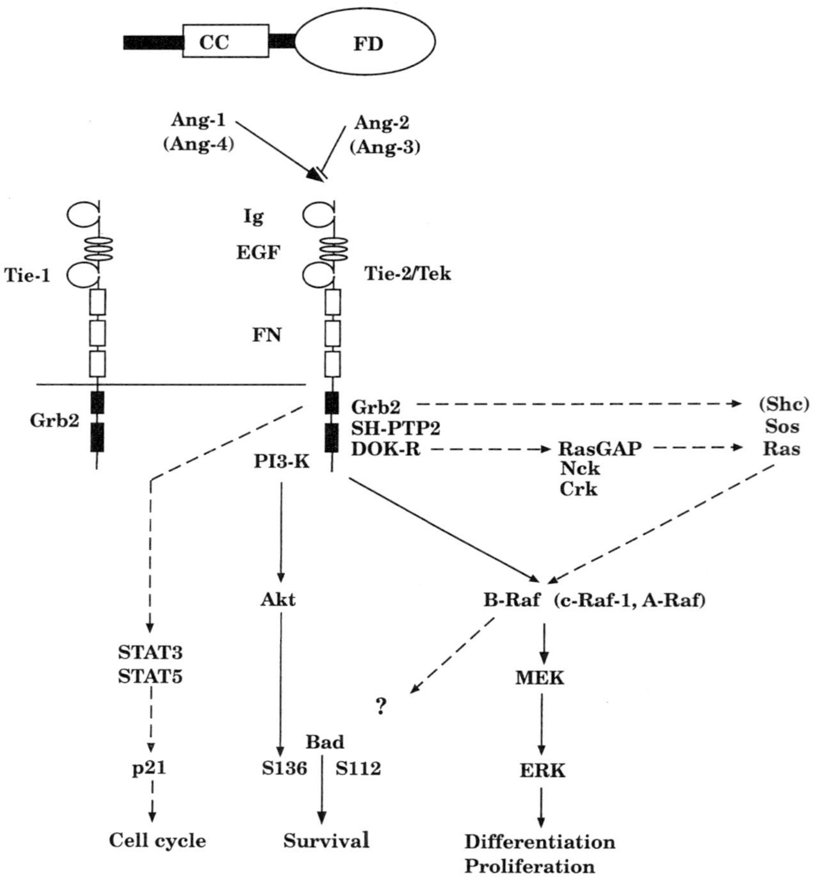

Figure 1 Schematic structures of the Tie receptor tyrosine kinases, their angiopoietin ligands, possible downstream signal transducers, and endothelial effects. *Abbreviations: CC*, coiled-coil domain; *FD*, fibrinogen-like domain; *Ig*, immunoglobulin-like domain; *EGF*, epidermal growth factor domain; *FN*, fibronectin domain. Grb2, SH-PTP2, STAT, B-Raf and DOK-R are explained in the text. Tek is involved in signaling cell survival by Bad phosphorylation via the PI3-K/Akt and possibly the B-Raf pathways. Tek may trigger the ERK pathway through Grb2/(Shc)/Sos/Ras. This pathway also may be regulated through Dok-R/RasGAP. The STAT3/ STAT5 by Tek may regulate the cell cycle through cyclin kinase inhibitors.

mation is the most common developmental vascular anomaly in humans, and the lesions are usually located in the skin. They are composed of dilated and serpiginous channels with vessel walls varying in the thickness of the smooth muscle cell (SMC) layer. Vikkula et al. (16) have shown that an arginine-to-tryptophan substitution in the kinase domain of Tie-2 cosegregates with the phenotype of VMs. They also demonstrated that this mutation results in increased activity of Tie-2 tyrosine kinase in vitro. Ultrastructural analyses of mice deficient for the Tie-2 agonistic ligand Ang-1 have revealed a defect in SMC and pericyte (PC) recruitment, resulting in an abnormal vasculature. These findings suggest that the Tie-2 signaling pathway is critical for endothelial cell (EC)-SMC/PC interaction in vascular development (16, 17).

III. REGULATION OF Tie EXPRESSION

Tie-1 and Tie-2 are first expressed in embryonic angioblasts, and upon their differentiation, expression continues throughout the developing embryonic endothelium, with the exception of the liver sinusoidal ECs (Table 1) (2–5, 9). However, careful comparisons have shown that the expression of the VEGF receptors precedes the appearance of Tie-1 mRNA in the embryos (18, 19). Although both Tie-1 and Tie-2 are down-regulated in the quiescent endothelium of several organs after development, these receptors can be detected in most adult endothelia and are particularly abundant in the endothelium of the lung (2), perhaps correlating with the rapid turnover rate of the lung ECs. Consistent with their roles in neovascularization, the Tie-1 and Tie-2 mRNAs are up-regulated in physiological angiogenesis associated with the development of corpus luteum and in wound healing (20).

The genomic regulatory regions of Tie-1 and Tie-2 necessary for the targeting of gene expression specifically to the endothelium have been identified (21, 22). A 1.2 kb Tek promoter is able to direct heterologous gene expression to embryonic endothelium in the early developmental stages (22). However, an additional EC-specific enhancer discovered in the first intron of the Tie-2 gene is needed to target transgene expression also to adult endothelium (23). In the case of Tie-1, a short 0.8 kb upstream region is sufficient for EC-specific expression throughout development and in adult animals (21). However, this promoter is down-regulated considerably in the endothelia of several organs after the postnatal period.

Despite much effort to determine the specific transcription factors interacting with endothelial promoters, the mechanisms that direct gene expression in the endothelium are still poorly understood. Neither Tie-1 nor Tie-2 contain classic promoter elements such as TATA or CAAT boxes. Progressive deletions and site-directed mutations of the Tie-1 and Tie-2 promoter/enhancer regions

Table 1 The Phenotypes of Tie and Angiopoietin Transgenic and Gene Targeted Mice

Receptor/ growth factor	Onset of expression	Gene targeting	Lethality	Phenotype	Reference
Tie-1	E8.0	LacZ in first coding exon	E13.5–14.5	Hemorrhages and edema, impaired vessel integrity	Puri et al., 1995
				Tie-1-negative cells selected against in organs vascularized by angiogenesis	Partanen et al., 1996
		PGKneobpA in first coding exon	P0	Hemorrhages and edema as a result of impaired vessel integrity; endocardial cells affected	Sato et al., 1995
Tie-2	E7.5	Kinase-dead Tie-2 under β-actin or polyoma virus promoter	~E9.5	Enlarged perivascular cavity, heart small, endocardium degenerated; hemorrhages in yolk sac cavity	Dumont et al., 1994
		LacZ in first coding exon		Heart underdeveloped, no trabeculae; fewer endothelial cells, hemorrhages	Dumont et al., 1994
		LacZ in second coding exon		Vasodilation and malformation of the vascular network; no capillary sprouts into neuroectoderm	Sato et al., 1995
Ang-1	E9.0	LacZ in first coding exon	E12.5	Endocardium immature, heart devoid of trabeculae, interactions between myocardium and endocardium altered; vessels more uniform and straighter branches, relatively rounded endothelial cells separated from underlying matrix	Suri et al., 1996
		Overexpression of Ang-1 under the K14 promoter in the basal layer of epidermis	Viable	Hypervascularization with increased branching of vessels	Suri et al., 1998
Ang-2		Overexpression of Ang-2 under Tie-2 promoter	E9.5–10.5	Mimics Ang-1 null phenotype, detachment of the endothelium from the underlying mesenchyme prominent	Maisonpierre et al., 1997
		Overexpression of Ang-2 under K14 promoter	E14	Embryonic lethality	Yancopoulos et al., pers. com.
		Null mice	P0-D3	Peri-/postnatal lethality	

showed that the critical EC-specific elements correspond to the Ets transcription factor-binding sites (23, 24). The Ets proteins are implicated in the regulation of gene expression during many important biological processes, such as cell growth, differentiation, and transformation. Several Ets proteins can bind to the same Ets binding sites, and it has been suggested that the expression of specific target genes in vivo is regulated by tissue-specific expression of particular Ets proteins (25). Among members of the Ets transcription factor family tested, NERF-2, which is expressed in ECs, showed the strongest transactivation of the Tie promoters (24). As Ets binding sites are conserved also in many other endothelial cell specific gene promoters, it is highly likely that members of the Ets factor family play an important role in vascular development.

Tie-2 also may be a target for hypoxic activation by the hypoxia-inducible factor-1α (HIF-1α)-related transcription factor HIF-2/EPAS1/HRF. Hypoxia-inducible factor-2 is expressed in the endothelium, and its cotransfection strongly induces Tie-2 promoter/enhancer activity (26). Although Tie-1 protein is also up-regulated by hypoxia, the effect of HIF-2 on Tie-1 gene expression remains to be determined (27).

A. Angiopoietin Ligands of Tie-2

The first Tie-2 ligand, Ang-1, was identified from human neuroepithelioma and mouse myoblast cell lines (11). Ang-1 is a novel endothelial regulatory factor that has been reported to promote angiogenic remodeling by vascular sprouting as well as vessel maturation and stabilization. Another related ligand, Ang-2, isolated using low-stringency screening of human and mouse cDNA libraries with the mouse Ang-1 as a probe, shows considerable homology with Ang-1. Ang-2 also was shown to bind to the Tie-2 receptor, but it did not induce its phosphorylation in ECs. Moreover, substantial excess of Ang-2 blocked Ang-1 activity, suggesting that the natural role of Ang-2 may be to antagonize the activation of Tie-2. However, more recent experiments have shown that Ang-2 can also exert agonistic activity (Duncan Stewart, personal communication).

Both Ang-1 and Ang-2 are widely expressed in embryonic tissues, Ang-1 signal being most prominent in the myocardium and Ang-2 in the dorsal aorta and developing aortic branches. Although Ang-1 appears to be widely expressed in adults, Ang-2 is selectively expressed in tissues subject to physiological angiogenesis, for example, in the ovary, uterus, and placenta (12). In these tissues, the expression of Ang-2 may block the constitutive Tie-2 activation signals, leading to local vessel destabilization (12, 28, 29). This effect may contribute to either new angiogenesis in the presence of vascular endothelial growth factor (VEGF) or vessel regression in the absence of VEGF. Both Ang-1 and Ang-2 map to human chromosome 8 (30), but so far there is no evidence that these genes would be linked to a human disease.

Using homology-based cloning approaches, mouse Ang-3 and human Ang-4 have been isolated (13). Both of these proteins bind to Tie-2; Ang-3 appears to act as an antagonist, whereas Ang-4 is an agonist. Several more distant angiopoietin homologues (Ang-X and Ang-Y), which do not bind to the Tie-2 receptor, were also cloned (13, 31, 32). Although the structural divergence between Ang-3 and Ang-4 is more extensive than that of human and mouse Ang-1 and Ang-2, chromosomal localization studies suggest that they represent the mouse and human counterparts of the same gene locus.

The structure of angiopoietins can be divided into N-terminal, coiled-coil, and fibrinogen-like domains (Fig. 1) (11). A mostly α-helical coiled-coil segment is thought to promote the multimerization of the ligand chains. The fibrinogen-like domain belongs to a family of structurally related molecules including ficolin-α, -β, tenascin, and fibrinogens β and γ. The fibrinogen-like domain represents the most conserved region of angiopoietins and comprises their receptor-binding portion (13). Determinants of the agonist versus antagonist roles of angiopoietins may reside within this domain, and multimerization of the fibrinogen-like domains appears to be needed for the active Tie-2 ligands. In addition, fibrinogen-like domains of the angiopoietins have one structural feature that distinguishes the angiopoietins from their more distant homologues. Specifically, all four angiopoietins have a pattern of three closely spaced cysteine residues, whereas Ang-X has two of these residues and all other fibrinogen-like domains have only the last one. The angiopoietins and angiopoietin-related proteins identified so far do not bind to the Tie-1 receptor. However, the possibility that angiopoietins induce heterodimerization of Tie-1 and Tie-2 should be addressed in future studies.

B. Tie-2 Signal Transduction

Several signal transduction molecules have been identified downstream of Tie-2. Using an autophosphorylated soluble Tie-2 kinase domain to probe a mouse embryo expression library, two signaling molecules were identified—Grb2 and SH-PTP2—which associated with specific phosphopeptides of the Tie-2 C-terminus (33). Also, Tie-1 was found to bind Grb2 (D. Dumont, personal communication). Jones et al. used the Tie-2 tyrosine kinase domain in yeast two hybrid system to isolate a novel protein related to the c-Abl-oncoprotein- and RasGAP (Ras GTPase activating protein)-associated DOK protein, which they named DOK-R (34). DOK-R binds to Tie-2 in a phosphotyrosine-dependent manner and is phosphorylated by Tie-2 in vitro (34). DOK-R also binds Nck and Crk adaptor proteins. It is also of considerable interest that DOK-R binds to GTPase-activating protein (RasGAP), as RasGAP knock-out embryos have vascular defects resembling those of Tie-2 null embryos (35). Thus, one of the important signals from the activated Tie-2 receptor may influence the Ras pathway via RasGAP.

Recently, Kontos et al. used a cell line transfected with a chimeric fms/Tie-2 tyrosine kinase receptor and showed that stimulation of this receptor by CSF-1 activates phosphoinositol-3 kinase (PI3-K), which in turn activates the Akt serine kinase implicated in cell survival (36, 37). Activated Akt phosphorylates a Bcl-2 family member, the Bad protein at serine 136 (38, 39). Phosphorylation of Bad at serine 136 and 112 has been reported to prompt Bad association with the 14-3-3 proteins and to inhibit the association of Bad with $BclX_L$, resulting in a cell survival signal (40).

We observed that phosphorylated, activated Tie-2 binds to the B-Raf serine kinase and phosphorylates it, resulting in increased B-Raf kinase activity. Tie-2 and B-Raf also cooperated to induce proliferation of chick embryo neuroretina cells (Y. Gunji, J. Lauren, A. Denouel-Galy, A. Eychene, K. Alitalo, unpublished data). These observations put B-Raf as one important downstream signaling partner of Tie-2. We have also demonstrated that Tie-2 can activate STAT3 and STAT5, but the biological significance of this signaling pathway needs further study (41).

Although ligands of Tie-1 are not known, it is possible that Tie-1 participates in Ang/Tie-2 complex formation by heterodimerization. It is also interesting that protein kinase-C activating tumor promoter and tumor necrosis factor-α treatment of endothelial cells leads to cleavage and release of soluble Tie-1 from the cell surface (42). The physiological relevance of this observation for Tie-1/Tie-2 function is not known.

C. Roles of Tie-1, Tie-2 and Angiopoietins in Vascular Development and in the Hematopoietic System

In contrast to the early defects in vasculogenesis in mice deficient of VEGF or its receptors, embryos lacking Tie-1, Tie-2, or Ang-1 exhibit defects somewhat later in angiogenesis, vascular remodeling, and blood vessel integrity (14, 43, 44). The phenotypes of the gene-targeted and transgenic mice are summarized in Table 1. Tie-2 null embryos showed abnormal development of the heart and vasculature. Embryos homozygous for a targeted mutation in Tie-2 died at E9.5 and Ang-1 null mice died at E12.5 because of disrupted vascular remodeling and EC survival, although the early formation of ECs was normal (14, 43, 44). The defects in Ang-1 null embryos were largely similar but somewhat milder than in the Tie-2 null embryos, consistent with the existence of other, functionally redundant angiopoietins. The null embryos failed to form an elaborated trabeculation of the heart ventricular wall, and the endocardium was weakly associated with the myocardium. They also lacked capillary invasion into the neuroectoderm, which occurs by sprouting angiogenesis.

Dumont et al. reported that in Tie-2 null embryos, the number of ECs was reduced, further suggesting the role of Tie-2 in survival signaling (14). This role is compatible with the observation that overexpression of Ang-1 in transgenic mice under the K14 promoter, which targets gene products to the basal layer of the epidermis, yielded a hypervascular phenotype (45). Considering the association of Tie-2 and B-Raf in Ang-1-stimulated cells, the recently reported phenotype of the B-Raf-deficient mice is intriguing, because these mice died in utero because of defects in vascular EC differentiation and survival. Thus, the phenotypes of B-Raf- and Tie-2-deficient embryos exhibit some striking similarities (14, 44, 46), which could indicate that they are components of overlapping signal transduction pathways.

Transgenic mice specifically overexpressing Ang-2 in their blood vessels under the Tie-2 promoter showed a phenotype mimicking the lack of Ang-1 or its receptor (12). Embryonic death at E9.5–10.5 was associated with heart abnormalities precisely mimicking those previously observed in embryos lacking Ang-1 or Tie-2. These effects of Ang-2 in vivo, together with the results of the Tie-2 receptor phosphorylation studies, support the idea that Ang-2 is an antagonist of Ang-1. Most of the Ang-2 null mice died perinatally or within a couple of days after birth, whereas mice defective of another putative antagonistic ligand, Ang-3, seem to be viable (T. Sato, G. Yancopoulos, personal communications). The existence of two antagonistic ligands and the different effects of the loss of function mutations further suggest the importance of fine tuning of Tie-2 activity.

Mice deficient for Tie-1 died between E13.5 and birth and displayed edema and hemorrhage as a result of poor structural integrity of the endothelium and a relative lack of angiogenic sprouting in certain organs (44, 47). The ECs of Tie-1 null embryos seemed to be "electron light" because of numerous intracellular and transcellular holes (48). Plasma and blood cells extravasated through the ECs because of altered internal structure of the ECs, resulting in edema and hemorrhage. Partanen et al. carried out analysis of Tie-1 function in chimeric mouse embryos and adults (49). Their study supports the conclusion that Tie-1 is required for embryonic angiogenesis and EC proliferation/survival at later stages of development. Selection against ECs lacking Tie-1 is continuous and this selection is especially strong in those parts of the vasculature formed by sprouting angiogenesis. The requirement for Tie-1 in various EC populations varies, and thus the mechanisms of organ-specific vascularization seem to differ (49, 50). It is possible that the functions of Tie receptors and their ligands are associated with the period of remodeling and pruning (51) of the primary vascular plexus and acquisition of pericytic coating after the long-range sprouting of the ECs. There is experimental evidence that the ECs are vulnerable to apoptotic stimuli during this period (52), when the primary angiogenic stimulus in the form of VEGF has been down-regulated, but before the vessels have obtained an outer layer of pericytes with the deposition of critical matrix molecules in between the ECs and pericytes, which apparently provide survival signals and structural integrity for the vessels.

Although the Tie-1 receptor was initially cloned from human leukemia cells and found to be expressed in a large fraction of hematopoietic progenitor cells as well as in developing megakaryoblasts, the role of the Tie receptors and their ligands in the hematopoietic system is still unknown (53–55). It should be noted that in the fetal liver, Ang-1 was expressed in clusters of three to four cells that did not represent cells of the endothelial lineage, smooth muscle cells, or associated pericytes within liver parenchyma but were rather possible sites of hemopoiesis. Ang-2-positive cells in the fetal liver were likely to be ECs or closely associated pericytes. Interestingly, the mRNAs encoding Ang-1 and its receptor Tie-2 are abundant in human megakaryoblastic leukemia cell lines (56). Unlike VEGFR-2-deficient embryos, Tie-1 and Tie-2 knock-out embryos had hematopoietic cells, and the contribution of Tie-2-/- cells to the hematopoietic lineages was unaltered (49, 57). It is interesting that recent experiments indicate that a circulating blood cell population possesses features of EC progenitors (58), but it is not known whether they represent the Tie- and Tie-2-positive progenitor cell population, which could have a dual differentiation capacity.

D. Roles of Tie-1, Tie-2, and Angiopoietins in Tumor Angiogenesis

Vascular endothelial growth factor and its receptors, VEGFR-1 and VEGFR-2, are necessary for tumor angiogenesis (59–61). Although the functions of Tie-1, Tie-2, and Ang:s in tumor angiogenesis remains a subject of speculation, several observations suggest that these receptors also are involved. The Tie-1 protein is detected in the vascular endothelium of breast cancers (62), and its mRNA expression increases in the endothelium of new blood vessels in brain tumors, melanomas of the skin, and their brain metastases when compared to the weak Tie-1 expression in normal skin and brain capillaries (63, 64). Tie-1 also is up-regulated in arteriovenous malformations, where the direct connection from arteries to the venous system results in dilated veins that appear ''arterialized'' with thickened walls due to the proliferation of perivascular fibroblasts (65).

The potential importance of Tie-2 in pathological vascular growth was suggested by inhibition studies using soluble extracellular domains of Tie-2 (66). In glioblastomas, which are highly vascularized tumors and overexpress VEGF, Tie-2 was up-regulated in the tumor endothelium (67). A cell type-specific up-regulation of the Tie-2 ligands also was reported during glioma progression. Although Ang-1 mRNA was expressed by the tumor cells, Ang-2 mRNA was expressed in a subset of the tumor ECs. These findings further favor a recently proposed model that local expression of Ang-2 might promote angiogenesis in the presence of VEGF (17). Local Ang-2 expression might lead to SMC/PC dropoff, which is thought to be a requirement for the sensitivity of ECs to angiogenic inducers, such as VEGF (17). Down-regulation of Ang-2, which was observed in larger vessels in glioma, may permit physical interaction of ECs with SMC/PC, leading to inhibition of EC proliferation and maturation of the vascular wall. In addition, Ang-1 has been reported to induce vascular sprouting in vitro and to block vascular permeability in vivo (68). These findings suggest that Ang-1 acts synergistically with Ang-2 and VEGF in angiogenesis, but antagonistically with VEGF in vascular permeability (69, 70).

REFERENCES

1. Partanen J, Armstrong E, Mäkelä TP, Korhonen J, Sandberg M, Renkonen R, Knuutila S, Huebner K, Alitalo K. A novel endothelial cell surface receptor tyrosine kinase with extracellular epidermal growth factor homology domains. Mol Cell Biol 1992; 12:1698–1707.
2. Korhonen J, Polvi A, Partanen J, Alitalo K. The mouse *tie* receptor tyrosine kinase gene: Expression during embryonic angiogenesis. Oncogene 1994; 9:395–403.
3. Sato TN, Qin Y, Kozak CA, Audus KL. *Tie-1* and *Tie-2* define a new class of putative receptor tyrosine kinase genes expressed in early embryonic vascular system. Proc Natl Acad Sci U S A 1993; 90:9355–9358.
4. Maisonpierre PC, Goldfarb M, Yancopoulos GD, Gao G. Distinct rat genes with related profiles of expression define a TIE receptor tyrosine kinase family. Oncogene 1993; 8:1631–1637.
5. Dumont DJ, Yamaguchi TP, Conlon RA, Rossant J, Breitman ML. *tek*, A novel tyrosine kinase gene located on mouse chromosome 4, is expressed in endothelial cells and their presumptive precursors. Oncogene 1992; 7:1471–1480.
6. Horita K, Yagi T, Kohmura N, Tomooka Y, Ikawa Y, Aizawa S. A novel tyrosine kinase, *hyk*, expressed in murine embryonic stem cells. Biochem Biophys Res Comm 1992; 189:1747–1753.
7. Iwama A, Hamaguchi I, Hashiyama M, Murayama Y, Yasunaga K, Suda T. Molecular cloning and characterization of mouse TIE and TEK receptor tyrosine kinase genes and their expression in hematopoietic stem cells. Biochem Biophys Res Commun 1993; 195:301–309.
8. Runting AS, Stacker SA, Wilks AF. *tie2*, A putative protein tyrosine kinase from a new class of cell surface receptor. Growth Factors 1993; 9:99–105.
9. Schnürch H, Risau W. Expression of tie-2, a member of a novel family of receptor tyrosine kinases, in the endothelial cell lineage. Development 1993; 119:957–968.
10. Dumont DJ, Gradwohl GJ, Fong G-H, Auerbach R, Breitman ML. The endothelial-specific receptor tyrosine kinase, *tek*, is a member of a new subfamily of receptors. Oncogene 1993; 8:1293–1301.
11. Davis S, Aldrich TH, Jones PF, Acheson A, Compton DL, Jain V, Ryan TE, Bruno J, Raziejewski C, Maisonpierre PC, Yancopoulos GD. Isolation of angiopoietin-1, a ligand for the TIE2 receptor, by secretion-trap expression cloning. Cell 1997; 87: 1161–1169.

12. Maisonpierre PC, Suri C, Jones PF, Bartunkova S, Wiegand SJ, Radziejewski C, Compton D, McClain J, Aldrich TH, Papadopoulos N, Daly TJ, Davis S, Sato TN, Yancopoulos GD. Angiopoietin-2, a natural antagonist for Tie2 that disrupts in vivo angiogenesis. Science 1997; 277:55–60.
13. Valenzuela DM, Griffiths J, Rojas J, Aldrich TH, Jones PF, Zhou H, McClain J, Copeland NG, Gilbert DJ, Jenkins NA, Huang T, Papadopoulos N, Maisonpierre PC, Davis S, Yancopoulos GD. Angiopoietins 3 and 4: Diverging gene counterparts in mice and humans. Proc Natl Acad Sci U S A 1999; 96:1904–1909.
14. Dumont DJ, Gradwohl G, Fong G-H, Puri MC, Gertsenstein M, Auerbach A, Breitman ML. Dominant-negative and targeted null mutations in the endothelial receptor tyrosine kinase, *tek*, reveal a critical role in vasculogenesis of the embryo. Genes Dev 1994; 8:1897–1909.
15. Gallione CJ, Pasyk KA, Boon LM, Lennon F, Johnson DW, Helmbold EA, Markel DS, Vikkula M, Mulligen JM, Warman ML. A gene for familial venous malformation maps to chromosome 9p in a second large kindred. J Med Genetics 1995; 32: 197–199.
16. Vikkula M, Boon LM, Carraway KL, Cavert JT, Diamonti JA, Goumnerov B, Pasy KA, Marchuk DA, Warman ML, Cantley LC, Mulliken JB, Olsen BR. Vascular dysmorphogenesis caused by an activating mutation in the receptor tyrosine kinase TIE2. Cell 1996; 87:1181–1190.
17. Folkman J, D'Amore PA. Blood vessel formation: What is its molecular basis? Cell 1996; 87:1153–1155.
18. Dumont DJ, Fong G-H, Puri M, Gradwohl G, Alitalo K, Breitman ML. Vascularization of the mouse embryo: A study of flk-1, tek, tie and VEGF expression during development. Mech Dev 1995; 203:80–92.
19. Yamaguchi T, Dumont D, Conion R, Breitman M, Rossant J. Flk-1, an flt-related receptor tyrosine kinase is an early marker for endothelial cell precursors. Development 1993; 118:489–498.
20. Korhonen J, Partanen J, Armstrong E, Vaahtonen A, Elenius K, Jalkanen M, Alitalo K. Enhanced expression of the tie receptor tyrosine kinase in endothelial cells during neovascularization. Blood 1992; 80:2548–2555.
21. Korhonen J, Lahtinen I, Halmekytö M, Alhonen L, Jänne J, Dumont D, Alitalo K. Endothelial specific gene expression directed by the *tie* gene promoter in vivo. Blood 1995; 86:1828–1835.
22. Schlaeger TM, Qin Y, Fujiwara Y, Magram J, Sato TN. Vascular endothelial cell lineage-specific promoter in transgenic mice. Development 1995; 121:1989–1098.
23. Schlaeger TM, Bartunkova S, Lawitts JA, Teichmann G, Risau W, Deutsch U, Sato TN. Uniform vascular-endothelial cell-specific gene expression in both embryonic and adult transgenic mice. Proc Natl Acad Sci U S A 1997; 94:3058–3063.
24. Iljin K, Dube A, Kontusaari S, Lahtinen I, Oettgen P, Alitalo K. Role of Ets factors in the activity and endothelial cell specificity of the mouse Tie gene promoter. FASEB J 1999; 13:377–386.
25. Karim FD, Urness LD, Thummel CS, Klemsz MJ, Mckercher SR, Celada A, van Beveren C, Maki RA, Gunter CV, Nye JA, Graves BJ. The ETS-domain: A new DNA-binding motif that recognizes a purine-rich core DNA sequence. Genes Dev 1990; 4:1451–1453.

26. Tian H, McKnight SL, Russel DW. Endothelial PAS domain protein 1 (EPAS1), a transcription factor selectively expressed in endothelial cells. Genes Dev 1997; 11: 72–78.
27. McCarthy MJ, Crowther M, Bell PRF, Brindle NPJ. The endothelial receptor tyrosine kinase tie-1 is upregulated by hypoxia and vascular growth factor. FEBS Lett 1998; 423:334–338.
28. Hanahan D. Signaling vascular morphogenesis and maintenance. Science 1997; 277: 48–50.
29. Wong AL, Haroon ZA, Werner S, Dewhirst MW, Greenberg CS, Peter KG. Tie-2 expression and phosphorylation in angiogenic and quiescent adult tissues. Circ Res 1997; 81:567–574.
30. Kukk E, Lymboussaki A, Taira S, Kaipainen A, Jeltsch M, Joukov V, Alitalo K. VEGF-C receptor binding and pattern of expression with VEGFR-3 suggest a role in lymphatic vascular development. Development 1997; 122:3829–3837.
31. Kim I, Kwak HJ, Ahn JE, So J-N, Liu M, Koh KN, Koh GY. Molecular cloning and characterization of a novel angiopoietin family protein, angiopoietin-3. FEBS Lett 1999; 443:353–356.
32. Peek R, van Gelderen BE, Bruinenberg M, Kijlstra A. Molecular cloning of a new angiopoietin like factor from the human cornea. Invest Ophthalmol Vis Sci 1998; 39:1782–1788.
33. Huang L, Turck C, Rao P, Peter K. GRB2 and SH-PTP2: Potentially important endothelial signaling molecules downstream of the TEK/TIE2 receptor tyrosine kinase. Oncogene 1995; 11:2097–2103.
34. Jones N, Dumont DJ. The Tek/Tie-2 receptor signals through a novel Dok-related docking protein, Dok-R. Oncogene 1998; 17:1097–1108.
35. Henkemeyer M, Rossi DJ, Holmyard DP, Puri MC, Mbamalu G, Harpal K, Shih TS, Jacks T, Pawson T. Vascular system defects and neuronal apoptosis in mice lacking ras GTPase-activating protein. Nature 1995; 377:695–701.
36. Kontos C, Stauffer T, Yang W-P, York J, Huang L, Blanar M, Meyer T, Peter K. Tyrosine 1101 of Tie2 is major site of association of p85 and is required for activation of phosphatidylinositol 3-kinase and Akt. Mol Cell Biol 1998; 18:4131–4140.
37. Franke T, Yang SI, Chen TO, Datta K, Kazlauskas A, Morrison DK, Kaplan DR, Tsichlis PN. The protein kinase encoded by the Akt proto-oncogene is a target of the PDGF-activated phosphatidylinositol 3-kinase. Cell 1995; 81:727–736.
38. Datta SR, Dudek H, Tao X, Masters S, Fu H, Gotoh Y, Greenberg ME. Akt phosphorylation of Bad couples survival signals to the cell-intrinsic death machinery. Cell 1997; 91:231–241.
39. del Peso L, Gonzalez-Garcia M, Page C, Herrera R, Nunez G. Interleukin-3-induced phosphorylation of Bad through the protein kinase Akt. Science 1997; 278:687–689.
40. Zah J, Harada H, Yang E, Jockel J, Korsmeyer SJ. Serine phosphorylation of death agonist Bad in response to survival factor results in binding to 14-3-3 not Bcl-X. Cell 1996; 87:619–628.
41. Korpelainen EI, Karkkainen M, Gunji Y, Vikkula M, Alitalo K. Endothelial receptor tyrosine kinases activate the STAT signaling pathway: Mutant Tie-2 causing venous malformations signals a distinct STAT activation response. Oncogene 1999; 18:1–8.

42. Yabkowitz R, Meyer S, Black T, Elliott G, Merewether A, Yamane K. Inflammatory cytokines and vascular endothelial growth factor stimulate the release of soluble tie receptor from human endothelial cells via metalloprotease activation. Blood 1999; 93:1969–1979.
43. Suri C, Jones PF, Patan S, Bartunkova S, Maisonpierre PC, Davis S, Sato TN, Yancopoulos GD. Requisite role of angiopoietin-1, a ligand for the TIE2 receptor, during embryonic angiogenesis. Cell 1997; 87:1161–1169.
44. Sato TN, Tozawa Y, Deutsch U, Wolburg-Buchholz K, Fujiwara Y, Gendron-Maguire M, Gridley T, Wolburg H, Risau W, Qin Y. Distinct roles of the receptor tyrosine kinases Tie-1 and Tie-2 in blood vessel formation. Nature 1995; 376:70–74.
45. Suri C, McClain J, Thurston G, McDonald DM, Zhou H, Oldmixon EH, Sato TN, Yancopoulos GD. Increased vascularization in mice overexpressing angiopoietin-1. Science 1998; 282:468–471.
46. Wojnowski L, Zimmer AM, Beck TW, Hahn H, Bernal R, Rapp UR, Zimmer A. Endothelial apoptosis in B-Raf-deficient mice. Nat Genet 1997; 16:293–297.
47. Puri MC, Rossant J, Alitalo K, Bernstein A, Partanen J. The receptor tyrosine kinase TIE is required for integrity and survival of vascular endothelial cells. EMBO J 1995; 14:5884–5891.
48. Patan S. TIE1 and TIE2 receptor tyrosine kinases inversely regulate embryonic angiogenesis by the mechanism of intussusceptive microvascular growth. Microvasc Res 1998; 56:1–21.
49. Partanen J, Puri MC, Schwartz L, Fischer K-D, Bernstein A, Rossant J. Cell autonomous functions of the receptor tyrosine kinsae TIE in a late phase of angiogenic capillary growth and endothelial cell survival during murine development. Development 1996; 122:3013–3021.
50. Pardanaud L, Yassine F, Dieterlen-Lièvre F. Relationship between vasculogenesis, angiogenesis and haemopoiesis during avian ontogeny. Development 1989; 105: 473–485.
51. Benjamin LE, Keshet E. Conditional switching of vascular endothelial growth factor (VEGF) expression in tumors: Induction of endothelial cell shedding and regression of hemangioblastoma-like vessels by VEGF withdrawal. Proc Natl Acad Sci U S A 1997; 94:8761–8766.
52. Alon T, Hemo I, Itin A, Pe'er J, Stone J, Keshet E. Vascular endothelial growth factor acts as a survival factor for newly formed retinal vessels and has implications for retinopathy of prematurity. Nat Med 1995; 1:1024–1028.
53. Partanen J, Mäkelä TP, Alitalo R, Lehväslaiho H, Alitalo K. Putative tyrosine kinases expressed in K-562 human leukemia cells. Proc Natl Acad Sci U S A 1990; 87:8913–8917.
54. Armstrong E, Korhonen J, Silvennoinen O, Cleveland JL, Lieberman MA, Alitalo R. Expression of tie receptor tyrosine kinase in leukemia cell lines. Leukemia 1993; 7:1585–1591.
55. Hashiyama M, Iwama A, Ohshiro K, Kurozumi K, Yasunaga KS, Masuho Y, Matsuda I, Yamaguchi N, Suda T. Predominant expression of a receptor tyrosine kinase, TIE, in hematopoietic stem cells and B-cells. Blood 1996; 87:93–101.
56. Kukk E, Wartiovaara U, Gunji Y, Kaukonen J, Buhring HJ, Rappold I, Matikainen MT, Vihko P, Partanen J, Palotie A, Alitalo K, Alitalo R. Analysis of Tie receptor

tyrosine kinase in hematopoietic progenitor and leukemia cells. Br J Haematol 1997; 98:195–203.
57. Shalaby F, Rossant J, Yamaguchi TP, Gertsenstein M, Wu XF, Breitman ML, Schuh AC. Failure of blood island formation and vasculogenesis in Flk-1-deficient mice. Nature 1995; 376:62–66.
58. Asahara T, Murohara T, Sullivan A, Silver M, van der Zee R, Li T, Witzenbichler B, Schatteman G, Isner JM. Isolation of putative progenitor endothelial cells for angiogenesis. Science 1997; 275:964–967.
59. Plate KH, Breier G, Weich HA, Risau W. Vascular endothelial growth factor is a potential tumor angiogenesis factor in human gliomas *in vivo*. Nature 1992; 359: 845–848.
60. Kim KJ, Li B, Winer J, Armanini M, Gillett N, Phillips HS, Ferrara N. Inhibition of vascular endothelial growth factor induced angiogenesis suppresses tumour growth in vivo. Nature 1993; 362:841–844.
61. Millauer B, Shawver L, Plate K, Risau W, Ullrich A. Glioblastoma growth inhibited in vivo by a dominant-negative Flk-1 mutant. Nature 1994; 367:576–579.
62. Salven P, Joensuu H, Heikkilä P, Matikainen MT, Wasenius VM, Alanko A, Alitalo K. Endothelial Tie growth factor receptor provides antigenic marker for assessment of breast cancer angiogenesis. Br J Cancer 1996; 74:69–72.
63. Kaipainen A, Vlaykova T, Hatva E, Böhling T, Jekunen A, Pyrhönen S, Alitalo K. Enhanced expression of the Tie receptor tyrosine kinase gene in the vascular endothelium of metastatic melanomas. Cancer Res 1994; 54:6571–6577.
64. Hatva E, Kaipainen A, Mentula P, Jääskeläinen J, Paetau A, Haltia M, Alitalo K. Expression of endothelial cell-specific receptor tyrosine kinases and growth factors in human brain tumors. Am J Pathol 1995; 146:368–378.
65. Hatva E, Jääskelainen J, Hirvonen H, Alitalo K, Haltia M. Tie endothelial cell-specific receptor tyrosine kinase is upregulated in the vasculature of arteriovenous malformations. J Neuropathol Exp Neurol 1996; 55:1124–1133.
66. Lin P, Polverini P, Dewhirst M, Shan S, Rao PS, Peters K. Inhibition of tumor angiogenesis using a soluble receptor establishes a role for Tie-2 in pathologic vascular growth. J Clin Invest 1997; 100:2072–2078.
67. Stratmann A, Risau W, Plate KH. Cell type-specific expression of angiopoietin-1 and angiopoietin-2 suggests a role in glioblastoma angiogenesis. Am J Pathol 1998; 153:1459–1466.
68. Koblizek TI, Weiss C, Yancopoulos GD, Deutsch U, Risau W. Angiopoietin-1 induces sprouting angiogenesis in vitro. Curr Biol 1998; 8:529–532.
69. Thurston G, Suri C, Smith K, McClain J, Sato TN, Yancopoulos GD, McDonald DM. Leakage-resistant blood vessels in mice transgenically overexpressing angiopoietin-1. Science 1999; 286:2511–2514.
70. Thurston G, Rudge JS, Ioffe E, Zhou H, Ross L, Croll SD, Glazer N, Holash J, McDonald DM, Yancopoulos GD. Angiopoietin-1 protects the adult vasculature against plasma leakage. Nat Med 2000; 6:460–463.

13
Vascular Endothelial Growth Factor Receptors

Arja Kaipainen, Eija Korpelainen, and Kari Alitalo
Haartman Institute, University of Helsinki, Helsinki, Finland

I. INTRODUCTION

A. Molecular Characterization

The specific angiogenic effects of the (vascular endothelial growth factor) VEGFs are based on their effects on vascular endothelium through high-affinity receptors located on endothelial cell surfaces. To date, three endothelial-specific receptor tyrosine kinases with structural and functional similarities to the platelet-derived growth factor (PDGF)-receptor family (subclass III) have been identified. These three VEGF receptors VEGFR-1, -2, and -3 were originally named flt (fms-like tyrosine kinase); KDR (kinase insert-domain-containing receptor)/FLK-1 (fetal liver kinase-1); and FLT4, respectively (1). These receptors have seven immunoglobulin-like loops in their extracellular domain and a tyrosine kinase domain split by a kinase insert. Vascular endothelial growth factor binds both VEGFR-1 and VEGFR-2, but it is not known whether these receptors heterodimerize (2–6). The active form of VEGF is a homodimer, and the main isoforms (consisting of 121, 165, 189, and 206 amino acid residues) display a similar ability to induce endothelial cell proliferation (6–9). The second immunoglobulin homology domain of these receptors is critical for ligand binding. The deletion of the second immunoglobulin-like domain of VEGFR-1 completely abolishes the binding of VEGF (10). There are only a few reports concerning the relative binding of different forms of VEGF. However, Soker et al. have shown that the semaphorin/collapsin receptor neuropilin-1 selectively binds $VEGF_{165}$ by the exon 7-encoded sequences (11, 12). Vascular endothelial growth factor-B and PlGF (placenta growth factor) bind only VEGFR-1, and VEGF-C and VEGF-D can interact with both VEGFR-2 and VEGFR-3 (13–20). Vascular endothelial growth factor forms heterodimers with VEGF-B and PlGF, and natural PlGF/VEGF heterodimers from a rat glioma cell line showed mitogenic activity toward endothelial cells (14, 17, 21). In addition to the high-affinity receptors, certain splice isoforms of VEGFs also bind heparan sulfate proteoglycans (HSPG) on the cell surface and in the pericellular matrix. Unlike for the fibroblast growth factors, HSPG binding is not required for ligand or receptor activation.

Human genes encoding VEGFR-1, -2, and -3 are located in chromosomal regions 13q12–q13, 4q11–q13, and 5q33–q35, respectively (22–25). Mouse homologues for VEGFR-1 and -2 have been mapped to chromosome 5 (23, 26, 27). A theory has been suggested for the evolution of the class III receptor tyrosine kinases (RTKs), in which an ancestral chromosome accommodating a seven and a five immunoglobulin homology domain-containing receptor (of subclass III) underwent a *cis*- and subsequent *trans*-duplication, resulting in the present gene family (23).

VEGFR-1 gene was first cloned from a human placental cDNA library (28), followed by the cloning of the mouse and rat homologues (29–32). VEGFR-2 gene was cloned from a human endothelial cell cDNA library (4, 26). Mouse (6, 27, 32, 33), rat (34), and quail (35) homologues also have been isolated. Vascular endothelial growth factor receptor-3 was cloned from human erythroleukemia cell and placental cDNA libraries (22, 36–38). Mouse (29) and quail (designated Quek2) (35) homologues of VEGFR-3 were subsequently identified from embryonic cDNA libraries. VEGFR-3 shows approximately 35% amino acid identity with VEGFR-1 and -2 in the extracellular domain and about 80% in the tyrosine kinase domain (36).

The VEGFR-1 receptor is a 180 kDa transmembrane glycoprotein, but its mRNA also can be spliced to produce a shorter soluble protein, lacking the seventh immunoglobulin-like domain as well as the transmembrane and intracellular domains (28, 39). This RNA splicing variant, originally detected in human umbilical vein endothelial cell (HUVEC) cDNA library encodes 31 unique amino acid residues before terminating in a stop codon (39). Another possible, alternatively spliced form differing in the COOH terminal region was reported by de Vries et al. (3). VEGFR-2 is a 200 kDa protein, and no alternatively spliced forms have been reported for this receptor. In VEGFR-3, alternative 3′ polyadenylation signals result in a 4.5 kb transcript and a more prevalent 5.8 kb transcript. The latter encodes 65 additional amino acid residues and is the major form detected in tissues. After its biosynthesis, the glycosylated 195 kDa VEGFR-3 on the cell surface is proteolytically cleaved at Arg472-Ser473, but the two chains remain linked by disulfide bonds (16, 36, 40) (Fig. 1).

Because hypoxia is a major regulator of VEGF expression, the regulation of the VEGFR genes by hypoxia has been investigated (41, 42), but the results

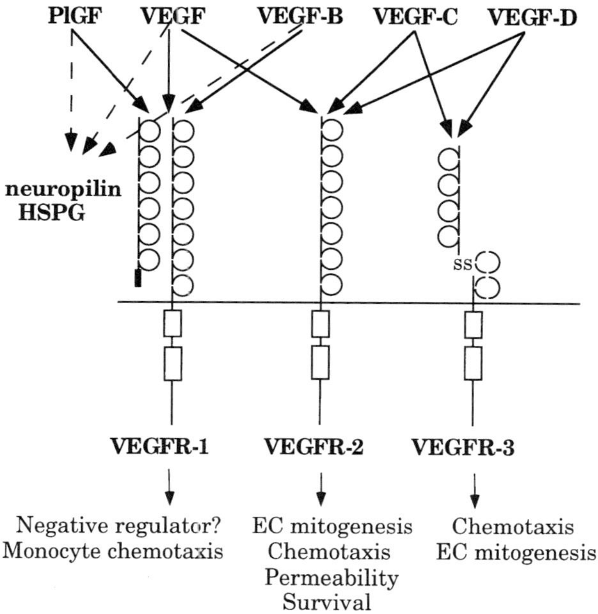

Figure 1 VEGFR interactions and signaling responses. *Abbreviations: VEGF*, vascular endothelial growth factor; *VEGFR*, vascular endothelial growth factor receptor; *PlgF*, placenta growth factor; *HSPG*, heparan sulfate proteoglycans; *EC*, endothelial cell.

remain controversial (43–46). However when adult mice were exposed to hypoxia, expression of VEGFR-1, but not VEGFR-2, was induced in endothelial cells of lung, heart, brain, kidney, and liver (47). These in vivo data support in vitro data of VEGFR-1 up-regulation by a hypoxia-inducible enhancer element located in its promoter (45).

B. VEGFR Signaling

Signaling pathways responsible for the biological activities of the VEGF family members are beginning to be elucidated. There is increasing evidence that VEGF stimulates some of the main signal transduction pathways, such as the phospholipase C-γ-protein kinase C (PLC-γ-PKC) pathway and the mitogen-activated protein kinase (MAPK) pathway (48–51). As most signal transduction studies have been carried out using endothelial cells that express more than one type of

VEGFR, it is not possible to attribute the results to a particular receptor. Attempts to study signal transduction by individual receptors using transfected cells have been compromised by the lack of a proper cellular background, which has turned out to be an important factor in VEGFR signaling. The heterogeneity of endothelial cells is another variable in the signal transduction studies. As a result, the signaling mechanisms discovered may offer possible targets for therapeutic intervention.

Like other receptor tyrosine kinases, VEGFRs are thought to dimerize upon ligand binding and undergo transautophosphorylation. Both VEGFR-2 and VEGFR-3 show strong tyrosine phosphorylation when stimulated with their respective ligands (6, 15, 52), but VEGFR-1 autophosphorylation is less obvious and has been reported only in transfected cells (3, 48, 52, 53). Four autophosphorylation sites have been detected in the bacterially expressed cytoplasmic domain of VEGFR-2 (54). Phosphorylated tyrosine residues serve to control the kinase activity of the receptor and to create docking sites for cytoplasmic signaling molecules, which are often substrates for the kinase. These molecules, either adapters or enzymes themselves, link VEGFRs to the signaling pathways discussed below.

Activation of MAP kinase in response to VEGF has been observed in both bovine brain capillary endothelial cells and rat liver sinusoidal endothelial cells (48, 50). It is likely to be mediated by VEGFR-2, as this receptor, but not VEGFR-1, can activate MAPK when transfected into NIH-3T3 fibroblasts (55). Interestingly, MAPK activation was delayed and the mitogenic response was weaker in fibroblasts than in endothelial cells, suggesting involvement of cell type-specific signaling mechanism(s) (55). The role of Ras remains to be elucidated. Seetharam et al. (48) observed activation of the guanine nucleotide exchange factor Sos in endothelial cells, but phosphorylation of the adapter protein Shc was barely detectable (48). Interestingly, activation of MAPK in bovine brain capillary endothelial cells by VEGF was selectively inhibited by the 16 kD N-terminal fragment of prolactin, an antiangiogenic factor that also inhibited the proliferation of these cells (50). Several investigators have reported phosphorylation of the Ras GTPase-activating protein (GAP) after VEGF stimulation in endothelial cells (48, 49, 52). This phosphorylation also has been observed in NIH-3T3 fibroblasts and porcine aortic endothelial cells transfected with VEGFR-1, whereas in contrast, these cells showed no clear MAPK activation or proliferation in response to VEGF (48, 52).

Recently, the PLC-γ-PKC pathway has been implicated in the mitogenic action of VEGF. Several groups have reported the VEGF-induced phosphorylation and activation of PLC-γ (48–51, 55) resulting in hydrolysis of phosphatidyl inositol 4,5-bisphosphate to diacylglycerols (DAGs) and inositol 1,4,5-trisphosphate (IP3). Inositol 1,4,5-trisphosphate is likely to be responsible for the increase in intracellular Ca^{2+} after VEGF stimulation (3, 56), whereas DAG activates PKC. Vascular endothelial growth factor selectively activates Ca^{2+}-sensitive PKC isoforms α and β2 in bovine aortic endothelial cells (BAEC), and the mitogenic effect of VEGF could be inhibited by a PKC-β selective inhibitor LY333531 in these cells (51). Interestingly, PKC has been implicated in VEGF-induced MAPK activation in VEGFR-2-transfected NIH-3T3 fibroblasts (55). Xia et al. have reported activation of the phosphoinositol-3 kinase (PI3-K) in response to VEGF and showed that this is not required for mitogenesis or activation of PKC (51). Recently PI3-K was implicated in antiapoptotic signaling (57, 58), and it is tempting to speculate that it may play a role in VEGF-delivered survival signals in immature vessels (59). Both PLC-γ and PI3-K activation in response to VEGF has been studied in porcine aortic endothelial cells transfected with either VEGFR-1 or VEGFR-2. In both cases, VEGF failed to activate PLC-γ and PI3-K (52). The reason for this discrepancy is not clear at present, but it may be due to different cellular backgrounds.

Signal transduction by VEGFR-3 was first studied using CSF-1R/VEGFR-3 chimeras, as VEGF-C—the natural ligand for VEGFR-3—was cloned only recently (15). When expressed in fibroblasts, the chimeric receptor underwent tyrosine phosphorylation and elicited a mitogenic response in response to CSF-1 (60–62). Only the chimera containing the cytoplasmic tail of the long isoform of VEGFR-3 was able to mediate anchorage-independent growth in soft agar and tumorigenicity in nude mice (61, 62), suggesting that the two isoforms have different signal transduction properties. The longer form exhibited higher autophosphorylation capacity (62), possibly because of the additional tyrosyl autophosphorylation sites present in its C-terminus (60). Although both forms bound to and phosphorylated Shc, phosphorylation levels were higher in cells expressing the long isoform (60–62). This difference was attributed to the Tyr1337 residue in the long isoform, as mutation of this residue to phenylalanine reduced Shc phosphorylation to the level of the short isoform (62). It is interesting that the same mutation also abolished colony growth in soft agar and tumorigenicity in nude mice (62), suggesting that Shc may be involved in mediating these responses. The authors hypothesize that although both isoforms can bind Shc through its SH2 domain, the crucial interaction is mediated by Tyr1337 and the phosphotyrosine binding (PTB) domain of Shc. Pajusola et al. (60) showed that activation of the long VEGFR-3 form also led to the phosphorylation of a 130 kD protein associated with Shc. Both isoforms were able to bind Grb2 in an inducible manner, and this interaction was mediated by the SH2 domain of Grb2 (60, 62). Similarly, both isoforms bound to GST-SH2(PLC-γ) fusion protein upon stimulation (60, 61). In contrast, no interaction was observed between the PI3-K SH2 domain and the two isoforms, and no PI3-K acivity could be detected in receptor immunoprecipitates (61).

C. Expression of VEGF Receptors in Tumors

VEGFR-1 and VEGFR-2 are expressed in vascular endothelium, whereas VEGFR-3 is found mainly in lymphatic endothelium (63, 64). Only a few melanomas and leukemias have been shown to aberrantly express any of these receptors (22, 65–67). Although the detailed molecular basis of the ''angiogenic switch'' is unknown, a prime candidate for the main inducer of tumor angiogenesis is VEGF. VEGF is expressed in all tumor cells studied and its receptor, VEGFR-2, is expressed by tumor-associated vasculature, suggesting a paracrine interaction (e.g., in the brain tumors listed in Table 1) (1). VEGFR-2 expression is most prominent in endothelia at the borders of the tumors, whereas VEGF mRNA is found around necrotic areas. Tumor hypoxia up-regulates VEGF expression, which in turn appears to induce VEGFR-2 expression in the endothelium (44, 68).

Autocrine VEGF ligand and receptor expression was shown to occur in angiosarcomas (69). Expression of VEGF and its receptors correlates with the degree of vascularization of many tumors (68, 70–76) and both have been shown to be good prognostic indicators of metastatic risk (77–79). Studies in animal models have illustrated the dependence of tumor vascularization and progression on VEGFR-2 signaling; a retrovirus encoding a dominant negative mutant of VEGFR-2 used to infect endothelial target cells in vivo was found to prevent

Table 1 In Situ Hybridization of VEGF and Its Receptors in Brain Tumors

No.	Tissue	VEGF	VEGFR2	VEGFR1	VEGFR3	vWF
1	Control brain, samples 1,2	−/+	−	−/+	−	−/+
2	Grade II oligoastrocytoma	+	−	+	−	−
3	Grade III astrocytoma	+	++	++	−	++
4	GBM, samples 1–3	*/+++	*/++	+++	−	*/++
5	Tissue next to GBM	+++	+	++	−	++
6	Grade I meningeoma	−/++	−/++	−/++	−	+
7	Grade II meningeoma	++	++	++	−	++
8	Melanoma metastasis	++	++	+++	−	++
9	Tissue next to metastasis	++	+	+	−	++
10	HP, samples 1–4	+/++	+/++	++	−	+/++
11	HB, EC	−	+++	++++	−	++
	HB, SC	++++	++	++	−	−

Adapted from Refs. 73, 76.

Abbreviations: *VEGF*, vascular endothelial growth factor; *VEGFR*, vascular endothelial growth factor receptor; −/+, signal indistinguishable from background; +, low level of expression; ++ to ++++ increasing level of expression; * not studied; *vWf*, von Willebrand factor; *GBM*, glioblastoma multiforme; *HP*, hemangiopericytoma; *HB*, hemangioblastoma; *EC*, endothelial cell; *SC*, stromal cell.

glioblastoma vascularization and growth in nude mice (80). Later, the study was extended to other types of tumors as well and in most cases, tumor growth was inhibited (81). Because the dominant negative VEGFR-2 could inhibit angiogenesis in vivo, compounds that reduce the tyrosine kinase activity of VEGFR-2 also should block its activity. Strawn et al. (82) have shown that two VEGFR-2 kinase inhibitors, SU1433 and SU1498, can prevent angiogenesis in chorioallantoic membrane assays.

The extent of VEGFR-1 involvement in tumor angiogenesis is unknown, but the receptor is not consistently up-regulated in tumors. The soluble VEGFR-1 form is composed of the six N-terminal extracellular ligand-binding domains generated by alternative transcription (39). The ability of soluble VEGFR-1 protein to inhibit tumor growth is presumably the result of paracrine inhibition of tumor angiogenesis in vivo, because tumor cell proliferation is not affected in vitro (83). The soluble form probably acts as a physiological down-regulator of VEGF by sequestering VEGF and by functioning in a dominant negative fashion, forming inactive heterodimers with full-length VEGF receptors (39, 83).

So far, little is known about VEGFR-3 expression in tumor angiogenesis or lymphangiogenesis. However, VEGFR-3 is increased in lymphatic endothelium in metastatic lymph nodes and lymphangiomas (63). Overexpression of VEGF-C in the basal keratinocytes of transgenic mice induces the formation of hyperplastic lymphatic vessels (84), a phenomenon typical for lymphangiomas. The receptor is absent from vascular endothelia of various brain tumors (73, 76). Interestingly, VEGFR-3 monoclonal antibody specifically stains endothelial cells of lymphatic vessels and blood vessels in hemangioma, spindle cells in Kaposi's sarcoma, vessels around lymphoma and in situ breast carcinoma (85, 86).

D. The Biological Roles of VEGFRs During Vascular Development

The significance of VEGFR-signaling recently has been demonstrated using gene-targeted animals. In all cases, disruption of signaling through endothelial-specific receptor tyrosine kinases is lethal. In targeted null mutants of VEGFR-2, early differentiation of both endothelial cells and primitive hematopoietic cells is severely blocked, and no blood vessels are formed (87). Thus, VEGFR-2 may be first expressed in putative hemangioblasts from the AGM (aorta-gonad-mesonephros) region of mouse embryos, and this marker may allow the isolation of these cells (88, 89). VEGF may regulate their endothelial differentiation. Of mature hematopoietic cells, only monocytes have been shown to contain VEGFR-1 (90). In contrast, mouse embryos homozygous for a targeted mutation of the VEGFR-1 locus develop endothelial cells in both embryonic and extraembryonic locations, but they do not form normal vascular channels (91). Therefore, a consecutive expression of the two VEGF receptors appears to be necessary for controlled early vascular development. In the VEGFR-3 knock-out mice, vasculogenesis and angiogenesis occur, but the organization of large vessels is abnormal and embryos die at embryonic day 9.5 because of cardivascular failure (92). Thus, VEGFR-3 is necessary for proper cardiovascular blood vessel development before its expression shifts to the lymphatic endothelium.

REFERENCES

1. Klagsbrun M, D'Amore P. Vascular endothelial growth factor and its receptors. Cytokine Growth Factor Rev 1996; 7:259–270.
2. Vaisman N, Gospodarowicz D, Neufeld G. Characterization of the receptors for vascular endothelial growth factor. J Biol Chem 1990; 265:19461–19466.
3. DeVries C, Escobedo JA, Ueno H, Houck K, Ferrara N, Williams LT. The *fms*-like tyrosine kinase, a receptor for vascular endothelial growth factor. Science 1992; 255: 989–991.
4. Terman BI, Dougher-Vermazen M, Carrion ME, Dimitrov D, Armellino DC, Gospodarowicz D, Böhlen P. Identification of the KDR tyrosine kinase as a receptor for vascular endothelial cell growth factor. Biochem Biophys Res Comm 1992; 187:1579–1586.
5. Gitay-Goren H, Soker S, Vlodavsky I, Neufeld G. The binding of vascular endothelial growth factor to its receptors is dependent on cell surface-associated heparin-like molecules. J Biol Chem 1992; 267:6093–6098.
6. Millauer B, Wizigmann-Voos S, Schnürch H, Martinez R, Moller N-PH, Risau W, Ullrich A. High affinity VEGF binding and developmental expression suggest Flk-1 as a major regulator of vasculogenesis and angiogenesis. Cell 1993; 72:835–846.
7. Tischer E, Mitchell R, Hartman T, Silva M, Gospodarowicz D, Fiddes JC, Abraham JA. The human gene for vascular endothelial growth factor. Multiple protein forms are encoded through alternative exon splicing. J Biol Chem 1991; 266:11947–11954.
8. Houck KA, Ferrara N, Winer J, Cachianes G, Li B, Leung DW. The vascular endothelial growth factor family—identification of a fourth molecular species and characterization of alternative splicing of RNA. Mol Endocrinol 1991; 5:1806–1814.
9. Ferrara N, Houck K, Jakeman L, Leung DW. Molecular and biological properties of the vascular endothelial growth factor family of proteins. Endocrine Rev 1992; 13:18–32.
10. Davis-Smyth T, Chen H, Park J, Presta LG, Ferrara N. The second immunoglobulin-like domain of the VEGF tyrosine kinase receptor Flt-1 determines ligand binding and may initiate a signal transduction cascade. EMBO J 1996; 15:4919–4927.
11. Soker S, Fidder H, Neufeld G, Klagsbrun M. Characterization of novel vascular endothelial growth factor (VEGF) receptors on tumor cells that bind VEGF165 via its exon 7-encoded domain. J Biol Chem 1996; 271:5761–5767.
12. Soker S, Takashima S, Miao HQ, Neufeld G, Klagsbrun M. Neuropilin-1 is expressed by endothelial and tumor cells as an isoform-specific receptor for vascular endothelial growth factor. Cell 1998; 92:735–745.

13. Kendall RL, Wang G, DiSalvo J, Thomas KA. Specificity of vascular endothelial cell growth factor receptor ligand binding domains. Biochem Biophys Res Comm 1994; 201:326–330.
14. Park JE, Chen HH, Winer J, Houck KA, Ferrara N. Placental growth factor. Potentiation of vascular endothelial growth factor bioactivity, *in vitro* and *in vivo*, and high affinity binding to Flt-1 but not to Flk-1/KDR. J Biol Chem 1994; 269:25646–25654.
15. Joukov V, Pajusola K, Kaipainen A, Chilov D, Lahtinen I, Kukk E, Saksela O, Kalkkinen N, Alitalo K. A novel vascular endothelial growth factor, VEGF-C, is a ligand for the Flt4 (VEGFR-3) and KDR (VEGFR-2) receptor tyrosine kinases. EMBO J 1996; 15:290–298.
16. Lee J, Gray A, Yuan J, Louth S-M, Avraham H, Wood W. Vascular endothelial growth factor-related protein: A ligand and specific activator of the tyrosine kinase receptor Flt4. Proc Natl Acad Sci U S A 1996; 93:1988–1992.
17. Olofsson B, Pajusola K, Kaipainen A, Von Euler G, Joukov V, Saksela O, Orpana A, Pettersson RF, Alitalo K, Eriksson U. Vascular endothelial growth factor B, a novel growth factor for endothelial cells. Proc Natl Acad Sci U S A 1996a; 93: 2576–2581.
18. Olofsson B, Korpelainen E, Pepper MS, Mandriota SJ, Aase K, Kumar V, Gunji Y, Jeltsch MM, Shibuya M, Alitalo K, Eriksson U. Vascular endothelial growth factor B (VEGF-B) binds to VEGF receptor-1 and regulates plasminogen activator activity in endothelial cells. Proc Natl Acad Sci U S A 1998; 95:11709–11714.
19. Orlandini M, Marconcini L, Ferruzzi R, Oliviero S. Identification of a c-fos-induced gene that is related to the platelet-derived growth factor/vascular endothelial growth factor family. Proc Natl Acad Sci U S A 1996; 93:11675–11680.
20. Achen MG, Jeltsch M, Kukk E, Mäkinen T, Vitali A, Wilks AF, Alitalo K, Stacker SA. Vascular endothelial growth factor D (VEGF-D) is a ligand for the tyrosine kinases VEGF receptor 2 (Flk1) and VEGF receptor 3 (Flt4). Proc Natl Acad Sci U S A 1998; 95:548–553.
21. DiSalvo J, Bayne ML, Conn G, Kwok PW, Trivedi PG, Soderman DD, Palisi PM, Sullivan KA, Thomas KA. Purification and characterisation of a naturally occurring vascular endothelial growth factor. Placenta growth factor heterodimer. J Biol Chem 1995; 270:7717–7723.
22. Aprelikova O, Pajusola K, Partanen J, Armstrong E, Alitalo R, Bailey SK, McMahon J, Wasmuth J, Huebner K, Alitalo K. FLT4, a novel class III receptor tyrosine kinase in chromosome 5q33-qter. Cancer Res 1992; 52:746–748.
23. Rosnet O, Stephenson D, Mattei M-G, Marchetto S, Shibuya M, Chapman VM, Birnbaum D. Close physical linkage of the FLT1 and FLT3 genes on chromosome 13 in man and chromosome 5 in mouse. Oncogene 1993; 8:173–179.
24. Spritz RA, Strunk KM, Lee ST, Lu-Kuo JM, Ward DC, Le Paslier D, Altherr MR, Dorman TE, Moir DT. A YAC contig spanning a cluster of human type III receptor protein tyrosine kinase genes (PDGFRA-KIT-KDR) in chromosome segment 4q12. Genomics 1994; 22:431–436.
25. Sait SN, Dougher-Vermazen M, Shows TB, Terman BI. The kinase insert domain receptor gene (KDR) has been relocated to chromosome 4q11—>q12. Cytogenet Cell Genet 1995; 70:145–146.

26. Terman BI, Carrion ME, Kovacs E, Rasmussen BA, Eddy RL, Shows TB. Identification of a new endothelial cell growth factor receptor tyrosine kinase. Oncogene 1991; 6:1677–1683.
27. Matthews W, Jordan CT, Gavin M, Jenkins NA, Copeland NG, Lemischka IR. A receptor tyrosine kinase cDNA isolated from a population of enriched primitive hematopoetic cells and exhibiting close genetic linkage to c-kit. Proc Natl Acad Sci U S A 1991; 88:9026–9030.
28. Shibuya M, Yamaguchi S, Yamane A, Ikeda T, Tojo A, Matsushime H, Sato M. Nucleotide sequence and expression of a novel human receptor type tyrosine kinase gene (flt) closely related to the fms family. Oncogene 1990; 5:519–524.
29. Finnerty H, Kelleher K, Morris GE, Bean K, Merberg DM, Kriz R, Morris JC, Sookdeo H, Turner KJ, Wood C, R. Molecular cloning of murine FLT and FLT4. Oncogene 1993; 8:2293–2298.
30. Choi K, Wall C, Hanratty R, Keller G. Isolation of a gene encoding a novel receptor tyrosine kinase from differentiated embryonic stem cells. Oncogene 1994; 9:1261–1266.
31. Yamane A, Seetharam L, Yamaguchi S, Gotoh N, Takahashi T, Neufeld G, Shibuya M. A new communication system between hepatocytes and sinusoidal endothelial cells in liver through vascular endothelial growth factor and Flt tyrosine kinase receptor family (Flt-1 and KDR/Flk-1). Oncogene 1994; 9:2683–2690.
32. Macchiarini P, Fontanini G, Hardin MJ, Squartini F, Angeletti CA. Relation of neovascularisation to metastasis of non-small-cell lung cancer. Lancet 1992; 340: 145–146.
33. Oelrichs RB, Reid HH, Bernard O, Ziemiecki A, Wilks AF. *NYK/FLK*-1: A putative receptor protein tyrosine kinase isolated from E10 embryonic neuroepithelium is expressed in endothelial cells of the developing embryo. Oncogene 1993; 8:11–18.
34. Sarzani R, Arnaldi G, De Pirro R, Moretti P, Schiaffino S, Rappelli A. A novel endothelial tyrosine kinase cDNA homologous to platelet-derived growth factor receptor dDNA. Biochem Biophys Res Commun 1992; 186:706–714.
35. Eichmann A, Marcelle C, Bréant C, Le Douarin NM. Two molecules related to the VEGF receptor are expressed in early endothelial cells during avian embryonic development. Mech Dev 1993; 42:33–48.
36. Pajusola K, Aprelikova O, Korhonen J, Kaipainen A, Pertovaara L, Alitalo R, Alitalo K. FLT4 receptor tyrosine kinase contains seven immunoglobulin-like loops and is expressed in multiple human tissues and cell lines. Cancer Res 1992; 52: 5738–5743.
37. Galland F, Karamysheva A, Mattei M-G, Rosnet O, Marchetto S, Birnbaum D. Chromosomal localization of FLT4, a novel receptor-type tyrosine kinase gene. Genomics 1992; 13:475–478.
38. Galland F, Karamysheva A, Pebusque M-J, Borg J-P, Rottapel R, Dubreuil P, Rosnet O, Birnbaum D. The *FLT4* gene encodes a transmembrane tyrosine kinase related to the vascular endothelial growth factor receptor. Oncogene 1993; 8:1233–1240.
39. Kendall RL, Thomas KA. Inhibition of vascular endothelial cell growth factor activity by an endogenously encoded soluble receptor. Proc Natl Acad Sci U S A 1993; 90:10705–10709.

40. Pajusola K, Aprelikova O, Armstrong E, Morris S, Alitalo K. Two human FLT4 receptor tyrosine kinase isoforms with distinct carboxyterminal tails are produced by alternative processing of primary transcripts. Oncogene 1993; 8:2931–2937.
41. Brogi E, Schatteman G, Wu T, Kim EA, Varticovski L, Keyt B, Isner JM. Hypoxia-induced paracrine regulation of vascular endothelial growth factor receptor expression. J Clin Invest 1996; 97:469–476.
42. Waltenberger J, Mayr U, Pentz S, Hombach V. Functional upregulation of the vascular endothelial growth factor receptor KDR by hypoxia. Circulation 1996; 94:1647–1654.
43. Sandner P, Wolf K, Bergmaier U, Gess B, Kurtz A. Induction of VEGF and VGEF recpetor gene expression by hypoxia: Divergent regulation *in vivo* and *in vitro*. Kidney Int 1997; 51:448–453.
44. Kremer C, Breier G, Risau W, Plate KH. Up-regulation of flk-1/vascular endothelial growth factor receptor 2 by its ligand in a cerebral slice culture system. Cancer Res 1997; 57:3852–3859.
45. Gerber HP, Condorelli F, Park J, Ferrara N. Differential transcriptional regulation of the two vascular endothelial growth factor receptor genes. J Biol Chem 1997; 272:23659–23667.
46. Marti HH, Wenger RH, Rivas LA, Straumann U, Digicaylioglu M, Henn V, Yonekawa Y, Bauer C, Gassmann M. Erythropoietin gene expression in human, monkey and murine brain. Eur J Neurosci 1996; 8:666–676.
47. Marti HH, Risau W. Systemic hypoxia changes the organ-specific distribution of vascular endothelial growth factor and its receptors. Proc Natl Acad Sci 1998; 95: 15809–15814.
48. Seetharam L, Gotoh N, Maru Y, Neufeld G, Yamaguchi S, Shibuya M. A unique signal transduction from FLT tyrosine kinase, a receptor for vascular endothelial growth factor (VEGF). Oncogene 1995; 10:135–147.
49. Guo D, Jia Q, Song HY, Warren RS, Donner DB. Vascular endothelial cell growth factor promotes tyrosine phosphorylation of mediators of signal transduction that contain SH2 domains. Association with endothelial cell proliferation. J Biol Chem 1995; 270:6729–6733.
50. D'Angelo G, Struman I, Martial J, Weiner RI. Activation of mitogen-activated protein kinases by vascular endothelial growth factor and basic fibroblast growth factor in capillary endothelial cells is inhibited by the antiangiogenic factor 16-kDa N-terminal fragment of prolactin. Proc Natl Acad Sci U S A 1995; 92:6374–6378.
51. Xia P, Aiello LP, Ishii H, Jiang ZY, Park DJ, Robinson GS, Takagi H, Newsome WP, Jirousek MR, King GL. Characterization of vascular endothelial growth factor's effect on the activation of protein kinase C, its isoforms, and endothelial cell growth. J Clin Invest 1996; 98:2018–2026.
52. Waltenberger J, Claesson-Welsh L, Siegbahn A, Shibuya M, Heldin C-H. Different signal transduction properties of KDR and Flt1, two receptors for vascular endothelial growth factor. J Biol Chem 1994; 269:26988–26995.
53. Sawano A, Takahashi T, Yamaguchi S, Aonuma M, Shibuya M. Flt-1 but not KDR/Flk-1 tyrosine kinase is a receptor for placenta growth factor, which is related to vascular endothelial growth factor. Cell Growth Differ 1996; 7:213–221.
54. Dougher-Vermazen M, Hulmes JD, Böhlen P, Terman BI. Biological activity and

phosphorylation sites of the bacterially expressed cytosolic domain of the KDR VEGF-receptor. Biochem Biophys Res Commun 1994; 205:728–738.
55. Takahashi T, Shibuya M. The 230 kDa mature form of KDR/Flk-1 activates the PLC-gamma pathway and partially induces mitotic signals in NIH3T3 fibroblasts. Oncogene 1997; 14:2079–2089.
56. Plouet J, Moukadiri H. Specific binding of vasculotropin to bovine brain capillary endothelial cells. Biochimie 1990; 72:51–55.
57. Kauffmann-Zeh A, Rodriquez-Viciana P, Ulrich E, Gilbert C, Coffer P, Downward J, Evan G. Suppression of c-Myc-induced apoptosis by Ras signalling through PI(3)K and PKB. Nature 1997; 385:544–548.
58. Kennedy SG, Wagner AJ, Conzen SD, Jordan J, Bellacosa A, Tsichlis PN, Hay N. The PI3-kinase/Akt signalling pathway delivers an anti-apoptotic signal. Genes Dev. 1997; 11:701–713.
59. Alon T, Hemo I, Itin A, Pe'er J, Stone J, Keshet E. Vascular endothelial growth factor acts as a survival factor for newly formed retinal vessels and has implications for retinopathy of prematurity. Nat Med. 1995; 1:1024–1028.
60. Pajusola K, Aprelikova O, Pelicci G, Weich H, Claesson-Welsh L, Alitalo K. Signalling properties of FLT4, a proteolytically processed receptor tyrosine kinase related to two VEGF receptors. Oncogene 1994; 9:3545–3555.
61. Borg J-P, deLapeyrière O, Noguchi T, Rottapel R, Dubreuil P, Birnbaum D. Biochemical characterization of two isoforms of FLT4, a VEGF receptor-related tyrosine kinase. Oncogene 1995; 10:973–984.
62. Fournier E, Dubreuil P, Birnbaum D, Borg JP. Mutation at tyrosine residue 1337 abrogates ligand-dependent transforming capacity of the FLT4 receptor. Oncogene 1995; 11:921–931.
63. Kaipainen A, Korhonen J, Mustonen T, van Hinsbergh VM, Fang G-H, Dumont D, Breitman M, Alitalo K. Expression of the fms-like tyrosine kinase FLT4 gene becomes restricted to endothelium of lymphatic vessels during development. Proc Natl Acad Sci U S A 1995; 92:3566–3570.
64. Wilting J, Birkenhäger R, Eichmann A, Kurz H, Martiny-Baron G, Marmé D, McCarthy JEG, Christ B, Weich HA. VEGF121 induces proliferation of vascular endothelial cells and expression of flk-1 without affecting lymphatic vessels of the chorioallantoic membrane. Dev Biol 1996; 176:76–85.
65. Liu B, Earl HM, Baban D, Shoaibi M, Fabra A, Kerr DJ, Seymour LW. Melanoma cell lines express VEGF receptor KDR and respond to exogenously added VEGF. Biochem Biophys Res Comm 1995; 217:721–727.
66. Cohen T, Gitay-Goren H, Sharon R, Shibuya M, Halaban R, Levi B-Z, Neufeld G. VEGF121, a vascular endothelial growth factor (VEGF) isoform lacking heparin binding ability, requires cell-surface heparan sulfates for efficient binding to the VEGF receptors of human melanoma cells. J Biol Chem 1995; 270:11322–11326.
67. Fiedler W, Graeven U, Süleyman E, Verago S, Kilic N, Stockschläder M, Hossfeld DK. Vascular endothelial growth factor, a possible paracrine growth factor in human acute myeloid leukemia. Blood 1997; 89:1870–1875.
68. Plate KH, Breier G, Weich HA, Risau W. Vascular endothelial growth factor is a potential tumour angiogenesis factor in human gliomas *in vivo*. Nature 1992; 359: 845–848.

69. Hashimoto M, Ohsawa M, Ohnishi A, Naka N, Hirota S, Kitamura Y, Aozasa K. Expression of vascular endothelial growth factor and its receptor mRNA in angiosarcoma. Lab Invest 1995; 73:859–863.
70. Brown LF, Berse B, Jackman RW, Tognazzi K, Manseau EJ, Dvorak HF, Senger DR. Increased expression of vascular permeability factor (vascular endothelial growth factor) and its receptors in kidney and bladder carcinomas. Am J Pathol 1993; 143:1255–1262.
71. Brown LF, Berse B, Jackman RW, Tognazzi K, Manseau EJ, Senger DR, Dvorak HF. Expression of vascular permeability factor (vascular endothelial growth factor) and its receptors in adenocarcinomas of the gastrointestinal tract. Cancer Res 1993; 53:4727–4735.
72. Brown LF, Berse B, Jackman RW, Tognazzi K, Guidi AJ, Dvorak HF, Senger DR, Connolly JL, Schnitt SJ. Expression of vascular permeability factor (vascular endothelial growth factor) and its receptors in breast cancer. Hum Pathol 1995; 26:86–91.
73. Hatva E, Kaipainen A, Mentula P, Jääskeläinen J, Paetau A, Haltia M, Alitalo K. Expression of endothelial cell-specific receptor tyrosine kinases and growth factors in human brain tumors. Am J Pathol 1995; 146:368–378.
74. Takahashi Y, Kitadai Y, Bucana CD, Cleary KR, Ellis LM. Expression of vascular endothelial growth factor and its receptor, KDR, correlates with vascularity, metastasis, and proliferation of human colon cancer. Cancer Res 1995; 55:3964–3968.
75. Warren RS, Yuan H, Matli MR, Gillett NA, Ferrara N. Regulation by vascular endothelial growth factor of human colon cancer tumorigenesis in a mouse model of experimental liver metastasis. J Clin Invest 1995; 95:1789–1797.
76. Hatva E, Bohling T, Jaaskelainen J, Persico MG, Haltia M, Alitalo K. Vascular growth factors and receptors in capillary hemangioblastomas and hemangiopericytomas. Am J Pathol 1996; 148:763–775.
77. Weidner N. Tumor angiogenesis: Review of current applications in tumor prognostication. Sem Diag Pathol 1993; 10:302–313.
78. Weidner N. Intratumor microvessel density as a prognostic factor in cancer [comment]. Am J Pathol 1995; 147:9–19.
79. Weidner N, Semple JP, Welch WR, Folkman J. Tumor angiogenesis and metastasis—correlation in invasive breast carcinoma. N Engl J Med 1991; 324:1–8.
80. Millauer B, Shawver L, Plate K, Risau W, Ullrich A. Glioblastoma growth inhibited in vivo by a dominant-negative Flk-1 mutant. Nature 1994; 367:576–579.
81. Millauer B, Longhi MP, Plate KH, Shawver LK, Risau W, Ullrich A, Strawn LM. Dominant-negative inhibition of Flk-1 suppresses the growth of many tumor types in vivo. Cancer Res 1996; 56:1615–1620.
82. Strawn LM, McMahon G, App H, Schreck R, Kuchler WR, Longhi MP, Hui TH, Tang C, Levitzki A, Gazit A, Chen I, Keri G, Orfi L, Risau W, Flamme I, Ullrich A, Hirth KP, Shawver LK. Flk-1 as a target for tumor growth inhibition. Cancer Res 1996; 56:3540–3545.
83. Goldman CK, Kendall RL, Cabrera G, Soroceanu L, Heike Y, Gillespie GY, Siegal GP, Mao X, Bett AJ, Huckle WR, Thomas KA, Curiel DT. Paracrine expression of a native soluble vascular endothelial growth factor receptor inhibits tumor growth, metastasis, and mortality rate. Proc Natl Acad Sci U S A 1998; 95:8795–8800.

84. Jeltsch M, Kaipainen A, Joukov V, Meng X, Lakso M, Rauvala H, Swartz M, Fukumura D, Jain R, Alitalo K. Vascular endothelial growth factor-C induces specific hyperplasia of lymphatic vessels in transgenic mice. Science 1997; 276: 1423–1425.
85. Jussila L, Valtola R, Partanen TA, Salven P, Heikkilä P, Matikainen M, Renkonen R, Kaipainen A, Detmar M, Tschachler E, Alitalo R, Alitalo K. Lymphatic endothelium and Kaposi's sarcoma spindle cells detected by antibodies against the vascular endothelial growth factor receptor-3. Cancer Res 1998; 58:1599–1604.
86. Lymboussaki A, Partanen TA, Olofsson B, Thomas-Crusells J, Fletcher CD, de Waal RM, Kaipainen A, Alitalo K. Expression of the vascular endothelial growth factor C receptor VEGFR-3 in lymphatic endothelium of the skin and in vascular tumors. Am J Pathol 1998; 153:395–403.
87. Shalaby F, Rossant J, Yamaguchi TP, Gertsenstein M, Wu XF, Breitman ML, Schuh AC. Failure of blood island formation and vasculogenesis in Flk-1-deficient mice. Nature 1995; 376:62–66.
88. Kennedy M, Firpo M, Choi K, Wall C, Robertson S, Kabrun N, Keller G. A common precursor for primitive erythropoiesis and definitive haematopoiesis. Nature 1997; 386:488–493.
89. Medvinsky A, Dzierzak E. Definitive hematopoiesis is autonomously initiated by the AGM region. Cell 1996; 86:897–906.
90. Clauss M, Gerlach M, Gerlach H, Brett J, Wang F, Familetti PC, Pan Y-CE, Olander JV, Connolly DT, Stern D. Vascular permeability factor: A tumor-derived polypeptide that induces endothelial cell and monocyte procoagulant activity and promotes monocyte migration. J Exp Med 1990; 172:1535–1545.
91. Fong GH, Rossant J, Gertsenstein M, Breitman ML. Role of the Flt-1 receptor tyrosine kinase in regulating the assembly of vascular endothelium. Nature 1995; 376: 66–70.
92. Dumont DJ, Jussila L, Taipale J, Lymboussaki A, Mustonen T, Pajusola K, Breitman M, Alitalo K. Cardiovascular failure in mouse embryos deficient in VEGF receptor-3. Science 1998; 282:946–949.

14

Regulation of Vascular Endothelial Growth Factor (VEGF) Expression

Ilan Stein and Eli Keshet
The Hebrew University–Hadassah Medical School, Jerusalem, Israel

I. GENERAL CONSIDERATIONS

The pivotal role that vascular endothelial growth factor (VEGF) plays as an initiator of neovascularization and its diverse biological activities are described in detail elsewhere in this book (see Chapter 11) and will not be reiterated here.

As a mediator of angiogenesis, VEGF acts in a paracrine fashion, that is, it is produced and secreted from the tissue toward which new blood vessels extend. A resultant VEGF gradient is "sensed" by nearby endothelial cells expressing cognate receptors, and transduction of the signal culminates in the induction of endothelial cell proliferation, migration, and tube formation. In principle, VEGF-mediated angiogenesis is likely to be regulated at both the ligand and receptor levels. In addition, VEGF-mediated responses might be modulated through regulated expression of natural inhibitors of angiogenesis. Although some studies suggest that regulation of VEGF receptors contributes significantly to the control of angiogenesis, current thought is that the main regulation is at the level of ligand expression. This is clearly seen in cases of compensatory angiogenesis in which the transition from a state of prolonged vascular quiescence to a swift angiogenic response is underlined by up-regulation of VEGF expression. This notion is also supported by findings that experimental overexpression of VEGF in different systems, including a system of developmental angiogenesis (1), results in an augmented angiogenic response (2, 3).

The fact that expression of VEGF is tightly regulated in vivo is reflected in many studies that show that a deviation from the normal levels of VEGF is detrimental to the vasculature. Perhaps the most dramatic case is the finding that a reduction of VEGF gene dosage by one half (in mice heterozygous for an inactivating mutation in VEGF) leads to severe vascular defects and early embryonic lethality (4, 5). Another example for the deleterious consequences of imbalances in VEGF expression are seen in the diabetic retina, where excessive production of VEGF during a process aimed to reinforce a compromised vascular system leads to a pathological vessel growth and retinopathy (6–8). Conversely, unscheduled down-regulation of VEGF expression results in obliteration of the newly formed vascular plexus (9).

To appreciate fully the multiple modes of VEGF regulation, it is important to note that VEGF is implicated in all major forms of neovascularization. Recent studies using mice with a deficient VEGF/VEGF receptor system have clearly shown that VEGF plays an essential role in vasculogenesis as well in sprouting and nonsprouting forms of angiogenesis. Likewise, VEGF plays a role in developmentally programmed neovascularization, in nonprogrammed angiogenesis in tumors, and in repair angiogenesis. The latter is defined as the formation of new blood vessels in the fully developed organism to compensate for injured or occluded vessels. Obviously, the triggers of these diverse forms of neovascularization are different. Thus, embryonic neovascularization, distinguished by formation of precise spatial vascular patterns, is governed by yet unidentified developmental cues; physiological angiogenesis is mostly driven by hormonal triggers or by the physiological consequences of tissue ischemia; and pathological angiogenesis is often triggered in a nonprogrammed fashion, primarily by stochastic genetic changes in tumors. Regulation of VEGF, according to the different triggers of neovascularization is discussed below.

The last section is concerned with molecular mechanisms of VEGF regulation, distinguishing transcriptional and posttranscriptional levels of regulation.

II. DEVELOPMENTAL, PHYSIOLOGICAL, AND PATHOLOGICAL SETTINGS OF VEGF INDUCTION

A. Developmental Regulation

During early embryonic development, VEGF is expressed predominantly by trophoblast and maternally derived cells. Later in development, VEGF expression is induced in a unique spatial manner, mostly in the endoderm juxtaposed to flk-1-positive mesodermal cells (10–12), suggesting that VEGF acts in a paracrine manner to induce vasculogenesis. A key unanswered question concerns the nature of signals that induce expression of VEGF in a unique spatial pattern. By analogy to other growth factors induced in a developmentally restricted cue, it is likely that VEGF is a downstream target of a yet unidentified signaling system.

In vitro studies have shown that VEGF expression is induced by several cytokines and growth factors (see below), including growth factors like basic fibroblast growth factor (bFGF) and transforming growth factor-alpha (TGF-α), which are themselves developmentally regulated. It is possible, therefore, that these growth factors mediate developmental regulation of VEGF.

Vascular endothelial growth factor also is involved in a non spatially patterned developmental angiogenesis—primarily expansion of the microvasculature during organogenesis. Examples include the formation of brain vessels by sprouting from perineural vessels in response to VEGF produced in the periventricular layer of the brain (10) and formation of the retina vasculature in response to VEGF produced by retinal glial cells (13). In the retinal system, subpathological levels of hypoxia caused by the onset of neuronal activity is detected by strategically located populations of neuroglia, first astrocytes, then Müller cells. In response, they secrete VEGF, inducing formation of the superficial and deep layers of retinal vessels, respectively (13). It appears, therefore, that at least some VEGF-mediated processes in the embryo are driven by hypoxia.

B. Hormonal Regulation

Angiogenesis is generally a quiescent process in the adult, healthy organism. A significant exception is the female reproductive system, in which the need for additional vasculature is constantly imposed by the periodic evolution of transient ovarian structures, such as ovarian follicles and corpora lutea (CL). Also, the endometrium undergoes a complex process of vascular proliferation, destruction, and regeneration with each menstrual cycle in preparation for implantation. Because these processes are initiated and controlled by cyclic release of hormones, it is assumed that neovascularization of these tissues is mediated by a hormonally regulated angiogenic factor.

In four processes of hormonally regulated angiogenesis, VEGF was found to be expressed in spatial and temporal proximity to the forming vasculature. Specifically, during follicular neovascularization, VEGF is induced by interstitial and peripheral theca layers; during formation of the CL vasculature, VEGF is produced by lutein cells; during neovascularization of the endometrium, VEGF is expressed throughout the endometrial stroma; and during vascularization of the decidua, VEGF is expressed in the decidua basalis (14–17). Altogether, VEGF was found to be expressed in at least 10 different steroidogenic or steroid-responsive cell types in vivo. Furthermore, in some cells up- regulation of VEGF expression is concurrent with the acquisition of steroidogenic activity, and expression in other cell types is restricted to a particular stage of the ovarian cycle (15).

Direct inducibility of uterine VEGF mRNA by 17β-estradiol (E2) was demonstrated in rats (18, 19). This steroid also induced VEGF expression in isolated human endometrial cells in vitro (20) and in endometrial carcinoma cell lines

(21). Interestingly, in all these cases, E2 induced VEGF expression within 1 hour, which is one of the most rapid physiological responses to estrogen.

The dynamic pattern of VEGF expression during the ovarian cycle suggests that VEGF expression is subjected to the regulatory role of gonadotropins. This is corroborated by evidence that suppression of gonadotropin secretion diminishes the increase in VEGF expression (22). Conversely, the use of a nonphysiological large dose of gonadotropins during ovulation induction therapy leads to excessive production of VEGF in the CL and, by virtue of its activity as a vascular permeability factor, to development of the ovarian hyperstimulation syndrome (OHSS). The latter is underlined by the shift of body fluids from the vascular bed into the extravascular space (23).

Another clinically important setting of hormonal VEGF regulation is hormone-dependent tumors. Examples include some thyroid cancers in which secretion of VEGF is stimulated by thyroid-stimulating hormone (TSH) (24) and androgen-dependent tumors in which withdrawal of androgen (by castration) inhibits tumor VEGF production (25). These findings may have important implications for antihormone tumor therapy, as they suggest the tumor vasculature as an additional target.

C. Regulation by Cytokines/Growth Factors

Regulation of VEGF expression by other cytokines and growth factors has been the subject of many in vitro studies. The list of cytokine and growth factors that up-regulate VEGF expression in a variety of cultured cells is extensive and includes the following: interleukin-1β (IL-1β), IL-6, epidermal growth factor (EGF), keratinocyte growth factor (KGF), insulin-like growth factor 1 (IGF-1), bFGF, platelet-derived growth factor-B (PDGF-B), TGF-α, TGF-β1, and tumor necrosis factor-α (TNF-α) (26–34).

The physiological or pathological significance of a given cytokine's potential to augment VEGF expression in cultured cells, most of them transformed, is unclear especially because in many cases, the in vivo pattern of VEGF expression is not coincidental with that of the given cytokine. Nevertheless, it is likely that at least some of these cytokines/growth factors function under certain pathological conditions. Notably, cytokines are likely to effect VEGF expression in the wound site, where expression of VEGF is significantly elevated in the hyperproliferative epithelium during wound healing. At least four cytokines present at the wound site (EGF, TGF-β1, KGF, and TNF-α) were shown to up-regulate VEGF in cultured human keratinocytes (29). Thus, in addition to their role in inducing re-epithelialization, these factors may indirectly promote neovascularization by up-regulating VEGF expression. A second example is at sites of atherosclerotic lesions, where factors like IL-1β and PDGF-BB are abundant and capable of inducing VEGF expression by smooth muscle cells. It is possible, therefore, that these factors accelerate progression of atherosclerotic lesions by promoting the development of new blood vessels (26, 32). A third example is highly malignant gliomas that overexpress EGF receptors and respond to EGF by increasing VEGF production (28). In this case, the EGF-VEGF regulatory link may contribute to a more angiogenic tumor phenotype.

D. Regulation by Hypoxia and Nutritional Stress

It has long been thought that that the driving force of compensatory angiogenesis is the condition of oxygen and nutrient deprivation resulting from insufficient perfusion. It is now well established that VEGF is the key angiogenic factor linking ischemia and compensatory angiogenesis. Here we focus on conditions of stress conducive for VEGF induction and on physiological and pathological settings of stress-induced, VEGF-mediated angiogenesis.

Initial findings have demonstrated that VEGF expression is up-regulated in hypoxic microenvironments of tumors whenever the rapid increase in tumor mass is not matched by accompanying neovascularization (35, 36). Experimental occlusion of particular vessels leads to up-regulation of VEGF expression in the region serviced by these vessels. For example, occlusion of major retinal vessels results in up-regulated VEGF expression in the ischemic retina (7). Occlusion of a major coronary artery leads to up-regulation of VEGF expression, specifically in the ischemic territory of the heart muscle, suggesting a role in natural formation of collaterals (37).

A large number of in vitro studies have shown that VEGF is hypoxia inducible in all cell types examined (35, 38–41). These findings are consistent with the putative role of VEGF in directing growth of vascular sprouts toward most, if not all, ischemic tissues. The possibility of an autocrine hypoxic response is suggested by findings that VEGF is also up-regulated in cultured endothelial cells exposed to hypoxia (40, 42) and that a newly discovered hypoxia-inducible transcription factor is preferentially expressed in endothelial cells in vivo (43). Yet, the physiological significance of these findings is not clear, considering the fact that endothelial cells are the cells closest to the oxygen source.

Although all cell types subjected to hypoxia eventually up-regulate VEGF expression, certain types of cells may function as specialized "hypoxia sensors," that is, cells with a lower threshold of hypoxic response than other cells within the same tissue. Specifically, astrocytes up-regulate VEGF production already at subpathological, developmentally generated levels of hypoxia (13) and are the first cells to respond to experimentally produced mild retinal ischemia (8). Neuronal cells up-regulate VEGF production only upon further increase in the level of hypoxia. Such hypoxic conditions may develop as a result of functional deterioration of retinal vessels, as in the case of proliferative diabetic retinopathy (PDR), obliteration of immature retinal vessels, as in the case of retinopathy of prematurity (ROP), and vascular occlusions, as in the case of a central retinal vein occlusion (CRVO). Hypoxic conditions resulting in up-regulated VEGF expression by the bulk of retinal cells lead to its excessive production and to accumulation of large amounts of VEGF in the vitreous, and result in retinopathy-associated vasculopathic growth (6–8, 44, 45).

In addition to hypoxia, acute glucose deprivation (an accompaniment of vascular insufficiency) also leads to VEGF induction (46). A fundamental question surrounds the conditions of stress that are conducive to VEGF induction. Multicell spheroids were used to simulate a clonal cell population in which gradients of oxygen, glucose, and other nutrients created a continuum of different microenvironments. Results uncovered a complex combinatorial relationship of oxygen and glucose deficiencies leading to VEGF induction. Importantly, VEGF is not induced in overstressed, metabolically compromised cells (46, 47). These findings suggest that the magnitude of the angiogenic response may depend on the nature of the insult (e.g., ischemia resulting from an abrupt vs. gradual occlusion of a major vessel). Different forms of stress also may account for the observation that the degree of collateral growth is highly variable among individuals.

Hypoxia-induced microvascular expansion operates to match vascular density to changes in oxygen supply. The other side of the coin in this process is hyperoxia-induced vascular regression. Neovascularization is often accompanied by a process of vascular "pruning," that is, elimination of some newly formed vascular loops. This process is induced after the initiation of flow through the newly formed vascular network and is thought to result from excess oxygen reaching the tissue (48). Exposure of an immature vascular system to hyperoxia leads to exaggerated vascular pruning and is, in fact, the cause of vascular obliteration associated with ROP. Studies have shown that vascular pruning is also mediated by VEGF, although in this case by its activity as a survival factor for immature vessels. Thus, vessels regress when hyperoxia suppresses VEGF expression to a level lower than the one required to sustain newly formed vessels (9).

E. Regulation of VEGF in Tumors

In many tumors, VEGF production is significantly increased relative to the nontransformed cell counterpart. This has been shown for tumors of diverse origins and in cases too numerous to specify here. Analysis of certain human tumors has suggested a gross correlation between augmented VEGF expression and increased tumor vascularity. Thus, VEGF is considered a major contributor to tumor angiogenesis; hence, it is a possible target for antiangiogenic tumor therapy. The role of VEGF in tumor angiogenesis is described in part 4 (Part 4: Regulation of Angiogenesis, p xx). Here we highlight one aspect of VEGF regulation in tumors, namely, the relative contributions of genetic versus environmental factors. Tumor angiogenesis is generally viewed as a consequence of a genetic ''angiogenic switch,'' that is, a stochastic genetic change that leads to up-regulated expression of a positive angiogenesis stimulator (49). With regard to VEGF, some of the most commonly encountered genetic changes detected in human cancers, such as activating mutations in *ras* and mutations in the P53 tumor suppressor gene, are accompanied by marked up-regulation of VEGF expression and a loss of the ability to potentiate protein kinase C (PKC)-induced VEGF expression, respectively (50, 51). Thus, enhanced VEGF-mediated angiogenesis might accompany common mutations in oncogenes and tumor suppressors rather than be the result of independent mutations taking place during tumor progression.

Irrespective of the above genetic changes, tumor cells, like their normal counterparts, are able to ''sense'' ischemia and respond by up-regulating VEGF expression. Therefore, stress-induced angiogenesis is an important component of tumor neovascularization, independent of angiogenic activities produced by a genetic switch. Indeed, in situ analyses of tumor biopsies have shown that VEGF is up-regulated in hypoxic tumor regions to a level significantly higher than in normoxic regions (35, 36). A compelling piece of evidence for the importance of stress-induced angiogenesis is the finding that when the ability to up-regulate VEGF by hypoxia is prevented (through the use of cells lacking the obligatory hypoxia-inducible factor [HIF]-1 partner, aryl hydrocarbon receptor nuclear translocator (ARNT, [see below]), tumor growth is greatly retarded (P. Ratcliffe, personal communication).

III. MECHANISMS OF VEGF REGULATION

Of the different modes of VEGF regulation described above, information is scanty regarding the mechanism of regulation by hormones or other cytokines/growth factors. Experiments using phorbol esters and cyclic adenosine monophosphate (cAMP) analogues indicated that VEGF mRNA expression is stimulated by both the PKC and PKA-mediated pathways (52). A limited promoter analysis has suggested the involvement of particular transcription factors in the cytokine/growth factor response, specifically, the requirement for AP-2-dependent binding and transactivation in the response to TGFα (53), and the role of SP-1 in the response to TNFα (54). However, a more comprehensive structure-function analysis of the VEGF promoter/enhancer is required to elucidate the mechanisms of its regulation by these factors.

In contrast, recent studies have provided important insights into the mechanism of VEGF regulation by hypoxia. The increase in steady-state levels of VEGF mRNA under hypoxic conditions is the result of both transcriptional activation and mRNA stabilization. It appears that hypoxia has no effect on alternative splicing of the primary transcript and there is no evidence for hypoxia-regulated translation of VEGF.

Transcriptional regulation of VEGF is mediated by the transcription factor, HIF-1 (55). Vascular endothelial growth factor shares with other HIF-1-regulated genes—notably genes whose products are involved in systemic (e.g., erythropoietin), local (inducible-NO synthase), and cellular (e.g., glycolytic enzymes) responses to hypoxia—consensus HIF-1 binding sequences in its promoter. The sequence TACGTGGG (spanning nucleotides -917 to -910 relative to the mouse VEGF transcription start site) is required for HIF-1 binding and for the hypoxic response. Mutations in this sequence prevent HIF-1 binding and abolish the majority of hypoxia inducibility (56). Also, inhibition of HIF-1 binding by preventing heterodimerization of HIF-1 with its obligatory partner, ARNT, abolishes a significant fraction (but not all) of hypoxia-inducible VEGF (56–58). It appears, therefore, that accumulation of HIF-1 protein under hypoxia is essential for transcriptional activation of VEGF under this stress. Interestingly, hypoxia does not increase production of HIF-1 protein but leads to stabilization of the otherwise extremely labile protein (59). The mechanism by which factor(s) that accumulate under hypoxic conditions prevent rapid degradation of HIF-1 is unknown.

It is not known whether VEGF expression is also regulated by the hypoxia-inducible transcription factor endothelial PAS-domain protein 1 (EPAS-1). EPAS-1 may play a role in the cross-talk between endothelial cells and smooth muscle cells or pericytes because it induces expression of tie-2 (43) and because the latter endothelial cell-specific receptor and its newly discovered ligand, angiopoietin-1 (60) are likely to function at the step of vascular remodeling (61, 62).

Considerable gaps still remain in our understanding of oxygen sensing, per se, and the pathway of signal transduction culminating in accumulation of hypoxia-inducible transcription factors. The molecular nature of the "oxygen sensor" is beyond the scope of this review. It is sufficient to mention that the proposition that the sensor is a heme protein is consistent with findings that expression of VEGF (as well as of other hypoxia-regulated genes) also is induced by transition metals like cobalt (63) and iron chelators (64). Other agents that increase expression of VEGF mRNA, including hydrogen peroxide (65), adenosine (66), and reactive oxygen species (67) also are thought to interject at some point in the oxygen sensing/transduction pathway.

Another level of regulation is hypoxia-induced stabilization of VEGF mRNA (68–70). The intrinsically short half-life of VEGF mRNA (approximately 30 minutes) is significantly extended under both hypoxia and hypoglycemia. This response is mediated by 3′-untranslated region (3′-UTR) sequences, as a VEGF 3′-UTR element confers hypoxia inducibility to a surrogate gene in vivo (71). It is assumed that posttranscriptional regulation of VEGF is mediated by hypoxia-augmented binding of yet unidentified protein(s) to its 3′-UTR. Initial studies have identified three adenylate-uridilate-rich RNA elements within the VEGF 3′-

UTR that form hypoxia-inducible RNA-protein complexes with unknown proteins of 32, 28, and 17kD (72, 73).

An important link between posttranscriptional regulation of VEGF and the von Hippel-Lindau (VHL) tumor suppressor gene was uncovered. Tumors developing in patients with the autosomal dominantly inherited VHL disease and in sporadic cases of VHL loss (predominantly hemangioblastoma and renal carcinoma) are distinguished by their hypervascularity. Not surprisingly, VEGF is highly expressed in these tumors even under normoxic conditions (74, 75). Reintroduction of a wild-type VHL gene into tumor cells lacking a functional VHL gene suppresses the elevated constitutive production of VEGF without affecting VEGF transcription initiation or elongation (as would have been suggested by VHL-elongin association) (75, 76). These results suggest that formation of a highly vascular stroma in VHL tumors is the result of a perturbed VHL-mediated, posttranscriptional regulation of VEGF.

REFERENCES

1. Flamme I, von Reutern M, Drexler HC, Syed S, Ali S, Risau W. Overexpression of vascular endothelial growth factor in the avian embryo induces hypervascularization and increased vascular permeability without alterations of embryonic pattern formation. Dev Biol 1995; 171:399–414.
2. Zhang HT, Craft P, Scott PA, Ziche M, Weich HA, Harris AL, Bicknell R. Enhancement of tumor growth and vascular density by transfection of vascular endothelial cell growth factor into MCF-7 human breast carcinoma cells. J Natl Cancer Inst 1995; 87:213–219.
3. Benjamin LE, Keshet E. Conditional switching of vascular endothelial cell growth factor (VEGF) expression in tumors: Induction of endothelial cell shedding and regression of hemangioblastoma-like vessels by VEGF withdrawl. Proc Natl Acad Sci U S A 1997; 94:8761–8766.
4. Carmeliet P, Ferreira V, Breier G, Pollefeyt S, Kieckens L, Gertsenstein M, Fahrig M, Vandenhoeck A, Harpal K, Eberhardt C, Declercq C, Pawling J, Moons L, Collen D, Risau W, Nagy A. Abnormal blood vessel development and lethality in embryos lacking a single VEGF allele. Nature 1996; 380:435–439.
5. Ferrara N, Carver Moore K, Chen H, Dowd M, Lu L, O'Shea KS, Powell Braxton L, Hillan KJ, Moore MW. Heterozygous embryonic lethality induced by targeted inactivation of the VEGF gene. Nature 1996; 380:439–442.
6. Aiello LP, Avery RL, Arrigg PG, Keyt BA, Jampel HD, Shah ST, Pasquale LR, Thieme H, Iwamoto MA, Park JE, Nguyen HV, Aiello LM, Ferrara N, King L. Vascular endothelial growth factor in ocular fluid of patients with diabetic retinopathy and other retinal disorders. N Engl J Med 1994; 331:1480–1487.
7. Miller JW, Adamis AP, Shima DT, D'Amore PA, Moulton RS, O'Reilly MS, Folkman J, Dvorak HF, Brown LF, Berse B, Yeo T-K, Yeo K-T. Vascular endothe-

lial growth factor/vascular permeability factor is temporally and spatially correlated with ocular angiogenesis in a primate model. Am J Pathol 1994; 145:574–584.
8. Pe'er J, Shweiki D, Itin A, Hemo I, Gnessin H, Keshet E. Hypoxia-induced expression of vascular endothelial growth factor by retinal cells is a common factor in neovascularizing ocular diseases. Lab Invest 1995; 72:638–645.
9. Alon T, Hemo I, Itin A, Pe'er J, Stone J, Keshet E. Vascular endothelial growth factor acts as a survival factor for newly formed retinal vessels and has implications for retinopathy of prematurity. Nat Med 1995; 1:1024–1028.
10. Breier G, Albrecht U, Sterrer S, Risau W. Expression of vascular endothelial growth factor during embryonic angiogenesis and endothelial cell differentiation. Development 1992; 114:521–532.
11. Jakeman LB, Armanini M, Phillips HS, Ferrara N. Developmental expression of binding sites and messenger ribonucleic acid for vascular endothelial growth factor suggests a role for this protein in vasculogenesis and angiogenesis. Endocrinology 1993; 133:848–859.
12. Dumont DJ, Fong GH, Puri MC, Gradwohl G, Alitalo K, Breitman ML. Vascularization of the mouse emryo: A study of flk-1, tek, tie, and vascular endothelial growth factor expression during development. Dev Dyn 1995; 203:80–92.
13. Stone J, Itin A, Alon T, Pe'er J, Gnessin H, Chan Ling T, Keshet E. Development of retinal vasculature is mediated by hypoxia-induced vascular endothelial growth factor (VEGF) expression by neuroglia. J Neurosci 1995; 15:4738–4747.
14. Ravindranath N, Little Ihrig L, Phillips HS, Ferrara N, Zeleznik AJ. Vascular endothelial growth factor messenger ribonucleic acid expression in the primate ovary. Endocrinology 1992; 131:254–260.
15. Shweiki D, Itin A, Neufeld G, Gitay Goren H, Keshet E. Patterns of expression of vascular endothelial growth factor (VEGF) and VEGF receptors in mice suggest a role in hormonally regulated angiogenesis. J Clin Invest 1993; 91:2235–2243.
16. Li XF, Gregory J, Ahmed A. Immunolocalisation of vascular endothelial growth factor in human endometrium. Growth Factors 1994; 11:277–282.
17. Chakraborty I, Das SK, Dey SK. Differential expression of vascular endothelial growth factor and its receptor mRNAs in the mouse uterus around the time of implantation. J Endocrinol 1995; 147:339–352.
18. Cullinan Bove K, Koos RD. Vascular endothelial growth factor/vascular permeability factor expression in the rat uterus: Rapid stimulation by estrogen correlates with estrogen-induced increases in uterine capillary permeability and growth. Endocrinology 1993; 133:829–837.
19. Hyder SM, Stancel GM, Chiappetta C, Murthy L, Boettger Tong HL, Makela S. Uterine expression of vascular endothelial growth factor is increased by estradiol and tamoxifen. Cancer Res 1996; 56:3954–3960.
20. Shifren JL, Tseng JF, Zaloudek CJ, Ryan IP, Meng YG, Ferrara N, Jaffe RB, Taylor RN. Ovarian steroid regulation of vascular endothelial growth factor in the human endometrium: Implications for angiogenesis during the menstrual cycle and in the pathogenesis of endometriosis. J Clin Endocrinol Metab 1996; 81:3112–3118.
21. Charnock Jones DS, Sharkey AM, Rajput Williams J, Burch D, Schofield JP, Fountain SA, Boocock CA, Smith SK. Identification and localization of alternately spliced mRNAs for vascular endothelial growth factor in human uterus and estrogen

regulation in endometrial carcinoma cell lines. Biol Reprod 1993; 48:1120–1128.

22. Dissen GA, Lara HE, Fahrenbach WH, Costa ME, Ojeda SR. Immature rat ovaries become revascularized rapidly after autotransplantation and show a gonadotropin-dependent increase in angiogenic factor gene expression. Endocrinology 1994; 134: 1146–1154.
23. McClure N, Healy DL, Rogers PA, Sullivan J, Beaton L, Haning RV Jr, Connolly DT, Robertson DM. Vascular endothelial growth factor as capillary permeability agent in ovarian hyperstimulation syndrome. Lancet 1994; 344:235–236.
24. Soh EY, Sobhi SA, Wong MG, Meng YG, Siperstein AE, Clark OH, Duh QY. Thyroid-stimulating hormone promotes the secretion of vascular endothelial growth factor in thyroid cancer cell lines. Surgery 1996; 120:944–947.
25. Joseph IB, Isaacs JT. Potentiation of the antiangiogenic ability of linomide by androgen ablation involves down-regulation of vascular endothelial growth factor in human androgen-responsive prostatic cancers. Cancer Res 1997; 57:1054–1057.
26. Li J, Perrella MA, Tsai JC, Yet SF, Hsieh CM, Yoshizumi M, Patterson C, Endege WO, Zhou F, Lee ME. Induction of vascular endothelial growth factor gene expression by interleukin-1 beta in rat aortic smooth muscle cells. J Biol Chem 1995; 270: 308–312.
27. Cohen T, Nahari D, Cerem LW, Neufeld G, Levi BZ. Interleukin 6 induces the expression of vascular endothelial growth factor. J Biol Chem 1996; 271:736–741.
28. Goldman CK, Kim J, Wong WL, King V, Brock T, Gillespie GY. Epidermal growth factor stimulates vascular endothelial growth factor production by human malignant glioma cells: A model of glioblastoma multiforme pathophysiology. Mol Biol Cell 1993; 4:121–133.
29. Frank S, Hubner G, Breier G, Longaker MT, Greenhalgh DG, Werner S. Regulation of vascular endothelial growth factor expression in cultured keratinocytes. Implications for normal and impaired wound healing. J Biol Chem 1995; 270:12607–12613.
30. Warren RS, Yuan H, Matli MR, Ferrara N, Donner DB. Induction of vascular endothelial growth factor by insulin-like growth factor 1 in colorectal carcinoma. J Biol Chem 1996; 271:29483–29488.
31. Stavri GT, Zachary IC, Baskerville PA, Martin JF, Erusalimsky JD. Basic fibroblast growth factor upregulates the expression of vascular endothelial growth factor in vascular smooth muscle cells. Synergistic interaction with hypoxia. Circulation 1995; 92:11–14.
32. Stavri GT, Hong Y, Zachary IC, Breier G, Baskerville PA, Yla Herttuala S, Risau W, Martin JF, Erusalimsky JD. Hypoxia and platelet-derived growth factor-BB synergistically upregulate the expression of vascular endothelial growth factor in vascular smooth muscle cells. FEBS Lett 1995; 358:311–315.
33. Pertovaara L, Kaipainen A, Mustonen T, Orpana A, Ferrara N, Saksela O, Alitalo K. Vascular endothelial growth factor is induced in response to transforming growth factor-beta in fibroblastic and epithelial cells. J Biol Chem 1994; 269:6271–6274.
34. Ryuto M, Ono M, Izumi H, Yoshida S, Weich HA, Kohno K, Kuwano M. Induction of vascular endothelial growth factor by tumor necrosis factor alpha in human glioma cells. Possible roles of SP-1. J Biol Chem 1996; 271:28220–28228.

35. Shweiki D, Itin A, Soffer D, Keshet E. Vascular endothelial growth factor induced by hypoxia may mediate hypoxia-initiated angiogenesis. Nature 1992; 359:843–845.
36. Plate KH, Breier G, Weich HA, Risau W. Vascular endothelial growth factor is a potential tumor angiogenesis factor in human gliomas in vivo. Nature 1992; 359:845–848.
37. Banai S, Shweiki D, Pinson A, Chandra M, Lazarovici G, Keshet E. Upregulation of vascular endothelial growth factor expression induced by myocardial ischaemia: Implications for coronary angiogenesis. Cardiovasc Res 1994; 28:1176–1179.
38. Minchenko A, Bauer T, Salceda S, Caro J. Hypoxic stimulation of vascular endothelial growth factor expression in vitro and in vivo. Lab Invest 1994; 71:374–379.
39. Freeman MR, Schneck FX, Gagnon ML, Corless C, Soker S, Niknejad K, Peoples GE, Klagsbrun M. Peripheral blood T lymphocytes and lymphocytes infiltrating human cancers express vascular endothelial growth factor: A potential role for T cells in angiogenesis. Cancer Res 1995; 55:4140–4145.
40. Liu Y, Cox SR, Morita T, Kourembanas S. Hypoxia regulates vascular endothelial growth factor gene expression in endothelial cells. Identification of a 5′ enhancer. Circ Res. 1995; 77:638–643.
41. Shima DT, Adamis AP, Ferrara N, Yeo KT, Yeo TK, Allende R, Folkman J, D'Amore PA. Hypoxic induction of endothelial cell growth factors in retinal cells: Identification and characterization of vascular endothelial growth factor (VEGF) as the mitogen. Mol Med 1995; 1:182–193.
42. Namiki A, Brogi E, Kearney M, Kim EA, Wu T, Couffinhal T, Varticovski L, Isner JM. Hypoxia induces vascular endothelial growth factor in cultured human endothelial cells. J Biol Chem 1995; 270:31189–31195.
43. Tian HL, McKnight SL, Russell DW. Endothelial PAS domain protein 1 (EPAS), a transcriptional factor selectively expressed in endothelial cells. Genes DEV 1997; 11:72–82.
44. Adamis AP, Miller JW, Bernal MT, D'Amico DJ, Folkman J, Yeo TK, Yeo KT. Increased vascular endothelial growth factor levels in the vitreous of eyes with proliferative diabetic retinopathy. Am J Ophthalmol 1994; 118:445–450.
45. Pe'er J, Folberg R, Itin A, Gnessin H, Hemo I, Keshet E. Upregulated expression of vascular endothelial growth factor in proliferative diabetic retinopahty. Br J Ophthalmol 1996; 80:241–245.
46. Shweiki D, Neeman M, Itin A, Keshet E. Induction of vascular endothelial growth factor expression by hypoxia and by glucose deficiency in multicell spheroids: Implications for tumor angiogenesis. Proc Natl Acad Sci U S A 1995; 92:768–772.
47. Waleh NS, Brody MD, Knapp MA, Mendonca HL, Lord EM, Koch CJ, Laderoute KR, Sutherland RM. Mapping of the vascular endothelial growth factor-producing hypoxic cells in multicellular tumor spheroids using a hypoxia-specific marker. Cancer Res 1995; 55:6222–6226.
48. Ashton N. Retinal vascularization in health and disease. Am J Opththalmol 1957; 44:7–17.
49. Hanahan D, Folkman J. Patterns and emerging mechanisms of the angiogenic switch during tumorigenesis. Cell 1996; 86:353–364.
50. Rak J, Mitsuhashi Y, Bayko L, Filmus J, Shirasawa S, Sasazuki T, Kerbel RS. Mu-

tant ras oncogenes upregulate VEGF/VPF expression: Implications for induction and inhibition of tumor angiogenesis. Cancer Res 1995; 55:4575–4580.

51. Kieser A, Weich HA, Brandner G, Marme D, Kolch W. Mutant p53 potentiates protein kinase C induction of vascular endothelial growth factor expression. Oncogene 1994; 9:963–969.
52. Claffey KP, Wilkison WO, Spiegelman BM. Vascular endothelial growth factor. Regulation by cell differentiation and activated second messenger pathways. J Biol Chem 1992; 267:16317–16322.
53. Gille J, Swerlick RA, Caughman SW. Transforming growth factor-α-induced transcriptional activation of the vascular permeability factor (VPF/VEGF) gene requires AP-2-dependent DNA binding and transactivation. EMBO J 1997; 6:750–759.
54. Ryuto M, Ono M, Izumi H, Yoshida S, Weich HA, Kohno K, Kuwano M. Induction of vascular endothelial growth factor by tumor necrosis factor alpha in human glioma cells. Possible roles of SP-1. J Biol Chem 1996; 271:28220–28228.
55. Semenza GL. Transcriptional regulation by hypoxia-inducible factor 1. Trends Cardiovas Med 1996; 6:151–157.
56. Forsythe JA, Jiang BH, Iyer NV, Agani F, Leung SW, Koos RD, Semenza GL. Activation of vascular endothelial growth factor gene transcription by hypoxia-inducible factor 1. Mol Cell Biol 1996; 16:4604–4613.
57. Salceda S, Beck I, Caro J. Absolute requirement of aryl hydrocarbon receptor nuclear translocator protein for gene activation by hypoxia. Arch Biochem Biophys 1996; 334:389–394.
58. Wood SM, Gleadle JM, Pugh CW, Hankinson O, Ratcliffe PJ. The role of the aryl hydrocarbon receptor nuclear translocator (ARNT) in hypoxic induction of gene expression. Studies in ARNT-deficient cells. J Biol Chem 1996; 271:15117–15123.
59. Huang LE, Arany Z, Livingston DM, Bunn HF. Activation of hypoxia-inducible transcription factor depends primarily upon redox-sensitive stabilization of its alpha subunit. J Biol Chem 1996; 271:32253–32259.
60. Davis S, Aldrich TH, Jones PF, Acheson A, Compton DL, Jain V, Ryan TE, Bruno J, Radziejewski C, Maisonpierre PC, Yancopoulos GD. Isolation of angiopoietin-1, a ligand for the TIE2 receptor, by secretion-trap expression cloning. Cell 1996; 87:1161–1169.
61. Suri C, Jones PF, Patan S, Bartunkova S, Maisonpierre PC, Davis S, Sato TN, Yancopoulos GD. Requisite role of angiopoietin-1, a ligand for the TIE2 receptor, during embryonic angiogenesis. Cell 1996; 87:1171–1180.
62. Vikkula M, Boon LM, Carraway KL, Calvert JT, Diamonti AJ, Goumnerov B, Pasyk KA, Marchuk DA, Warman ML, Cantley LC, Mulliken JB, Olsen BR. Vascular dysmorphogenesis caused by an activating mutation in the receptortyrosine kinase TIE2. Cell 1996; 87:1181–1190.
63. Ladoux A, Frelin C. Cobalt stimulates the expression of vascular endothelial growth factor mRNA in rat cardiac cells. Biochem Biophys Res Commun 1994; 204:794–798.
64. Beerepoot LV, Shima DT, Kuroki M, Yeo KT, Voest EE. Up-regulation of vascular endothelial growth factor production by iron chelators. Cancer Res 1996; 56:3747–3751.
65. Brauchle M, Funk JO, Kind P, Werner S. Ultraviolet B and H2O2 are potent inducers

of vascular endothelial growth factor expression in cultured keratinocytes. J Biol Chem 1996; 271:21793–21797.

66. Hashimoto E, Kage K, Ogita T, Nakaoka T, Matsuoka R, Kira Y. Adenosine as an endogenous mediator of hypoxia for induction of vascular endothelial growth factor mRNA in U-937 cells. Biochem Biophys Res Commun 1994; 204:318–324.
67. Kuroki M, Voest EE, Amano S, Beerepoot LV, Takashima S, Tolentino M, Kim RY, Rohan RM, Colby KA, Yeo KT, Adamis AP. Reactive oxygen intermediates increase vascular endothelial growth factor expression in vitro and in vivo. J Clin Invest 1996; 98:1667–1675.
68. Shima DT, Deutsch U, D'Amore PA. Hypoxic induction of vascular endothelial growth factor (VEGF) in human epithelial cells is mediated by increases in mRNA stability. FEBS Lett 1995; 370:203–208.
69. Ikeda E, Achen MG, Breier G, Risau W. Hypoxia-induced transcriptional activation and increased mRNA stability of vascular endothelial growth factor in C6 glioma cells. J Biol Chem 1995; 270:19761–19766.
70. Stein I, Neeman M, Shweiki D, Itin A, Keshet E. Stabilization of vascular endothelial growth factor mRNA by hypoxia and hypoglycemia and coregulation with other ischemia-induced genes. Mol Cell Biol 1995; 15:5363–5368.
71. Damert A, Machein M, Breier G, Fujita MQ, Hanahan D, Risau W, Plate KH. Upregulation of vascular endothelial growth factor expression in a rat glioma is conferred by two distinct hypoxia-driven mechanisms. Cancer Res 1997; 57:3860–3864.
72. Levy AP, Levy NS, Goldberg MA. Post-transcriptional regulation of vascular endothelial growth factor by hypoxia. J Biol Chem 1996; 271:2746–2753.
73. Levy AP, Levy NS, MA Goldberg. Hypoxia-inducible protein binding to vascular endothelial growth factor mRNA and its modulation by the von Hippel-Lindau protein. J Biol Chem 1996; 271:25492–25497.
74. Wizigmann Voos S, Breier G, Risau W, Plate KH. Up-regulation of vascular endothelial growth factor and its receptors in von Hippel-Lindau disease-associated and sporadic hemangioblastomas. Cancer Res 1995; 55:1358–1364.
75. Gnarra JR, Zhou S, Merrill MJ, Wagner JR, Krumm A, Papavassiliou E, Oldfield EH, Klausner RD, Linehan WM. Post-transcriptional regulation of vascular endothelial growth factor mRNA by the product of the VHL tumor suppressor gene. Proc Natl Acad Sci U S A 1996; 93:10589–10594.
76. Iliopoulos O, Levy AP, Jiang C, Kaelin WG Jr, Goldberg MA. Negative regulation of hypoxia-inducible genes by the von Hippel-Lindau protein. Proc Natl Acad Sci U S A 1996; 93:10595–10599.

15
Fibroblast Growth Factors

David A. Moscatelli and Daniel B. Rifkin
New York University School of Medicine, New York, New York

I. INTRODUCTION

The fibroblast growth factors (FGF) were originally characterized as potent endothelial cell mitogens. Fibroblast growth factors induce an angiogenic response in endothelial cells in culture and will initiate blood vessel growth when administered in model systems in animals. However, the roles of the FGFs in natural angiogenesis in vivo have been less well documented. This review will outline current knowledge about the biochemical properties of the FGFs and their receptors and will evaluate the evidence for their roles in angiogenesis.

II. HISTORY OF FGFs

Fibroblast growth factor was originally identified as an activity in pituitary extracts that stimulated the proliferation of Balb/c 3T3 cells (1, 2). The mitogenic activity was partially purified from bovine pituitary and brain and was found to be due to a molecule with a molecular weight of 14–16 kDa with a basic isoelectric point (3, 4). Shortly afterward, evidence accumulated that a second 3T3 cell mitogen with an acidic isoelectric point occurred in brain (5, 6). The mitogenic activity of these FGFs was not restricted to fibroblasts, and stimulated many cell types including endothelial cells (7). Although small amounts of both the basic and the acidic mitogen were purified by conventional chromatography methods (8, 9), further characterization was aided by observations made by investigators purifying angiogenesis factors. Because both angiogenic factors and the FGFs were mitogenic for endothelial cells, they were suspected to be closely related.

The discovery that an endothelial cell mitogen from a tumor extract bound strongly to heparin (10) suggested that heparin affinity columns might be used for the purification of the FGFs. Indeed, both basic and acidic FGF bound strongly to heparin affinity columns, with acidic FGF eluting at 1 M NaCl and basic FGF eluting at 1.5 M NaCl (11–13). Complete characterization of the FGFs was greatly facilitated by the use of heparin affinity columns. In addition, heparin affinity columns, by permitting a simple and rapid purification of FGFs, helped demonstrate that mitogenic activities and angiogenic factors identified in a variety of tissues were all due to either basic or acidic FGF. This reduced a large list of poorly characterized mitogens to synonyms for basic and acidic FGF.

However, the apparent simplicity of the FGF family did not last. Up to now, 12 other polypeptides with amino acid sequence homology to basic and acidic FGF have been identified. These related molecules are the products of the *int*-2 (FGF-3), *hst/K-fgf* (FGF-4), FGF-5, and FGF-6 proto-oncogenes (14–18); keratinocyte growth factor (FGF-7) (19), androgen-induced growth factor (FGF-8) (20, 21), glial growth factor (FGF-9) (22); and the recently identified FGF-10 (23) and FGF homologous factors (24). With the discovery of the extent of the FGF family, acidic and basic FGF were renamed FGF-1 and FGF-2, respectively. The related molecules that have been characterized also have mitogenic activity and bind tightly to heparin affinity columns, suggesting that these 14 polypeptides constitute a family of heparin-binding growth factors. Further complexity arises because some members of the family also exist in multiple forms arising from alternate splicing of the message or initiation of translation at alternative codons. As the angiogenic properties of these other FGF family members, in general, have not been well defined, this review will be limited to FGF-1 and FGF-2.

A. FGF-2

Fibroblast growth factor-2 was originally purified from bovine pituitary as a 146 amino acid protein with a molecular weight of 16.5 kDa and an isoelectric point of 9.6 (25). Molecules with identical properties were purified from bovine brain, retina, and adrenal, and human brain (12, 26–29). Smaller forms containing truncations at the amino terminal end, but still retaining biological activity, were isolated from corpus luteum, adrenal, and testes (30, 31). At least some of the truncated forms seem to arise from proteolysis that occurs during the extraction procedure (32), and, with careful isolation in the presence of protease inhibitors, FGF-2 molecules even larger than 146 amino acids have been obtained (33, 34). However, it is possible that some proteolytic processing of FGF-2 occurs in vivo.

When both bovine and human FGF-2 cDNA were cloned, an AUG codon was found in the proper context to initiate translation of a protein of 155 amino acids, and no in-frame AUG codons were found upstream (35, 36). Therefore, translation was predicted to initiate at this AUG codon and to result in an 18 kDa protein. However, larger forms of FGF-2 were purified from human placenta and from guinea pig brain (37, 38). These higher molecular weight forms of FGF-2 have been shown to arise from the use of three upstream CUG codons as alternate initiation codons for translation. Translation from these codons occurs through the process of internal ribosomal entry (39). Thus, human FGF-2 is expressed in four forms: an 18 kDa form (155 amino acids) generated by initiation at the AUG codon and 22, 22.5, and 24 kDa forms (196, 201, and 210 amino acids) arising from the CUG codons (40, 41). The high-molecular-weight forms of FGF-2 contain the same amino acid sequence as the 18 kDa form but have, in addition, N-terminal extensions of varying lengths. Both 18 kDa and higher molecular weight forms are expressed in brain (38, 42) and a number of different cell lines (43–45). The relative amounts of the individual forms of FGF-2 have been reported to vary in response to cell stress, during development, and among different tissues in the adult (46–51).

The alternate forms of FGF-2 have different subcellular distributions. Both the 155 amino acid form of FGF-2 and the higher molecular weight forms lack a typical signal sequence for secretion and are mainly retained within the cell. The 155 amino acid form is primarily located in the cytosol, whereas the higher molecular weight forms are present in the nuclear and ribosomal fractions (43, 52, 53). These results suggest that the higher molecular weight forms of FGF-2 contain a nuclear translocation sequence. Indeed, when the N-terminal extension of the higher molecular weight forms is grafted to normally cytoplasmic proteins, it is able to drive these recombinant proteins to the nucleus (54, 55). Interestingly, the N-terminal extension of FGF-2 is not able to direct nuclear translocation of FGF-1 due to the presence of a cytosolic retention domain in FGF-1 (56). The N-terminal extensions in the higher molecular weight forms of FGF-2 contain several stretches of alternating glycine and arginine residues. Some of the arginine residues in these sequences are methylated (57, 58), as has been described for other nuclear proteins. Inhibition of arginine methylation blocks the nuclear accumulation of the high-molecular-weight forms of FGF-2 (59). Thus, arginine methylation may provide a nuclear retention signal for high-molecular-weight FGF-2.

The significance of nuclear forms of FGF-2 is not clear. Overexpression of either 18 kDa FGF-2 or the high-molecular-weight forms has been reported to have distinct effects on cell growth and integrin and FGF receptor expression (60–62). High-level expression of the high-molecular-weight forms causes transformation of NIH 3T3 cells in a manner that does not involve activation of the FGF receptor, whereas transformation of NIH 3T3 cells by overexpression of 18 kDa FGF-2 requires activation of the receptor (60). Thus, 18 kDa FGF-2 stimulates cells through an autocrine mechanism, whereas high-molecular-weight FGF-2 stimulates cells through an intracrine mechanism. Low-level expression of high molecular weight FGF-2 results in slow growth with a high incidence of multinucleate cells (63, 64). Interestingly, trout and Xenopus FGF-2 cDNA have a stop codon in frame just before the AUG for initiation of translation of 18 kDa FGF-2 and, therefore, high-molecular-weight FGF-2 forms cannot be synthesized in these organisms (65). As low levels of 18 kDa FGF-2 also are found in the nucleus, perhaps 18 kDa FGF-2 performs the nuclear functions of FGF-2 in trout and Xenopus. The N-terminal extension found in mammalian FGF-2 may have evolved to provide more efficient targeting of FGF-2 to the nucleus.

The amino acid sequence of 18 kDa FGF-2 is highly conserved among species with 89% to 95% identity among human, bovine, ovine, and rat FGF-2s (35, 36, 66–68). Xenopus FGF-2 is more divergent but still shares 84% homology with human FGF-2 (69). This low level of divergence suggests that there may be functional importance for many regions of FGF-2. There seems to be more variation in the N-terminal extensions of the high-molecular-weight forms of FGF-2 (57, 70), suggesting that these regions are less functionally restricted. Additional information about biologically active sequences in FGF-2 can be obtained by comparing it to other members of the FGF family. However, the homology to other members of the family extends over almost the entire sequence of FGF-2, from amino acids 28 to 150 of the 155 amino acid form. X-ray crystallographic and nuclear magnetic resonance (NMR) studies of FGF-2 structure have revealed that the molecule is composed of a threefold repeat of a four-stranded antiparallel beta-meander and has a structure similar to interleukin-1 (71–75). In keeping with the homology data, the first 19 and last 3 amino acids are disordered (71).

Fibroblast growth factor-2 contains four cysteine residues, and two of these are conserved among all members of the FGF family, suggesting that they may have important functions in the biology of the FGFs. However, none of the cysteines are necessary for biological activity, because in vitro mutagenesis of the cysteine residues to serine does not alter the mitogenic activity of FGF-2 (76, 77).

The heparin-binding and receptor-binding regions of FGF-2 have been mapped based on the ability of synthetic peptides representing different amino acid sequences in FGF-2 to bind radiolabeled heparin, to block binding of radiolabeled FGF-2 to its receptor, and to act as agonists or antagonists of FGF-2 biological activity (78). The receptor-binding activity was found in two regions, amino acids 33–77 and 115–124 of the 155 amino acid form. The inclusion of C-terminal sequences in the 115–124 peptide increased its potency. Heparin binding was strongest in these same regions, but lower heparin-binding capacity was found in other sequences, suggesting that heparin-binding sites are distributed throughout the molecule. From crystallographic data, a highly charged surface composed of lysine 128, arginine 129, lysine 134, lysine 138, and lysine 144 that formed a potential heparin-binding site was identified (73). In some crystals, sulfate and selenate ions were found to bind to asparagine 36, arginine 129, and lysine 134, suggesting that these residues formed part of the heparin-binding site (71, 72). In cocrystals of FGF-2 with a heparin hexasaccharide, asparagine-36, arginine-129, lysine-134, and glutamine-143 were found to form the primary interactions with the hexasaccharide (79). The hexasaccharide also interacted with an additional binding site formed by lysine-35, asparagine-110, and lysine-144. Site-directed mutagenesis identified 11 amino acids throughout the FGF-2 molecule as contributing to the energy of the FGF-heparin interaction (80). In keeping with the crystallography results, asparagine 36, arginine 129, lysine 134, and glutamine 143 contributed the most energy to the binding. Thus, the primary heparin-binding site is composed of discontinuous residues arranged on one side of the molecule.

The receptor-binding sequences in FGF-2 also have been further defined. Site-directed mutation of FGF-2 has identified two potential receptor-interacting sites. The higher affinity interaction involves a cluster of solvent exposed hydrophobic amino acids (tyrosine-33, tyrosine-112, leucine-149, and methionine-151) and two polar residues (arginine-53 and asparagine-110) on one face of the molecule (81). In addition, mutation of glutamic acid 105 has been found to alter receptor binding (82). Thus, the primary receptor-binding site is composed of a cluster of residues on one surface of the molecule rather than a continuous peptide sequence. A secondary receptor-binding site with approximately 250-fold lower affinity and located on a different face of the molecule is composed of amino acids lysine-119, tyrosine-120, and tryptophane-123 (81). This corresponds to one of the receptor-binding regions identified from the earlier studies with synthetic peptides (78). Mutations in the secondary binding site had little effect in receptor competition binding assays, but greatly diminished biological activity of FGF-2 (81, 82). Not all of these residues may be necessary for effective binding of FGF-2 to its receptor, as FGF-2 molecules missing the first 69 or last 46 amino acids have been reported to have biological activity (83, 84).

Fibroblast growth factor-2 has been found in all organs and tissues examined (85). It is synthesized by cultured fibroblasts, endothelial cells, glial cells, and smooth muscle cells (86–92), and, as these cell types are ubiquitous, they may be the source of FGF-2 in the organs. However, a variety of other cultured cells, including a number of tumor cell lines (86, 93–95), also synthesize FGF-2, raising the possibility that expression of FGF-2 is wide-spread in vivo or that expression of high levels of FGF-2 is an adaptation to culture. Immunolocalization studies of normal adult tissue have shown that FGF-2 is indeed produced by a variety of cell types, including skeletal, cardiac, and smooth muscle and epithelial cells of sweat glands, trachea, bronchi, colon, and endometrial glands (96). Fibroblast growth factor-2 is also found in the endothelial cells of some, but not all, blood vessels (96, 97). In adults, mRNA is expressed in much higher levels in brain than in other tissues (67). In normal brain, high-level expression is restricted to discrete areas, where it is present mainly in neuronal cell bodies, but lower level expression is found throughout the tissue, where it seems to be associated with glial cells (98–100). In injured brain, the expression of FGF-2 increases in the area of injury and seems to be associated with reactive astrocytes (99). Normally the amount of FGF-2 found in circulation is low, but increased levels are found in the serum from cancer patients and patients with limb ischemia (101–103).

B. FGF-1

Fibroblast growth factor-1 was isolated originally as a 154 amino acid protein in addition to truncated forms of 140 and 134 amino acids (104–107). The primary translation product for human FGF-1 is 155 amino acids (108). There appear to be no N-terminal extended forms of FGF-1, as a termination codon is found at position −1 to the AUG initiation codon. However, the existence of alternate 5′ untranslated exons in FGF-1 mRNAs has been described (109, 110). These sequences are involved in tissue-specific transcription of the molecule (111, 112), but none alters the size of the expressed protein.

Fibroblast growth factor-1 has 55% amino acid sequence identity to 18 kDa FGF-2. Homology extends over the entire sequence of the molecule except for the 18 N-terminal amino acids and a 2 amino acid insert at positions 117 and 118. Like FGF-2, FGF-1 has a β-trefoil crystal structure (74, 113). The first 24 and last 2 amino acids are disordered and have no particular interaction with the rest of the molecule (113, 114).

Fibroblast growth factor-1 contains three cysteine residues that, like the cysteine residues in FGF-2, do not seem to be necessary for biological activity. Crabb et al. reported that FGF-1 in which these residues have been reduced and carboxymethylated still retains biological activity (115). In contrast, Jaye et al. have reported that quantitative alkylation of cysteine residues abolishes the receptor-binding activity (116). Finally, the studies of Linemeyer et al. (117) have shown that disulfide bond formation between the cysteines is incompatible with biological activity in FGF-1. These studies showed that cysteine residues in brain-derived and recombinant FGF-1 are normally reduced, that formation of intramolecular disulfide bonds results in an inactive molecule, and that reduction of the disulfide bonds restores activity. In addition, site-directed mutation of any of the cysteine residues to serine results in an FGF-1 with high biological activity (117). Together these investigations suggest that the cysteine residues are not necessary for biological activity, but modification of the cysteines may hinder the formation of biologically active conformations of FGF-1.

Attempts to map binding regions of FGF-1 have identified two sites. A synthetic peptide corresponding to residues 50–73 of the primary translation product competed with FGF-1 for heparin binding (118). This region is homologous to one of the regions identified for heparin binding in FGF-2. A second binding region was indicated by chemical modification experiments. Methylation of lysine residues in FGF-1 caused a reduction in its affinity for heparin, receptor affinity, and biological potency (119). The alteration in activity was correlated with the modification of lysine-133. Site-directed mutation of this lysine to glutamic acid resulted in an FGF-1 with a lower affinity for heparin and reduced mitogenicity but no alteration in its receptor affinity or ability to stimulate early responses in cells (120). Thus, this residue seems to be important in heparin interactions, but not in receptor binding. In keeping with these results, cocrystals of FGF-1 with sulfate ions have demonstrated potential heparin-binding sites at asparagine-33, lysine-133, and lysine-128 (113). These amino acids have positions equivalent to amino acids in FGF-2 that contribute to its heparin-binding site. Like FGF-2, residues that contribute to heparin binding in FGF-1 are likely to be distributed throughout the molecule.

The residues identified as contributing to the higher affinity receptor-binding site of FGF-2 are all conserved in FGF-1, except for a leucine for methionine substitution at position 150 (113). The residues that contribute to the lower affinity receptor-binding site in FGF-2 are included in a five-residue surface loop. Except for tryptophane-122, these residues are not conserved in FGF-1. In addition, this loop in FGF-1 contains a two amino acid insertion. Replacement of the five residues in this loop in FGF-2 with the seven residues of the FGF-1 loop confers FGF-1–like receptor interactions to FGF-2 (121). These residues are critical to receptor discrimination between FGF family members.

Fibroblast growth factor-1 appears to have a more limited distribution than FGF-2. It has been found in neural tissue, kidney, prostate, and cardiac muscle (9, 115, 122–126). Immunolocalization studies have detected FGF-1 in neurons in discrete regions of the cerebrum and cerebellum (127). It has also been identified in cultured vascular smooth muscle cells (92, 128).

III. SECRETION OF FGFs

Fibroblast growth factor-1 and all isoforms of FGF-2 lack a signal sequence that would direct the newly synthesized molecules to the classic protein secretion pathway. The absence of a signal sequence for secretion makes it difficult to understand the mode of action of the FGFs in vivo. How are these molecules released to exert their effects in vivo? It has been proposed that they are released from dead or dying cells (129, 130) and, thus, may be primarily involved in responses to tissue destruction. In a variation on this, it has been suggested that FGF-2 is released through small, nonlethal disruptions of the plasma membrane (131–133). Such disruptions may occur during cell migration (131) or by the action of complement on the plasma membrane (134). However, there is increasing evidence that, despite the lack of a signal sequence, low levels of the growth factor are released by healthy cells. In cultured endothelial cells, which both synthesize and have receptors for FGF-2, basal levels of protease production and DNA synthesis are inhibited by neutralizing antibodies to FGF-2 (135, 136). These results suggest that the cells release small amounts of FGF-2 that can activate their own FGF receptors in an autocrine manner. An alternative explanation is that, in mass culture experiments, the death of a minute percentage of the cells releases enough FGF-2 to cause these results, and that healthy cells release no FGF-2. This possibility was eliminated in experiments in which the migration of single cells expressing different amounts of FGF-2 was investigated (137). Cell movement was shown to be proportional to the content of FGF-2 and could be inhibited by antibodies to FGF-2, indicating that the cells were responding to their own FGF-2 that was released to a space accessible to the antibodies. As only a single cell was present in each well during this experiment, the FGF-2 had to be released from the responding cell. Additional evidence for release of FGF from healthy cells comes from experiments with COS cells transfected with the cDNA for FGF-2. These cells quantitatively release pulse-labeled FGF-2 in an energy-dependent manner (138). Thus, it appears that healthy cells release biologically significant amounts of FGF-2. Release of FGF-2 was not blocked by inhibitors of the classic endoplasmic reticulum-Golgi secretory pathway (138, 139). Release of FGF-2 was enhanced by calcium ionophore and inhibited by methylamine, low temperature, and serum-free conditions (139). These treatments affect exocytosis, suggesting that an FGF-2 release involves an atypical exocytotic pathway.

The release of FGF-1 has some unique characteristics compared to the release of FGF-2. Release of FGF-1 is accelerated under stress conditions, including heat shock, serum starvation, and transformation of cells with the human immunodeficiency virus-1 TAT protein (140–142), whereas the release of FGF-2 is not (56). Under stress conditions, FGF-1 was released into the medium in a biologically inactive form but could be recovered in an active form after ammonium sulfate fractionation or reduction. Formation of disulfide-linked dimers of FGF-1 seems to be important in this process, and mutation of cysteine 30 inhibited release of FGF-1 (143, 144), suggesting that the dimers required for release are formed by disulfide bonds using this cysteine. In addition, a region of FGF-1 near the C-terminus that binds phospholipids is required for release through the heat shock-induced pathway (143, 144). Inhibitors of the endoplasmic reticulum-Golgi secretion pathway, exocytosis, and multidrug resistance proteins did not inhibit, but stimulated, release of FGF-1 under stress conditions (143). Fibroblast growth factor-1 release is also increased by exposure of endothelial cells to oxidized low density lipoprotein (145), but release does not seem to be through the stress-induced pathway.

IV. FGF RECEPTORS

Receptors for FGF-2 were initially identified from the binding of radioactive FGF-2 and from crosslinking labeled FGF-2 to receptors with bifunctional crosslinking agents. Scatchard analysis of the binding of ^{125}I-FGF-2 to several cell types suggested that a single class of high-affinity receptors existed (146–148). However, a number of different sizes of FGF-2 receptors were identified by crosslinking studies. Most investigators reported the presence of two receptors with molecular weights of 130,000 and 150,000 (146, 147), although in some cell types only one receptor was identified (149, 150). Binding of labeled FGF-1 to cells also indicated a single class of high-affinity binding sites and identified receptors of similar molecular weights (151–153). In several cell types, the binding of labeled FGF-2 was competed with unlabeled FGF-1, and the binding of labeled FGF-1 was competed with unlabeled FGF-2, suggesting that in these cells the two growth factors bound to the same receptor (147, 154, 155). These studies implied that the members of the FGF family may interact with overlapping affinities for the same family of receptors.

The relationship of FGF receptors was partially resolved with the cloning and sequencing of the receptors. Five protein receptors for FGFs have been described. Four are closely related molecules that form a family of transmembrane tyrosine kinase receptors (156, 157). The fifth is a cysteine-rich transmembrane protein with no intrinsic tyrosine kinase activity (158).

The cysteine-rich FGF receptor binds both FGF-1 and FGF-2 with high affinity (158). Interestingly, this molecule also has been identified separately as a transmembrane protein specific to the medial cisternae of the Golgi apparatus (159) and as a cell surface ligand for E-selectin (160). These observations suggest that the molecule may cycle between the cell surface and the Golgi, and may thereby further modulate the distribution of the FGFs between extra- and intracellular compartments. Indeed, overexpression of the cysteine-rich FGF receptor in CHO cells reduces the cellular content of both FGF-1 and FGF-2 (161).

The four tyrosine kinase FGF receptors all share a similar structure: an extracellular portion containing three immunoglobulin-like domains and a stretch of acidic amino acids, a transmembrane region, and an intracellular portion consisting of a long juxtamembrane domain and a split tyrosine kinase domain (162–165). However, each of the receptors can exist in multiple forms that arise from alternative splicing of the primary transcript. An important splicing event for FGF receptors 1, 2, and 3 involves the second half of the third immunoglobulin-like domain. Two alternate exons can be spliced at this site, generating membrane-bound receptors that have different ligand binding affinities (166–171). All receptor isoforms generated by this splicing event bind FGF-1 with high affinity. Receptor isoforms incorporating the IIIc exon bind FGF-2 with high affinity, whereas those incorporating the IIIb exon bind FGF-2 with much lower affinity (172).

For FGF receptor 1, a third possible exon can occur in the second half of the third immunoglobulin-like domain. Transcripts including this exon encode a truncated secreted receptor that binds FGF-2 (173). Secreted receptors also can be generated by proteolytic degradation of the receptor near its transmembrane region (174). Secreted receptor molecules have been found in blood and the basement membrane of endothelial cells (175, 176); it is not clear if these molecules are generated by alternate splicing or proteolysis. The secreted receptors may act as carriers of FGFs or may modulate FGF activity by competing with cell-surface receptors.

Another splicing event can generate receptor isoforms missing the first of the three immunoglobulin-like domains (177–180). Isoforms of FGF receptor-1 having two immunoglobulin-like domains have been reported to have higher affinity for FGF-1 than receptor isoforms with three immunoglobulin-like domains (181). Alternative splicing in the tyrosine kinase region of FGF receptor-1 can generate isoforms with inactive kinase domains (182). Overexpression of these receptor isoforms diminishes the activity of FGF receptor-1 isoforms with the intact kinase domains (183). Other described splicing events generate receptor isoforms that lack the stretch of acidic amino acids (184), contain a two amino acid insert in the intracellular juxtamembrane region, or have alternate C-terminal tails (180, 185). The functional significance of these last splicing events has not been determined. Thus, a combination of splicing events can produce FGF receptors with a variety of affinities for FGFs and a variety of activities.

As with other tyrosine kinase receptors, ligand binding to the FGF receptors results in receptor dimerization and transphosphorylation (186). Seven tyrosine residues in the cytoplasmic domain of FGF receptor-1 have been identified as sites of autophosphorylation (187). Phosphorylation of one of these tyrosines regulates binding of phospholipase Cγ1 to the receptor (188). Phospholipase Cγ1 binding to activated FGF receptor-1 results in its phosphorylation and activation (189). However, replacement of the tyrosine in the phospholipase Cγ1 binding site with phenylalanine abrogates phospholipase Cγ1 binding, phosphorylation, and activation, but has little effect on a number of biological responses to FGFs (190–193). Indeed, only two of the phosphorylated tyrosines are required for FGF receptor signaling (187), and these are located in the activation loop of the tyrosine kinase domain (194). Activated FGF receptors also phosphorylate Shc and a novel membrane-anchored adapter protein, FRS2. These proteins, in turn, bind to and phosphorylate grb-2 and SOS, leading to activation of the *ras* signaling pathway (Fig. 1) (195, 196). Other signaling molecules that are phosphorylated as a result of activation of the FGF receptor are 80K-H, *src*, and cortactin (197, 198). The role of these molecules in FGF signaling is not clear, but signaling

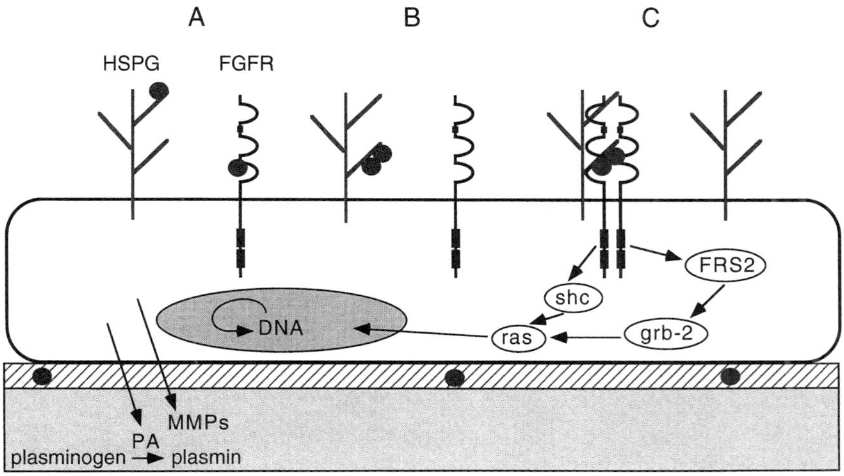

Figure 1 Fibroblast growth factor effects on endothelial cells. Fibroblast growth factor (*closed circles*) binds to heparan sulfate proteoglycans (HSPG) on cell surface or in the extracellular matrix or directly to receptor (FGFR) monomers (**A**). Binding of FGF to heparan sulfates potentiates FGF dimerization (**B**). Each member of an FGF dimer can bind to an FGF receptor, causing receptor dimerization and activation (**C**). Activated FGF receptors phosphorylate FRS2 and shc. Phosphorylated FRS2 recruits grb-2, causing activation of the *ras* signaling pathway. Activation of the *ras* signaling pathway results in DNA replication, cell proliferation, and increased expression of plasminogen activator (PA) and matrix metalloproteinases (MMPs). Plasminogen activator converts plasminogen to plasmin, which, in turn, activates pro-MMps. Plasmin and MMPs degrade basement membrane (*hatched area*) and underlying extracellular matrix (*gray area*), allowing the endothelial cell to penetrate the surrounding tissue.

requires long-term activation of the receptor and the pattern of phosphorylated proteins changes throughout this process (199, 200).

V. INTERACTION WITH HEPARAN SULFATES

Although signal transduction occurs through binding to receptors, the actions of FGFs are influenced also through their interactions with heparan sulfates. As expected from its high affinity for heparin, FGF-2 added exogenously to cultured cells binds to heparinlike molecules produced by the cells (89, 148, 201). These molecules have been identified as heparan sulfate proteoglycans (HSPG) present on the cell surface and in the extracellular matrix (202, 203). Fibroblast growth factor-2 interacts with the heparan sulfate moieties of these molecules (202) and efficient binding depends on the presence of N-sulfate groups (204). The core protein of the proteoglycan has little effect on the binding of FGF-2 to the heparan sulfate moieties, and FGF-2 has been reported to bind to the cell surface proteoglycans syndecan-1, -2, -3, and -4, glypican-1 and -3, betaglycan, and CD44, and to the extracellular matrix proteoglycan perlecan (205–211). Fibroblast growth factor-2 also has been shown to bind to heparinlike molecules in basement membranes in vivo (212) and to be present in isolated basement membranes (213).

Because FGF-1 also binds strongly to heparin, it is likely that FGF-1 also interacts with heparinlike molecules in the extracellular matrix. Indeed, FGF-1 has been shown to bind to extracellular matrix molecules produced by cells (153, 214, 215) and to basement membranes in vivo (212). Although FGF-1 and FGF-2 bind to the same proteoglycans in 3T3 cells (215), in some tissues different proteoglycans may bind either FGF-1 or FGF-2 exclusively (216). The ability of some proteoglycans to bind FGF-1 uniquely may reflect the fact that FGF-1 binds with high affinity to different polysaccharide sequences than FGF-2 (217).

Fibroblast growth factor-2 has a lower affinity for these heparan sulfates ($2 - 600 \times 10^{-9}$ M) (148, 204, 218) than for its cell surface receptors ($2 - 5 \times 10^{-11}$ M) (148, 149, 163), and binding to the HSPGs does not preclude FGF-2 from binding to receptors (148, 219). In contrast, the binding of FGF-2 to heparan sulfates confers several biological advantages to the growth factor. (a) FGF-2 bound to heparin or heparan sulfates is protected from proteolysis and thermal denaturation (202, 220, 221); (b) the heparan sulfate-bound FGF-2 serves as a reserve of growth factor that can support long-term responses to FGF-2 after a brief exposure to the growth factor (200, 222); (c) the heparan sulfates of the tissues may provide a means to localize FGF-2 to a particular site, limiting its diffusion (223); (d) soluble heparan sulfates can act as carriers of FGF-2 and, by preventing its interaction with fixed heparan sulfates in the tissues, assure its dissemination away from its site of release (223); these soluble heparan sulfates are generated by the action of proteases or heparinases on the fixed heparan sulfate proteoglycans (203, 224); and (e) FGF-2 can be internalized through its interaction with cell surface heparan sulfates, clearing excess active molecules from the cell surface, perhaps helping to dampen the response to FGF-2 (225–227).

In some cells, the biological activity of FGF-1 is greatly potentiated by the addition of heparin (151, 228, 229) or HSPG (214). It is not entirely clear how this potentiation occurs, but it could be related to some of the effects described above for the interaction of FGF-2 with heparin and heparan sulfates. Like FGF-2, FGF-1 is protected from thermal denaturation and proteolytic degradation by heparin (220, 230) and, therefore, may be more stable in a complex with heparin or HSPG. In addition, interaction of FGF-1 with heparin seems to alter the conformation of the protein, inasmuch as addition of heparin increases the binding of FGF-1 to specific monoclonal antibodies (151). Nuclear magnetic resonance studies of FGF-1 in solution have shown that heparin stabilizes the molecule (231). This change in conformation also may be responsible for the approximately two-fold greater affinity of FGF-1 for its receptor in the presence of heparin on cells that produce their own heparan sulfates (151, 232).

In addition to the above activities, heparan sulfates play a critical role in signal transduction through the FGF receptors. Cells expressing FGF receptors, but devoid of heparan sulfates, do not respond to FGF-1 or FGF-2 in the absence of heparin or heparan sulfate (233, 234). Initial experiments suggested that this requirement for heparin in biological responses to FGF reflected a requirement for heparin in the binding of FGFs to their receptors (233, 235). However, titration of the binding of radiolabeled FGF-2 to FGF receptor-1 expressed on cells lacking heparan sulfates revealed that FGF-2 bound to receptors in the absence of added heparin. Addition of heparin or heparan sulfates increased the affinity of FGF-2 for its receptor by fivefold (236). Similar results were obtained when binding of unlabeled FGF-2 to the purified extracellular domain of FGF receptor-1 was measured by differential calorimetry (237). Fibroblast growth factor-2 also bound to its receptor in the absence of heparin in this system, but addition of heparin increased binding affinity tenfold. In addition, measurement of the binding of unlabeled FGF-1 to the extracellular domain of FGF receptor-2 by differential calorimetry showed that heparin was not necessary for FGF-1 binding and did not affect the affinity of the interaction (238). Heparin or heparan sulfates increase the affinity of FGF-2 for its receptors by decreasing the dissociation rate of the FGF-2 receptor complex (236, 239, 240). These results suggest that trimolecular complexes of FGF-2, receptor, and heparan sulfate are formed and that these complexes are more stable than complexes of FGF-2 and receptor alone.

The role of heparan sulfates in FGF signaling has been elusive. It was initially proposed that binding of FGF-2 to heparin or heparan sulfate altered its conformation, converting FGF-2 to a receptor-competent form (241). However, FGF-2 cocrystallized with heparin trisaccharides or hexasaccharides was found to have the same crystal structure as FGF-2 alone, suggesting that there is no significant alteration of FGF-2 conformation on binding heparin (79, 242). A second model for the role of heparin in potentiating FGF-2 bioactivity is that it causes growth factor dimerization, and the dimerized growth factors each bind to a receptor molecule, causing receptor dimerization (Fig. 1) (238). This model is based on the observation that heparin can cause dimerization of FGF-1 and FGF-2 in vitro (238, 243). In addition, when FGF receptor was expressed in mutant CHO cells lacking heparan sulfates, crosslinked dimers of the receptor could not be obtained after addition of FGF-1 and crosslinking reagent. In contrast, if FGF receptors were expressed in wild-type CHO cells expressing heparan sulfates, or if exogenous heparin was added to the mutant CHO cells expressing receptors, crosslinked dimers of the receptor were observed. This model has been slightly modified recently. Analysis of the crystal packing of FGF-2 has identified faces that may interact strongly enough to give dimers (244). The faces of FGF-2 that interact with heparin are in the correct position to promote interaction between the dimerization motifs when two FGF-2 molecules bind to the same heparin molecule. This interpretation suggests that FGF-2 may dimerize in the absence of heparin, but heparin potentiates the dimerization. However, the crystal structure of FGF-2 in complex with the extracellular portion of FGF receptor-1 shows that the FGF-2 molecules do not directly interact in the complex and sit on opposite sides of a receptor dimer, suggesting that ligand dimerization is not directly related to receptor binding (245).

Another recent model arose from experiments to identify sequences in heparin and heparan sulfates that promote the activity of FGF-2. Heparin sequences that bind to FGF-2 are at least 5 sugar residues in length and have N-sulfated glucosamine groups and at least one 2-O-sulfated iduronic acid (246–248). However, heparin sequences longer than those required to bind FGF-2 (dodecasaccharides or longer) are necessary for promoting biological responses to FGF-2 (249). This finding, together with the observation of a putative heparin-binding region in FGF receptor-1 (250), led to the proposal that heparin or heparan sulfates must bind to both the growth factor and the receptor to promote a biological response. However, the affinity of the unoccupied receptor for heparin appears to be low. A number of investigators have reported that partially purified extracellular domain of FGF receptor-1 or FGF receptor-2 does not bind to heparin affinity columns in the absence of ligand (234, 238, 243). In addition, intact FGF receptor-1 does not bind to endothelial cell, 3T3 cell, or CHO cell heparan sulfates in the absence of ligand (251). In contrast, an interaction between heparin and purified extracellular domain of FGF receptor-1 was detected by differential calorimetry (237). The affinity of the receptor for heparin was about 200-fold lower than the affinity of FGF-2 for heparin. Therefore, the heparin-binding region of the unoccupied receptor may interact with heparin too weakly to detect under physiological conditions. The crystal structure of FGF-2 in complex with the extracellular domain of FGF receptor-1 shows that receptor-ligand dimers are formed through interactions of each FGF-2 molecule with two receptor molecules and interactions between the receptor extracellular domains (245). In these receptor-ligand dimers, a positively charged channel is formed from residues contributed by both ligand and receptor. This channel has a length and size to accommodate a heparin dodecasaccharide. Thus, heparin may act to stabilize receptor-ligand dimers.

VI. THE ROLE OF FGFs IN TUMOR FORMATION

Because FGF-1 and FGF-2 are found widely in adult tissues and receptors for FGF are found on many cells that synthesize FGF-1 or FGF-2, formation of tumors through an autocrine loop involving these growth factors is a possibility.

However, several investigations have demonstrated that FGF-2 and FGF-1 have low oncogenic potential. Although high-level expression of these growth factors in cultured normal cells caused the cells to acquire some transformed properties, such as altered morphology, increased growth rate, and the ability to grow in soft agar, injection of these cells into animals led to the formation of only minute, nonprogressing tumors (252–255). Furthermore, cell transformation by unmodified FGF-2 required expression of FGF-2 at levels 100 times greater than those observed in the highest producing normal cell line; lower level production resulted in a nontransformed morphology (255). The poor transforming ability and tumorigenicity of these molecules is related to their inefficient release from the cell, as expression of FGF-1 or FGF-2 to which a secretory signal sequence has been fused results in cell lines that have a transformed phenotype with lower levels of FGF expression and that are highly tumorigenic (256–258). Similarly, FGF-4, which contains a signal sequence, is highly oncogenic, but deletion of the signal sequence decreased its oncogenicity (259). The lack of signal sequence may keep these factors sequestered inside cells, limiting their action by physically separating them from their receptors.

Interestingly, overexpression of intact FGF-1 in a bladder tumor cell line decreases the time required to form tumors when these cells are implanted in mice (260). The effects of FGF-1 expression on tumor development is apparently not due to the ability of released FGF-1 to induce vascularization of the tumor, as overexpression of FGF-2 in the bladder tumor cells has no effect on tumor progression (261). As the bladder tumor cells have receptors that recognize FGF-1 but not FGF-2 (262), the ability of FGF-1 to promote tumorigenesis may be the result of autocrine stimulation of the tumor cells. Thus, although expression of FGF-1 or FGF-2 may not be sufficient to induce tumor growth, it may contribute to tumor progression.

VII. ANGIOGENIC PROPERTIES

One of the major roles proposed for the FGFs in vivo is in the induction of new blood vessel growth or angiogenesis (263). Angiogenesis occurs physiologically in the development of the vascular system during embryonic, fetal, and adolescent growth, during the normal cycling of the female reproductive system, and during the healing of wounds. Angiogenesis also contributes to several pathologies either directly, as in diabetic retinopathy, or indirectly by supporting the growth of pathological tissues, as in rheumatoid arthritis and tumor growth. Neovascularization occurs from capillaries and is initiated when the capillary endothelial cells penetrate through their basement membranes, migrate toward the source of angiogenic inducer, and proliferate, forming new cords of endothelial cells that eventually develop into capillaries (264). The FGFs have effects on cultured endothelial cells that are consistent with a role in this process. Fibroblast growth factor-2 induces an invasive phenotype in cultured endothelial cells (265), enabling them to penetrate basement membranes in vitro (266). The ability to penetrate the basement membrane relies on the increased production of the proteolytic enzymes plasminogen activator and collagenase in response to FGF-2 (Fig. 1) (94, 266, 267). In addition, both FGF-1 and FGF-2 are chemotactic for endothelial cells (267, 268), suggesting that these factors support the directed growth of capillaries during angiogenesis. Finally, FGF-1 and FGF-2 stimulate endothelial cell proliferation (269). Thus, FGF-1 and FGF-2 have properties expected for angiogenic factors and, indeed, induce angiogenesis in vivo in a number of model systems (270–275).

However, the roles of the FGFs and their receptors in physiological angiogenesis in vivo have been difficult to sort out, not only because of the overlapping biological properties of the members of the FGF family, but also because similar biological effects are induced by unrelated growth factors. For example, FGF receptor-1 was first identified as a gene that is up-regulated in endothelial cells forming tubes in vitro (276), so it might be expected to have a critical role in angiogenesis in vivo. However, knock out of the FGF receptor-1 gene is lethal at embryonic stages but has no effect on early vascular development (277, 278). Although FGF receptor-1 is expressed on some cultured endothelial cells and in aortic endothelial cells in vivo (166, 279–281), expression of FGF receptor-2 has been detected in other endothelial cells (280). Thus, it is possible that vascular development is mediated through other FGF receptors in FGF receptor-1 knockout mice or that FGF receptor-1 mediates angiogenesis at specific sites at later stages of development.

In several studies, administration of neutralizing antibodies to FGF-2 has had no effect on tumor growth in animals, suggesting that these antibodies had no effect on tumor angiogenesis (282, 283). Furthermore, knock out of the FGF-2 gene has no effect on vascular development, retinal neovascularization, or tumor growth (284–286) (C. Basilico, personal communication). It is possible that the role of FGF-2 is filled by other members of the FGF family in these systems.

However, it appears that endogenous FGF-2 is important in some instances of angiogenesis. Collagen sponges were implanted subcutaneously in rats, and the effect of antibodies to FGF-2 on the subsequent formation of granulation tissue in these sponges was investigated (287). When a pellet that slowly released neutralizing antibody to FGF-2 was included in the sponge, vascularization of the sponge and granulation tissue formation were inhibited. In addition, treatment of animals with antibodies to FGF-2 gives a small reduction in growth of gliomas (288–290), and treatment of melanomas with antisense FGF-2 constructs inhibits melanoma growth (291). Where studied, these treatments seem to exert their affects, at least in part, through the inhibition of angiogenesis. Thus, FGFs may have a role in the vascularization of certain types of tumors or may contribute to angiogenesis in wound healing.

VIII. CONCLUSIONS

Although FGFs are potent angiogenic factors when administered to animals, the role of FGFs in physiological angiogenesis is unclear. Part of the confusion may be due to the incredible redundancy of the FGF system, where a large family of growth factors interacts with overlapping specificity with a variety of alternately spliced receptors. Thus, inhibition of the action of FGF-2 may still allow FGF-1 or other family members to mediate angiogenic responses. Perhaps the true role of FGFs in angiogenesis will be revealed in animals carrying knock outs of both FGF-1 and FGF-2 genes.

ACKNOWLEDGMENTS

This work was supported by grants from the National Institutes of Health.

REFERENCES

1. Armelin HA. Pituitary extracts and steroid hormones in the control of 3T3 cell growth. Proc Natl Acad Sci U S A 1973; 70:2702–2706.
2. Gospodarowicz D. Localization of a fibroblast growth factor and its effect alone and with hydrocortisone on 3T3 cell growth. Nature 1974; 249:123–127.
3. Gospodarowicz D. Purification of a fibroblast growth factor from bovine pituitary. J Biol Chem 1975; 250:2515–2520.
4. Gospodarowicz D, Bialecki H, Greenburg G. Purification of the fibroblast growth factor activity from bovine brain. J Biol Chem 1978; 253:3736–3743.
5. Maciag T, Cerundolo J, Ilsley S, Kelley PR, Forand R. An endothelial cell growth factor from bovine hypothalamus: Identification and partial characterization. Proc Natl Acad Sci U S A 1979; 76:5674–5678.
6. Thomas KA, Riley MC, Lemmon SK, Baglan NC, Bradshaw RA. Brain fibroblast growth factor. Nonidentity with myelin basic protein fragments. J Biol Chem 1980; 255:5517–5520.
7. Gospodarowicz D, Greenburg G, Bialecki H, Zetter BR. Factors involved in the modulation of cell proliferation in vivo and in vitro: The role of fibroblast and epidermal growth factors in the proliferative response of mammalian cells. In Vitro 1978; 14:85–118.

8. Bohlen P, Baird A, Esch F, Ling N, Gospodarowicz D. Isolation and partial molecular characterization of pituitary fibroblast growth factor. Proc Natl Acad Sci U S A 1984; 81:5364–5368.
9. Thomas KA, Rios-Candelore M, Fitzpatrick S. Purification and characterization of acidic fibroblast growth factor from bovine brain. Proc Natl Acad Sci U S A 1984; 81:357–361.
10. Shing Y, Folkman J, Sullivan R, Butterfield C, Murray J, Klagsbrun M. Heparin affinity: Purification of a tumor-derived capillary endothelial cell growth factor. Science 1984; 223:1296–1299.
11. Klagsbrun M, Shing Y. Heparin affinity of anionic and cationic capillary endothelial cell growth factors: Analysis of hypothalamus-derived growth factors and fibroblast growth factors. Proc Natl Acad Sci U S A 1985; 82:805–809.
12. Gospodarowicz D, Cheng J, Lui GM, Baird A, Bohlen P. Isolation of brain fibroblast growth factor by heparin-sepharose affinity chromatography: Identity with pituitary fibroblast growth factor. Proc Natl Acad Sci U S A 1984; 81:6963–6967.
13. Maciag T, Mehlman T, Friesel R, Schreiber AB. Heparin binds endothelial cell growth factor, the principal endothelial cell mitogen in bovine brain. Science 1984; 225:932–935.
14. Dickson C, Peters G. Potential oncogene product related to growth factors. Nature (London) 1987; 326:833.
15. Delli Bovi P, Curatola AM, Kern FG, Greco A, Ittmann M, Basilico C. An oncogene isolated by transfection of Kaposi's sarcoma DNA encodes a growth factor that is a member of the FGF family. Cell 1987; 50:729–737.
16. Taira M, Yoshida T, Miyagawa K, Sakamoto H, Terada M, Sugimura T. cDNA sequence of human transforming gene hst and identification of the coding sequence required for transforming activity. Proc Natl Acad Sci U S A 1987; 84:2980–2984.
17. Zhan X, Botes B, Hu X, Goldfarb M. The human FGF-5 oncogene encodes a novel protein related to fibroblast growth factors. Mol Cell Biol 1988; 8:3487–3495.
18. Marics I, Adelaide J, Raybaud F, Mattei M, Coulier F, Planche J, DeLapeyriere O, Birnbaum D. Characterization of the hst-related FGF-6 gene, a new member of the fibroblast growth factor gene family. Oncogene 1989; 4:335–340.
19. Finch PW, Rubin JS, Miki T, Ron D, Aaronson SA. Human KGF is FGF-related with properties of a paracrine effector of epithelial cell growth. Science 1989; 245: 752–755.
20. Tanaka A, Miyamoto K, Minamino N, Takeda M, Sato B, Matsuo H, Matsumoto K. Cloning and characterization of an androgen-induced growth factor essential for the androgen-dependent growth of mouse mammary carcinoma cells. Proc Natl Acad Sci U S A 1992; 89:8928–8932.
21. Kouhara H, Koga M, Kasayama S, Tanaka A, Kishimoto T, Sato B. Transforming activity of a newly cloned androgen-induced growth factor. Oncogene 1994; 9: 455–462.
22. Naruo K, Seko C, Kuroshima K, Matsutani E, Sasada R, Kondo T, Kurokawa T. Novel secretory heparin-binding factors from human glioma cells (glia-activating factors) involved in glial cell growth. J Biol Chem 1993; 268:2857–2864.
23. Yamasaki M, Miyake A, Tagashira S, Itoh N. Structure and expression of the rat

mRNA encoding a novel member of the fibroblast growth factor family. J Biol Chem 1996; 271:15918–15921.

24. Smallwood PM, Munoz-Sanjuan I, Tong P, Macke JP, Hendry SHC, Gilbert DJ, Copeland NG, Jenkins NA, Nathans J. Fibroblast growth factor (FGF) homologous factors: new members of the FGF family implicated in nervous system development. Proc Natl Acad Sci U S A 1996; 93:9850–9857.
25. Esch F, Baird A, Ling N, Ueno N, Hill F, Denoroy L, Klepper R, Gospodarowicz D, Bohlen P, Guillemin R. Primary structure of bovine pituitary basic fibroblast growth factor (FGF) and comparison with the amino-terminal sequence of bovine brain acidic FGF. Proc Natl Acad Sci U S A 1985; 82:6507–6511.
26. Baird A, Esch F, Gospodarowicz D, Guillemin R. Retina- and eye-derived endothelial cell growth factors: Partial molecular characterization and identity with acidic and basic fibroblast growth factors. Biochemistry 1985; 24:7855–7860.
27. Gospodarowicz D, Baird A, Cheng J, Lui GM, Esch F, Bohlen P. Isolation of fibroblast growth factor from bovine adrenal gland: Physicochemical and biological characterization. Endocrinology 1986; 118:82–90.
28. Bohlen P, Esch F, Baird A, Jones KL, Gospodarowicz D. Human brain fibroblast growth factor. Isolation and partial chemical characterization. FEBS Lett 1985; 185:177–181.
29. Gimenez-Gallego G, Conn G, Hatcher VB, Thomas KA. Human brain-derived acidic and basic fibroblast growth factors: Amino terminal sequences and specific mitogenic activities. Biochem Biophys Res Commun 1986; 135:541–548.
30. Gospodarowicz D, Cheng J, Lui GM, Baird A, Esch F, Bohlen P. Corpus luteum angiogenic factor is related to fibroblast growth factor. Endocrinology 1985; 117: 2383–2391.
31. Ueno N, Baird A, Esch F, Ling N, Guillemin R. Isolation and partial characterization of basic fibroblast growth factor from bovine testis. Mol Cell Endocrinol 1987; 49:189–194.
32. Klagsbrun M, Smith S, Sullivan R, Shing Y, Davidson S, Smith JA, Sasse J. Multiple forms of basic fibroblast growth factor: Amino-terminal cleavages by tumor cell- and brain cell-derived acid proteinases. Proc Natl Acad Sci U S A 1987; 84: 1839–1843.
33. Story MT, Esch F, Shimasaki S, Sasse J, Jacobs SC, Lawson RK. Amino-terminal sequence of a large form of basic fibroblast growth factor isolated from human benign prostatic hyperplastic tissue. Biochem Biophys Res Commun 1987; 142: 702–709.
34. Ueno N, Baird A, Esch F, Ling N, Guillemin R. Isolation of an amino terminal extended form of basic fibroblast growth factor. Biochem Biophys Res Commun 1986; 138:580–588.
35. Abraham JA, Whang JL, Tumolo A, Mergia A, Friedman J, Gospodarowicz D, Fiddes JC. Human basic fibroblast growth factor: Nucleotide sequence and genomic organization. EMBO J 1986; 5:2523–2528.
36. Abraham JA, Mergia A, Whang JL, Tumolo A, Friedman J, Hjerrild KA, Gospodarowicz D, Fiddes JC. Nucleotide sequence of a bovine clone encoding the angiogenic protein, basic fibroblast growth factor. Science 1986; 233:545–548.

37. Sommer A, Brewer MT,Thompson RC, Moscatelli D, Presta M, Rifkin DB. A form of human basic fibroblast growth factor with an extended amino terminus. Biochem Biophys Res Commun 1987; 144:543–550.
38. Moscatelli D, Joseph-Silverstein J, Manejias R, Rifkin DB. M_r 25,000 heparin-binding protein from guinea pig brain is a high molecular weight form of basic fibroblast growth factor. Proc Natl Acad Sci U S A 1987; 84:5778–5782.
39. Vagner S, Gensac M, Maret A, Bayard F, Amalric F, Prats H, Prats A. Alternative translation of human fibroblast growth factor 2 mRNA occurs by internal entry of ribosomes. Mol Cell Biol 1995; 15:35–44.
40. Florkiewicz RZ, Sommer A. The human bFGF gene encodes four polypeptides: Three initiate translation from non-AUG codons. Proc Natl Acad Sci U S A 1989; 86:3978–3981.
41. Prats H, Kaghad M, Prats AC, Klagsbrun M, Lelias JM, Liauzun P, Chalon P, Tauber JP, Amalric F, Smith JA, Caput D. High molecular mass forms of basic fibroblast growth factor are initiated by alternative CUG codons. Proc Natl Acad Sci U S A 1989; 86:1836–1840.
42. Presta M, Rusnati M, Maier JAM, Ragnotti G. Purification of basic fibroblast growth factor from rat brain: Identification of a Mr 22,000 immunoreactive form. Biochem Biophys Res Commun 1988; 155:1161–1172.
43. Renko M, Quarto N, Moromoto T, Rifkin DB. Nuclear and cytoplasmic localization of different basic fibroblast growth factor species. J Cell Physiol 1990; 144:108–114.
44. Iberg N, Rogelj S, Fanning P, Klagsbrun M. Purification of 18-and 22-kDa forms of basic fibroblast growth factor from rat cells transformed by the *ras* oncogene. J Biol Chem 1989; 19951–19955.
45. Tsuboi R, Sato Y, Rifkin DB. Correlation of cell migration, cell invasion, receptor number, proteinase production, and basic fibroblast growth factor levels in endothelial cells. J Cell Biol 1990; 110:511–517.
46. Giordano S, Sherman L, Lyman W, Morrison R. Multiple molecular weight forms of basic fibroblast growth factor are developmentally regulated in the central nervous system. Dev Biol 1992; 152:293–303.
47. Liu L, Doble BW, Kardami E. Perinatal phenotype and hypothyroidism are associated with elevated levels of 21.5 to 22-kDa basic fibroblast growth factor in cardiac ventricles. Dev Biol 1993; 157:507–516.
48. Dono R, Zeller R. Cell type-specific nuclear transportation of fibroblast growth factor-2 isoforms during chicken kidney and limb morphogenesis. Dev Biol 1994; 163:316–330.
49. Riese J, Zeller R, Dono R. Nucleo-cytoplasmic translocation and secretion of fibroblast growth factor-2 during avian gastrulation. Mech Dev 1995; 49:13–22.
50. Coffin JD, Florkiewicz RZ, Neumann J, Mort-Hopkins T, Dorn GW, Lightfoot P, German R, Howles PN, Kier A, O'Toole BA, Sasse J, Gonzalez AM, Baird A, Doetschman T. Abnormal bone growth and selective translational regulation in basic fibroblast growth factor (FGF-2) transgenic mice. Mol Biol Cell 1995; 6:1861–1873.
51. Vagner S, Touriol C, Galy B, Audigier S, Gensac M, Amalric F, Bayard F, Prats H, Prats A. Translation of CUG- but not AUG-initiated forms of human fibroblast

growth factor 2 is activated in transformed and stressed cells. J Cell Biol 1996; 135:1391–1402.

52. Klein S, Morimoto T, Rifkin DB. Characterization of fibroblast growth factor-2 binding to ribosomes. Growth Factors 1996; 13:219–228.
53. Florkiewicz RZ, Baird A, Gonzalez A-M. Multiple forms of bFGF: Differential nuclear and cell surface localization. Growth Factors 1991; 4:265–275.
54. Bugler B, Amalric F, Prats H. Alternative initiation of translation determines cytoplasmic or nuclear localization of basic fibroblast growth factor. Mol Cell Biol 1991; 11:573–577.
55. Quarto N, Finger FP, Rifkin DB. The NH2-terminal extension of high molecular weight bFGF is a nuclear targeting signal. J Cell Physiol 1991; 147:311–318.
56. Shi J, Friedman S, Maciag T. A carboxyl-terminal domain in fibroblast growth factor (FGF)-2 inhibits FGF-1 release in response to heat shock in vitro. J Biol Chem 1997; 272:1142–1147.
57. Sommer A, Moscatelli D, Rifkin DB. An amino-terminally extended and post-translationally modified form of a 25kD basic fibroblast growth factor. Biochem Biophys Res Commun 1989; 160:1267–1274.
58. Burgess WH, Bizik J, Mehlman T, Quarto N, Rifkin DB. Direct evidence for methylation of arginine residues in high molecular weight forms of basic fibroblast growth factor. Cell Regulation 1991; 2:87–93.
59. Pintucci G, Quarto N, Rifkin DB. Methylation of high molecular weight fibroblast growth factor-2 determines post-translational increases in molecular weight and affects its intracellular distribution. Mol Biol Cell 1996; 7:1249–1258.
60. Bikfalvi A, Klein S, Pintucci G, Quarto N, Mignatti P, Rifkin DB. Differential modulation of cell phenotype by different molecular weight forms of basic fibroblast growth factor: Possible intracellular signaling by the high molecular weight forms. J Cell Biol 1995; 129:233–243.
61. Klein S, Bikfalvi A, Birkenmeier TM, Giancotti FG, Rifkin DB. Integrin regulation by endogenous expression of 18-kDa fibroblast growth factor-2. J Biol Chem 1996; 271:22583–22590.
62. Estival A, Monzat V, Miquel K, Gaubert F, Hollande E, Korc M, Vaysse N, Clemente F. Differential regulation of fibroblast growth factor (FGF) receptor-1 mRNA and protein by two molecular forms of basic FGF. Modulation of FGFR-1 mRNA stability. J Biol Chem 1996; 271:5663–5670.
63. Pasumarthi KBS, Kardami E, Cattini PA. High and low molecular weight fibroblast growth factor-2 increase proliferation of neonatal rat cardiac myocytes but have differential effects on binucleation and nuclear morphology. Evidence for both paracrine and intracrine actions of fibroblast growth factor-2. Circ Res 1996; 78:126–136.
64. Quarto N, Talarico D, Florkiewicz R, Rifkin DB. Selective expression of high molecular weight basic fibroblast growth factor confers a unique phenotype to NIH 3T3 cells. Cell Regulation 1991; 2:699–708.
65. Hata J, Takeo J, Segawa C, Yamashita S. A cDNA encoding fish fibroblast growth factor-2, which lacks alternative translation initiation. J Biol Chem 1997; 272: 7285–7289.
66. Simpson RJ, Moritz RL, Lloyd CJ, Fabri LJ, Nice EC, Rubira MR, Burgess AW.

Primary structure of ovine pituitary basic fibroblast growth factor. FEBS Lett 1987; 224:128–132.

67. Shimasaki S, Emoto N, Koba A, Mercado M, Shibata F, Cooksey K, Baird A, Ling N. Complementary DNA cloning and sequencing of rat ovarian basic fibroblast growth factor and tissue distribution study of its mRNA. Biochem Biophys Res Commun 1988; 157:256–263.
68. Kurokawa T, Seno M, Igarashi K. Nucleotide sequence of rat basic fibroblast growth factor cDNA. Nucl Acids Res 1988; 16:5201.
69. Kimelman D, Abraham JA, Haaparanta T, Palisi TM, Kirschner MW. The presence of fibroblast growth factor in the frog egg: Its role as a natural mesoderm inducer. Science 1988; 242:1053–1056.
70. Brigstock DR, Klagsbrun M, Sasse J, Farber PA, Iberg N. Species-specific high molecular weight forms of basic fibroblast growth factor. Growth Factors 1990; 4: 45–52.
71. Eriksson AE, Cousens LS, Weaver LH, Matthews BW. Three-dimensional structure of human basic fibroblast growth factor. Proc Natl Acad Sci U S A 1991; 88: 3441–3445.
72. Eriksson AE, Cousens LS, Matthews BW. Refinement of the structure of human basic fibroblast growth factor at 1.6 Å resolution and analysis of presumed heparin binding sites by selenate substitution. Protein Sci 1993; 2:1274–1284.
73. Zhang J, Cousens LS, Barr PJ, Sprang SR. Three-dimensional structure of human basic fibroblast growth factor, a structural homolog of interleukin 1β. Proc Natl Acad Sci U S A 1991; 88:3446–3450.
74. Zhu X, Komiya H, Chirino A, Faham S, Fox GM, Arakawa T, Hsu BT, Rees DC. Three-dimensional structures of acidic and basic fibroblast growth factors. Science 1991; 251:90–93.
75. Moy F, Seddon A, Bohlen P, Powers R. High-resolution solution structure of basic fibroblast growth factor determined by multidimensional heteronuclear magnetic resonance spectroscopy. Biochemistry 1996; 35:13552–13561.
76. Seno M, Sasada R, Iwane M, Sudo K, Kurokawa T, Ito K, Igarashi K. Stabilizing basic fibroblast growth factor using protein engineering. Biochem Biophys Res Commun 1988; 151:701–708.
77. Fox GM, Schiffer SG, Rohde MF, Tsai LB, Banks AR, Arakawa T. Production, biological activity, and structure of recombinant basic fibroblast growth factor and an analog with cysteine replaced by serine. J Biol Chem 1988; 263:18452–18458.
78. Baird A, Schubert D, Ling N, Guillemin R. Receptor-and heparin-binding domains of basic fibroblast growth factor. Proc Natl Acad Sci U S A 1988; 85:2324–2328.
79. Faham S, Hileman RE, Fromm JR, Linhardt RJ, Rees DC. Heparin structure and interactions with basic fibroblast growth factor. Science 1996; 271:1116–1120.
80. Thompson LD, Pantoliano MW, Springer BA. Energetic characterization of the basic fibroblast growth factor-heparin interaction: Identification of the heparin-binding domain. Biochemistry 1994; 33:3831–3840.
81. Springer BA, Pantoliano MW, Barbera FA, Gunyuzlu PL, Thompson LD, Herblin WF, Rosenfeld SA, Book GW. Identification and concerted function of two receptor binding surfaces on basic fibroblast growth factor required for mitogenesis. J Biol Chem 1994; 269:26879–26884.

82. Zhu H, Ramnarayan K, Anchin J, Miao WY, Sereno A, Millman L, Zheng J, Balaji VN, Wolff ME. Glu-96 of basic fibroblast growth factor is essential for high affinity receptor binding. Identification by structure-based site-directed mutagenesis. J Biol Chem 1995; 270:21869–21874.
83. Seddon A, Decker M, Muller T, Armellino D, Kovesdi I, Gluzman Y, Bohlen P. Structure/activity relationships in basic FGF. Ann N Y Acad Sci 1991; 638:98–108.
84. Seno M, Sasada R, Kurokawa T, Igarashi K. Carboxyl-terminal structure of basic fibroblast growth factor significantly contributes to its affinity for heparin. Eur J Biochem 1990; 188:239–245.
85. Baird A, Esch F, Mormede P, Ueno N, Ling N, Bohlen P, Ying S-Y, Wehrenberg WB, Guillemin R. Molecular characterization of fibroblast growth factor: Distribution and biological activities in various tissues. Recent Prog Horm Res 1986; 42: 143–205.
86. Moscatelli D, Presta M, Joseph-Silverstein J, Rifkin DB. Both normal and tumor cells produce basic fibroblast growth factor. J Cell Physiol 1986; 129:273–276.
87. Connolly DT, Stoddard BL, Harakas NK, Feder J. Human fibroblast-derived growth factor is a mitogen and chemoattractant for endothelial cells. Biochem Biophys Res Commun 1987; 144:705–712.
88. Schweigerer L, Neufeld G, Friedman J, Abraham JA, Fiddes JC, Gospodarowicz D. Capillary endothelial cells express basic fibroblast growth factor, a mitogen that promotes their own growth. Nature 1987; 325:257–259.
89. Vlodavsky I, Folkman J, Sullivan R, Fridman R, Ishai-Michaeli R, Sasse J, Klagsbrun M. Endothelial cell-derived basic fibroblast growth factor: Synthesis and deposition into subendothelial extracellular matrix. Proc Natl Acad Sci U S A 1987; 84:2292–2296.
90. Hatten ME, Lynch M, Rydel RE, Sanchez J, Joseph-Silverstein J, Moscatelli D, Rifkin DB. In vitro neurite extension by granule neurons is dependent upon astroglial-derived fibroblast growth factor. Dev Biol 1988; 125:280–289.
91. Gospodarowicz D, Ferrara N, Haaparanta T, Neufeld G. Basic fibroblast growth factor: Expression in cultured bovine vascular smooth muscle cells. Eur J Cell Biol 1988; 46:144–151.
92. Weich HA, Iberg N, Klagsbrun M, Folkman J. Expression of acidic and basic fibroblast growth factors in human and bovine vascular smooth muscle cells. Growth Factors 1990; 2:313–320.
93. Klagsbrun M, Sasse J, Sullivan R, Smith JA. Human tumor cells synthesize an endothelial cell growth factor that is structurally related to basic fibroblast growth factor. Proc Natl Acad Sci U S A 1986; 83:2448–2452.
94. Presta M, Moscatelli D, Joseph-Silverstein J, Rifkin DB. Purification from a human hepatoma cell line of a basic fibroblast growth factor-like molecule that stimulates capillary endothelial cell plasminogen activator production, DNA synthesis, and migration. Mol Cell Biol 1986; 6:4060–4066.
95. Schweigerer L, Neufeld G, Mergia A, Abraham JA, Fiddes JC, Gospodarowicz D. Basic fibroblast growth factor in human rhabdomyosarcoma cells: Implications for the proliferation and neovascularization of myoblast-derived tumors. Proc Natl Acad Sci U S A 1987; 84:842–846.

96. Cordon-Cardo C, Vlodavsky I, Haimovitz-Friedman A, Hicklin D, Fuks Z. Expression of basic fibroblast growth factor in normal tissues. Lab Invest 1990; 63:832–840.
97. Hanneken A, Lutty GA, McLeod DS, Robey F, Harvey AK, Hjelmeland LM. Localization of basic fibroblast growth factor to the developing capillaries of the bovine retina. J Cell Physiol 1989; 138:115–120.
98. Pettmann B, Labourdette G, Weibel M, Sensenbrenner M. The brain fibroblast growth factor (FGF) is localized in neurons. Neurosci Lett 1986; 68:175–180.
99. Finklestein SP, Apostolides PJ, Caday CG, Prosser J, Philips MF, Klagsbrun M. Increased basic fibroblast growth factor (bFGF) immunoreactivity at the site of focal brain wounds. Brain Res 1988; 460:253–259.
100. Emoto N, Gonzalez A-M, Walicke PA, Wada E, Simmons DM, Shimasaki S, Baird A. Basic fibroblast growth factor (FGF) in the central nervous system: Identification of specific loci of basic FGF expression in the rat brain. Growth Factors 1989; 2:21–29.
101. Fujimoto K, Ichimori Y, Kakizoe T, Okajima E, Sakamoto H, Sugimura T, Terada M. Increased serum levels of basic fibroblast growth factor in patients with renal cell carcinoma. Biochem Biophys Res Commun 1991; 180:386–392.
102. Sliutz G, Tempfer C, Obermair A, Dadak C, Kainz C. Serum evaluation of basic FGF in breast cancer patients. Anticancer Res 1995; 15:2675–2677.
103. Rohovsky S, Kearney M, Pieczek A, Rosenfield K, Schainfeld R, D'Amore P, Isner J. Elevated levels of basic fibroblast growth factor in patients with limb ischemia. Am Heart J 1996; 132:1015–1019.
104. Gimenez-Gallego G, Rodkey J, Bennett C, Rios-Candelore M, DiSalvo J, Thomas K. Brain-derived acidic fibroblast growth factor: Complete amino acid sequence and homologies. Science 1985; 230:1385–1388.
105. Esch F, Ueno N, Baird A, Hill F, Denoroy L, Ling N, Gospodarowicz D, Guillemin R. Primary structure of bovine brain acidic fibroblast growth factor (FGF). Biochem Biophys Res Commun 1985; 133:554–562.
106. Burgess WH, Mehlman T, Marshak DR, Fraser BA, Maciag T. Structural evidence that endothelial cell growth factor β is the precursor of both endothelial cell growth factor α and acidic fibroblast growth factor. Proc Natl Acad Sci U S A 1986; 83:7216–7220.
107. Harper JW, Strydom DJ, Lobb RR. Human class 1 heparin- binding growth factor: Structure and homology to bovine acidic brain fibroblast growth factor. Biochemistry 1986; 25:4097–4103.
108. Jaye M, Howk R, Burgess W, Ricca G, Chiu I-M, Ravera MW, O'Brien SJ, Modi WS, Maciag T, Drohan WN. Human endothelial cell growth factor: cloning, nucleotide sequence, and chromosomal localization. Science 1986; 233:541–545.
109. Crumley G, Dionne CA, Jaye M. The gene for human acidic fibroblast growth factor encodes two upstream exons alternatively spliced to the first coding exon. Biochem Biophys Res Commun 1990; 171:7–13.
110. Chiu I-M, Wang W-P, Lehtoma K. Alternative splicing generates two forms of mRNA coding for human heparin-binding growth factor 1. Oncogene 1990; 5:755–762.
111. Myers RL, Payson RA, Chotani MA, Deaven LL, Chiu I-M. Gene structure and

differential expression of acidic fibroblast growth factor mRNA: Identification and distribution of four different transcripts. Oncogene 1993; 8:341–349.
112. Myers RL, Ray SK, Eldridge R, Chotani MA, Chiu I-M. Functional characterization of the brain-specific FGF-1 promoter, FGF-1.B. J Biol Chem 1995; 270:8257–8266.
113. Blaber M, DiSalvo J, Thomas KA. X-ray crystal structure of human acidic fibroblast growth factor. Biochemistry 1996; 35:2086–2094.
114. Romero A, Pineda-Lucena A, Gimenez-Gallego G. X-ray structure of native full-length human fibroblast-growth factor at 0.25-nm resolution. Eur J Biochem 1996; 241:453–461.
115. Crabb JW, Armes LG, Carr SA, Johnson CM, Roberts GD, Bordoli RS, McKeehan WL. Complete primary structure of prostatropin, a prostate epithelial cell growth factor. Biochemistry 1986; 25:4988–4993.
116. Jaye M, Burgess WH, Shaw AB, Drohan WN. Biological equivalence of natural bovine and recombinant human α-endothelial cell growth factors. J Biol Chem 1987; 262:16612–16617.
117. Linemeyer DL, Menke JG, Kelly LJ, DiSalvo J, Soderman D, Schaeffer M-T, Ortega S, Gimenez-Gallego G, Thomas KA. Disulfide bonds are neither required, present, nor compatible with full activity of human recombinant acidic fibroblast growth factor. Growth Factors 1990; 3:287–298.
118. Mehlman T, Burgess WH. Identification and characterization of heparin-binding proteins using a gel overlay procedure. Anal Biochem 1990; 188:159–163.
119. Harper JW, Lobb RR. Reductive methylation of lysine residues in acidic fibroblast growth factor: Effect on mitogenic activity and heparin affinity. Biochemistry 1988; 27:671–678.
120. Burgess WH, Shaheen AM, Ravera M, Jaye M, Donohue PJ, Winkles JA. Possible dissociation of the heparin-binding and mitogenic activities of heparin-binding (acidic fibroblast) growth factor-1 from its receptor-binding activities by site-directed mutagenesis of a single lyine residue. J Cell Biol 1990; 111:2129–2138.
121. Seddon AP, Aviezer D, Li L-Y, Böhlen P, Yayon A. Engineering of fibroblast growth factor: Alteration of receptor binding specificity. Biochemistry 1995; 34: 731–736.
122. D'Amore PA, Klagsbrun M. Endothelial cell mitogens derived from retina and hypothalamus: Biochemical and biological similarities. J Cell Biol 1984; 99:1545–1549.
123. Gautschi-Sova P, Jiang Z, Frater-Schroder M, Bohlen P. Acidic fibroblast growth factor is present in nonneural tissue: isolation and chemical characterization from bovine kidney. Biochemistry 1987; 26:5844–5847.
124. Casscells W, Speir E, Sasse J, Klagsbrun M, Allen P, Lee M, Calvo B, Chiba M, Haggroth L, Folkman J, Epstein SE. Isolation, characterization, and localization of heparin-binding growth factors in the heart. J Clin Invest 1990; 85:433–441.
125. Quinkler W, Maasberg M, Bernotat-Danielowski S, Luthe N, Sharma HS, Schaper W. Isolation of heparin-binding growth factors from bovine, porcine and canine hearts. Eur J Biochem 1989; 181:67–73.
126. Sasaki H, Hoshi H, Hong Y-M, Suzuki T, Kato T, Sasaki H, Saito M, Youki H, Karube K, Konno S, Onodera M, Saito T, Aoyagi S. Purification of acidic fibroblast

growth factor from bovine heart and its localization in the cardiac myocytes. J Biol Chem 1989; 264:17606–17612.
127. Wilcox BJ, Unnerstall JR. Expression of acidic fibroblast growth factor mRNA in the developing and adult rat brain. Neuron 1991; 6:397–409.
128. Winkles JA, Friesel R, Burgess WH, Howk R, Mehlman T, Weinstein R, Maciag T. Human vascular smooth muscle cells both express and respond to heparin-binding growth factor I (endothelial cell growth factor). Proc Natl Acad Sci U S A 1987; 84:7124–7128.
129. Gajdusek CM, Carbon S. Injury-induced release of basic fibroblast growth factor from bovine aortic endothelium. J Cell Physiol 1989; 139:570–579.
130. Brooks R, Burrin J, Kohner E. Characterization of release of basic fibroblast growth factor from bovine retinal endothelial cells in monolayer cultures. Biochem J 1991; 276:113–120.
131. McNeil PL, Muthukrishnan L, Warder E, D'Amore PA. Growth factors are released by mechanically wounded endothelial cells. J Cell Biol 1989; 109:811–822.
132. Muthukrishnan L, Warder E, McNeil P. Basic fibroblast growth factor is efficiently released from a cytolsolic storage site through plasma membrane disruptions of endothelial cells. J Cell Physiol 1991; 148:1–16.
133. Ku P, D'Amore P. Regulation of basic fibroblast growth factor (bFGF) gene and protein expression following its release from sublethally injured endothelial cells. J Cell Biochem 1995; 58:328–343.
134. Benzaquen L, Nicholson-Weller A, Halperin J. Terminal complement proteins C5b-9 release basic fibroblast growth factor and platelet-derived growth factor from endothelial cells. J Exp Med 1994; 179:985–992.
135. Sato Y, Rifkin DB. Autocrine activities of basic fibroblast growth factor: Regulation of endothelial cell movement, plasminogen activator synthesis, and DNA synthesis. J Cell Biol 1988; 107:1199–1205.
136. Sakaguchi M, Kajio T, Kawahara K, Kato K. Antibodies against basic fibroblast growth factor inhibit the autocrine growth of pulmonary artery endothelial cells. FEBS Lett 1988; 233:163–166.
137. Mignatti P, Morimoto T, Rifkin DB. Basic fibroblast growth factor released by single, isolated cells stimulates their migration in an autocrine manner. Proc Natl Acad Sci U S A 1991; 88:11007–11011.
138. Florkiewicz R, Majack R, Buechler R, Florkiewicz E. Quantitative export of FGF-2 occurs through an alternative, energy-dependent, non-ER/Golgi pathway. J Cell Physiol 1995; 162:388–399.
139. Mignatti P, Morimoto T, Rifkin DB. Basic fibroblast growth factor, a protein devoid of a secretory signal sequence, is released by cells via a pathway independent of the endoplasmic reticulum-Golgi complex. J Cell Physiol 1992; 151:81–93.
140. Jackson A, Friedman S, Zhan X, Engleka KA, Forough R, Maciag T. Heat shock induces the release of fibroblast growth factor 1 from NIH 3T3 cells. Proc Natl Acad Sci U S A 1992; 89:10691–10695.
141. Shin J, Opalenik S, Wehby J, Mahesh V, Jackson A, Tarantini F, Maciag T, Thompson J. Serum-starvation induces the extracellular appearance of FGF-1. Biochim Biophys Acta 1996; 1312:27–38.

142. Opalenik S, Shin J, Wehby J, Mahesh V, Thompson J. The HIV-1 TAT protein induces the expression and extracellular appearance of acidic fibroblast growth factor. J Biol Chem 1995; 270:17457–17467.
143. Jackson A, Tarantini F, Gamble S, Friedman S, Maciag T. The release of fibroblast growth factor-1 from NIH 3T3 cells in response to temperature involves the function of cysteine residues. J Biol Chem 1995; 270:33–36.
144. Tarantini F, Gamble S, Jackson A, Maciag T. The cysteine residue responsible for the release of fibroblast growth factor-1 residues in a domain independent of the domain for phosphatidylserine binding. J Biol Chem 1995; 270:29039–29042.
145. Ananyeva N, Tjurmin A, Berliner J, Chisolm G, Liau G, Winkles J, Haudenschild C. Oxidized LDL mediates the release of fibroblast growth factor-1. Arterioscler Thromb Vasc Biol 1997; 17:445–453.
146. Neufeld G, Gospodarowicz D. The identification and partial characterization of the fibroblast growth factor receptor of baby hamster kidney cells. J Biol Chem 1985; 260:13860–13868.
147. Olwin BB, Hauschka SD. Identification of the fibroblast growth factor receptor of Swiss 3T3 cells and mouse skeletal muscle myoblasts. Biochemistry 1986; 25: 3487–3492.
148. Moscatelli D. High and low affinity binding sites for basic fibroblast growth factor on cultured cells: Absence of a role for low affinity binding in the stimulation of plasminogen activator production by bovine capillary endothelial cells. J Cell Physiol 1987; 131:123–130.
149. Moenner M, Chevallier B, Badet J, Barritault D. Evidence and characterization of the receptor to eye-derived growth factor I, the retinal form of basic fibroblast growth factor, on bovine epithelial lens cells. Proc Natl Acad Sci U S A 1986; 83: 5024–5028.
150. Neufeld G, Gospodarowicz D. Identification of the fibroblast growth factor receptor in human vascular endothelial cells. J Cell Physiol 1988; 136:537–542.
151. Schreiber AB, Kenney J, Kowalski WJ, Friesel R, Mehlman T, Maciag T. Interaction of endothelial cell growth factor with heparin: Characterization by receptor and antibody recognition. Proc Natl Acad Sci U S A 1985; 82:6138–6142.
152. Friesel R, Burgess WH, Mehlman T, Maciag T. The characterization of the receptor for endothelial cell growth factor by covalent ligand attachment. J Biol Chem 1986; 261:7581–7584.
153. Kan M, DiSorbo D, Hou J, Hoshi H, Mansson P-E, McKeehan WL. High and low affinity binding of heparin-binding growth factor to a 130-kDa receptor correlates with stimulation and inhibition of growth of a differentiated human hepatoma cell. J Biol Chem 1988; 263:11306–11313.
154. Neufeld G, Gospodarowicz D. Basic and acidic fibroblast growth factors interact with the same cell surface receptors. J Biol Chem 1986; 261:5631–5637.
155. Hoshi H, Kan M, Chen J-K, McKeehan W. Comparative endocrinology-paracrinology-autocrinology of human adult large vessel endothelial and smooth muscle cells. In Vitro Cell Dev Biol 1988; 24:309–320.
156. Jaye M, Schlessinger J, Dionne CA. Fibroblast growth factor receptor tyrosine ki-

nases: Molecular analysis and signal transduction. Biochim Biophys Acta 1992; 1135:185–199.
157. Johnson DE, Williams LT. Structural and functional diversity in the FGF receptor multigene family. Adv Cancer Res 1993; 60:1–41.
158. Burrus LW, Zuber ME, Lueddecke BA, Olwin BB. Identification of a cysteine-rich receptor for fibroblast growth factors. Mol Cell Biol 1992; 12:5600–5609.
159. Gonatas JO, Mezitis SG, Stieber A, Fleischer B, Gonatas NK. MG-160. A novel sialoglycoprotein of the medial cisternae of the Golgi apparatus. J Biol Chem 1989; 264:636–653.
160. Steegmaier M, Levinovitz A, Isenmann S, Borges E, Lenter M, Kocher HP, Kleuser B, Vestweber D. The E-selectin-ligand ESL-1 is a variant of a receptor for fibroblast growth factor. Nature 1995; 373:615–620.
161. Zuber ME, Zhou Z, Burrus LW, Olwin BB. Cysteine-rich FGF receptor regulates intracellular FGF-1 and FGF-2 levels. J Cell Physiol 1997; 170:217–227.
162. Lee PL, Johnson DE, Cousens LS, Fried VA, Williams LT. Purification and complementary DNA cloning of a receptor for basic fibroblast growth factor. Science 1989; 245:57–60.
163. Dionne CA, Crumley G, Bellot F, Kaplow JM, Searfoss G, Ruta M, Burgess WH, Jaye M, Schlessinger J. Cloning and expression of two distinct high-affinity receptors cross-reacting with acidic and basic fibroblast growth factors. EMBO J 1990; 9:2685–2692.
164. Keegan K, Johnson DE, Williams LT, Hayman MJ. Isolation of an additional member of the fibroblast growth factor receptor family, FGFR-3. Proc Natl Acad Sci U S A 1991; 88:1095–1099.
165. Partanen J, Makela TP, Eerola E, Korhonen J, Hirvonen H, Claesson-Welsh L, Alitalo K. FGFR-4, a novel acidic fibroblast growth factor receptor with a distinct expression pattern. EMBO J 1991; 10:1347–1354.
166. Johnson DE, Lu J, Chen H, Werner S, Williams LT. The human fibroblast growth factor receptor genes: A common structural arrangement underlies the mechanisms for generating receptor forms that differ in their third immunoglobulin domain. Mol Cell Biol 1991; 11:4627–4624.
167. Werner S, Duan D-SR, de Vries C, Peters KG, Johnson DE, Williams LT. Differential splicing in the extracellular region of fibroblast growth factor receptor 1 generates receptor variants with different ligand-binding specificities. Mol Cell Biol 1992; 12:82–88.
168. Dell KR, Williams LT. A novel form of fibroblast growth factor receptor-2. Alternative splicing of the third immunoglobulin-like domain confers ligand binding specificity. J Biol Chem 1992; 267:21225–21229.
169. Miki T, Bottaro DP, Fleming TP, Smith CL, Burgess WH, Chan AM-L, Aaronson SA. Determination of ligand-binding specificity by alternative splicing: Two distinct growth factor receptors encoded by a single gene. Proc Natl Acad Sci U S A 1992; 89:246–250.
170. Chellaiah AT, McEwen DG, Werner S, Xu J, Ornitz DM. Fibroblast growth factor receptor (FGFR) 3. Alternative splicing in immunoglobulin-like domain III creates a receptor highly specific for acidic FGF/FGF-1. J Biol Chem 1994; 269:11620–11627.

171. Avivi A, Yayon A, Givol D. A novel form of FGF receptor-3 using an alternative exon in the immunoglobulin domain III. FEBS Lett 1993; 330:249–252.
172. Ornitz DM, Xu J, Colvin JS, McEwen DG, MacArthur CA, Coulier F, Gao G, Goldfarb M. Receptor specificity of the fibroblast growth factor family. J Biol Chem 1996; 271:15292–15297.
173. Duan D-SR, Werner S, Williams LT. A naturally occurring secreted form of fibroblast growth factor (FGF) receptor 1 binds basic FGF in preference over acidic FGF. J Biol Chem 1992; 267:16076–16080.
174. Levi E, Fridman R, Miao H, Ma Y, Yayon A, Vlodavsky I. Matrix metalloproteinase 2 releases active soluble ectodomain of fibroblast growth factor receptor 1. Proc Natl Acad Sci U S A 1996; 93:7069–7074.
175. Hanneken A, Ying W, Ling N, Baird A. Identification of soluble forms of the fibroblast growth factor receptor in blood. Proc Natl Acad Sci U S A 1994; 91:9170–9174.
176. Hanneken A, Maher PA, Baird A. High affinity immunoreactive FGF receptors in the extracellular matrix of vascular endothelial cells—implications for the modulation of FGF-2. J Cell Biol 1995; 128:1221–1228.
177. Johnson DE, Lee PL, Lu J, Williams LT. Diverse forms of a receptor for acidic and basic fibroblast growth factors. Mol Cell Biol 1990; 10:4728–4736.
178. Reid HH, Wilks AF, Bernard O. Two forms of the basic fibroblast growth factor receptor-like mRNA are expressed in the developing mouse brain. Proc Natl Acad Sci U S A 1990; 87:1596–1600.
179. Mansukhani A, Moscatelli D, Talarico D, Levytska V, Basilico C. A murine fibroblast growth factor (FGF) receptor expressed in CHO cells is activated by both basic FGF and Kaposi FGF. Proc Natl Acad Sci U S A 1990; 87:4378–4382.
180. Champion-Arnaud P, Ronsin C, Gilbert E, Gesnel MC, Houssaint E, Breathnach R. Multiple mRNAs code for proteins related to the BEK fibroblast growth factor receptor. Oncogene 1991; 6:979–987.
181. Wang F, Kan M, Yan G, Xu J, McKeehan WL. Alternately spliced NH_2-terminal immunoglobulin-like loop I in the ectodomain of the fibroblast growth factor (FGF) receptor 1 lowers affinity for both heparin and FGF-1. J Biol Chem 1995; 270: 10231–10235.
182. Hou J, Kan M, McKeehan K, McBride G, Adams P, McKeehan WL. Fibroblast growth factor receptors from liver vary in three structural domains. Science 1991; 251:665–668.
183. Shi E, Kan M, Xu J, Wang F, Hou J, McKeehan WL. Control of fibroblast growth factor receptor kinase signal transduction by heterodimerization of combinatorial splice variants. Mol Cell Biol 1993; 13:3907–3918.
184. Miki T, Fleming TP, Bottaro DP, Rubin JS, Ron D, Aaronson SA. Expression cDNA cloning of the KGF receptor by creation of a transforming autocine loop. Science 1991; 251:72–75.
185. Hattori Y, Odagiri H, Nakatani H, Miyagawa K, Naito K, Sakamoto H, Katoh O, Yoshida T, Sugimura T, Terada M. K-*sam*, an amplified gene in stomach cancer, is a member of the heparin-binding growth factor receptor genes. Proc Natl Acad Sci U S A 1990; 87:5983–5987.
186. Bellot F, Crumley G, Kaplow JM, Schlessinger J, Jaye M, Dionne CA. Ligand-

induced transphosphorylation between different FGF receptors. EMBO J 1991; 10: 2849–2854.

187. Mohammadi M, Dikic I, Sorokin A, Burgess WH, Jaye M, Schlessinger J. Identification of six novel autophosphorylation sites on fibroblast growth factor receptor 1 and elucidation of their importance in receptor activation and signal transduction. Mol Cell Biol 1996; 16:977–989.
188. Mohammadi M, Honegger AM, Rotin D, Fischer R, Bellot F, Li W, Dionne CA, Jaye M, Rubinstein M, Schlessinger J. A tyrosine-phosphorylated carboxy-terminal peptide of the fibroblast growth factor receptor (flg) is a binding site for the SH2 domain of phospholipase C-γ1. Mol Cell Biol 1991; 11:5068–5078.
189. Burgess WH, Dionne CA, Kaplow U, Mudd R, Friesel R, Zilberstein A, Schlessinger J, Jaye M. Characterization and cDNA cloning of phospholipase cγ-a major substrate for heparin-binding growth factor-1 (acidic fibroblast growth factor)-activated tyrosine kinase. Mol Cell Biol 1990; 10:4770–4777.
190. Mohammadi M, Dionne CA, Li W, Li N, Spivak T, Honegger AM, Jaye M, Schlessinger J. Point mutation in FGF receptor eliminates phosphatidylinositol hydrolysis without affecting mitogenesis. Nature 1992; 358:681–684.
191. Peters KG, Marie J, Wilson E, Ives HE, Escobedo J, Del Rosario M, Mirda D, Williams LT. Point mutation of an FGF receptor abolishes phosphatidylinositol turnover and Ca^{2+} flux but not mitogenesis. Nature 1992; 358:678–681.
192. Spivak-Kroizman T, Mohammadi M, Hu P, Jaye M, Schlessinger J, Lax I. Point mutation in the fibroblast growth factor receptor eliminates phosphatidylinositol hydrolysis without affecting neuronal differentiation of PC12 cells. J Biol Chem 1994; 269:14419–14423.
193. Roghani M, Mohammadi M, Schlessinger J, Moscatelli D. Induction of urokinase-type plasminogen activator by fibroblast growth factor (FGF)-2 is dependent on expression of FGF receptors and does not require activation of phospholipase Cγ1. J Biol Chem 1996; 271:31154–31159.
194. Mohammadi M, Schlessinger J, Hubbard S. Structure of the FGF receptor tyrosine kinase domain reveals a novel autoinhibitory mechanism. Cell 1996; 86:577–587.
195. Kouhara H, Hadari Y, Spivak-Kroizman T, Schilling J, Bar-Sagi D, Lax I, Schlessinger J. A lipid-anchored Grb2-binding protein that links FGF-receptor activation to the Ras/MAPK signaling pathway. Cell 1997; 89:693–702.
196. Wang J, Xu H, Li H, Goldfarb M. Broadly expressed SNT-like proteins link FGF receptor stimulation to activators of Ras. Oncogene 1996; 13:721–729.
197. Zhan X, Plourde C, Hu X, Friesel R, Maciag T. Association of fibroblast growth factor receptor-1 with c-src correlates with association between c-src and cortactin. J Biol Chem 1994; 269:20221–20224.
198. Goh K, Lim Y, Ong S, Siak C, Cao X, Tan Y, Guy G. Identification of p90, a prominent tyrosine-phosphorylated protein in fibroblast growth factor-stimulated cells, as 80K-H. J Biol Chem 1996; 271:5832–5838.
199. Zhan X, Hu X, Friesel R, Maciag T. Long term growth factor exposure and differential tyrosine phosphorylation are required for DNA synthesis in BALB/c 3T3 cells. J Biol Chem 1993; 268:9611–9620.
200. Flaumenhaft R, Moscatelli D, Saksela O, Rifkin DB. The role of extracellular matrix in the action of basic fibroblast growth factor: Matrix as a source of growth

factor for long-term stimulation of plasminogen activator production and DNA synthesis. J Cell Physiol 1989; 140:75–81.

201. Baird A, Ling N. Fibroblast growth factors are present in the extracellular matrix produced by endothelial cells in vitro: Implications for a role of heparinase-like enzymes in the neovascular response. Biochem Biophys Res Commun. 1987; 142: 428–435.
202. Saksela O, Moscatelli D, Sommer A, Rifkin DB. Endothelial cell-derived heparan sulfate binds basic fibroblast growth factor and protects it from proteolytic degradation. J Cell Biol 1988; 107:743–751.
203. Saksela O, Rifkin DB. Release of basic fibroblast growth factor-heparan sulfate complexes from endothelial cells by plasminogen activator-mediated proteolytic activity. J Cell Biol 1990; 110:767–775.
204. Bashkin P, Doctrow S, Klagsbrun M, Svahn CM, Folkman J, Vlodavsky I. Basic fibroblast growth factor binds to subendothelial extracellular matrix and is released by heparitinase and heparin-like molecules. Biochemistry 1989; 28:1737–1743.
205. Kiefer MC, Stephans JC, Crawford K, Okino K, Barr PJ. Ligand-affinity cloning and structure of a cell surface heparan sulfate proteoglycan that binds basic fibroblast growth factor. Proc Natl Acad Sci U S A 1990; 87:6985–6989.
206. Chernouscv MA, Carey DJ. N-syndecan (syndecan-3) from neonatal rat brain binds basic fibroblast growth factor. J Biol Chem 1993; 268:16810–16814.
207. Steinfeld R, Van Den Berghe H, David G. Stimulation of fibroblast growth factor receptor-1 occupancy and signaling by cell surface-associated syndecans and glypican. J Cell Biol 1996; 133:405–416.
208. Song H, Shi W, Filmus J. OCI-5/rat glypican-3 binds to fibroblast growth factor-2 but not to insulin-like growth factor-2. J Biol Chem 1997; 272:7574–7577.
209. Andres JL, DeFalcis D, Noda M, Massague J. Binding of two growth factor families to separate domains of the proteoglycan betaglycan. J Biol Chem 1992; 267:5927–5930.
210. Bennett KL, Jackson DG, Simon JC, Tanczos E, Peach R, Modrell B, Stamenkovic I, Plowman G, Aruffo A. CD44 isoforms containing exon V3 are responsible for the presentation of heparin-binding growth factor. J Cell Biol 1995; 128:687–698.
211. Aviezer D, Hecht D, Safran M, Eisinger M, David G, Yayon A. Perlecan, basal lamina proteoglycan, promotes basic fibroblast growth factor-receptor binding, mitogenesis, and angiogenesis. Cell 1994; 79:1005–1013.
212. Jeanny J-C, Fayein N, Moenner M, Chevallier B, Barritault D, Courtois Y. Specific fixation of bovine brain and retinal acidic and basic fibroblast growth factors to mouse embryonic eye basement membranes. Exp Cell Res 1987; 171:63–75.
213. Folkman J, Klagsbrun M, Sasse J, Wadzinski M, Ingber D, Vlodavsky I. A heparin-binding angiogenic protein—basic fibroblast growth factor—is stored within basement membrane. Am J Pathol 1988; 130:393–400.
214. Gordon PB, Choi HU, Conn G, Ahmed A, Ehrmann B, Rosenberg L, Hatcher VB. Extracellular matrix heparan sulfate proteoglycans modulate the mitogenic capacity of acidic fibroblast growth factor. J Cell Physiol 1989; 140:584–592.
215. Brown KJ, Hendry IA, Parish CR. Acidic and basic fibroblast growth factor bind with differing affinity to the same heparan sulfate proteoglycan on BALB/c 3T3

cells: Implications for potentiation of growth factor action by heparin. J Cell Biochem 1995; 58:6–14.

216. Nurcombe V, Ford MD, Wildschut JA, Bartlett PF. Developmental regulation of neural response to FGF-1 and FGF-2 by heparan sulfate proteoglycan. Science 1993; 260:103–106.
217. Ishihara M. Structural requirements in heparin for binding and activation of FGF-1 and FGF-4 are different from that for FGF-2. Glycobiology 1994; 4:817–824.
218. Vigny M, Ollier-Hartmann MP, Lavigne M, Fayein N, Jeanny JC, Laurent M, Courtois Y. Specific binding of basic fibroblast growth factor to basement membrane-like structures and to purified heparan sulfate proteoglycan of the EHS tumor. J Cell Physiol 1988; 137:321–328.
219. Moscatelli D. Metabolism of receptor-bound and matrix-bound basic fibroblast growth factor by bovine capillary endothelial cells. J Cell Biol 1988; 107:753–759.
220. Gospodarowicz D, Cheng J. Heparin protects basic and acidic FGF from inactivation. J Cell Physiol 1986; 128:475–484.
221. Sommer A, Rifkin DB. Interaction of heparin with human basic fibroblast growth factor: Protection of the angiogenic protein from proteolytic degradation by a glycosaminoglycan. J Cell Physiol 1989; 138:215–220.
222. Presta M, Maier JAM, Rusnati M, Ragnotti G. Basic fibroblast growth factor is released from endothelial extracellular matrix in a biologically active form. J Cell Physiol 1989; 140:68–74.
223. Flaumenhaft R, Moscatelli D, Rifkin DB. Heparin and heparan sulfate increase the radius of diffusion and action of bFGF. J Cell Biol 1990; 111:1651–1659.
224. Ishai-Michaeli R, Eldor A, Vlodavsky I. Heparanase activity expressed by platelets, neutrophils, and lymphoma cells releases active fibroblast growth factor from extracellular matrix. Cell Regul 1990; 1:833–842.
225. Gannoun-Zaki L, Pieri I, Badet J, Moenner M, Barritault D. Internalization of basic fibroblast growth factor by Chinese hamster lung fibroblast cells: Involvement of several pathways. Exp Cell Res 1991; 197:272–279.
226. Roghani M, Moscatelli D. Basic fibroblast growth factor is internalized through both receptor-mediated and heparan sulfate-mediated mechanisms. J Biol Chem 1992; 267:22156–22162.
227. Rusnati M, Urbinati C, Presta M. Internalization of basic fibroblast growth factor (bFGF) in cultured endothelial cells: Role of the low affinity heparin-like bFGF receptors. J Cell Physiol 1993; 154:152–161.
228. Uhlrich S, Lagente O, Lenfant M, Courtois Y. Effect of heparin on the stimulation of non-vascular cells by human acidic and basic FGF. Biochem Biophys Res Commun 1986; 137:1205–1213.
229. Mueller SN, Thomas KA, Di Salvo J, Levine EM. Stabilization by heparin of acidic fibroblast growth factor mitogenicity for human endothelial cells in vitro. J Cell Physiol 1989; 140:439–448.
230. Rosengart TK, Johnson WV, Friesel R, Clark R, Maciag T. Heparin protects heparin-binding growth factor-I from proteolytic inactivation in vitro. Biochem Biophys Res Commun 1988; 152:432–440.
231. Pineda-Lucena A, Jimenez M, Lozano R, Nieto J, Santoro J, Rico M, Gimenez-

Gallego G. Three-dimensional structure of acidic fibroblast growth factor in solution: Effects of binding to a heparin functional analog. J Mol Biol 1996; 264: 162–178.

232. Kaplow JM, Bellot F, Crumley G, Dionne CA, Jaye M. Effect of heparin on the binding affinity of acidic FGF for the cloned human FGF receptors, flg and bek. Biochem Biophys Res Commun 1990; 172:107–112.

233. Rapraeger AC, Krufka A, Olwin BB. Requirement of heparan sulfate for bFGF-mediated fibroblast growth and myoblast differentiation. Science 1991; 252:1705–1708.

234. Ornitz DM, Yayon A, Flanagan JG, Svahn CM, Levi E, Leder P. Heparin is required for cell-free binding of basic fibroblast growth factor to a soluble receptor and for mitogenesis in whole cells. Mol Cell Biol 1992; 12:240–247.

235. Yayon A, Klagsbrun M, Esko JD, Leder P, Ornitz DM. Cell surface, heparin-like molecules are required for binding of basic fibroblast growth factor to its high affinity receptor. Cell 1991; 64:841–848.

236. Roghani M, Mansukhani A, Dell'Era P, Bellosta P, Basilico C, Rifkin DB, Moscatelli D. Heparin increases the affinity of basic fibroblast growth factor for its receptor but is not required for binding. J Biol Chem 1994; 269:3976–3984.

237. Pantoliano MW, Horlick RA, Springer BA, Van Dyk DE, Tobery T, Wetmore DR, Lear JD, Nahapetian AT, Bradley JD, Sisk WP. Multivalent ligand-receptor binding interactions in the fibroblast growth factor system produce a cooperative growth factor and heparin mechanism for receptor dimerization. Biochemistry 1994; 33: 10229–10248.

238. Spivak-Kroizman T, Lemmon MA, Dikic I, Ladbury JE, Pinchasi D, Huang J, Jaye M, Crumley G, Schlessinger J, Lax I. Heparin-induced oligomerization of FGF molecules is responsible for FGF receptor dimerization, activation, and cell proliferation. Cell 1994; 79:1015–1024.

239. Moscatelli D. Basic fibroblast growth factor (bFGF) dissociates rapidly from heparan sulfates but slowly from receptors. Implications for mechanisms of bFGF release from pericellular matrix. J Biol Chem 1992; 267:25803–25809.

240. Nugent MA, Edelman ER, Kinetics of basic fibroblast growth factor binding to its receptor and heparan sulfate proteoglycan: A mechanism for cooperativity. Biochemistry 1992; 31:8876–8883.

241. Klagsbrun M, Baird A. A dual receptor system is required for basic fibroblast growth factor activity. Cell 1991; 67:229–231.

242. Ornitz DM, Herr AB, Nilsson M, Westman J, Svahn C-M, Waksman G. FGF binding and FGF receptor activation by synthetic heparan-derived di- and trisaccharides. Science 1995; 268:432–436.

243. Ornitz DM, Leder P. Ligand specificity and heparin dependence of fibroblast growth factor receptors 1 and 3. J Biol Chem 1992; 267:16305–16311.

244. Venkataraman G, Sasisekharan V, Herr AB, Ornitz DM, Waksman G, Cooney CL, Langer R, Sasisekharan R. Preferential self-association of basic fibroblast growth factor is stabilized by heparin during receptor dimerization and activation. Proc Natl Acad Sci U S A 1996; 93:845–850.

245. Plotnikov AN, Schlessinger J, Hubbard SR, Mohammadi M. Structural basis for FGF receptor dimerization and activation. Cell 1999; 98:641–650.

246. Turnbull JE, Fernig DG, Ke Y, Wilkinson MC, Gallagher JT. Identification of the basic fibroblast growth factor binding sequence in fibroblast heparan sulfate. J Biol Chem 1992; 267:10337–10341.
247. Ishihara M, Tyrrell DJ, Stauber GB, Brown S, Cousens LS, Stack RJ. Preparation of affinity-fractionated, heparin-derived oligosaccharides and their effects on selected biological activities mediated by basic fibroblast growth factor. J Biol Chem 1993; 268:4675–4683.
248. Tyrrell DJ, Ishihara M, Rao N, Horne A, Kiefer MC, Stauber GB, Lam LH, Stack RJ. Structure and biological activities of a heparin-derived hexasaccharide with high affinity for basic fibroblast growth factor. J Biol Chem 1993; 268:4684–4689.
249. Aviezer D, Levy E, Safran M, Svahn C, Buddecke E, Schmidt A, David G, Vlodavsky I, Yayon A. Differential structural requirements of heparin and heparan sulfate proteoglycans that promote binding of basic fibroblast growth factor to its receptor. J Biol Chem 1994; 269:114–121.
250. Kan M, Wang F, Xu J, Crabb JW, Hou J, McKeehan WL. An essential heparin-binding domain in the fibroblast growth factor receptor kinase. Science 1993; 259: 1918–1921.
251. Richard C, Liuzzo JP, Moscatelli D. Fibroblast growth factor-2 can mediate cell attachment by linking receptors and heparan sulphate proteoglycans on neighboring cells. J Biol Chem 1995; 270:24188–24196.
252. Jaye M, Lyall RM, Mudd R, Schlessinger J, Sarver N. Expression of acidic fibroblast growth factor cDNA confers growth advantage and tumorigenesis to Swiss 3T3 cells. EMBO J 1988; 7:963–969.
253. Neufeld G, Mitchell R, Ponte P, Gospodarowicz D. Expression of human basic fibroblast growth factor cDNA in baby hamster kidney-derived cells results in autonomous cell growth. J Cell Biol 1988; 106:1385–1394.
254. Sasada R, Kurokawa T, Iwane M, Igarashi K. Transformation of mouse BALB/c 3T3 cells with human basic fibroblast growth factor cDNA. Mol Cell Biol 1988; 8:588–594.
255. Quarto N, Talarico D, Sommer A, Florkiewicz R, Basilico C, Rifkin DB. Transformation by basic fibroblast growth factor requires high levels of expression: Comparison with transformation by *hst*/K-*fgf*. Oncogene Res 1989; 5:101–110.
256. Rogelj S, Weinberg RA, Fanning P, Klagsbrun M. Basic fibroblast growth factor fused to a signal peptide transforms cells. Nature (London) 1988; 331:173–175.
257. Blam S, Mitchell R, Tischer E, Rubin JS, Silva M, Silver S, Fiddes JC, Abraham JA, Aaronson SA. Addition of growth hormone secretion signal to basic fibroblast growth factor results in cell transformation and secretion of aberrant forms of the protein. Oncogene 1988; 3:129–136.
258. Forough R, Zhan X, MacPhee M, Friedman S, Engleka KA, Sayers T, Wiltrout RH, Maciag T. Differential transforming abilities of non-secreted and secreted forms of human fibroblast growth factor-1. J Biol Chem 1993; 268:2960–2968.
259. Talarico D, Basilico C. The K-fgf/hst oncogene induces transformation through an autocrine mechanism that requires extracellular stimulation of the mitogenic pathway. Mol Cell Biol 1991; 11:1138–1145.
260. Jouanneau J, Moens G, Bourgeois Y, Poupon M, Thiery J. A minority of carcinoma

cells producing acidic fibroblast growth factor induces a community effect for tumor progression. Proc Natl Acad Sci U S A 1994; 91:286–290.

261. Jouanneau J, Plouet J, Moens G, Thiery J. FGF-2 and FGF-1 expressed in rat bladder carcinoma cells have similar angiogenic potential but different tumorigenic properties in vivo. Oncogene 1997; 14:671–676.

262. Savagner P, Valles A, Jouanneau J, Yamada K, Thiery J. Alternative splicing in fibroblast growth factor receptor 2 is associated with induced epithelial-mesenchymal transition in rat bladder carcinoma cells. Mol Biol Cell 1994; 5:851–862.

263. Folkman J, Klagsbrun M. Angiogenic factors. Science 1987; 235:442–447.

264. Ausprunk DH, Folkman J. Migration and proliferation of endothelial cells in preformed and newly formed blood vessels during tumor angiogenesis. Microvasc Res 1977; 14:53–65.

265. Montesano R, Vassalli J, Baird A, Guillemin R, Orci L. Basic fibroblast growth factor induces angiogenesis in vitro. Proc Natl Acad Sci U S A 1986; 83:7297–7301.

266. Mignatti P, Tsuboi R, Robbins E, Rifkin DB. In vitro angiogenesis on the human amniotic membrane: Requirement for basic fibroblast growth factor-induced proteinases. J Cell Biol 1989; 108:671–682.

267. Moscatelli D, Presta M, Rifkin DB. Purification of a factor from human placenta that stimulates capillary endothelial cell protease production, DNA synthesis, and migration. Proc Natl Acad Sci U S A 1986; 83:2091–2095.

268. Terranova VP, DiFlorio R, Lyall RM, Hic S, Friesel R, Maciag T. Human endothelial cells are chemotactic to endothelial cell growth factor and heparin. J Cell Biol 1985; 101:2330–2334.

269. Gospodarowicz D, Ferrara N, Schweigerer L, Neufeld G. Structural characterization and biological functions of fibroblast growth factor. Endocrine Rev 1987; 8: 95–114.

270. Shing Y, Folkman J, Haudenschild C, Lund D, Crum R, Klagsbrun M. Angiogenesis is stimulated by a tumor-derived endothelial cell growth factor. J Cell Biochem 1985; 29:275–287.

271. Thomas KA, Rios-Candelore M, Gimenez-Gallego G, DiSalvo J, Bennett C, Rodkey J, Fitzpatrick S. Pure brain-derived acidic fibroblast growth factor is a potent angiogenic vascular endothelial cell mitogen with sequence homology to interleukin 1. Proc Natl Acad Sci U S A 1985; 82:6409–6413.

272. Lobb RR, Alderman EM, Fett JW. Induction of angiogenesis by bovine brain class 1 heparin-binding growth factor. Biochemistry 1985; 19:4969–4973.

273. Hayek A, Culler FL, Beattie GM, Lopez AD, Cuevas P, Baird A. An in vivo model for study of the angiogenic effects of basic fibroblast growth factor. Biochem Biophys Res Commun 1987; 147:876–880.

274. Thompson JA, Anderson KD, DiPietro JM, Zwiebel JA, Zametta M, Anderson WF, Maciag T. Site-directed neovessel formation in vivo. Science 1988; 241:1349–1352.

275. Thompson JA, Haudenschild CC, Anderson KD, DiPietro JM, Anderson WF, Maciag T. Heparin-binding growth factor 1 induces the formation of organoid neovascular structures in vivo. Proc Natl Acad Sci U S A 1989; 86:7928–7932.

276. Ruta M, Howk R, Ricca G, Drohan W, Zabelshansky M, Laureys G, Barton DE,

Francke U, Schlessinger J, Givol D. A novel protein tyrosine kinase gene whose expression is modulated during endothelial cell differentiation. Oncogene 1988; 3: 9–15.
277. Yamaguchi TP, Harpal K, Henkemeyer M, Rossant J. *fgfr*-1 is required for embryonic growth and mesodermal patterning during mouse gastrulation. Genes Dev 1994; 8:3032–3044.
278. Deng C-X, Wynshaw-Boris A, Shen MM, Daugherty C, Ornitz DM, Leder P. Murine FGFR-1 is required for early postimplantation growth and axial organization. Genes Dev 1994; 8:3045–3057.
279. Peters KG, Werner S, Chen G, Williams LT. Two FGF receptor genes are differentially expressed in epithelial and mesenchymal tissues during limb formation and organogenesis in the mouse. Development 1992; 114:233–243.
280. Bastaki M, Nelli E, Dell'Era P, Rusnati M, Molinari-Tosatti M, Parolini S, Auerbach R, Rucco L, Possati L, Presta M. Basic fibroblast growth factor-induced angiogenic phenotype in mouse endothelium. A study of aortic and microvascular endothelial cell lines. Arterioscler Thromb Vasc Biol 1997; 17:454–464.
281. Liaw L, Schwartz S. Comparison of gene expression in bovine aortic endothelium in vivo versus in vitro. Differences in growth regulatory molecules. Arterioscler Thromb 1993; 13:985–993.
282. Matsuzaki K, Yoshitake Y, Matuo Y, Sasaki H, Nishikawa K. Monoclonal antibodies against heparin-binding growth factor II/basic fibroblast growth factor that block its biological activity: Invalidity of the antibodies for tumor angiogenesis. Proc Natl Acad Sci U S A 1989; 86:9911–9915.
283. Dennis P, Rifkin D. Studies on the role of basic fibroblast growth factor in vivo: Inability of neutralizing antibodies to block tumor growth. J Cell Physiol 1990; 144:84–98.
284. Ortega S, Ittmann M, Tsang S, Ehrlich M, Basilico C. Neuronal defects and delayed wound healing in mice lacking fibroblast growth factor 2. Proc Natl Acad Sci U S A 1998; 95:5672–5677.
285. Zhou M, Sutliff R, Paul R, Lorenz J, Hoying J, Haudenschild C, Yin M, Coffin J, Kong L, Kranias E, Luo W, Boivin G, Duffy J, Pawlowski S, Doetschman T. Fibroblast growth factor 2 control of vascular tone. Nat Med 1998; 4:201–207.
286. Ozaki H, Okamoto N, Ortega S, Chang M, Ozaki K, Sadda S, Vinores M, Derevjanik N, Zack D, Basilico C, Campochiaro P. Basic fibroblast growth factor is neither necessary nor sufficient for the development of retinal neovascularization. Am J Pathol 1998; 153:757–765.
287. Broadley KN, Aquino AM, Woodward SC, Buckley-Sturrock A, Sato Y, Rifkin DB, Davidson JM. Monospecific antibodies implicate basic fibroblast growth factor in normal wound repair. Lab Invest 1989; 61:571–575.
288. Gross J, Herblin W, Dusak B, Czerniak P, Diamond M, Sun T, Eidsvoog K, Dexter D, Yayon A. Effects of modulation of basic fibroblast growth factor on tumor growth in vivo. J Natl Cancer Inst 1993; 85:121–131.
289. Takahashi J, Fukumoto M, Kozai Y, Ito N, Oda Y, Kikuchi H, Hatanaka M. Inhibition of cell growth and tumorigenesis of human glioblastoma cells by a neutralizing antibody against human basic fibroblast growth factor. FEBS Lett 1991; 288: 65–71.

290. Stan A, Nemati M, Pietsch T, Walter G, Dietz H. In vivo inhibition of angiogenesis and growth of the human U-87 malignant glial tumor by treatment with an antibody against basic fibroblast growth factor. J Neurosurg 1995; 82:1044–1052.
291. Wang Y, Becker D. Antisense targeting of basic fibroblast growth factor and fibroblast growth factor receptor-1 in human melanomas blocks intratumoral angiogenesis and tumor growth. Nat Med 1997; 3:887–893.

16
Role of Proangiogenic Cytokines and Inhibitors of Neovascularization in Tumor Angiogenesis

Peter J. Polverini
University of Minnesota School of Dentistry, Minneapolis, Minnesota

Robert M. Strieter
University of Michigan Medical School, Ann Arbor, Michigan

I. INTRODUCTION

Angiogenesis, the formation of new capillary blood vessels, is one of the most fundamental biological processes encountered in mammalian organisms. Angiogenesis is a rare event in adult tissues where its expression is restricted to several important physiological processes. In contrast, angiogenesis is widely encountered in a number of disease settings and is central to the pathogenesis of solid tumor development. A diverse array of cytokines from multiple cellular sources function to sustain the growth and progression of tumors by providing them with a readily available supply of new microvessels. Many of these mediators are produced by tumor cells as well as by resident host cells and inflammatory cells populations that are recruited to the tumor site. These cytokines influence virtually every aspect of the angiogenic cascade and many of them have overlapping and sometimes opposing functions. It is now well accepted that tumor angiogenesis reflects a competition among cytokines that, on the one hand, function to promote angiogenesis and, on the other hand, suppress the angiogenic response. Several lines of evidence support the view that neovascularization of tumors occurs when the dynamic equilibrium that governs the orderly production of proangiogenic and angiostatic cytokines becomes disrupted in favor of those members that promote angiogenesis. In this chapter, I will describe the function of several cytokine families in the process of tumor angiogenesis and the mechanism by which the dynamic equilibrium between stimulators and inhibitors becomes distorted and leads to unwarranted angiogenesis.

II. NEOPLASIA IS AN ANGIOGENESIS-DEPENDENT DISEASE

A substantial amount of work over the last 25 to 30 years has firmly established that solid tumors are ''angiogenesis dependent'' (1–4). This premise, first proposed by Folkman, was based on several key observations. First, tumors implanted in avascular or poorly vascularized organs or tissues grow ever so slowly, as small 1 to 2 mm^3 spheres or as thin wafers. Under these circumstances, tumors are able to acquire essential, albeit limited nutrients by diffusion from the surrounding environment (5, 6). Tumors are able to survive in this dormant state for prolonged periods but are unable to grow progressively. However, as the advancing edge of the tumor approaches adjacent microvessels, ''angiogenic factors'' released from the tumor stimulate endothelial cells to grow and migrate toward the tumor and organize into a capillary network. This switch from the relatively quiescent prevascular stage to the more dynamic vascular phase is accompanied by exponential growth and eventual spread of the tumor to more distant sites (7). These observations have been validated in human tumors. For example, human retinoblastomas that metastasize to the vitreous or the anterior chamber of the eye remain avascular until they settle on the richly vascular iris or retina and become vascularized. Carcinoma of the ovary metastasizes to the peritoneum as avascular spheres that fail to grow until they become vascularized. The appearance of neovascularization at the base of melanomas that enter the vertical growth phase and the red ''blush'' that is associated with cervical and oral carcinoma herald the onset of rapid growth and increased metastatic potential. An increase in the number of new capillaries in certain types of breast and prostate cancer correlates with malignant and metastatic potential and, thus, is of considerable prognostic significance (8).

III. ANGIOGENESIS IS ACQUIRED EARLY IN THE MULTISTEP CARCINOGENIC PROCESS

It is now well established that tumors evolve through a series of steps (9, 10). This model emerged from studies of the mechanism of chemical carcinogen-induced liver and skin cancer and is now a universally accepted model for human tumor development. The first step in the carcinogenic process is the emergence of ''initiated'' cells: cells that have become committed to neoplastic development as a result of one or more genetic mutations. During the promotion phase, initiated cell populations undergo selective clonal expansion and acquire new or altered phenotypic traits indicative of progression toward malignancy. Although the initiation step is thought to occur within hours or days after exposure to carcinogens, promotion occurs over months or years. During progression, cells undergo malignant conversion and acquire properties such as invasion and metastasis that characterize malignant behavior. It is during the multistep carcinogenic process that cells acquire altered or new phenotypic traits that enable them to evade host defense and become established as "new autonomous growths." Although the carcinogenic process can be analyzed in some detail in vitro and the presumptive neoplastic progenitors in some cases identified in experimental model systems in vivo, this is not the case for human cancers. We have not yet developed strategies or identified the appropriate biomarkers that allow for the identification of populations of cells that we can say unequivocally are the committed progenitors of human cancers. From a clinical standpoint, the earliest lesions we are able to identify are premalignant ones. These represent altered cell populations with morphological and functional alterations that indicate they have acquired one or more steps in the carcinogenic process. One of the earliest and perhaps most significant properties expressed by preneoplastic cell populations is their ability to elicit an angiogenic response.

Although angiogenesis can be acquired at any time during the carcinogenic process, angiogenic activity is often a predictable feature of preneoplastic cells and is one of the earliest indications that a cell population has become committed to malignancy (1). One of the earliest observations demonstrating the angiogenic potential of preneoplastic cells was a series of studies from the Gullino laboratory, then at the National Cancer Institute. Using a series of murine breast cell lines derived from mouse strains that exhibited either a high or low incidence of spontaneous mammary tumors, these investigators showed that mammary cells derived from mice at risk for developing mammary carcinomas consistently were able to stimulate angiogenesis when implanted into the rabbit cornea, whereas cells derived from mice with a low incidence of spontaneous tumors exhibited little or no angiogenic activity (11–13).

Similarly, Polverini et al. (14) showed that cloned populations of preneoplastic keratinocytes derived from carcinogen-treated, non–tumor-bearing hamster buccal pouches were potently angiogenic, yet not tumorigenic when introduced into nude mice or neonatal hamsters. The same situation appears to hold true for many human tumors and their preneoplastic progenitors. Brem and colleagues (15) and Jensen et al. (16) examined a series of human breast lesions of varying malignant potential. They observed a strong correlation between the angiogenic activity of a particular breast lesion and its malignant potential that preceded morphological and functional changes indicative of neoplastic transformation. Chodak (17) in examining the urine of patients with neoplastic and nonneoplastic lesions of the bladder for the presence of endothelial cell migration-stimulating activity, was able to distinguish between benign and premalignant conditions as well as detect the emergence of recurrent tumors. Thus, it would appear that expression of angiogenic activity may be predictive of malignant potential acquired early in the carcinogenic process and that is independent of other transformation-linked traits. It is important to remember, however, that although angiogenesis is necessary for tumorigenicity it is, by itself, not sufficient. Furthermore, the capacity of tumors to induce angiogenesis does not always correlate with either malignant potential or frank malignancy. As an example, adrenal adenomas are benign tumors that are potently angiogenic but rarely undergo malignant conversion.

Tumors induce angiogenesis by a variety of mechanisms. Tumor cells produce diffusible angiogenic mediators that directly activate endothelial cells, stimulating them to grow, migrate directionally, and organize into sprouts. They elaborate cytokines, which attract and activate macrophages (18, 19), mast cells (20), and neutrophils (21), which in turn elaborate angiogenic factors. They also are able to block the production of or become refractory to inhibitors of angiogenesis (22, 23). They produce enzymes that release angiogenic factors sequestered in the extracellular matrix (24), and they stimulate adjacent normal tissues to make enzymes such as stromelysins (25) and collagenases (26, 27) that can be activated to promote angiogenesis.

IV. TUMOR ANGIOGENESIS REFLECTS A SHIFT IN THE NET BALANCE BETWEEN STIMULATORS AND INHIBITORS OF ANGIOGENESIS

It is now generally agreed that growth of tumors depends in part on the relative concentration of proangiogenic and angiostatic mediators produced by tumor cells or tumor-associated host cells (2, 22, 28–33). A recent study by O'Rielly et al. (31) showed that a disruption in the net balance between positive and negative regulators of angiogenesis can have a profound effect on tumor growth and metastasis. There is considerable experimental and clinical evidence that a primary tumor mass can maintain its metastases in a dormant state by inhibiting their growth. The mechanism underlying the suppressive effects of primary tumors on metastases has been the subject of much controversy and speculation for years. In an elegant series of experiments, O'Reilly et al. (31) provided a compelling explanation for this phenomenon. The authors found that when a primary tumor was implanted and allowed to grow in mice, metastases were suppressed. However, upon removal of the primary tumor, occult metastases emerged and rapidly vascularized. Serum from mice bearing primary tumors was found to contain an "inhibitory factor" that blocked endothelial cell proliferation and induced endothelial cell apoptosis. Purification of this inhibitory factor revealed a 38 kDa plasminogen fragment they termed "angiostatin." Systemic administration of angiostatin potently blocked neovascularization and growth of metastases. More recent work from the Folkman laboratory has revealed the existence of still other potent endogenous inhibitors of angiogenesis (33). These data further emphasize the importance of how an imbalance in a normally finely tuned angiogenesis regulatory system can have significant and often deleterious consequences for the host organism.

V. TUMOR ANGIOGENESIS IS MEDIATED BY PROANGIOGENIC CYTOKINES AND INHIBITORS OF NEOVASCULARIZATION

Tumor cells communicate with one another and their neighboring stromal cells through a complex network of extracellular signals. These signaling molecules include hormones and components of the extracellular matrix along with a large number of cytokines and soluble growth factors, as well as their antagonists and soluble receptors. Many of these molecules are produced by tumor cells as well as a number of accessory cell populations that normally populate tumors. The net effect of these functionally diverse pleotrophic cytokines is to regulate the growth and biological activities of tumor cells, suppress the antitumor activity of infiltrating host cells, and enhance the establishment of the stromal compartment that is conducive to tumor growth by stimulating both the deposition of matrix proteins and the sustained development of a new microvascular network.

A large number of cytokines influence the various components of the angiogenic response (4, 34–38) (Tables 1 and 2). The majority of the proangiogenic mediators are proteins, and many of them are growth factors that induce endothelial cells to divide, migrate toward the inducing stimulus, and differentiate into tubular structures. These include, among others, vascular endothelial growth factor, acidic and basic fibroblast growth factor (aFGF, bFGF), transforming growth factor α and β, epidermal growth factor, tumor necrosis factor, platelet-derived endothelial growth factor, pleiotropin, hepatocyte growth factor/scatter factor, the interferons, platelet factor 4, and a number of interleukins (39). Most are secreted by a variety of cells, including endothelial cells themselves, in response to exogenous or endogenous stimuli. They are produced locally and function in an autocrine or paracrine manner. These mediators can stimulate angiogenesis directly by interacting with receptors on the endothelial cell surface, or indirectly by attracting and activating accessory cells, such as inflammatory macrophages, and inducing them to produce angiogenic mediators (19, 40). Others, such as copper, may function as cofactors in key interstitial enzyme systems or, in the case of plasminogen activator, can activate latent enzymes such as transforming

Table 1 Proangiogenic Cytokines

Growth factors
Acidic fibroblast growth factor (aFGF)
Basic fibroblast growth factor (bFGF)
CXC chemokines (ELR motif containing)
Epidermal growth factor (EGF)
Interleukin 1 (IL-1)
Interleukin 2 (IL-2)
Midkine
Platelet-derived endothelial cell growth factor
Pleiotrophin
Scatter factor/hepatocyte growth factor (SF/HGF)
Transforming growth factor-alpha (TGF-α)
Transforming growth factor-beta (TGF-β)
Tumor necrosis factor-alpha (TNF-α)
Vascular endothelial growth factor/vascular permeability factor (VEGF/VPF)
Other proteins and peptides
Angiogenin
Angiotensin II
Ceruloplasm
Fibrin
Human angiogenic factor
Plasminogen activator
Polyamines
Substance P
Urokinase
Carbohydrates and lipids
12(R)-hydroxyeicosatrienoic acid (compound D)
Hyaluronan fragments
Lactic acid
Monobutyrin
Prostaglandins E1 and E2

growth factor-β to reveal its angiogenic (or angiostatic) activity (41). Still others play a key role in stabilizing or enhancing the function of stimulatory molecules normally sequestered in the extracellular matrix surrounding blood vessels, as heparin does, which when bound to bFGF, facilitates its interaction with high affinity receptors on the endothelial cell surface (4, 42).

Although the mediators responsible for inducing new capillary growth have been the subject of extensive investigation (4, 34, 43), only recently has attention focused on the mechanisms and mediators responsible for the timely down-regu-

Table 2 Endogenous Inhibitors of Angiogenesis

Angiostatic steroids and sulfated polysaccharides
Eosinophilic major basic protein
High-molecular-weight hyaluronan
Interferons
Interleukin-1
Laminin peptides
Placental RNase (angiogenin) inhibitor
Platelet factor 4
IP10
Prostaglandin synthesis inhibitors
Protamine
Somatostatin
Thrombospondin 1 and 2
Tissue inhibitors of metalloproteinases
Vitamin A and retinoids
Vitreous fluid

lation of angiogenesis (28, 34, 35, 44). A common property of these inhibitors is that almost all can influence the ability of cells to produce, interact with, or degrade their extracellular matrix (45–49). Alterations in the organization and composition of the extracellular matrix have a profound effect on the growth and function of endothelial cells and on determining whether endothelial cells will differentiate and organize into a three-dimensional capillary network (23, 47).

An important feature of the angiogenic cytokines is that, with rare exception (i.e., vascular endothelial cell growth factor [VEGF]), none are endothelial cell-specific and thus unique to the process of angiogenesis. Most of these mediators have a wide range of functions and target cells. This is perhaps one of the most remarkable feature of the angiogenic response, that is, the ability of endothelial cells to respond in an identical fashion to a phylogenetically diverse array of mediators. It would appear that the angiogenic phenotype has evolved as a highly conserved response without the need for its own mediator system. Endothelial cells are able to use whatever growth stimulators and inhibitors are available to them to produce new capillaries. For example, during embryonic development, basic fibroblast growth factor (bFGF) (50) has been shown to be the principal mediator of vasculogenesis and angiogenesis. In contrast, in adult organisms, this same mediator has a much more restricted role in physiological angiogenic responses, and an entirely different complement of angiogenic mediators come into play as, for example, in wound repair (18, 37, 40, 51). Whether angiogenic stimulators and inhibitors are tissue- or process-specific is the subject of much speculation. Clearly, the great redundancy in positive and negative regulators capable of orchestrating an angiogenic response attests to its fundamental importance in pathophysiological processes.

VI. EXAMPLES OF CYTOKINE FAMILIES THAT MEDIATE TUMOR ANGIOGENESIS

A. Basic Fibroblast Growth Factor

One of the most extensively studied mediators shown to stimulate tumor angiogenesis is bFGF (52–55). Basic fibroblast growth factor belongs to a family of heparin-binding growth factors. This single-copy gene is able to encode multiple isoforms of bFGF, most of which are able to mediate angiogenesis. Basic fibroblast growth factor can to influence a number of properties of endothelial cells directly and induce them to divide, migrate from their parent vessel, and degrade their extracellular matrix. Its versatility as an angiogenic cytokine is further enhanced by its ability modulate the function of accessory cell populations that accumulate within tumors. Expression and export of bFGF have been shown to be directly linked to the transition from hyperplasia to neoplasia in a transgenic mouse model system and are major players in stimulating angiogenesis in several human tumors (56–60). In addition to functioning as a direct mitogen, several lines of evidence show that bFGF can up-regulate urokinase-type plasminogen activator expression and release bFGF that is stored in the basement membrane surrounding blood vessels (42, 61). Thus, increased fibrinolytic activity along with the capacity to export large amounts of bFGF collectively contribute to the angiogenic phenotype that is mediated by bFGF.

Another mechanism by which bFGF can influence tumor angiogenesis is by inducing endogenous expression of bFGF in quiescent endothelial cells (62, 63). Several studies have shown that tumor cells of different origin release molecules that are able to interact with endothelial cells and up-regulate the expression of bFGF, which in turn stimulates the fibrinolytic potential of endothelial cells in an autocrine manner. In addition, interleukin (IL)-2 and thrombin induce bFGF expression in endothelial cells. This autocrine mechanism may serve to amplify further the angiogenic response at the tumor site, further ensuring that an angiogenic response will proceed unabated (52). A third mechanism by which bFGF can influence tumor angiogenesis is by suppressing certain homeostatic properties of endothelial cells that normally function to guard against unwarranted angiogenesis. Chen et al. (64) and Polverini (23) have shown that bFGF and scatter factor (SF), another recently recognized proangiogenic cytokine, can down-regulate expression of the angiogenesis inhibitory matrix molecule, thrombospondin-1, and further deplete tissue stores of this key angiogenesis regulatory molecule.

B. Scatter Factor and the *c-Met* Proto-oncogene

Scatter factor, also known as hepatocyte growth factor, is a potent mesenchymal cell-derived mitogenic cytokine. It was first reported to be angiogenic by Bussolino et al. (65). These authors showed that nanomolar concentrations of SF stimulated endothelial cell receptor kinase activity, cell proliferation, and motility. Scatter factor also was able to induce the repair of wounds in endothelial cell monolayers, and stimulate the scatter of endothelial cells grown in three-dimensional collagen gels and neovascularization in the rabbit cornea. This work was confirmed by Grant et al. (66), who reported that SF stimulated endothelial cell migration, proliferation, capillary tube formation in Matrigel, and angiogenesis in rat corneas.

Scatter factor was first identified by Stoker et al. (67) as a fibroblast derived cytokine that induced dispersion and spreading and enhanced the motility of normally cohesive epithelial cell populations (68–71). It is a heparin-binding glycoprotein consisting of a 60 kDa heavy a chain and a 30 kDa light b chain linked by disulfide bonds (72–74). Scatter factor is a member of the family of kringle-containing proteins and exhibits about 38% amino acid sequence homology to the proenzyme plasminogen (75). It has been demonstrated by functional, biochemical, and sequence analysis that SF and hepatocyte growth factor are one and the same protein and are indistinguishable ligands for the c-*met* proto-oncogene tyrosine kinase receptor (76–80)

In addition to stimulating cell motility, SF can influence the growth and differentiation of a variety of epithelial cell types including mammary and renal tubular epithelial cells, keratinocytes, bronchial epithelia, and biliary epithelial cells (81–83). Scatter factor also functions as a morphogen, where it induces kidney and mammary epithelial cells grown on collagen gels to organize rapidly into branching tubules and mammary duct-like structures, respectively (84, 85). Similarly, when vascular endothelial cells are grown on the reconstituted basement membrane, Matrigel, SF rapidly induces endothelial cells to organize into capillary-like tubes (66, 81) and is angiogenic in vivo (65, 66, 86).

The SF receptor, the *c-met* proto-oncogene, is a tyrosine kinase growth factor receptor that is found predominantly on epithelial cells and on some mesenchymal cells, that is, endothelial cells (87). Although mesenchymal in origin, endothelial cells display certain features of epithelial cells, including the formation of gap and tight junctions, a flattened squamous-like morphology, and the ability to organize into tubular structures. Thus, endothelial cells have the potential to serve as both a source and target of SF. The significance of this conversion of SF/*c-met* from a paracrine to an autocrine signaling system in tumor development and neovascularization has implications in the pathogenesis of Kaposi's sarcoma. Recently Naidu et al. (86) reported that SF is a major mediator of angiogenesis and can down-regulate production of the angiogenesis inhibitor, thrombospondin-1, by endothelial cells (23). In addition, Lamsus et al. (88) has demonstrated that SF is able to bind to a number of matrix molecules, including thrombospondin-1. This suggest that SF, in addition to mediating Kaposi's sarcoma angiogenesis directly, also may do so by blocking the production of thrombospondin-1 or sequestering this important angiogenic inhibitor from interacting with endothelial cells.

C. Mechanisms of Scatter Factor-Induced Angiogenesis

The production of SF by cells close to vascular endothelium originally lead Rosen and colleagues to speculate on a role for SF in angiogenesis (71, 73). They found that bovine aortic and human iliac artery smooth muscle cells produced SF in concentrations comparable to several lines of fibroblasts. Using a variety of assays that measure different aspects of motility, these workers subsequently found that SF was a potent stimulator of motility for both large and small vessel endothelial cell motility (71, 73, 89, 90). Using a microcarrier bead migration assay (71, 73, 90), they showed that stimulated migration was abolished in the presence of cyclohexamide but was unaffected by hydroxyurea, indicating a requirement for protein but not DNA synthesis. Also, agents that activate the adenylate cyclase signaling pathway, transforming growth factor-β, a variety of protein kinase inhibitor and antimicrofilament and antimicrotubule agents block SF induced migration. The detachment of endothelial cells from carrier beads and reattachment to culture surfaces appeared to require protein phosphorylation and an intact cytoskeletal system.

An important early step in the formation of new capillaries is the focal degradation by endothelial cells of the subendothelial basement membrane and their subsequent invasion across this matrix barrier. Both mouse and human SF are able to significantly enhance the proteolytic and invasive properties of endothelial cells. Not unexpectedly, treatment of endothelial cells with SF induces large increases in both secreted and cell-associated urokinase-type plasminogen activator activity (83, 66). Scatter factor is also mitogenic for endothelial cells (91) and can induce endothelial cells to differentiate into capillary-like structures in vitro. The ability of SF to induce endothelial cells to organize into vessel-like structures is consistent with its previously described morphogenetic-inducing potential, where it has been shown to induce kidney epithelial cells (84) and mammary epithelial cells to form duct-like structures in suspension culture (85). It would appear that SF is able to influence several endothelial cell functions that are associated with the angiogenic phenotype.

VII. THE PROANGIOGENIC AND ANGIOINHIBITORY PROPERTIES OF THE CXC CHEMOKINES

Recently, a new family of cytokines has been identified that appear to have proangiogenic and angiostatic activities (92–96). These cytokines are characterized as heparin-binding proteins that in their monomeric forms are all less than 10 kDa. This family displays four highly conserved cysteine amino acid residues, with the first two cysteines separated by one nonconserved amino acid residue. Because of their chemotactic properties and the presence of the CXC cysteine motif, these cytokines have been designated the CXC chemokine family. These chemokines are all clustered on human chromosome 4 and exhibit between 20% and 50% homology on the amino acid level (92–96).

At least 12 different CXC chemokines have been identified. These include platelet factor-4 (PF4), NH_2-terminal truncated form of platelet basic protein (PBP) [connective tissue activating protein-III (CTAP-III), beta-thromboglobulin (BTG), and neutrophil activating protein-2 (NAP-2)], IL-8, growth-related oncogenes α,β,γ (GROα, GROβ, GROγ) gamma–interferon-inducible protein (IP-10), monokine induced by gamma-interferon (MIG), epithelial neutrophil-activating protein-78 (ENA-78), and granulocyte chemotactic protein-2 (GCP-2) (Table 3) (92–99).

The CXC chemokines were all initially identified on the basis of their ability to induce neutrophil activation and chemotaxis (92–99). Interleukin-8 has been the most extensively studied CXC chemokine family member and is produced by an array of cells including monocytes, alveolar macrophages, neutro-

Table 3 CXC Chemokine Mediators of Angiogenesis

Angiogenic CXC chemokines containing the ERL motif
Interleukin-8 (IL-8)
Epithelila neutrophil-activating protein-78 (ENA-78)
Growth-related oncogene alpha (GROα)
Growth-related oncogene beta (GROβ)
Growth-related oncogene gamma (GROγ)
Granulocyte chemotactic protein-2 (GCP-2)
Platet basic protein (PBP)
Connective tissue-activating protein-III (CTAP-III)
Beta-thromboglobulin (βTG)
Neutrophil-activating protein-2 (NAP-2)
Angiostatic CXC chemokines lacking the ELR motif
Platelet factor-4 (PF4)
Gamma-interferon-inducible protein (IP-10)
Monokine induced by gamma-interferon (MIG)

phils, keratinocytes, mesangial cells, epithelial cells, hepatocytes, fibroblasts, and endothelial cells (92–96, 100). Although numerous in vivo and in vitro investigations have demonstrated the importance of IL-8 in acute inflammation as a chemotactic and activating factor for neutrophils, only recently has it become apparent that this CXC chemokine, as well as other members of the CXC chemokine family, may also function as mediators of angiogenesis.

One of the first studies implicating the CXC chemokines in angiogenesis was from the Strieter laboratory (101–103). These authors showed that recombinant IL-8 mediated both endothelial cell chemotactic and proliferative activity in vitro and angiogenic activity in corneal micropocket model in both rats and rabbits. Because macrophages are a major source of angiogenic activity in wounds and other chronic diseases (104), the investigators extended their studies to see whether IL-8 was an angiogenic factor liberated by activated human monocytes or by synovial macrophages isolated from rheumatoid arthritis synovial tissues (101). Conditioned media from both populations of mononuclear phagocytes induced significant chemotactic activity for endothelial cells. Furthermore, when these supernatants were exposed to neutralizing antibodies to IL-8 or IL-8 antisense oligonucleotides introduced into macrophages expressing IL-8, endothelial cell chemotaxis and angiogenic activity were significantly reduced (101). These findings demonstrated that IL-8 could function as a mediator of angiogenesis in pathological settings. Interestingly, another member of the CXC chemokine family, PF4, has been shown to have angiostatic properties (105) and is able to attenuate the growth of tumors in vivo (74). These observations would suggest that members of the CXC chemokine family can function as either angiogenic or angiostatic factors in regulating neovascularization.

Recent studies suggest that the proangiogenic and angiostatic effects of these chemokines can be attributed to specific domains within these molecules. Recently, both Hebert et al. (106) and Clark-Lewis et al. (107) have demonstrated an amino acid sequence in the primary structure of the CXC chemokine family that appears, in part, to account for the ability of these chemokines to function in neutrophil chemotaxis and activation. They demonstrated that the three amino acid residues that immediately preceded the first cysteine amino acid are critically important in binding and activating neutrophils. These amino acids, Glu-Leu-Arg, the ELR motif, are absent in those members of the CXC chemokine family (PF4, IP-10, and MIG) that have been reported to function as inhibitors of angiogenesis. Differences in amino acid composition may explain in part the disparity of angiogenic activity of the CXC chemokine family and lend support to the hypothesis that an imbalance in the expression of angiogenic and angiostatic CXC chemokines may be important in pathological angiogenic responses (108).

For example, Arenberg et al. (109) demonstrated that the introduction of IP10 into non–small-cell lung carcinomas in SCID mice impairs tumor growth and metastases by blocking tumor angiogenesis. These reports and others support the contention that members of the CXC chemokine family may exert disparate effects in mediating angiogenesis, and that the ELR motif is the putative domain that dictates the angiogenic activity of this family. The magnitude of the expression of either proangiogenic and angiostatic CXC chemokines during neovascularization may significantly contribute to the regulation of angiogenesis during tumor progression (110).

VIII. SUMMARY

It is now well established that angiogenesis is a highly regulated process that is under the control of both stimulatory and inhibitory molecules. Although the complement of positive and negative regulators of angiogenesis may vary in different physiological and pathological settings, the recognition of this dual mechanism of control is necessary if we are to gain a more thorough understanding of this complex process and its significance in disease. The recent elucidation of the cooperative interaction among positive and negative regulatory molecules during normal physiological angiogenesis and the apparent disruption of this program in tumors suggest that future studies of pathological angiogenesis must focus on the interaction of positive and negative regulators. The implications of these findings for the development of therapeutic strategies for the treatment of solid tumors and other angiogenesis-dependent disorders are obvious. The use of inhibitors of neovascularization for the treatment of solid tumors has long been envisioned as a possible mode of therapy (4, 32). Several examples already exist in which this approach has met with success (111, 112). As the tools of genetic engineering move from the bench to the bedside, and as the molecular and biochemical basis underlying the functional diversity of the mediators of angiogenesis are defined, it may be possible to up-or down-regulate angiogenic responses with exquisite precision. Regardless of the diverse settings in which angiogenesis is found and the great redundancy of mediator systems that participate in this process, the sorting out of the mechanisms that control the balanced production of positive and negative regulators of angiogenesis will no doubt prove to be a fruitful area of investigation. These mechanisms will ultimately have an impact on the treatment of angiogenesis-dependent diseases such as tumor development and progression.

REFERENCES

1. Folkman J. Tumor angiogenesis. Adv Cancer Res 1085a; 43:175–203.
2. Folkman J. Toward an understanding of angiogenesis: search and discovery. Perspect Biol Med 1985b; 9:10–36.

3. Schor AM, Schor SL. Tumor angiogenesis. J Pathol 1983; 141:385–413.
4. Folkman J, Klagsbrun M. Angiogenic factors. Science 1987; 235:442–447.
5. Folkman J, Cole P, Zimmerman S. Tumor behavior in isolated perfused organs: in vitro growth and metastasis of biopsy material in rabbit thyroid and canine intestinal segments. Ann Surg 1966; 164:491–502.
6. Gimbrone MA Jr, Leapman SB, Cotran RS, Folkman J. Tumor dormancy in vivo by prevention of neovascularization. J Exp Med 1972; 136:261–276.
7. Gimbrone MA Jr, Cotran RS, Leapman SB, Folkman J. Tumor growth and neovascularization: an experimental model using the rabbit cornea. J Natl Cancer Inst 1974; 52:413–427.
8. Weidner N, Semple JP, Welch WR, Folkman J. Tumor angiogenesis and metastasis-correlation in invasive breast carcinoma. N Engl J Med 1991; 324: 1–8.
9. Nowell PC. The clonal evolution of tumor cell populations. Science 1976; 194: 23–28.
10. Farber E, Cameron C. The sequential analysis of cancer development. Adv Cancer Res 1980; 31:125–225.
11. Brem SS, Gullino PM, Medina D. Angiogenesis: a marker for neoplastic transformation of mammary papillary hyperplasia. Science 1977; 195:880–882.
12. Gimbrone MA Jr, Gullino PM. Neovascularization induced by intraoccular xenographs of normal, preneoplastic, and neoplastic mouse mammary tissue. J Natl Cancer Inst 1976; 55:305–318.
13. Gimbrone MA Jr, Gullino PM. Angiogenic capacity of preneoplastic lesions of murine mammary gland as a marker of neoplastic transformation. Cancer Res 1976; 36:2611–2620.
14. Polverini PJ, Solt DB. Expression of the angiogenic phenotype by a subpopulation of keratinocytes from 7,12-Dimethylbenz(a)anthracene-initiated hamster pouch epithelium. Carcinogenesis 1988; 9:117–122.
15. Brem SS, Jensen HM, Gullino PM. Angiogenesis as a marker of preneoplastic lesions of the breast. Cancer 1978; 41:239–244.
16. Jensen HM, Chen I, DeVault MR, Lewis AE. Angiogenesis induced by normal breast tissue: a probable marker for precancer. Science 1982; 218:293–295.
17. Chodak GW, Scheiner CJ, Zetter BR. Urine from patients with transitional-cell carcinoma stimulates migration of capillary endothelial cells. N Engl J Med 1981; 305:869–874.
18. Polverini PJ, Cotran RS, Gimbrone MA Jr, Unanue ER. Activated macrophages induce vascular proliferation. Nature 1977; 269:804–806.
19. Polverini PJ, Leibovich SJ. Induction of neovascularization in vivo and endothelial cell proliferation in vitro by tumor-associated macrophages. Lab Invest 1984; 51: 635–642.
20. Starkey JR, Crowle PK, Taubenberger S. Mast-cell-deficient W/Wv mice exhibit a decreased rate of tumor angiogenesis. Int J Cancer 1988; 42:48–52.
21. Welch DR, Schissel DJ, Howrey RP, Aeed PA. Tumor-elicited polymorphonuclear cells, in contrast to "normal" circulating polymorphonuclear cells, stimulate invasive and metastatic potentials of rat mammary adenocarcinoma cells. Proc Natl Acad Sci U S A 1989; 86:5859–5863.

22. Rastinejad F, Polverini PJ, Bouck NP. Regulation of the activity of a new inhibitor of angiogenesis by a cancer suppressor gene. Cell 1989; 56:345–355.
23. Polverini PJ. How the extracellular matrix and macrophages contribute to angiogenesis and vasoproliferative-dependent diseases. Eur J Cancer 1996; 32A:2430–2437.
24. Briozzo P, Badet J, Capony F, Pieri I, Montcourrier P, Barritault D, Rochefort H. MCF7 mammary cancer cells respond to bFGF and internalize it following its release from the extracellular matrix: a permissive role for cathepsin D. Exp Cell Res 1991; 194:252–259.
25. Polverini PJ. The pathophysiology of angiogenesis. Crit Rev Oral Biol Med 1995; 6:230–247.
26. van den Hooff A. Stromal involvement in malignant growth. Adv Cancer Res 1988; 50:159–196.
27. van den Hooff A. The role of stromal cells in tumor metastasis: a new link. Cancer Cells 1991; 3:186–187.
28. Bouck N. Tumor angiogenesis: role of oncogenes and tumor suppressor genes. Cancer Cells 1990; 2:179–185.
29. Bouck N. Angiogenesis: a mechanism by which oncogenes and tumor suppressor genes regulate tumorigenesis. In: Benz CC, Liu ET, eds. Oncogenes and Tumor Suppressor Genes in Human Malignancy. Boston: Kluwer, 1993:359–371.
30. Liotta LA, Steeg PS, Stetler-Stevenson WG. Cancer metastasis and angiogenesis: an imbalance of positive and negative regulation. Cell 1991; 64:327–336.
31. O'Reilly MS, Holmgren L, Shing Y, Chen C, Rosenthal RA, Moses M, Lane WS, Cao Y, Sage EH, Folkman J. Angiostatin: a novel angiogenesis inhibitor that mediates the suppression of metastases by Lewis lung carcinoma. Cell 1994; 79:315–328.
32. Hanahan D, Folkman J. Patterns and emerging mechanisms of the angiogenic switch during tumorigenesis. Cell 1996; 86:353–364.
33. Folkman J. New perspectives in clinical oncology from angiogenesis research. Eur J Cancer 1996; 32A:2534–2539.
34. Klagsbrun M, D'Amore PA. Regulators of angiogenesis. Annu Rev Physiol 1991; 53:217–239.
35. Moses MA, Langer R. Inhibitors of angiogenesis. Biotechnology 1991; 9:630–634.
36. Leibovich SL. Role of cytokines in the process of tumor angiogenesis. In: Human cytokines: Their role in disease and therapy. 1994:539–555.
37. Polverini PJ. Macrophage-induced angiogenesis: a review. In: Sorg C, ed. Macrophage-Derived Regulatory Factors. Basel: S. Karger, 1989:54–73.
38. DiPietro LA, Polverini PJ. Role of the macrophage in the positive and negative regulation of wound neovascularization. Behring Inst Mitt 1993; 92:238–247.
39. Leek RD, Harris AL, Lewis CE. Cytokine networks in solid human tumors: regulation of angiogenesis. J Leukoc Biol 1994; 423–435.
40. Sunderkotter C, Goebeler M, Schultze-Osthoff K, Bhardwaj R, Sorg C. Macrophage-derived angiogenesis factors. Pharmac Ther 1991; 51:195–216.
41. Roberts AB, Sporn MB. Regulation of endothelial cell growth, architecture, and matrix synthesis by TGF-β. Am Rev Respir Dis 1989; 140:1126–1128.
42. Vlodavski I, Folkman J, Sullivan R, Fridman R, Ishai-Michaeli R, Sasse J, Klags-

brun M. Endothelial cell-derived basic fibroblast growth factor: synthesis and deposition into subendothelial extracellular matrix. Proc Natl Acad Sci U S A 1987; 84:2292–2296.
43. Klagsbrun M, Folkman J. Peptide growth factors and their receptors. II. In: Sporn MB, Roberts AB, eds. Angiogenesis. Handbook of Experimental Pharmacology. Vol. 95. Berlin: Springer-Verlag, 1990:549–586.
44. Polverini PJ. Inhibitors of neovascularization: critical mediators in the coordinate regulation of angiogenesis. In: Maragoudakis ME, Gullino P, Lelkes PI, eds. Angiogenesis, Molecular Biology, Clinical Aspects. New York: Plenum, 1994:29–38.
45. Canfield AE, Schor AM, Schor SL, Grant ME. The biosynthesis of extracellular-matrix components by bovine retinal endothelial cells display distinctive morphological phenotypes. Biochem J 1986; 235:375–383.
46. Madri J, Pratt B, Tucker A. Phenotypic modulation of endothelial cells by transforming growth factor-β depends upon the composition and organization of the extrcellular matrix. J Cell Biol 1988; 106:1375–1384.
47. Maragoudakis ME, Sarmonika M, Panoutsacopoulou M. Inhibition of basement membrane biosynthesis prevents angiogenesis. J Pharmacol Exp Ther 1988; 244: 729–733.
48. Ingber D, Folkman J. Inhibition of angiogenesis through modulation of collagen metabolism. Lab Invest 1988; 59:44–51.
49. Ingber DE, Folkman J. Mechanochemical switching between growth and differentiation during fibroblast growth factor-stimulated angiogenesis in vitro. Role of the extracellular matrix. J Cell Biol 1989; 109:317–330.
50. Risau W. Embryonic angiogenesis factors. Pharmac Ther 1991; 51:371–376.
51. Sunderkotter C, Steinbrink K, Goebeler M, Bhardwaj R, Sorg C. Macrophages and angiogenesis. J Leukoc Biol 1994; 55:410–422.
52. Bassilico C, Moscatelli D. The FGF family of growth factors and oncogenes. Adv Cancer Res 1992; 59:115–165.
53. Gulandris A, Urbanati C, Rusanti M, Ziche M, Presta. Interaction of high molecular weight basic fibroblast growth factor (bFGF) with endothelium: biological activities and intracellular fate of human recombinant Mr 24,000 bFGF. J Cell Physiol 1994; 161:149–159.
54. Montesano R, Vassalli J-D, Baird A, Guillemin R, Orci L. Basic fibroblast growth factor induces angiogenesis in vitro. Proc Natl Acad Sci U S A 1986; 83:7297–7301.
55. Bussolino F, Albini A, Camussi G, Presta M, Vigietto G, Ziche M, Persico G. Role of soluable mediator in angiogenesis. Eur J Cancer 1996; 32A:2401–2412.
56. Kandell J, Bossy-Wetzei E, Radvanyi F, Klagsbrun M, Folkman J, Hanahan D. Neovascularization is associated with a switch to the export of bFGF in the multistep development of fibrosarcoma. Cell 1991; 66:1095–1104.
57. Nakamoto T, Chang C, Li A, Chodak GW. Basic fibroblast growth factor in human prostate cancer cells. Cancer Res 1992; 52:571–577.
58. Zagzag D, Miller DC, Sato Y, Rifkin DB, Burstein DE. Immunohistochemical localization of basic fibroblast growth factor in astrocytomas. Cancer Res 1990; 50: 7393–7398.
59. Takahashi JA, Mori H, Fukumoto M. Gene expression of fibroblast growth factors

in human gliomas and meningiomas: demonstration of a cellular source of basic fibroblast growth factor mRNA and peptide in tumor tissue. Proc Natl Acad Sci U S A 1990; 87:5710–5714.

60. Nguyen M, Watanabe H, Budson AE, Riche JP, Hayes DF, Folkman J. Elevated levels of an angiogenic peptide, basic fibroblast growth factor, in the urine of patients with a wide spectrum of cancers. J Natl Cancer Inst 1994; 86:356–361.
61. Vlodavsky I, Bar-Shavit R, Ishai-Michaeli R, Bashkin P, Fuks Z. Extracellular sequestration and release of fibroblast growth factor: a regulatory mechanism? Trends Biochem Sci 1991; 16:268–271.
62. Mignatti P, Morimoto T, Rifkin DB. Basic fibroblast growth factor released by single, isolated cells stimulates their migration in an autocrine manner. Proc Natl Acad Sci U S A 1991; 88:11007–11011.
63. Mignatti P, Morimoto T, Rifkin DB. Basic fibroblast growth factor, a protein devoid of a signal sequence, is released by cells via a pathway independent of the endoplasmic reticulum-golgi complex. J Cell Physiol 1992; 151:81–93.
64. Chen ZS, Caughman SW, Lawley TJ, Swerlick RA. Angiogenic factors decrease thrombospondin-1 expression in dermal microvascular endothelial cells. J Invest Dermatol 1996; 106:823A.
65. Bussolino F, DiRenzo MF, Ziche M, Bocchietto E, Olivero M, Naldini L, Gaudino G, Tamagnone L, Coffer A, Comoglio PM. Hepatocyte growth factor is a potent angiogenic factor which stimulates endothelial cell motility and growth. J Cell Biol 1992; 119:629–641.
66. Grant DS, Kleinman HK, Goldberg ID, Bhargava MM, Nickoloff BJ, Kinsella JL, Polverini PJ, Rosen EM. Scatter factor induces blood vessel formation in vivo. Proc Natl Acad Sci U S A 1993; 90:1937–1941.
67. Stoker M, Perryman M. An epithelial scatter factor released by embryo fibroblasts. J Cell Sci 1985; 77:209–233.
68. Stoker M. Junctional competence in clones of mammary epithelial cells, and modulation by conditioned medium. J Cell Physiol 1984; 171:174–183.
69. Stoker M, Perryman M. An epithelial scatter factor released by embryo fibroblasts. J Cell Sci 1985; 77:209–233.
70. Stoker M, Gherardi E, Perryman M, Gray J. Scatter factor is a fibroblast-derived modulator of epithelial cell motility. Nature 1987; 327:238–242.
71. Rosen EM, Goldberg ID, Kacinski BM, Buckholtz T, Vinter DW. Smooth muscle releases an epithelial scatter factor which binds to heparin. In Vitro Cell Dev Biol 1989; 25:163–173.
72. Gherardi E, Gray J, Stoker M, Perryman M, Furlong R. Purification of scatter factor, a fibroblast-derived basic protein which modulates epithelial interactions and movement. Proc Natl Acad Sci U S A 1989; 86:5844–5848.
73. Rosen EM, Meromsky L, Setter E, Vinter DW, Goldberg ID. Purification and migration-stimulating activities of scatter factor. Proc Soc Exp Biol Med 1990; 195: 34–43.
74. Weidner KM, Behrens J, Vandekereckhove J, Birchmeier W. Scatter factor: molecular characteristics and effect on invasiveness of epithelial cells. J Cell Biol 1990; 111:2097–2108.
75. Nakamura T, Nishizawa T, Hagiya M, Seki T, Shimonishi M, Sugimura A, Shimizu

S. Molecular cloning and expression of human hepatocyte growth factor. Nature 1989; 342:440–443.

76. Furlong RA, Takheara T, Taylor WG, Nakamura T, Rubin JS. Comparison of biologic and immunochemical properties indicate that scatter factor and hepatocyte growth factor are indistinguishable. J Cell Sci 1991; 100:173–177.
77. Weidner KM, Arakaki N, Vandekereckhove J, Weingart S, Hartmann G, Reider H, Fonatsch C, Tsubouchi H, Hishida T, Diakuhara Y, Birchmeier W. Evidence for the identity of human scatter factor and hepatocyte growth factor. Proc Natl Acad Sci U S A 1991; 88:7001–7005.
78. Bottaro DP, Rubin JS, Faletto DL, Chan AM, Kmiecik TE, Vande Woude GF, Aaronson SA. Identification of the hepatocyte growth factor receptor as the *c-met* proto-oncogene product. Science 1991; 251:802–804.
79. Naldini L, Tamagnone L, Vigna E, Sachs M, Hartmann L, Birchmeier W, Daikuhara Y, Tsubouchi H, Blasi F, Comoglio PM. Extracellular proteolytic cleavage by urokinase is required for activation of hepatocyte growth factor/scatter factor. EMBO J 1992; 11:4825–4833.
80. Bhargava M, Joseph A, Knesel J, Halaban R, Li Y, Pang S, Goldberg I, Setter E, Donovan MA, Zarnegar R, Michalopoulos GA, Nakamura T, Faletto D, Rosen EM. Scatter factor and hepatocyte growth factor: activities, properties, and mechanism. Cell Growth Differ 1992; 3:11–20.
81. Rubin JS, Chan AM-L, Bottaro DP, Burgess WH, Taylor WG, Cech AC, Hirschfield DW, Wong J, Miki T, Finch PW, Aaronson SA. A broad spectrum human lung fibroblast-derived mitogen is a variant of hepatocyte growth factor. Proc Natl Acad Sci U S A 1991; 88:415–419.
82. Kan M, Zhang GH, Zarnegar R, Michalapoulos G, Myoken Y, McKeehan WL, Stevens JL. Hepatocyte growth factor-hematopoietin A stimulates the growth of rat proximal tubular epithelial cells (rpte), rat non-parenchymal liver cells, human melanoma cells, mouse keratinocytes, and stimulates anchorage-independent growth of SV40-transformed rpte. Biochem Biophys Res Commun 1991; 174:331–337.
83. Rosen EM, Goldberg ID. Scatter factor and the c-met receptor: a paradigm for mesenchymal epithelial interaction. EXS 1997; 79:193–208.
84. Montesano R, Matsumoto K, Nakamura T, Orci L. Identification of a fibroblast-derived epithelial morphogen as hepatocyte growth factor. Cell 1991; 67:901–908.
85. Tsarfaty I, Resau JH, Rulong S, Keydar I, Faletto D, Vande Woude GF. The *met* proto-oncogene receptor and lumen formation. Science 1992; 257:1258–1261.
86. Naidu YM, Rosen EM, Zitnick R, Goldberg I, Park M, Naujokas M, Polverini PJ, Nickoloff BJ. Role of scatter factor in the pathogenesis of AIDS-related Kaposi's sarcoma. Proc Natl Acad Sci U S A 1994; 91:5281–5285.
87. Park M, Dean M, Kaul K, Braun MJ, Gonda MA, Vande Woude GF. Sequence of met proto-oncogene cDNA has features characteristic of the tyrosine kinase family of growth factor receptors. Proc Natl Acad Sci U S A 1987; 84:6379–6384.
88. Lamszus K, Joseph A, Jin L, Chowdhury S, Fuchs A, Polverini PJ, Goldberg ID, Rosen EM. Scatter factor binds to thrombospondin and other extracellular matrix components. Am J Pathol 1996; 149:805–820.

89. Rosen EM, Carley W, Goldberg ID. Scatter factor regulates vascular endothelial cells' motility. Cancer Invest 1990; 8:647–650.
90. Rosen EM, Mermsky L, Setter E, Vinter DW, Goldberg I. Smooth muscle-derived factor stimulates mobility of human tumor cells. Invasion Metastasis 1990; 10:49–64.
91. Morimoto A, Okamura K, Hamanaka R, Sato Y, Shima N, Higashio K, Kuwano M. Hepatocyte growth factor modulates migration and proliferation of human microvascular endothelial cells in culture. Biochem Biophys Res Commun 1991; 179: 1042–1049.
92. Baggiolini M, Dewald B, Waltz A. Interleukin-8 and related chemotactic cytokines. In: Gallin JI, Golgstein IM, Snyderman R, eds. Inflammation: Basic Principles and Clinical Correlates. New York: Raven Press Ltd, 1992.
93. Baggiolini M, Waltz A, Kunkel SL. Neutrophil activating peptide-1/interleukin 8, a novel cytokine that activates neutrophils. J Clin Invest 1989; 84:1045–1049.
94. Matsushima K, Oppenheim JJ. Interleukin 8 and MCAF: novel inflammatory cytokines inducible by IL-1 and TNF. Cytokine 1989; 2–13.
95. Miller MD, Krangel MS. Biology and biochemistry of the chemokines: a family of chemotactic and inflammatory cytokines. Crit Rev Immunol 1992; 12:17–46.
96. Oppenheim JJ, Zachariae OC, Mukaida N, Matsushima K. Properties of the novel proinflammatory supergene ''intercrine'' cytokine family. Annu Rev Immunol 1991; 9:617–648.
97. Farber JM. HuMIG: a new member of the chemokine family of cytokines. Biochem Biophys Res Comm 1993; 192:223–230.
98. Proost P, De Wolf-Peeters C, Conings R, Opdenakker G, Billiau A, Van Damme J. Identification of a novel granulocyte chemotactic protein (GCP-1) from human tumors: in vitro and in vivo comparison with natural forms of GROα, IP-10, and IL-8. J Immunol 1993; 150:1000–1010.
99. Walz A, Burgener R, Car B, Baggiolini M, Kunkel SL, Strieter RM. Structure and neutrophil-activating properties of a novel inflammatory peptide (ENA-78) with homology to IL-8. J Exp Med 1991; 174:1355–1362.
100. Strieter RM, Polverini PJ, Arenberg DA, Kunkel SL. The role of CXC chemokines as regulators of angiogenesis. Shock 1995; 4:155–160.
101. Koch AE, Polverini PJ, Kunkel SL, Harlow LA, Di Pietro LA, Elner VM, Elner SG, Strieter RM. Interleukin-8 (IL-8), as a macrophage-derived mediator of angiogenesis. Science 1992; 258:1798–1801.
102. Strieter RM, Kasahara K, Allen RM, Standiford TJ, Rolfe MW, Becker FS, Chensue SW, Kunkel SL. Cytokine-induced neutrophil-derived interleukin-8. Am J Pathol 1992; 141:397–407.
103. Strieter RM, Kunkel SL, Elner VM, Martinyl CL, Koch AE, Polverini PJ, Elner SG. Interleukin-8: a corneal factor that induces neovascularization. Am J Pathol 1992; 141:1279–1284.
104. Polverini PJ. Macrophage-induced angiogenesis: a review. In: Cytokines. Basel: S. Karger 1989:54–73.
105. Maione TE, Gray GS, Petro J, Hunt AJ, Donner AL, Bauer SI, Carson HF, Sharp RJ. Inhibition of angiogenesis by recombinant human platelet factor-4. Science 1990; 247:77–79.

106. Hebert CA, Vitangcol RV, Baker JB. Scanning mutagenesis of interleukin-8 identifies a cluster of residues required for receptor binding. J Biol Chem 1991; 266: 18989–18994.
107. Clark-Lewis I, Dewald B, Geiser T, Moser B, Baggiolini M. Platelet factor 4 binds to interleukin 8 receptors and activates neutrophils when its N terminus is modified with Glu-Leu-Arg. Proc Natl Acad Sci U S A 1993; 3574–3577.
108. Strieter RM, Polverini PJ, Kunkel SL, Arenberg DA, Burdick MD, Kasper J, Dzuiba J, Van Damme J, Walz A, Marriott D, Chan S-Y, Roczniak S, Shanafelt AB. The functional role of the "ELR" motif in CXC chemokine-mediated angiogenesis. J Biol Chem 1995; 270:27348–27357.
109. Strieter RM, Polverini PJ, Arenberg DA, Walz A, Opdenakker G, Van Damme J, Kunkel SL. The role of c-x-c chemokines as regulators of angiogenesis in lung cancer. J Leukocyte Biol 1995; 57:752–762.
110. Arenberg DA, Kunkel SL, Polverini PJ, Morris SB, Burdick MD, Glass MC, Taub DT, Iannettoni MD, Whyte RI, Strieter RM. Interferon-γ-inducible protein 10 (IP-10) is an angiostatic factor that inhibits human non–small-cell lung cancer (NSCLC) tumorigenesis and spontaneous metastasis. J Exp Med 1996; 184:981–992.
111. Orchard PJ, Smith CM II, Woods WG, Day DL, Dehner LP. Treatment of hemangioendotheliomas with alpha interferon. Lancet 1989; 2:565–567.
112. White CW, Wolf SJ, Korones DN, Sondheimer HM, Tosi MF, Yu A. Treatment of childhood angiomatous diseases with recombinant interferon alpha. J Pediatr 1991; 118:59–66.

17

The Link Between Oncogenes, Signal Transduction Therapy, and Tumor Angiogenesis

Robert S. Kerbel and Alicia Viloria-Petit
Sunnybrook and Women's College Health Science Centre, University of Toronto, Toronto, Ontario, Canada

Futoshi Okada
Cancer Institute, Hokkaido University School of Medicine, Sapporo, Hokkaido, Japan

Janusz Rak
Hamilton Civic Hospitals Research Centre, McMaster University, Hamilton, Ontario, Canada

I. POSITIVE AND NEGATIVE REGULATORS OF TUMOR ANGIOGENESIS

Folkman first put forward the hypothesis that the growth of solid tumors is "angiogenesis dependent" (1, 2) and, therefore, anticancer treatment strategies can be designed to include drugs that selectively target newly formed, immature blood vessels in tumors while leaving normal mature vessels elsewhere in the body unharmed (1, 2). This hypothesis has stood the test of time, at least in preclinical models of tumor growth and therapy (3, 4). There is now great interest, both in academic research laboratories and in the biotechnical/pharmaceutical industry, in the development of drugs that either inhibit or enhance angiogenesis, because of: (a) the possibility that resistance to certain angiogenesis inhibitors may not develop in tumor cells exposed to such drugs, even over prolonged periods (5–7); (b) the identification of a growing number of molecular targets on "activated" endothelial cells associated with newly formed blood vessel capillaries, such as acutely up-regulated receptor tyrosine kinases (8–10), integrins (11), and adhesion molecules (12, 13, 72); (c) the discovery of a number of potentially powerful endogenous protein inhibitors of angiogenesis that can cause tumor regressions (14); and that are usually internal fragments of higher molecular weight proteins (14); (d) a growing sense of urgency about the need to devise new and innovative anticancer strategies or drugs to replace or supplement the ones that have been used with such limited success for the past 50 years.

When Folkman first put forward his seminal hypothesis more than 25 years ago, he envisioned a scenario in which developing tumor masses remained microscopic and dormant as long as they were incompetent to induce angiogenesis (1, 2). Termination of this dormant phenotype, he suggested, was brought about by the induction and release of soluble and diffusable growth factor that he called "TAF"—tumor angiogenic factor (1, 2). Release of this hypothetical molecule into the extracellular environment would set in motion the various trains of events associated with the formation of new blood vessel capillaries sprouting from the mature and pre-existing host vasculature located in the vicinity of a TAF-producing tumor mass. These events include localized proteolysis of the basement membranes surrounding mature blood vessels, migration of endothelial cells through the newly created breach, endothelial cell proliferation, the formation of rudimentary tubes or vascular sprouts, and the joining of such newly formed vessels to form a vascular network (4, 15). It took about another 15 years before a molecule that could be equated with TAF was identified. It turned out to be basic fibroblast growth factor (bFGF), also known as FGF-2 (16, 17). Since then, at least a dozen more growth factors have been identified that have potential tumor angiogenesis-promoting activity (4). They include some growth factors also known to have mitogenic autocrine activity for tumor cells, such as transforming growth factor alpha (TGFα), and a number of tumor- or stromal cell-derived paracrine growth factors (for endothelial cells) including vascular endothelial cell growth factor (VEGF), which is also known as vascular permeability factor (VPF), scatter factor (SF), also known as hepatocyte growth factor (HGF), transforming growth factor beta (TGFβ), angiopoietin 1 and 2, platelet-derived growth factor (PDGF), and interleukin-8 (IL-8), among others (4). In addition to these growth factors, whose expression can be induced or up-regulated in tumor cells, there is a family of angiogenesis-inhibitory molecules, some of which are now known to be strongly down-regulated in tumor cells. Thrombospondin-1 is perhaps the best example of such an inhibitor (4). Noel Bouck and her colleagues first reported evidence that the wild-type *p53* gene is a positive regulator of thrombospondin expression; hence, inactivation of *p53* by mutational or deletion events can result in loss of thrombospondin expression (18). Indeed, this led Bouck to propose that a major consequence of inactivation of wild-type suppressor genes would be to facilitate tumor angiogenesis, primarily by eliminating or reducing the expression of endogenous inhibitors of angiogenesis (19). This would contribute (indirectly) to the tumor-promoting function of such genetic alterations, in addition to their direct effects on enhancing unrestricted cell proliferation and cell survival (4, 18).

II. THE CONNECTION OF ONCOGENES TO TUMOR ANGIOGENESIS

A survey of some of the growth factors up-regulated in tumor cells immediately suggests a possible role for oncogenes in tumor angiogenesis. For example, both TFGα and TGFβ, which are proangiogenic molecules in vivo (4), are known to be induced or up-regulated in mutant *ras* transformed cells (20, 21). The same is true for bFGF (22). Two other considerations led us, in 1995, to speculate that a major unappreciated function of oncogenes is to contribute to the angiogenic phenotype in tumors. First, it is known that the growth fraction of many solid tumors is very low (23, 24), in some cases surprisingly so, as in rapidly expanding metastatic prostate cancer deposits growing in the bone (25). The low fractions of solid tumors are thought to be a major source of the intrinsic resistance characteristics of such tumors to cytotoxic chemotherapeutic drugs, which generally target rapidly dividing cells (26). This presents an interesting paradox, given the emphasis that has been placed on aberrant cell-cycle regulation (''unrestricted cell proliferation'') as the predominant functional effect of most oncogenes on the transformed phenotype. For example, because metastatic prostatic cancers have tumor cell growth fractions in the range of only 2% (25), it is difficult to accept the idea that oncogenes that contribute to prostate cancer do so primarily, if at all, through their effects on *directly* promoting aberrant cell proliferation. It is worth pointing out that when tumor cells are grown in monolayer cell culture, it is not uncommon to encounter growth fractions in the range of 75%, far greater than what is ever observed in vivo (26). However, growth in vitro as three-dimensional multicellular spheroids can lead to a very significant reduction in the growth fraction (26), despite the presence of numerous inactivated tumor suppressor genes and mutant oncogenes in the cultured tumor cells. The predominant use of monolayer cell culture systems to study cancer biology in vitro has resulted in a somewhat distorted view of the relative importance and contribution of uncontrolled cell-cycle proliferation to the overall growth and expansion of solid tumors in vivo (26). The question that emerges is, how do oncogenes contribute to the ability of tumors to grow indefinitely in addition to, or instead of, promoting aberrant cell proliferation? Could an indirect mechanism of growth promotion be involved, namely induction of, or contribution to, angiogenesis?

A second paradoxical observation that caught our attention concerns the therapeutic effects of a new class of anticancer drugs generically known as signal transduction inhibitors. The best-known examples of such drugs include small-molecular-weight *Ras* farnesyltransferase inhibitors (FTIs) (27, 28) and monoclonal neutralizing antibodies to overexpressed cell surface-receptor tyrosine kinases such as the EGF receptor or *erb*B2/HER-2/neu (29, 30). In general, such drugs are considered to be cytostatic rather than cytotoxic agents, as they inhibit growth of target tumor cells in (monolayer) cell culture in the absence of any significant killing (27, 28, 31). Moreover the cytostatic effects are often modest, in the range of 30% to 60% inhibition at the highest drug concentrations (27, 28, 31). Consequently a reasonable prediction would be that such drugs would possess only modest antitumor effects in vivo when tested on established tumors, that is overt regressions of tumor mass would not be a feature of treatment with such drugs. Rather, tumors would be kept from expanding by an induced state of dormant growth. Surprisingly this is not necessarily the case (31–33). Regression of established experimental tumors in mice have been observed in some cases, for example, using *Ras* FTIs on certain transgenic ‘‘oncomouse’’ strains (32). Moreover, the extent and rapidity of tumor regressions can match, or even exceed, maximum tolerated doses of conventional cytotoxic anticancer drugs such as adriamycin (32).

How can such an unexpected discrepancy be accounted for? One possible explanation is that the agents may be found to be cytotoxic when tested against tumor cells grown in a solid tumor (multicellular) context, rather than in monolayer cell cultures, which is the usual way tumor cells are grown for drug testing studies in cell culture. Indeed there is evidence that *ras* oncogenes can function as potent survival factors by suppressing the massive levels of apoptosis of epithelial cells observed when such cells are grown nonphysiologically as multicellular spheroids (34). This probably explains why *Ras* FTIs can induce apoptosis in *ras*-transformed cells grown anchorage independently, but not in monolayer cell culture (35), and, as it now turns out, in vivo as well when tested on established solid tumors (36).

However, an alternative mechanism of cell killing by such signal transduction inhibitors could involve inhibition of tumor angiogenesis, as we first suggested in 1995 (37), and as schematically outlined in Figure 1. If it is supposed that activation of an oncogene such as *ras* leads to a marked induction in tumor cells of a paracrine-acting angiogenesis growth factor such as VEGF/VPF, treatment of such cells with a drug such as a Ras FTI could result in down-regulation/suppression of that tumor cell-derived angiogenesis factor. This in turn could endow the drug with potential antiangiogenic properties that could then lead to an increase in tumor cell apoptosis. This is because blocked angiogenesis often is associated with an increase in the levels of apoptotic cells detected in tumors (38, 39). Moreover, even modest (twofold to threefold) reductions in VEGF/VPF expression can be associated with profound degrees of tumor growth inhibition (40), as well as endothelial cell apoptosis (41, 42) leading to blood vessel destruction (41, 43).

In an effort to test these hypotheses, we initiated a series of experiments designed to determine, first whether mutant *ras* oncogenes, and subsequently other oncogenes, could act as inducers of VEGF/VPF gene and protein expression. Assuming such an association could be uncovered, we could then test the effects of various signal transduction antitumor inhibitory drugs for their effects

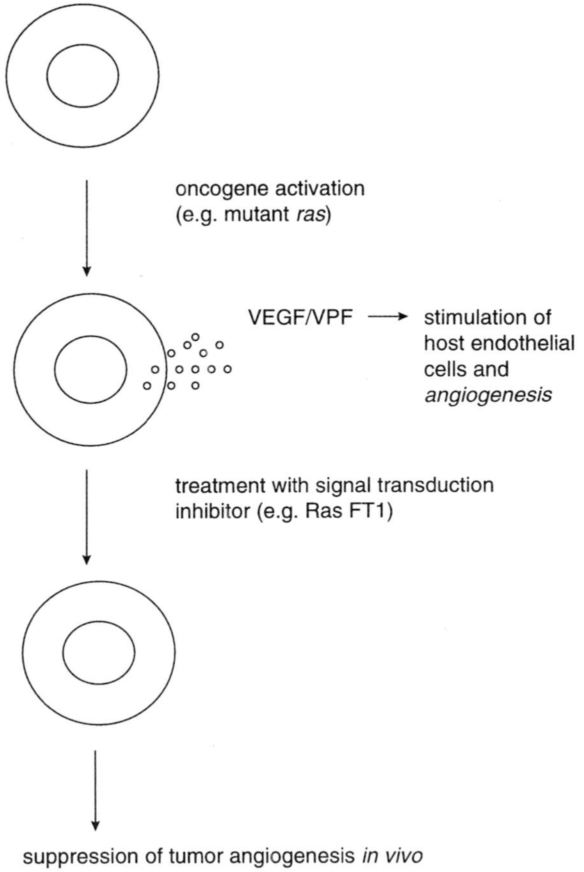

Figure 1 Outline of how oncogenes and signal transduction inhibitor drugs may contribute to induction and inhibition of tumor angiogenesis, respectively. Oncogene (e.g., *ras*) activation can lead to induction of Vascular endothelial growth factor/vascular permeability factor (VEGF/VPF), a potent mediator of angiogenesis. Vascular endothelial growth factor/vascular permeability factor cannot function as an autocrine growth factor for tumor cells, as tumor cells generally lack receptors for VEGF/VPF. In contrast, ''activated'' endothelial cells can express high levels of VEGF/VPF, perhaps due to the inductive effect of VEGF/VPF itself. Treatment of the VEGF/VPF-positive tumor cells with a signal transduction inhibitor, e.g. a Ras farnesyltransferase inhibitor (FTI), can lead to, among many other changes, a reduction in VEGF/VPF expression. This could, in turn, lead to a suppressed in vivo angiogenic response. Oncogene activation also could lead to expression of growth factors having both autocrine and paracrine/angiogenesis promoting functions (such as tumor growth factor [TGF]α) and down-regulation of angiogenesis inhibitory molecules, such as thrombospondin (see text).

on VEGF/VPF expression, both in vitro and in vivo, against appropriate target tumor cells. Our first experiments used intestinal epithelial cell line IEC-18 cells, a spontaneously immortalized cell line of rat intestinal epithelium totally incapable of forming tumors in nude mice (37). A number of clonal *ras*-transformed sublines were obtained by transfection of IEC-18 cells with a mutant human H-*ras* oncogene (37), all of which were found to be highly tumorigenic in nude mice, for example, the IEC-*ras*3, IEC-*ras*4 and IEC-*ras*7 cell lines (37). As shown in Figure 2, the parental IEC-18 cell line was essentially negative for VEGF/VPF gene expression, as assessed by Northern blotting experiments (37). In obvious contrast, the *ras*-transformed sublines were all strongly VEGF/VPF positive. This included a clone in which mutant H-*ras* was put under the control of heavy metal-inducible promoter, so long as the cells were exposed to zinc and cadmium (37), as shown in Figure 2. Similarly, IEC-18 cells transfected with a tetracyclin-regulated *ras* gene expression construct were VEGF/VPF mRNA positive in the absence of tetracyclin and negative in its presence (unpublished observations). At the time our results were published, Marmé and colleagues reported a virtually identical pattern of results using v-*ras*-(and v-*raf*)-transformed NIH 3T3 fibroblasts (44). Since then, a number of confirmatory reports have appeared, showing an association between *ras* expression—often, but not always mediated by mutant *ras* oncogene transfection—and induction or up-regulation of VEGF/VPF gene expression in mouse, rat, hamster, and human cells of variable origin (45–53). This is summarized in Table 1. In virtually all

Figure 2 Mutant *ras* oncogene regulates expression of vascular endothelial growth factor (VEGF) mRNA. In panel (**A**) a Northern blot of VEGF mRNA is shown of human HT1080 human fibrosarcoma cells (as a positive control), nontumorigenic rat intestinal epithelial cell line-18 (IEC-18 cells), and two clones of IEC-18, called *ras*-7 and *ras*-3, which were obtained by transfection of IEC-18 cells with a mutant human H-*ras* oncogene. These latter two lines are tumorigenic, and unlike IEC-18 cells, express abundant VEGF transcripts. MT-*ras* is a clone of IEC-18 which expresses its transfected mutant H-*ras* oncogene only when exposed to heavy metals such as zinc and cadmium, as the gene is under the control of a metallothionein promoter. Vascular endothelial growth factor mRNA is not expressed in this clone unless they are exposed to these metals, as shown in the upper panel. Panel (**B**) shows a Northern blot for VEGF mRNA in human DLD-1 and HCT-116 human colorectal carcinoma cells, each of which contains a single mutant K-*ras* allele. DKS-8 and Hkl-2 are sublines obtained from DLD-1 and HCT-116, respectively, in which the mutant K-*ras* allele has been disrupted by gene targeting (54). The DLD-1 and HCT-116 cell lines are tumorigenic in nude mice, whereas DKS-8 and Hkl-2 are not. The suppression of VEGF mRNA is matched by a down-regulation in VEGF protein released by the cells into the conditioned medium. The results are taken from Rak et al. (37).

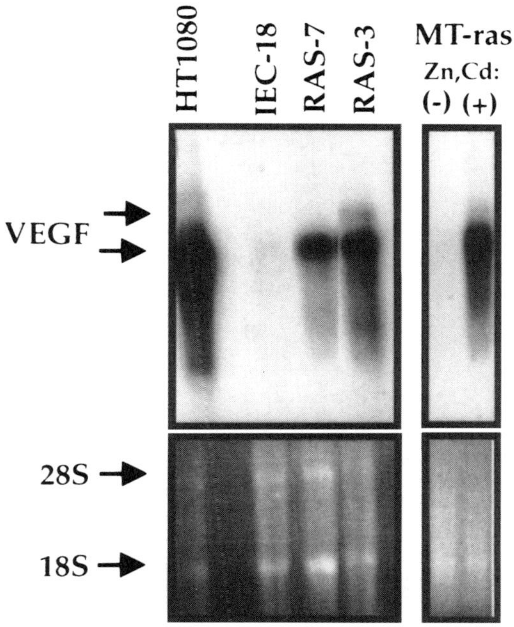
HT1080
IEC-18
RAS-7
RAS-3
MT-ras
Zn,Cd:
(-) (+)
VEGF
28S
18S

(A)

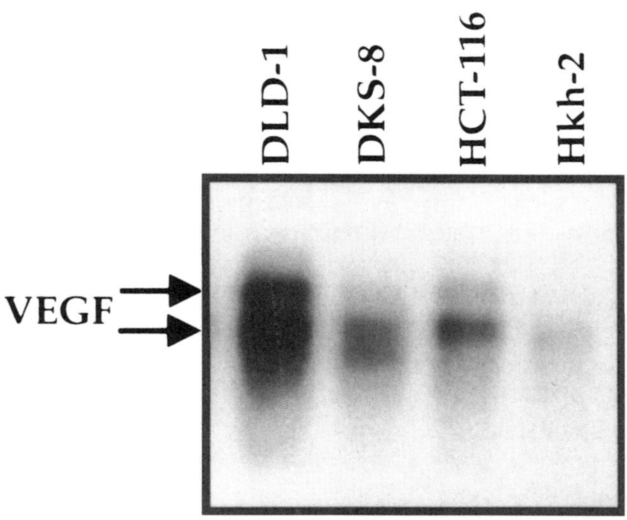
DLD-1
DKS-8
HCT-116
Hkh-2
VEGF

(B)

Table 1 Mutant *ras* Oncogene Induction or Up-regulation of VEGF/VPF

Cells/System	Reference[a]
H-ras-transformed intestinal epithelial cells	Ref. 37
v-ras-transformed NIH-3T3 cells	Ref. 44
H-ras in mouse squamous cell carcinomas	Ref. 47
H-ras-transformed NIH-3T3 cells	Ref. 46
H-ras-transformed endothelial cells	Ref. 51
H-ras in Li Fraumeni p53-human fibroblasts	Ref. 48
v-H-ras in human IMR-90 fibroblasts	Ref. 52
v-H-ras in NIH-3T3 cells	Ref. 53

[a]More recently, up-regulation of VEGF as a function of Ras activity has been shown by several other investigators (see Ref. 68 for review).

of these experiments, the increase in mRNA expression was matched by a commensurate increase in protein expression.

An alternative and complementary method to demonstrate a cause-and-effect relationship between oncogenic *ras* mutations and VEGF/VPF expression is to examine VEGF/VPF-positive human colorectal carcinomas that carry a single mutant K-*ras* allele and sublines of such tumors in which the dominantly acting mutant K-*ras* allele is disrupted by gene-targeting methods (37). Such sublines have been obtained by Shirasawa et al. from the highly tumorigenic HCT-116 and DLD-1 human colorectal carcinomas (54). It is remarkable that the sublines containing a disrupted K-*ras* allele were found to be nontumorigenic in nude mice (37, 43, 54) despite the retention of the numerous other genetic alterations normally associated with, and presumed to be causative of, advanced colon cancer. Could this profound loss in tumorigenicity be related, at least in part, to a significant suppression of VEGF/VPF expression in the mutant K-*ras* knock-out sublines? We have speculated that the answer to this is affirmative, based on several findings (43). First, the knock-out sublines were found to express an approximately fourfold reduction in VEGF/VPF mRNA (Fig. 2) and protein levels (37). Second, a similar reduction in VEGF/VPF expression mediated by transfection of HCT-116 or DLD-1 cells with a $VEGF_{121}$ antisense cDNA expression construct resulted in the derivation of several clones from each parent line that was suppressed twofold to fourfold for VEGF/VPF protein expression (43). All of these clones were profoundly suppressed in their tumor-forming ability in nude mice, but not in cell culture (Fig. 3). Third, if VEGF/VPF deficient mutant K-*ras* knock-out sublines were used as recipients for a $VEGF/VPF_{121}$ "sense" transfection procedure, a number of the VEGF/VPF-expressing variants showed a weak but detectable increase in tumor-forming ability in nude mice, but no growth advantage in tissue culture (Fig. 4) (43). These results, taken together,

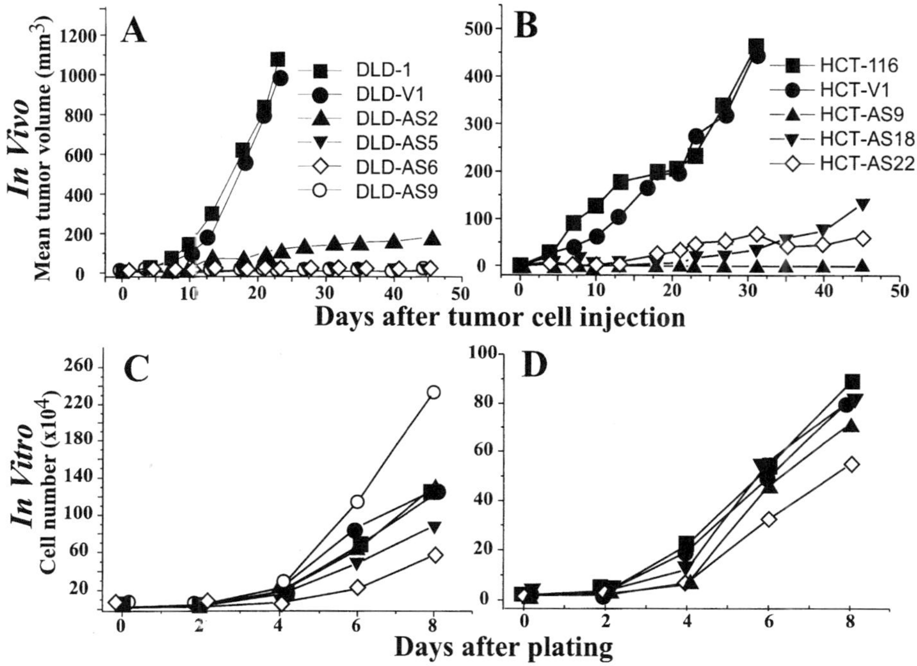

Figure 3 Up-regulated VEGF expression is *a necessary* condition for K-*ras*-dependent tumor formation by human colorectal cancer cells. DLD-1 (**A, C**) and HCT-116 (**B, D**) cell lines both derived from advanced colorectal cancer and both harboring a mutant K-*ras* allele were rendered VEGF deficient by transfection with an antisense $VEGF_{121}$ expression vector (clones designated as AS). As in the case of deletion of mutant K-*ras* itself, down-regulation of VEGF/vascular permeability factor (VPF) expression leads to a severe impairment of tumor-forming capacity of all sublines tested compared to their parental or vector transfected (*V*) counterparts (**A, B**). No consistent change in in vitro growth properties was observed in conjunction with antisense or control transfection (**C, D**).

suggest that *ras* oncogene-induced VEGF/VPF expression is necessary, but clearly not sufficient, for aggressive tumorigenic growth of these colorectal cancer cells in vivo. This conclusion would appear to make intuitive sense because knocking out the mutant *ras* allele would lead to suppression of numerous and different pro-cell transformation events involving, for example, growth, invasion, and survival, *in addition to angiogenesis*. Restoring some degree of VEGF/VPF expression would not affect these other vital transformed cell-associated phenotypes. Indeed, even the degree of angiogenesis competence that is restored by a $VEGF_{121}$ transfection method might be an underestimate, because other VEGF/VPF isoforms (e.g., $VEGF_{165}$) and additional proangiogenic growth factors (e.g.,

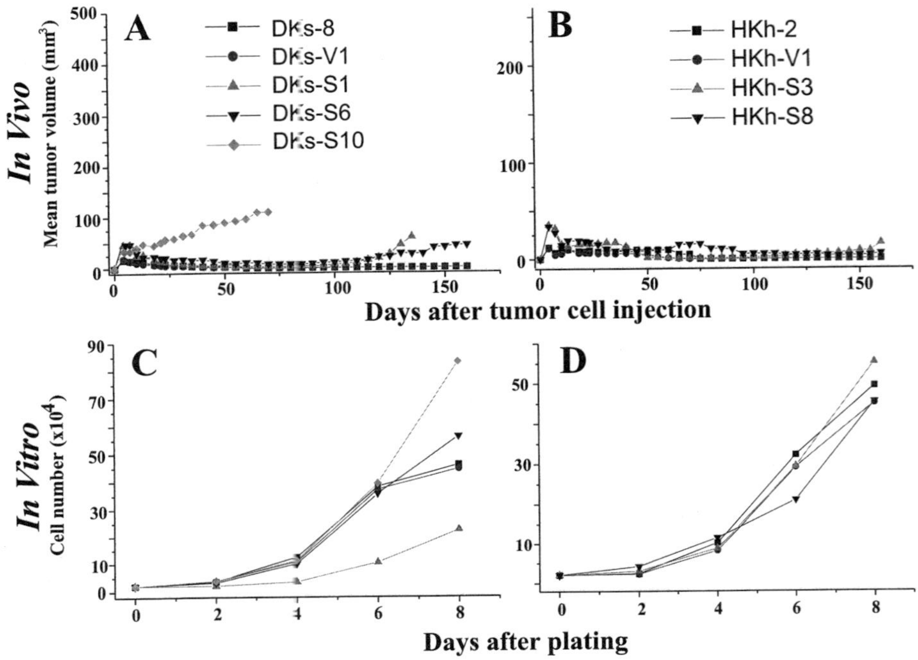

Figure 4 Up-regulation of vascular endothelial growth factor/vascular permeability factor (VEGF/VPF) expression is insufficient to fully rescue the tumorigenic phenotype in colorectal cancer cells (DKS-8 and Hkh-2) in which a mutant K-*ras* allele has been disrupted by homologous recombination. DKS-8 (**A, C**) and Hkh-2 (**B, D**) cell lines both derived from advanced colorectal cancer and both harboring a disrupted mutant K-*ras* allele, were engineered to re-express $VEGF_{121}$ (designated as sense -S) in excess to what was detectable in the case of their control transfected counterparts (designated as V) or parental cell lines DLD-1 and HCT-116, respectively. No consistent change in in vitro growth properties was observed in conjunction with this transfection (**C, D**); however, a weak but noticeable increase in tumor take accompanied re-expression of VEGF.

bFGF, IL-8, etc.) possibly suppressed in the knock-out sublines would not have their levels restored by transfection of a sense $VEGF/VPF_{121}$ cDNA expression construct (43).

More recently, we and others have found that other genetic alterations that effectively function as dominant oncogenes, for example, overexpression of the EGF and *erb*B2/neu/Her2 receptor tyrosine kinases, also are associated with induction or up-regulation of VEGF/VPF mRNA or protein expression (Figs. 5, 6) (55). This is consistent with the previous results of some other studies showing, for example, that TGFα or insulinlike growth factor (IGF)-1 can induce VEGF/

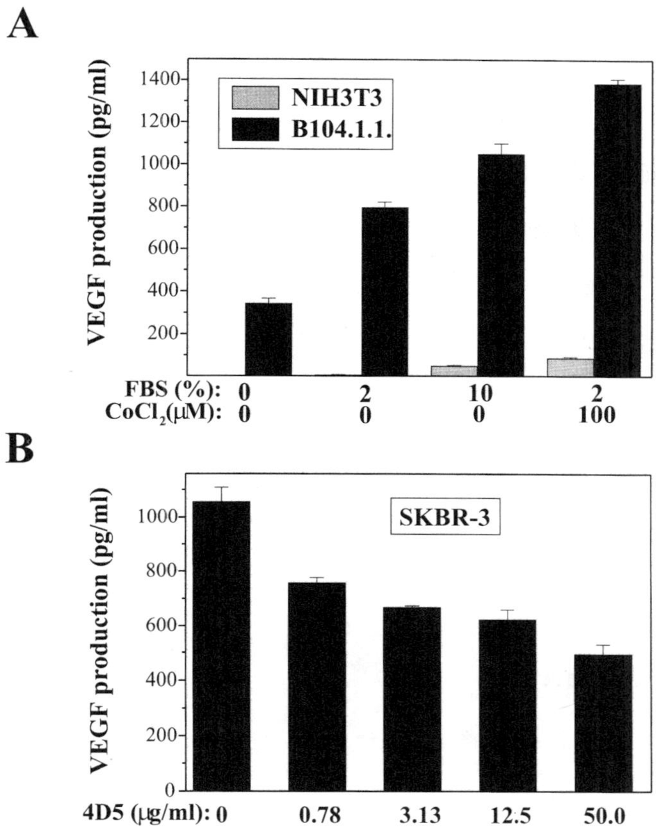

Figure 5 Vascular endothelial growth factor/vascular permeability factor immunoreactivity in conditioned medium of cells transformed with *erb*B-2/*neu* oncogene. **A**. Overexpression of mutant *erb*B-2 in NIH3T3 cells leads to an increase in constitutive VEGF/VPF production as well as hypersensitivity of the cells to serum and hypoxiamimetic treatment with cobalt chloride cells. **B**. Treatment of human breast cancer cells SKBR-3 with monoclonal anti-*erb*B-2/*neu* neutralizing antibody 4D7 leads to down-regulation of VEGF/VPF production (55).

VPF expression in vitro (56, 57). It is also now known that other classes of oncogenes, for example genes that encode transcription factors such as c-*fos* (45) or protein translational initiation factors such as elF-4e (58), can function as potent inducers of VEGF/VPF expression, both in vitro and in vivo (45). Thus a generic function of many oncogenes may be to promote tumor growth and survival *indirectly* through an angiogenesis-dependent mechanism, as well as *di-*

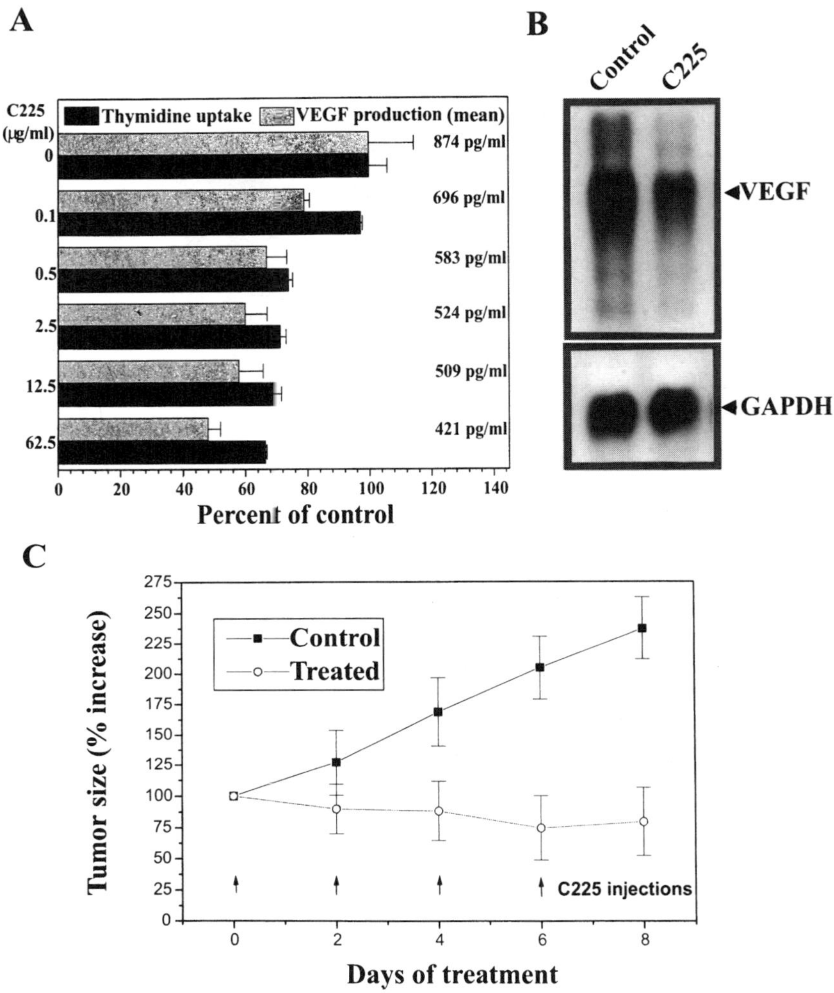

Figure 6 The inhibitory effect of epidermal growth factor receptor (EGFR) neutralizing antibody C225 on vascular endothelial growth factor (VEGF) production by squamous cell carcinoma cells A431 **A**. Inhibition of VEGF/vascular permeability factor (VPF) protein secretion. **B**. Inhibition of VEGF gene expression in vitro. **C**. Inhibition of tumor growth in vivo. This treatment also reduced VEGF/VPF expression and blood vessel counts in tumors of A431 cells (55).

rectly through their effects on enhancing intrinsic tumor cell proliferation and survival. This suggests that various signal transduction inhibitors being developed as anticancer drugs may function in vivo as de facto antiangiogenic agents.

III. SIGNAL TRANSDUCTION INHIBITORS AS ANTI-TUMOR AGENTS: DO THEY INHIBIT TUMOR ANGIOGENESIS IN VIVO?

This is a difficult question to answer in a definitive manner but the evidence obtained thus far would appear to indicate that one possible effect of administering a variety of signal transduction inhibitors to tumor-bearing mice would be to suppress VEGF/VPF expression, and in all probability a number of other proangiogenic growth factors as well, thereby endowing such drugs with the potential to block or suppress tumor growth, at least in part, by inhibiting the angiogenesis competence of the treated tumors.

Our first attempt at analyzing this question involved an examination of the effects of Ras FTI called L-739, 749 (37) on VEGF/VPF expression using VEGF/VPF-cultured *ras*-transformed IEC-18 cells as a target population in vitro (37). The results showed that one effect of drug treatment of such cells in vitro was down-regulation of VEGF/VPF expression (Fig. 7) (37). We have not yet determined whether a similar effect of the drug would be observed in vivo in drug-treated, tumor-bearing mice.

However, such an in vivo effect has been observed with a different class of antitumor signal transduction-inhibitory agent, namely monoclonal neutralizing antibodies to the human EGF receptor (55, 73). We had found that human A431 squamous carcinoma cells, which overexpress the EGF receptor, displayed reduced (up to twofold) levels of VEGF/VPF mRNA and protein in vitro after treatment in culture with varying concentrations of the EGF receptor-neutralizing antibody, which is known as C225 (Fig. 6) (31). We therefore attempted a similar treatment of A431 squamous carcinoma cells grown as subcutaneous xenografts in nude mice (55). For these experiments nude mice were injected with A431 cells and the tumors were allowed to grow for 3 to 4 weeks. One group of mice was injected four times with C225 intraperitoneally (one injection every 2 days) and the tumors were removed shortly after the last injection. They were assessed for their relative expression of VEGF/VPF protein by immunostaining, in comparison to the control mice. The results showed a rather striking down-regulation of VEGF/VPF expression in the A431 tumors removed from mice that had been given the C225 antibody (55). The level of reduction could not be quantitated with accuracy but would appear to exceed threefold (55). As discussed above, this level of suppression, when induced by an antisense method, can have profound

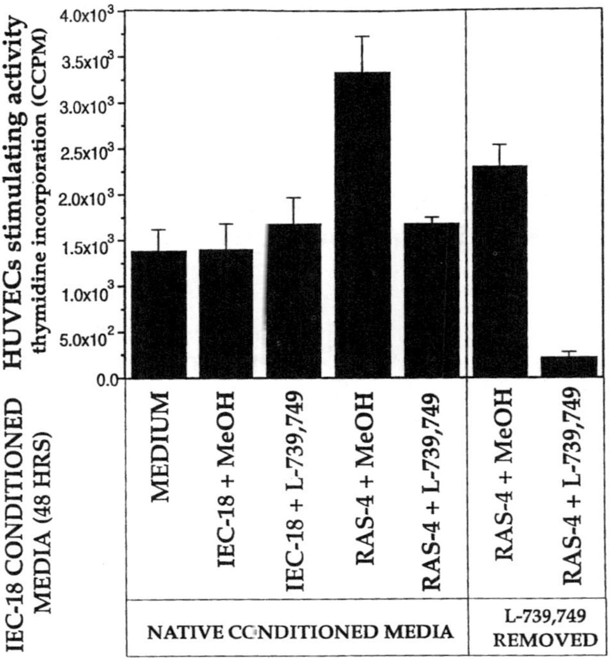

Figure 7 Reversal of *ras*-dependent up-regulation of VEGF/VPF by treatment with a farnesyl transferase inhibitor L-739, 749. Intestinal epithelial cell line (IEC)-18 parental cells or their *ras* transfectants (RAS-4) were treated with 25 μM L-739, 749 or the equivalent volume of vehicle (MeOH). The VEGF/VPF activity in conditioned medium was assayed against human umbilical endothelial cells (HUVECs). The endothelial stimulating activity of VEGF/VPF is lost from conditioned medium of *ras*-transformed cells upon treatment with L-739,749. The latter is also true for conditioned medium from which L-739,749 has been removed (37).

suppressive consequences on tumor growth in vivo in the absence of any antitumor effect in cell culture (40, 43).

Thus, it would seem reasonable to postulate that long-term therapy of tumors with agents such as C225 could lead to an indirect mechanism of suppression of tumor growth as a result of blocked angiogenesis. This may be true of many drugs designed to inhibit the expression of different classes of mutant or overexpressed oncoproteins. If so, it could help explain why such drugs appear to be more potent in vivo than one would anticipate from their behavior as antitumor drugs on cells grown in monolayer cell culture, where generally only modest and noncytotoxic effects are observed. In this respect, it would be interesting to determine whether the putative antiangiogenic effects of such agents can be separated from their direct antiproliferative effects on tumor cells. Are the drug concentrations and scheduling that are optimal for inhibiting (directly) tumor cell growth (or survival) the same as for inhibiting angiogenesis?

IV. INTERACTION OF ONCOGENES (AND TUMOR SUPPRESSOR GENES) AND ANGIOGENESIS INHIBITORS

The emphasis in this discussion has been on the idea that oncogenes can contribute to tumor angiogenesis primarily by virtue of their stimulatory effects on the expression of proangiogenic growth factors such as VEGF/VPF. However, as discussed earlier, the angiogenic switch is also affected by the loss of angiogenesis inhibitors, such as thrombospondin-1, as a result of inactivation of the *p53* gene (18). It is conceivable that oncogenes could contribute to the angiogenic switch by causing a similar down-regulation of various angiogenesis inhibitors. Indeed, several groups have reported that the levels of thrombospondin in *ras* oncogene transformed fibroblasts can be strongly suppressed (59, 60, 69). Likewise, inactivation of the von Hippel-Lindau suppressor gene can lead to a significant induction or up-regulation of VEGF/VPF gene and protein expression (61, 62). Hence it is becoming clear that mutant/deleted tumor suppressor genes and oncogenes can influence angiogenesis by acting in a pleiotrophic fashion (69).

V. INTERACTION OF ONCOGENES WITH PHYSIOLOGICAL REGULATORS OF TUMOR ANGIOGENESIS

One important and potent mediator of VEGF/VPF expression, both in vitro and in vivo is reduced oxygen concentrations, that is, hypoxia (63, 64). This effect of hypoxia is mediated both by a transcriptional effect and an increase in mRNA stability (65), the latter of which seems to be the more potent (65, 66). This has led to the view that physiological stresses such as hypoxia in solid tumors may be the major inducing influence of angiogenesis, rather than genetic changes per se (67). However it is becoming increasingly evident that a *combination* of genetic and egigenetic (i.e., hypoxia) changes can function synergistically to boost VEGF/VPF expression in tumor cells (46, 51, 55). This effect, as observed in mutant *neu* oncogene-transformed NIH 3T3 (B104.1.1) fibroblasts can be dramatic (Fig. 7) (55). The signaling pathways that are involved in this interaction are now being analyzed (46, 49). For example, in H-*ras*-transformed endothelial cells, VEGF/VPF expression can be down-regulated by wortmannin, a PI3 kinase inhibitor (51). Activation of PI3 kinase, but not MAP kinases, has also been implicated in combined oncogene-hypoxia induction of VEGF/VPF transcription in *ras*-transformed fibroblasts (49).

The impact of PI3K on activity of VEGF/VPF promoter can be mediated by up-regulation of a transcription factor known as hypoxia-inducible factor 1 (HIF-1) (49). This factor is composed of two functional subunits, including HIF-1 α and the beta subunit, which is also known as arylhydrocarbon-receptor nuclear translocator (ARNT) (71). In mouse embryos lacking ARNT expression, a number of hypoxia-inducible genes, including VEGF/VPF, cannot be switched on by low oxygen tension or glucose deprivation; hence, this important mode of angiogenic regulation is absent in most of the developing tissues. Interestingly, the sustained expression of VEGF/VPF in the gut of ARNT-/-embryos stands in contrast to this general pattern (71). This may suggest that in the intestine, the expression of VEGF/VPF may be independent of hypoxia in general or of ARNT in particular. In addition other than hypoxia regulators of HIF-1 activity (p53, IGF2) are of considerable interest (71). This is consistent with our observation that in the human colorectal cancer cell lines DLD-1 and HCT-116, the influence of hypoxia and *ras* on production of VEGF/VPF protein is less than synergistic and in some cases fairly minimal, at least as compared to the impact exerted by the oncogenic *ras* alone (Fig. 8). It is therefore possible that the degree of synergy between *ras* and various microenvironmental influences is somewhat cell-type dependent. It also has been suggested that efficient VEGF/VPF transcription under hypoxic conditions is dependent on activity of cytoplasmatic protein kinases such as *src* and *raf* (68). In particular, constitutively activated *v-src* oncogene has been postulated to stimulate HIF-1 gene expression and DNA-binding capacity and to thereby induce a hypoxialike up-regulation of VEGF/VPF transcription (71). On the other hand, both hypoxia and oncogenic *ras* also are known to up-regulate VEGF/VPF through nontranscriptional mechanisms such as an increase in mRNA stability (53). Although the exact molecular details of the latter effect remain unknown, the up-regulation of VEGF/VPF has been observed in cells expressing activated forms of *ras* (38, 45), *raf*-1 (45) and MEK-1 (unpublished data), suggesting a role of the classical MAPK pathway in control of VEGF/VPF production. Furthermore, in hyperplastic papillomas that develop in mice harboring v-H-*ras* transgene expression, VEGF/VPF was attenuated when the transgene was expressed on the *fos* -/- background, suggesting a role of c-*fos* and AP-1 transcription factors in *ras*-dependent VEGF/VPF expression. However, in human and rat intestinal epithelial cell lines expressing mutant K-*ras* or H-*ras* oncogenes, the constitutively elevated production of VEGF/VPF protein could not be reduced in the presence of MEK-1 inhibitor PD98059 but it was effectively down-regulated by treatment of these cells with high concentrations of PI3K inhibitor LY294002 (or with an antioxidant, N-acetyl-cysteine) pointing to the *ras*/PI3K pathway rather than *ras*/*raf*/MEK/MAPK pathway (69). It should be kept in mind that the consequences of activation of Ras and other signal transduc-

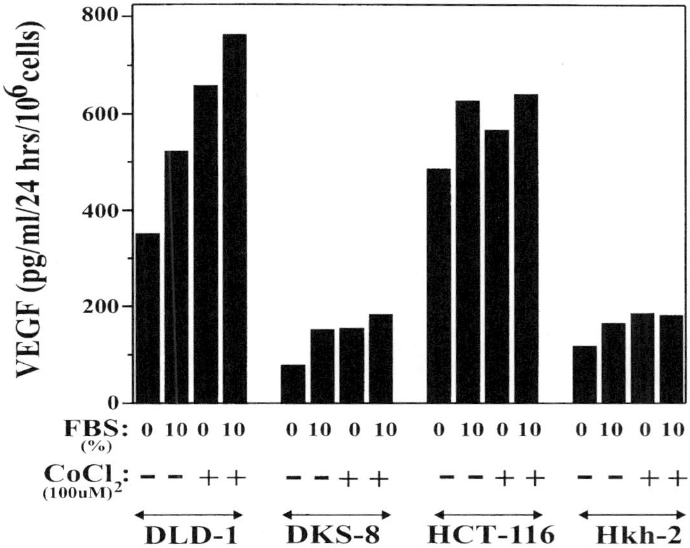

Figure 8 The requirement for K-*ras* oncogene expression for efficient upregulation of vascular epithelial growth factor/vascular permeability factor (VEGF/VPF) in human colorectal cancer cells. Two colorectal cancer cell lines DLD-1 and HCT-116 and their variants in which a mutant K-*ras* allele has been deleted by homologous recombination (DKS-8 and Hkh-2) were assayed for production of VEGF/VPF in the presence or absence of serum or hypoxia-mimetic agent cobalt chloride cells. In the absence of mutant K-*ras* expression, neither of these treatments was able to efficiently up-regulate VEGF production.

ing, and potentially oncogenic, proteins differ depending on cell type and a biological context (69). These specific circumstances may define the role of different signaling pathways in changes of VEGF/VPF expression and angiogenic capacity of cells affected by different types of transforming events.

VI. SUMMARY

We have tried to stress that mutant oncogenes or overexpressed, nonmutated proto-oncogenes, in addition to their direct effect on promoting aberrant tumor cell proliferation (and survival) may possess a crucial indirect means of stimulating tumor cell growth through regulation of angiogenesis. This effect would never be observed in tissue culture studies of oncogene function using pure cultures of tumor cells, and probably helps explain why the proangiogenic function of oncogenes has not been appreciated until recently. Indeed, the very first indication of a possible contributory role of oncogenes, such as *ras* and *myc*, to tumor angiogenesis was first reported by Thompson et al. in 1989, who used reconstituted organ cultures of the mouse prostate gland for their studies (71). This potentially important contribution of oncogenes to tumor growth and development may have an impact on how various signal transduction inhibitors that are now in early phase clinical trials, such as how monoclonal neutralizing antibodies to the human EGF receptor (53, 73) or farnesyl transferase inhibitors (37, 68) function in vivo as antitumor agents.

ACKNOWLEDGMENTS

We are grateful to Lynda Woodcock and Cassandra Cheng for their excellent secretarial assistance. R.S. Kerbel's angiogenesis-related research is supported by grants from the Medical Research Council of Canada and the National Institutes of Health, USA (CA41223). R.S. Kerbel is a Terry Fox Scientist of the National Cancer Institute of Canada.

REFERENCES

1. Folkman J. Tumor angiogenesis: Therapeutic implications. New Engl J Med 1971; 285:1182–1186.
2. Folkman J. Anti-angiogenesis: New concept for therapy of solid tumors. Ann Surg 1972; 175:409–416.
3. Folkman J. What is the evidence that tumors are angiogenesis-dependent? J Natl Canc Inst 1990; 82 4–6.
4. Bouck N, Stellmach V, Hsu SC. How tumors become angiogenic. Adv Cancer Res 1996; 69:135–174.
5. Kerbel RS. Inhibition of tumor angiogenesis as a strategy to circumvent acquired resistance to anti-cancer therapeutic agents. BioEssays 1991; 13:31–36.
6. Boehm T, Folkman J, Browder T, O'Reilly MS. Antiangiogenic therapy of experimental cancer does not induce acquired drug resistance. Nature 1997; 390:404–407.
7. Kerbel RS. A cancer therapy resistant to resistance. Nature 1997; 390:335–336.
8. Folkman J, D'Amore PA. Blood vessel formation: What is its molecular basis? Cell 1996; 87:1153–1155.
9. Terman BI, Dougher-Vermazen M. Biological properties of VEGF/VPF receptors. Cancer Metastasis Rev 1996; 15:159–163.
10. Thomas KA. Vascular endothelial growth factor, a potent and selective angiogenic agent. J Biol Chem 1996; 271:603–606.
11. Stromblad S, Cheresh DA. Cell adhesion and angiogenesis. Trends Cell Biol 1998; 6:462–46889.

12. Brooks PC. Cell adhesion molecules in angiogenesis. Cancer Metastasis Rev 1996; 15:187–194.
13. Bischoff J. Approaches to studying cell adhesion molecules in angiogenesis. Trends Cell Biol 1995; 5:69–74.
14. Folkman J. Angiogenesis inhibitors generated by tumors. Mol Med 1995; 1:120–122.
15. Hanahan D, Folkman J. Patterns and emerging mechanisms of the angiogenic switch during tumorigenesis. Cell 1996; 86:353–364.
16. Baird A, Klagsbrun M. The fibroblast growth factor family. Cancer Cells 1991; 3: 239–243.
17. Rak J, Kerbel RS. bFGF and tumor angiogenesis—back in the limelight? Nat Med 1997; 3:1083–1084.
18. Dameron KM, Volpert OV, Tainsky MA, Bouck N. Control of angiogenesis in fibroblasts by p53 regulation of thrombospondin-1. Science 1994; 265:1582–1584.
19. Bouck N. Tumor angiogenesis: The role of oncogenes and tumor suppressor genes. Cancer Cells 1990; 2:179–185.
20. Marshall CJ, et al. The involvement of activated ras in determining the transformed phenotype. Proc R Soc Lond B Biol Sci 1985; 226:99–106.
21. Roberts AB, Sporn MB, Assoian RK, Smith JM, Roche NS, Wakefield LM, Heine UI, Liotta LA, Falanga V, Kehrl JH, Fauci AS. Transforming growth factor type beta: Rapid induction of fibrosis and angiogenesis in vivo and stimulation of collagen formation in vitro. Proc Natl Acad Sci U S A 1986; 83:4167–4171.
22. Iberg N, Rogelj S, Fanning P, Klagsbrun M. Purification of 18-and 22-kDa forms of basic fibroblast growth factor from rat cells transformed by the ras oncogene. J Biol Chem 1989; 264:19951–19955.
23. Tannock I. Cell kinetics and chemotherapy: a critical review. Cancer Treat Rep 1978; 62:1117–1133.
24. Olive PL, Durand RE. Drug and radiation resistance in spheroids: Cell contact and kinetics. Cancer Metastasis Rev 1994; 13:121–138.
25. Berges RR, Vukanovic J, Epstein J, CarMichel M, Cisek L, Johnson DE, Veltri RW, Walsh CT, Isaacs JT. Implication of cell kinetic changes during the progression of human prostatic carcinoma. Clin Cancer Res 1995; 1:473–480.
26. St. Croix B, Florenes VA, Rak JW, Flanagan M, Bhattacharya N, Slingerland JM, Kerbel RS. Impact of the cyclin dependent kinase inhibitor $p27^{Kipl}$ on adhesion-dependent resistance of tumor cells to anticancer agents. Nat Med 1996; 2:1204–1210.
27. Kohl NE, Mosser SD, deSolms SJ, Giuliani EA, Pompliano DL, Graham SL, Smith RL, Scolnick EM, Oliff A, Gibbs JB. Selective inhibition of *ras*-dependent transformation by a farnesyltransferase inhibitor. Science 1993; 260:1934–1942.
28. James GL, Golstein JL, Brown MS, Rawson TE, Somers TC, McDowell RS, Crowley CW, Lucas BK, Levinson AD, Marsters JJC. Benzodiazepine peptidomimetics: Potent inhibitors of ras farnesylation in animal cells. Science 1993; 260:1937–1942.
29. Mendelsohn J, Fan Z. Epidermal growth factor receptor family and chemosensitization. J Natl Canc Inst 1997; 89:341–343.
30. Fendly BM, Winget M, Hudziak RM, Lipari MT, Napier MA, Ullrich A. Characterization of murine monoclonal antibodies reactive to either the human epidermal growth factor receptor or HER2/neu gene product. Cancer Res 1990; 50:1550–1558.

31. Goldstein NI, Prewett M, Zuklys K, Rockwell P, Mendelsohn J. Biological efficacy of a chimeric antibody to the epidermal growth factor receptor in a human tumor xenograft model. Clin Cancer Res 1995; 1:1311–1318.
32. Kohl NE, Omer CA, Conner MW, Anthony NJ, Davide JP, deSolms SJ, Giuliani EA, Gomez RP, Graham SL, Hamilton K, Handt LK, Hartman GD, Koblan KS, Kral AM, Miller PJ, Mosser SD, O'Neill TJ, Rands E, Schaber MD, Gibbs JB, Oliff A. Inhibition of farnesyltransferase induces regression of mammary and salivary carcinomas in *ras* transgenic mice. Nat Med 1995; 1:792–797.
33. Ohnishi Y, Nakamura H, Yoshimura M, Takuda Y, Iwasawa M, Ueyama Y, Tamaoki N, Shimamura K. Prolonged survival of mice with human gastric cancer treated with an anti-c-erbB-2 monoclonal antibody. Br J Cancer 1995; 71:969–973.
34. Rak J, Mitsuhashi Y, Erdos V, Huang S-N, Filmus J, Kerbel RS. Massive programmed cell death in intestinal epithelial cells induced by three-dimensional growth conditions: Suppression by expression of a mutant c-H-*ras* oncogene. J Cell Biol 1995; 131:1587–1598.
35. Lebowitz P, Sakamuro D, Prendergast GC. Farnesyl transferase inhibitors induce apoptosis of Ras-transformed cells denied substratum attachment. Cancer Res 1997; 57:708–713.
36. Barrington RE, Subler MA, Rands E, Omer CA, Miller PJ, Hundley JE, Koester SK, Troyer DA, Bearss DJ, Conner MW, Gibbs JB, Hamilton K, Koblan KS, Mosser SD, O'Neill TJ, Schaber MD, Senderak ET, Windle JJ, Oliff A, Kohl NE. A farnesyltransferase inhibitor induces tumor regression in transgenic mice harboring multiple oncogenic mutations by mediating alterations in both cell cycle control and apoptosis. Mol Cell Biol 1998; 18:85–92.
37. Rak J, Mitsuhashi Y, Bayko L, Filmus J, Sasazuki T, Kerbel RS. Mutant *ras* oncogenes upregulate VEGF/VPF expression: Implications for induction and inhibition of tumor angiogenesis. Cancer Res 1995; 55:4575–4580.
38. Folkman J. Clinical applications of research on angiogenesis. New Engl J Med 1995; 333:1757–1763.
39. O'Reilly MS, Holmgren L, Chen C, Folkman J. Angiostatin induces canal sustains dormancy of human tumors in mice. Nat Med 1996; 2:689–692.
40. Cheng SY, Huang HJ, Nagane M, Ji XD, Wang D, Shih CC, Arap W, Huang CM, Cavenee WK. Suppression of glioblastoma angiogenicity and tumorigenicity by inhibition of endogenous expression of vascular endothelial growth factor. Proc Natl Acad Sci U S A 1996; 93:8502–8507.
41. Benjamin LE, Keshet E. Conditional switching of vascular endothelial growth factor (VEGF) expression in tumors: Induction of endothelial cell shedding and regression of hemangioblastoma-like vessels by VEGF withdrawal. Proc Natl Acad Sci U S A 1997; 94:8761–8766.
42. Alon T, Hemo I, Itin A, Pe'er J, Stone J, Keshet E. Vascular endothelial growth factor acts as a survival factor for newly formed retinal vessels and has implications for retinopathy of prematurity. Nat Med 1995; 1:1024–1028.
43. Okada F, Rak J, St. Croix B, Lieubeau B, Kaya M, Roncari L, Sasazuki S, Kerbel RS. Impact of oncogenes on tumor angiogenesis: Mutant *K-ras* upregulation of VEGF/VPF is necessary but not sufficient for tumorigenicity of human colorectal carcinoma cells. Proc Natl Acad Sci U S A 1998; 95:3609–3614.

44. Grugel S, Finkenzeller G, Weindel K, Barleon B, Marmé D. Both v-Ha-ras and v-raf stimulate expression of the vascular endothelial growth factor in NIH 3T3 cells. J Biol Chem 1995; 270:25915–25919.
45. Saez E, Rutberg SE, Mueller E, Oppenheim H, Smoluk J, Yuspa SH, Spiegelman BM. c-*fos* is required for malignant progression for skin tumors. Cell 1995; 82:721–732.
46. Mazure NM, Chen EY, Yeh P, Laderoute KR, Giaccia AJ. Oncogenic transformation and hypoxia synergistically act to modulate vascular endothelial growth factor expression. Cancer Res 1996; 56:3436–3440.
47. Larcher F, Robles AI, Duran H, Murillas R, Quintanilla M, Cano A, Conti CJ, Jorcano JL. Up-regulation of vascular endothelial growth factor/vascular permeability factor in mouse skin carcinogenesis correlates with malignant progression state and activated H-ras expression levels. Cancer Res 1996; 56:5391–5396.
48. Volpert OV, Dameron KM, Bouck N. Sequential development of an angiogenic phenotype by human fibroblasts progressing to tumorigenicity. Oncogene 1997; 14: 1495–1502.
49. Mazure NM, Chen EY, Laderoute KR, Giaccia AJ. Induction of vascular endothelial growth factor by hypoxia is modulated by a phosphatidylinositol 3-kinase/Akt signaling pathway in Ha-ras-transformed cells through a hypoxia inducible factor-1 transcriptional element. Blood 1997; 90:3322–3331.
50. Lingen MW, DiPietro LA, Solt DB, Bouck NP, Polverini PJ. The angiogenic switch in hamster buccal pouch keratinocytes is dependent on TGFbeta-1 and is unaffected by ras activation. Carcinogenesis 1997; 18:329–338.
51. Arbiser JL, Moses MA, Fernandez CA, Ghiso N, Cao Y, Klauber N, Frank D, Brownlee M, Flynn E, Parangi S, Byers HR, Folkman J. Oncogenic H-ras stimulates tumor angiogenesis by two distinct pathways. Proc Natl Acad Sci U S A 1997; 94: 861–866.
52. Enholm B, Paavonen K, Ristimaki A, Kumar V, Gunji Y, Klefstrom J, Kivinen L, Laiho M, Olofsson B, Joukov V, Eriksson U, Alitalo K. Comparison of VEGF, VEGF-B, VEGF-C and Ang-1 mRNA regulation by serum, growth factors, oncoproteins and hypoxia. Oncogene 1997; 14:2475–2483.
53. White FC, Benehacene A, Scheele JS, Kamps M. VEGF mRNA is stabilized by ras and tyrosine kinase oncogenes, as well as by UV radiation—evidence for divergent stabilization pathways. Growth Factors 1997; 14:199–212.
54. Shirasawa S, Furuse M, Yokoyama N, Sasazuki T. Altered growth of human colon cancer cell lines disrupted at activated Ki-ras. Science 1993; 260:85–88.
55. Viloria-Petit AM, Rak J, Hung M-C, Rockwell P, Goldstein N, Kerbel RS. Neutralizing antibodies against EGF and ErbB-2/*neu* receptor tyrosine kinases down-regulate VEGF production by tumor cells *in vitro* and *in vivo* Angiogenic implications for signal transduction therapy of solid tumors. Am J Pathol 1997; 151:1523–1530.
56. Goldman CK, Kim J, Wong WL, King V, Brock T, Gillespie GY. Epidermal growth factor stimulates vascular endothelial growth factor production by human malignant glioma cells: A model of glioblastoma multiforme pathophysiology. Mol Biol Cell 1993; 4:121–133.
57. Goad DL, Rubin J, Wang H, Tashjian AH Jr, Patterson C. Enhanced expression of vascular endothelial growth factor in human SaOS-2 osteoblast-like cells and murine

osteoblasts induced by insulin-like growth factor I. Endocrinology 1996; 137:2262–2268.

58. Kevil CG, De Benedetti A, Payne DK, Coe LL, Laroux FS, Alexander JS. Translational regulation of vascular permeability factor by eukaryotic initiation factor 4E: Implications for tumor angiogenesis. Int J Cancer 1996; 65:785–790.
59. Zabrenetzky V, Harris CC, Steeg PS, Roberts DD. Expression of the extracellular matrix molecule thrombospondin inversely correlates with malignant progression in melanoma, lung and breast carcinoma cell lines. Int J Cancer 1994; 59:191–195.
60. Sheibani N, Frazier WA. Repression of thrombospondin-1 expression, a natural inhibitor of angiogenesis, in polyoma middle T transformed NIH3T3 cells. Cancer Lett 1996; 107:45–52.
61. Siemeister G, Weindel K, Mohrs K, Barleon B, Martiny-Baron G, Marme D. Reversion of deregulated expression of vascular endothelial growth factor in human renal carcinoma cells by von Hippel-Lindau tumor suppressor protein. Cancer Res 1996; 56:2299–2301.
62. Mukhopadhyay D, Knebelmann B, Cohen HT, Ananth S, Sukhatme VP. The von Hippel-Lindau tumor suppressor gene product interacts with Spl to repress vascular endothelial growth factor promoter activity. Mol Cell Biol 1997; 17:5629–5639.
63. Shweiki D, Itin A, Soffer D, Keshet E. Vascular endothelial growth factor induced by hypoxia may mediate hypoxia-initiated angiogenesis. Nature 1992; 359:843–845.
64. Shweiki D, Neeman M, Itin A, Keshet E. Induction of vascular endothelial growth factor expression by hypoxia and by glucose deficiency in multicell spheroids: Implications for tumor angiogenesis. Proc Natl Acad Sci U S A 1995; 92:768–772.
65. Ikeda E, Achen MG, Breier G, Risau W. Hypoxia-induced transcriptional activation and increased mRNA stability of vascular endothelial growth factor in C6 glioma cells. J Biol Chem 1995; 270:19761–19766.
66. Stein I, Neeman M, Shweiki D, Itin A, Keshet E. Stabilization of vascular endothelial growth factor mRNA by hypoxia and hypoglycemia and coregulation with other ischemia-induced genes. Mol Cell Biol 1995; 15:5363–5368.
67. D'Amore PA, Shima DT. Tumor angiogenesis: A physiological process or genetically determined? Cancer Metastasis Rev 1996; 15:205–212.
68. Rak J, et al. Oncogenes and angiogenesis: Signaling three dimensional tumor growth. J Invest Dermatology 2000. In Press.
69. Rak J, et al. Oncogenes and tumor angiogenesis: Differential modes of vascular endothelial growth factor upregulation in ras-transformed epithelial cells and fibroblasts. Cancer Res 2000; 60:490–498.
70. Lopez-Ocejo et al. Oncogenes and tumor angiogenesis: The HPV-16 E6 oncoprotein activates VEGF gene promoter in a p53-independent manner. Oncogene 2000; 19: 4611–4620.
71. Somenza GL. Hypoxia, clonal selection and the role of HIF-1 in tumor progression. Critical Rev Biochem Mol Biol 2000; 35:71–103.
72. St Croix B, et al. Genes expressed in human tumor endothelium. Science 2000; 289: 1197–1200.
73. Perrok F, et al. Anti-epidermal growth factor receptor antibody C225 inhibits angiogenesis in human transitional cell carcinoma growing orthotopically in nude mice. Clin Cancer Res 1999; 5:257–265.

18

Genetic Control of Angiogenesis by Tumor Suppressor Genes

Maartje Los and Emile E. Voest
University Medical Center Utrecht, Utrecht, The Netherlands

I. TUMOR SUPPRESSOR GENES

Tumorigenesis is a multistep process in which multiple genetic changes result in disturbance of the control of cell proliferation. Proliferation of normal cells is regulated by proto-oncogenes. Somatic mutations, in specific target tissues, can convert proto-oncogenes into active oncogenes. This event results in a potentiation of function, which leads to uncontrolled proliferation and, ultimately, to the development of a tumor. Tumor suppressor genes are a different class of genes involved in some forms of carcinogenesis. These genes are negative regulators of cell division. Loss of function of tumor suppressor genes by mutations or deletions results in deregulation of cell growth. This plays an important role in the development and progression of malignancies.

The role of tumor suppressor genes in cancer was first postulated by Knudson in 1971 in the so-called "two-hit theory" (1). He noticed that to inactivate tumor suppressor genes, both alleles had to be mutated. This hypothesis is applicable to hereditary and nonhereditary forms of cancer. This was noticed first in retinoblastoma. Both alleles of the retinoblastoma gene were inactivated. Other examples are Li-Fraumeni syndrome with mutations in the *p53* gene and von Hippel-Lindau (VHL) syndrome in which the VHL gene is mutated. Several tumor suppressor genes have been cloned so far and various putative tumor suppressor genes have been mapped (2).

It is well-known that the ability of a tumor to induce the proliferation of blood vessels has a profound effect on tumor growth and metastasis. That tumor growth is angiogenesis dependent was first proposed by Folkman in 1971 (3).

He showed that in tumor cells inoculated into isolated perfused organs, complete absence of angiogenesis was associated with restriction of tumor growth to a few millimeters in diameter.

Neovascularization of a tumor usually originates in a subset of cells, an angiogenic clone. The new vessels also contribute to the growth of the nonangiogenic tumor cells. The switch to the angiogenic phenotype is mediated by a balance between positive and negative regulators of angiogenesis. Different factors may determine whether tumor cells become angiogenic. These factors include environmental conditions (e.g., hypoxia) and genetic changes. The genetic control of angiogenesis may be mediated by oncogenes or tumor suppressor genes. In the previous chapter, the role of oncogenes was discussed. This chapter describes the role of the tumor suppressor genes VHL and *p53* in the regulation of angiogenesis. As far as we know, there are no studies that show a direct role for other tumor suppressor genes such as retinoblastoma susceptibility gene (Rb), Wilms' tumor gene (WT1), adenomatous polyposis coli gene (APC), deleted-in-colon-carcinoma gene (DCC), and neurofibromatosis type 1 gene (NF1) in the regulation of angiogenesis.

A. The von Hippel-Lindau Gene

von Hippel-Lindau disease is an autosomal dominant-inherited disorder, characterized by highly vascularized tumors: hemangioblastomas of the central nervous system and the retina, renal cell carcinomas, and pheochromocytomas (Fig. 1). Other manifestations of the disease are cysts in liver, pancreas, kidneys, and epididymis. Inactivation of the VHL gene also has been observed in sporadic renal cell cancer, sporadic hemangioblastoma, and colorectal cancer (4–6). The well-vascularized phenotype of tumors in VHL disease suggests that inactivation of the VHL tumor suppressor gene induces an angiogenic factor or down-regulates an angiogenic inhibitor.

The first evidence that an angiogenic factor is overexpressed in VHL-related tumors came from an immunohistochemical study of VHL disease-associated and sporadic hemangioblastomas. Vascular endothelial growth factor (VEGF) and its receptors: flt-1 and KDR were found to be up-regulated in these highly vascularized brain lesions (7). Furthermore, high expression levels of VEGF also could be demonstrated in VHL-related renal cell carcinoma (8).

That the regulation of VEGF indeed is mediated by the VHL gene was demonstrated by the following experiments. In vitro studies showed that 786-O human renal cell carcinoma cells, which lack the endogenous wild-type VHL gene, express high levels of VEGF mRNA and protein. Transfection of these cells with an expression vector containing the cDNA of the wild-type VHL gene resulted in a down-regulation of VEGF mRNA and protein (9–11). In KC-12 renal cell carcinoma cells, a cell line derived from a VHL patient, we also ob-

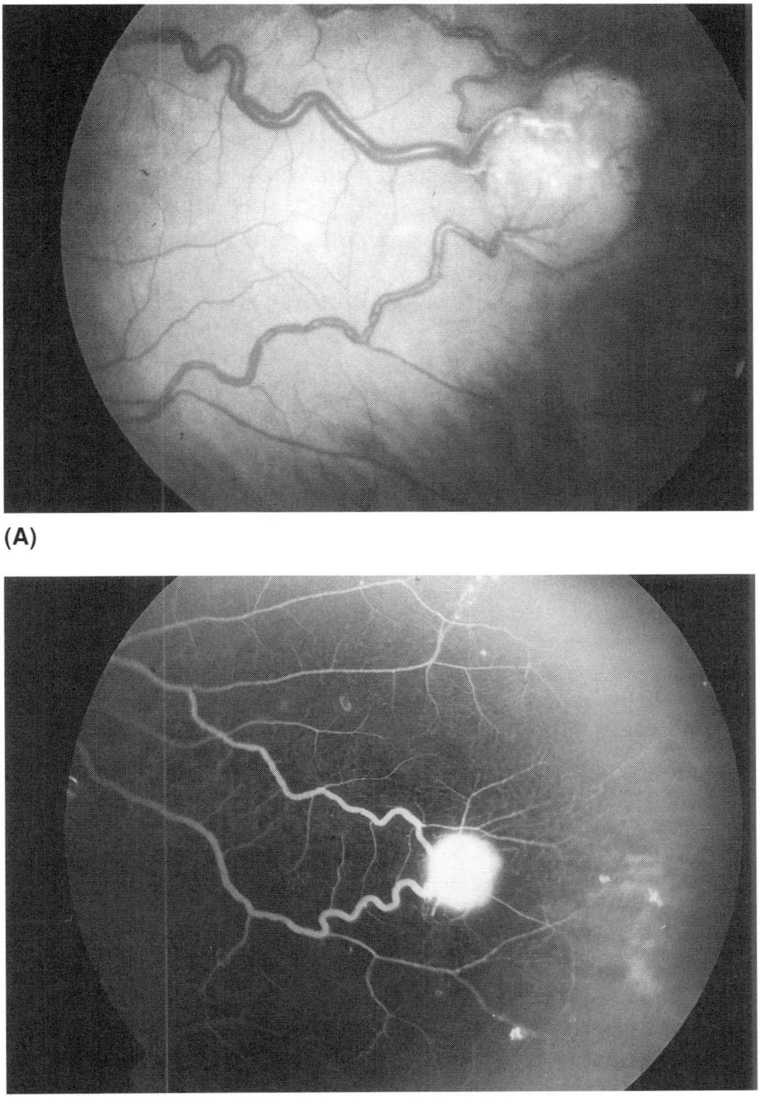

(A)

(B)

Figure 1 Angioma of the retina of a patient with von Hippel-Lindau disease, **A.** funduscopy. **B.** fluorescein angiogram.

served down-regulation of VEGF by introducing the wild-type VHL gene (Fig. 2) (data unpublished).

The mitogenic activity of conditioned media obtained from renal cell carcinoma cells with and without a functional VHL gene was tested on bovine capillary endothelial (BCE) cells. For in vitro proliferation, BCE cells depend on exogenous growth factors. Conditioned media of both cells, with and without functional VHL, could stimulate the proliferation of BCE cells. Neutralizing anti-VEGF monoclonal antibodies inhibited the mitogenic activity of conditioned media derived from cells without a functional VHL gene. The mitogenic activity of conditioned media from cells with wild-type VHL was not affected by anti-VEGF antibodies. Anti-basic fibroblast growth factor (bFGF) monoclonal antibodies had no effect on the mitogenic effects of either conditioned media. From these experiments, the investigators concluded that VEGF is a critical angiogenic factor in conditioned media of cells with a nonfunctional VHL gene (11).

In addition to VEGF, the VHL gene appears to play a crucial role in the regulation of other genes involved in angiogenesis. In vitro studies showed that the VHL gene product interacts with fibronectin (12). Fibronectin is an extracellular glycoprotein that binds members of the integrin family of cell-surface receptors. Mouse embryos lacking fibronectin develop severe defects in the vasculature (13). In VHL nullizygous mouse embryos, the assembly of the extracellular fibronectin matrix was grossly impaired compared to VHL +/+ and VHL +/− embryos.

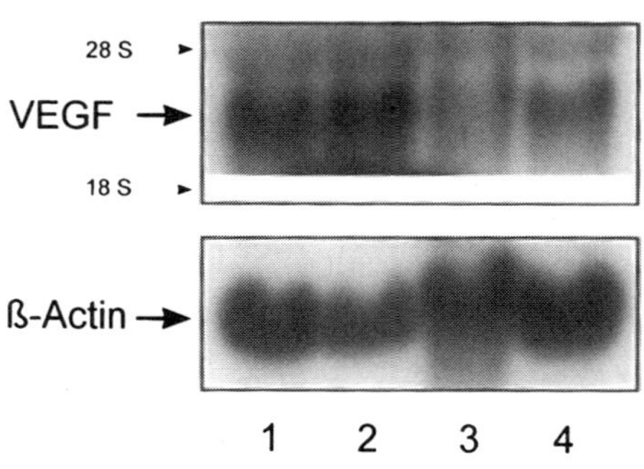

Figure 2 Northern blot analysis of vascular endothelial growth factor (VEGF) in von Hippel-Lindau (VHL) renal carcinoma cells. Total RNA (15 μg) from KC-12 cells lacking wild-type VHL (lane 1), KC-12 cells stably transfected with pCEP (Invitrogen) expression vector alone (lane 2), and KC-12 cells stably transfected with an expression vector encoding wild-type VHL: wild-type-10 (lane 3) and wild-type-6 (lane 4) were blotted and probed with ^{32}P-labeled cDNA fragments of VEGF and β-actin.

Recently, we showed that the expression of urokinase-type plasminogen activator (uPA) and plasminogen activator inhibitor 1 (PAI-1) is regulated by the VHL gene. In renal cell carcinoma cells lacking wild-type VHL, high levels of PAI-1 mRNA and protein were measured. Introduction of wild-type VHL resulted in a down-regulation of PAI-1. In contrast, uPA mRNA and protein levels were higher in cells with wild-type VHL compared to cells lacking a functional VHL gene (14).

More evidence that the VHL gene is involved in angiogenesis came from studies with the VHL knock-out mice. The VHL nullizygous embryos die between E10.5 and E12.5 because of the absence of normal embryonic vasculogenesis of the placenta. Subsequent hemorrhage in VHL −/− embryos caused necrosis and death (15).

In summary, several studies showed that the VHL tumor suppressor gene plays an important role in the regulation of different genes involved in angiogenesis. At present, it is unclear how the VHL gene product regulates these various genes and gene products. Different mechanisms of action have been proposed: interaction with transcription factors, regulation of mRNA stability, transcription elongation, and involvement in the degradation of proteins (16).

Several groups have shown that the VHL gene, in addition to VEGF, regulates other hypoxia-inducible mRNA such platelet-derived growth factor (PDGF)-B and glucose transporter 1 (GLUT-1) at the level of mRNA stability (10, 17). There is also evidence that VHL regulation of VEGF occurs at the level of transcription. It has been demonstrated that wild-type VHL can interact with the transcription factor Sp1, and that this interaction inhibits Sp1 activity. The VEGF promotor contains Sp1-binding sites and the VHL/Sp1 complex inhibits VEGF promotor activity (18, 19).

Three groups independently reported that the VHL gene is involved in transcription elongation. In vitro studies have shown that VHL can bind elongin B and C and that this complex is a negative regulator of the transcription elongation complex: elongin or SIII (20–22). Another protein binding to this complex is CUL2, a member of the cullin protein family. In yeast, cullins can target certain proteins for ubiquitination and degradation (23). There are no studies yet that show that genes involved in angiogenesis are regulated by VHL at levels of transcription elongation or protein degradation.

To investigate whether the in vitro data are supported by observations in patients with VHL disease, we tested body fluids of VHL patients for the presence of four different endothelial mitogens: VEGF, bFGF, interleukin-8 (IL-8), and endothelin-1 (ET-1). In 80% of the VHL patients, VEGF was detectable in aqueous fluid of the anterior chamber of their eyes. A strong positive correlation ($r = 0.90$) was found between age and ocular VEGF concentrations in aqueous humor of the eyes (Fig. 3). At comparable ages, VEGF levels in ocular fluid of

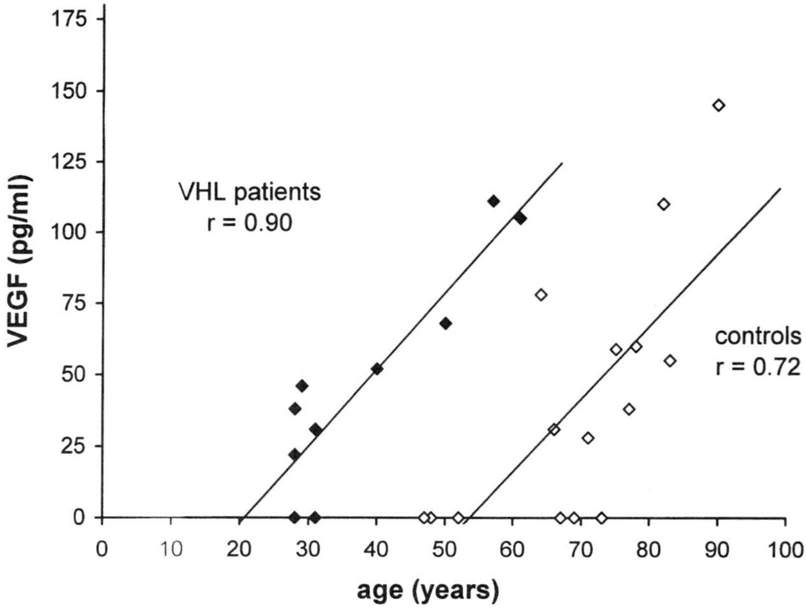

Figure 3 Correlation of VEGF concentrations, in aqueous humor of the anterior chamber of the eye, with age in patients with VHL disease and control individuals.

VHL patients were significantly higher than in unaffected individuals (8). A possible role for VEGF in the development of retinal angioma is supported by the observation that VEGF concentrations are elevated in the vitreous and anterior chamber fluid of patients with active retinal and anterior-segment neovascularization associated with several ocular diseases (24, 25).

Vascular endothelial growth factor, also known as vascular permeability factor (VPF), was originally recognized for its ability to increase permeability of the microvasculature for circulating plasma proteins. High concentrations of VEGF were found in guinea pig and in human tumor ascites fluids (26). Tumor ascites fluid accumulation might result from increased permeability of the blood vessels lining the peritoneal cavity as a result of VEGF production by tumor cells (27). High concentrations of VEGF were measured in glioblastoma cyst fluid, which suggests that increased vascular permeability leads to cyst formation (28). A frequent manifestation of VHL disease is the development of cysts in various organs. We measured a tenfold to sixteenfold increase in VEGF concentration in two independent renal cysts as compared with VEGF levels in peripheral blood samples (8). This suggests that VEGF plays a role in cyst formation.

The mean concentration of VEGF in the serum of VHL patients was higher than in matched controls but it did not reach significance. In contrast, lower levels of VEGF were found in the urine of VHL patients than in matched controls (8). The recent observation by Möhle et al. that thrombin-activated platelets release VEGF makes VEGF measurement in serum less reliable (29). In our study, no correlation was found in individual VEGF levels in body fluids and manifestations of the disease. This finding suggests that in addition to VEGF, other factors may be involved in the development of VHL-related tumors. However, no differences were observed between concentrations of bFGF, IL-8, and ET-1 in serum and urine in VHL patients and the matched control group (8). These in vivo findings support the in vitro observations that VEGF is regulated by the VHL gene and contributes to the well-vascularized phenotype of VHL tumors.

B. The *p53* Gene

p53 is a nuclear protein present in small amounts in normal cells. In general, *p53* serves as a molecular stress-responsive device. In response to DNA damage, *p53* levels increase rapidly. Accumulation of *p53* causes an arrest of the cell cycle in the G1 phase, rather than allowing it to go into S phase and replicate the damaged DNA. In this way *p53* allows cells extra time for repair mechanisms to act (30). If the repair fails, *p53* may trigger cell suicide by apoptosis. This was demonstrated by Clarke et al., who showed that *p53* was required for the induction of apoptosis in thymocytes exposed to ionizing radiation (31).

p53 contains an acidic domain near its N-terminus that is similar to those noted in well-characterized transcription factors. Therefore, it is thought that *p53* acts as a transcriptional regulator, enhancing the expression of genes with a specific *p53*-binding site and interacting with a variety of transcription factors to inhibit the expression of other genes (32).

Mutations of the *p53* tumor suppressor gene are the most frequently observed genetic changes in human cancers. The *p53* gene has been implicated in inherited and sporadic forms of cancer (33). Germline mutations in the *p53* gene are responsible for the Li-Fraumeni cancer syndrome. This is a rare autosomal dominant syndrome characterized by an elevated risk of early-onset breast cancer, childhood sarcomas, and other neoplasms. Fifty percent of the carriers of a mutated *p53* gene in families affected by the Li-Fraumeni syndrome will have a diagnosis of cancer by the age of 30 and 90% by the age of 65 (34).

The typical *p53* mutations are missense mutations, usually altering protein conformation. Mutant *p53* proteins have a much longer half-life than the wild-type proteins, resulting in accumulation of mutant proteins in tumors (35). Because *p53* mutations in malignant tumors are common, it was proposed by several groups that *p53* plays a role in the switch of tumor cells to the angiogenic phenotype.

C. *p53* and Thrombospondin-1

Thrombospondin-1 (TSP-1) is a potent inhibitor of neovascularization and appears to be partially under control of *p53*. The effect of *p53* on the expression of TSP-1 was studied in cultured fibroblasts from Li-Fraumeni patients (36). These cells have one wild-type and one mutant allele of the *p53* gene. At early passage, when the fibroblasts still have one mutant and one wild-type allele, the secretion of TSP-1 in media was high. On continued passage in culture, the fibroblasts lost their wild-type allele, which resulted in a significant decrease of secretion of TSP-1. Reintroduction of the wild-type *p53* gene into late-passage Li-Fraumeni fibroblasts restored both TSP-1 mRNA levels and the antiangiogenic phenotype.

p53 is frequently mutated in human breast carcinomas (37). In BT549 cells, a human breast carcinoma cell line, *p53* is mutated and these cells do not produce TSP-1 protein. Introduction of wild-type *p53* in BT549 cells resulted in secretion of TSP-1 (38). Furthermore, the investigators showed that conditioned medium of parental BT549 cells induced neovascularization in the rat cornea model and stimulated migration of capillary endothelial cells in a Boyden chamber assay. Interestingly, conditioned medium of BT549 cells expressing wild-type *p53* was not angiogenic in both assays (38).

In bladder carcinoma, TSP-1 expression was significantly associated with the *p53* expression status. An analysis of 163 transitional cell carcinomas of the bladder revealed that tumors with wild-type *p53* express high levels of TSP-1. Tumors with *p53* alterations were significantly more likely to express low levels of TSP (39). In this group of patients, TSP-1 expression was associated with disease recurrence and overall survival. Patients with low TSP-1 expression exhibited increased recurrence rates and decreased overall survival.

D. *p53* and VEGF

Inactivation of *p53* is a critical event in the conversion of an astrocytoma to a glioblastoma (40). Glioblastomas tend to be well vascularized and express high levels of the angiogenic factors bFGF and VEGF. Mukhopadhyay et al. described a regulatory role for *p53* in suppressing basal VEGF transcription (41). The investigators transfected wild-type *p53* and mutant *p53* into 293 cells (an adenovirus-transformed human fetal kidney cell line) and showed that wild-type *p53*, but not mutant *p53*, had a pronounced suppressive effect on VEGF gene expression. By use of a VEGF promoter-luciferase construct, the effect of wild-type and mutant *p53* on the VEGF promoter was analyzed. In 293 cells and U87 cells (human glioblastoma-astrocytoma cells), the VEGF promoter activity was significantly reduced in the presence of wild-type *p53*. Mutant *p53* did not affect promoter activity. It is known that *p53* specifically represses the activity of TATA promoters that do not contain a wild-type *p53* DNA-binding sequence (42). The VEGF promoter does not have a TATA box or a *p53*-binding sequence. The repression observed might therefore be mediated by other factors that activated by *p53*.

Kieser et al. tried to identify a mediator of the *p53* effects on VEGF. It has been recognized that expression of VEGF can be induced by tumor phorbol esters, such as 12-O-tetradecanoylphorbol-13-acetate (TPA), which activates protein kinase C (PKC) (43). This was tested in an NIH 3T3 cell line, which stably overexpresses the temperature-sensitive *p53*, displaying mutant phenotype at 37° C and wild-type phenotype at 32.5° C. The presence of mutant *p53* at 37° C in these cells augmented VEGF mRNA induction by TPA significantly compared to the presence of wild-type *p53* at 32.5° C. Mutant *p53* specifically increases TPA induction of VEGF without affecting the expression of other TPA-inducible genes. These data demonstrate that PKC is involved in the VEGF regulation by *p53* (44).

In human non–small-cell lung cancer (NSCLC) it has been observed, by immunohistochemistry, that expression of mutant *p53* is associated with high levels of VEGF protein (45–47). In NSCLC, a significant association also was found between expression of mutant *p53*, VEGF levels, and microvessel count (45).

The same observations were done in human colorectal cancers. Also in these tumors, accumulation of mutant *p53* is closely associated with higher VEGF expression levels and increased vessel count (48). Another study of 163 patients with colorectal tumors showed that patients with tumors that were positive for both mutant *p53* and VEGF had a significantly poorer prognosis as a result of the development of metastases, compared to patients with tumors negative for *p53* and VEGF (49, 50). In human colon cancer cell lines with the *p53* mutations KM12L.4 and SW620, transduction with an adenoviral vector containing the wild-type *p53* gene resulted in a decrease of VEGF mRNA and protein expression compared to controls. In these cell lines, no thrombospodin mRNA was detected, either before or after treatment with the adenoviral vector containing wild-type *p53* (51).

E. *p53* and Miscellaneous Factors Involved in Angiogenesis

The role of *p53* in the regulation of bFGF is less well characterized. One study showed an effect of *p53* on the regulation of the promotor of bFGF. The authors hypothesized that loss of normal function of *p53* activates the bFGF transcription, which results in tumor progression and stimulation of angiogenesis (52).

Matrix metalloproteinases (MMP) are a family of genes involved in the breakdown of the extracellular matrix components. This breakdown is important for physiological and pathological processes such as trophoblast implantation, wound healing, angiogenesis, and tumor cell invasion. The promotor of the human type IV collagenase, or MMP2, contains a *p53*-binding site. The observation that wild-type *p53*, but not *p53* mutants, induces MMP2 expression suggests a role for *p53* in the regulation of the breakdown of the extracellular matrix (53).

II. CONCLUSION

The switch of tumor cells to the angiogenic phenotype is regulated by both the microenvironment and changes in the genetic background of tumor cells. This chapter has provided strong support for a role of two tumor suppressor genes, *p53* and VHL, in the regulation of angiogenesis. It is expected that in the near future, the number of genes involved in the direct or indirect regulation of angiogenesis will increase. Insight into the specific mechanisms of genetic control of angiogenesis may lead to new treatment strategies to control neovascularization.

REFERENCES

1. Knudson AG. Mutation and cancer: Statistical study of retinoblastoma. Proc Natl Acad Sci U S A 1971; 68:820–823.
2. Knudson AG. Antioncogenes and human cancer. Proc Natl Acad Sci U S A 1993; 90:10914–10921.
3. Folkman J. Tumor angiogenesis: Therapeutic implications. N Engl J Med 1971; 285: 404.
4. Knudson AG. VHL gene mutations and clear cell renal carcinomas. Sci Am 1995; 1:180–181.
5. Kanno H, Kondo K, Ito S, Yamamoto I, Fujii S, Torigoe S, Sakai N, Hosaka M, Shuin T, Yao M. Somatic mutations of the von Hippel-Lindau tumor suppressor gene in sporadic central nervous system hemangioblastomas. Cancer Res 1994; 54: 4845–4847.
6. Zhuang Z, Emmert-Buck MR, Roth MJ, Gnarra J, Linehan WM, Liotta LA, Lubensky IA. Von Hippel-Lindau disease gene deletion detected in microdissected sporadic human colon carcinoma specimens. Hum Pathol 1996; 27:152–156.
7. Wizigmann-Voos S, Breier G, Risau W, Plate KH. Up-regulation of vascular endothelial growth factor and its receptors in von Hippel-Lindau disease-associated and sporadic hemangioblastomas. Cancer Res 1995; 55:1358–1364.
8. Los M, Aarsman CJ, Terpstra L, Wittebol-Post D, Lips CJM, Blijham GH, Voest EE. Elevated ocular levels of vascular endothelial growth factor in patients with von Hippel-Lindau disease. Ann Oncol 1997; 8:1015–1022.
9. Siemeister G, Weindel K, Mohrs K, Barleon B, Martiny Baron G, Marmé D. Reversion of deregulated expression of vascular endothelial growth factor in human renal

carcinoma cells by von Hippel-Lindau tumor suppressor protein. Cancer Res 1996; 56:2299–2301.

10. Iliopoulos O, Levy AP, Jiang C, Kaelin WGJ, Goldberg MA. Negative regulation of hypoxia-inducible genes by the von Hippel-Lindau protein. Proc Natl Acad Sci U S A 1996; 93:10595–10599.
11. Gnarra JR, Zhou S, Merrill MJ, Wagner JR, Krumm A, Papavassiliou E, Oldfield EH, Klausner RD, Linehan WM. Post-transcriptional regulation of vascular endothelial growth factor mRNA by the product of the VHL tumor suppressor gene. Proc Natl Acad Sci U S A 1996; 93:10589–10594.
12. Ohh M, Yauch RL, Lonergan KM, Whaley JM, Stemmer-Rachamimov AO, Louis DN, Gavin BJ, Kley N, Kaelin WGJ, Iliopoulos O. The von Hippel-Lindau tumor suppressor protein is required for proper assembly of an extracellular fibronectin matrix. Mol Cell 1998; 1:959–968.
13. George EL, Georges-Labouesse EN, Patel-King RS, Rayburn H, Hynes RO. Defects in mesoderm, neural tube and vascular development in mouse embryos lacking fibronectin. Development 1993; 119:1079–1091.
14. Los M, Zeamari S, Foekens JA, Gebbink MFBG, Voest EE. Regulation of the urokinase-type plasminogen activator system by the von Hippel Lindau tumor suppressor gene. Cancer Res 1999; 59:4440–4445.
15. Gnarra JR, Ward JM, Porter FD, Wagner JR, Devor DE, Grinberg A, Emmert-Buck MR, Westphal H, Klausner RD, Linehan WM. Defective placental vasculogenesis causes embryonic lethality in VHL-deficient mice. Proc Natl Acad Sci U S A 1997; 94:9102–9107.
16. Maher ER, Kaelin WG. von Hippel-Lindau disease. Medicine 1997; 76:381–391.
17. Levy AP, Levy NS, Goldberg MA. Hypoxia-inducible protein binding to vascular endothelial growth factor mRNA and its modulation by the von Hippel-Lindau protein. J Biol Chem. 1996; 271:25492–25497.
18. Pal S, Claffey KP, Cohen HT, Mukhopadhyay D. Activation of Sp1-mediated vascular permeability factor/vascular endothelial growth factor transcription requires specific interaction with protein kinase C zeta. J Biol Chem 1998; 273:26277–26280.
19. Mukhopadhyay D, Knebelmann B, Cohen HT, Ananth S, Sukhatme VP. The von Hippel-Lindau tumor suppressor gene product interacts with Sp1 to repress vascular endothelial growth factor promoter activity. Mol Cell Biol 1997; 17:5629–5639.
20. Aso T, Lane WS, Conaway JW, Conaway RC. Elongin (SIII): A multisubunit regulator of elongation by RNA polymerase II. Science 1995; 269:1439–1443.
21. Kibel A, Iliopoulos O, Decaprio JA, Kaelin WG. Binding of the von Hippel-Lindau tumor suppressor protein to Elongin B and C. Science 1995; 269:1444–1446.
22. Duan DR, Pause A, Burgess WH, Aso T, Chen DY, Garrett KP, Conaway RC, Conaway JW, Linehan WM, Klausner RD. Inhibition of transcription elongation by the VHL tumor suppressor protein. Science 1995; 269:1402–1406.
23. Pause A, Lee S, Worrell RA, Chen DY, Burgess WH, Linehan WM, Klausner RD. The von Hippel-Lindau tumor-suppressor gene product forms a stable complex with human CUL-2, a member of the Cdc53 family of proteins. Proc Natl Acad Sci U S A 1997; 94:2156–2161.
24. Aiello LP, Avery RL, Arrigg PG, Keyt BA, Jampel HD, Shah ST, Pasquale LR, Thieme H, Iwanoto MA, Park JE, Nguyen HV, Aiello LM, Ferrara N, King GL.

Vascular endothelial growth factor in ocular fluid of patients with diabetic retinopathy and other retinal disorders. N Engl J Med 1994; 331:1480–1487.
25. Adamis PA, Miller JW, Bernal M-T, D'Amico DJ, Folkman J, Yeo T-K, Yeo K-T. Increased vascular endothelial growth factor levels in the vitreous of eyes with proliferative diabetic retinopathy. Amer J Opthalmol 1994; 118:445–450.
26. Yeo K-T, Wang HH, Nagy JA, Sioussat TM, Ledbetter SR, Hoogewerf AJ, Zhou Y, Masse EM, Senger DR, Dvorak HF, Yeo T-K. Vascular permeability factor (vascular endothelial growth factor) in guinea pig and human tumor and inflammatory effusions. Cancer Res 1993; 53:2912–2918.
27. Nagy JA, Masse EM, Herzberg KT, Meyers MS, Yeo K-T, Yeo T-K, Sioussat TM, Dvorak HF. Pathogenesis of ascites tumor growth: Vascular permeability factor, vascular hyperpermeability, and ascites fluid accumulation. Cancer Res 1995; 55: 360–368.
28. Takano S, Yoskii Y, Kondo S, Suzuki H, Maruno T, Shirai S, Nose T. Concentration of vascular endothelial growth factor in serum and tumor tissue of brain tumor patients. Cancer Res 1996; 56:2185–2190.
29. Möhle R, Green D, Moore MAS, Nachman RL, Rafii S. Constitutive production and thrombin-induced release of vascular endothelial growth factor by human megakaryocytes and platelets. Proc Natl Acad Sci U S A 1997; 94:663–668.
30. Lane DP. p53, Guardian of the genome. Nature 1992; 358:15–16.
31. Clarke AR, Purdie CA, Harrison DJ, Morris RG, Bird CC, Hooper ML, Wyllie AH. Thymocyte apoptosis induced by p53-dependent and independent pathways. Nature 1993; 362:849–852.
32. Vogelstein B, Kinzler KW. p53 Function and dysfunction. Cell 1992; 70:523–526.
33. Harris CC, Hollstein M. Clinical implications of the p53 tumor-suppressor gene. N Engl J Med 1993; 329:1318–1327.
34. Srivastava S, Zou ZQ, Pirollo K, Blattner W, Chang EH. Germ-line transmission of a mutated p53 gene in a cancer-prone family with Li-Fraumeni syndrome. Nature 1990; 348:747–749.
35. Levine AJ, Momand J, Finlay CA. The p53 tumour suppressor gene. Nature 1991; 351:453–456.
36. Dameron KM, Volpert OV, Tainsky MA, Bouck N. Control of angiogenesis in fibroblasts by p53 regulation of thrombospondin-1. Science 1994; 265:1582–1584.
37. Cox LA, Chen G, Lee EY. Tumor suppressor genes and their roles in breast cancer. Breast Cancer Res Treat 1994; 32:19–38.
38. Volpert OV, Stellmach V, Bouck N. The modulation of thrombospondin and other naturally occurring inhibitors of angiogenesis during tumor progression. Breast Cancer Res Treat 1995; 36:119–126.
39. Grossfeld GD, Ginsberg DA, Stein JP, Bochner BH, Esrig D, Groshen S, Dunn M, Nichols PW, Taylor CR, Skinner DG, Cote RJ. Thrombospondin-1 expression in bladder cancer: Association with p53 alterations, tumor angiogenesis, and tumor progression. J Natl Cancer Inst 1997; 89:219–227.
40. Sidransky D, Mikkelsen T, Schwechheimer K, Rosenblum ML, Cavanee W, Vogelstein B. Clonal expansion of p53 mutant cells is associated with brain tumor progression. Nature 1992; 355:846–847.
41. Mukhopadhyay D, Tsiokas L, Sukhatme VP. Wild-type p53 and v-src exert opposing

influences on human vascular endothelial growth factor gene expression. Cancer Res 1995; 55:6161–6165.

42. Mack DH, Vartikar J, Pipas JM, Laimins LA. Specific repression of TATA-mediated but not initiator-mediated transcription by wild-type p53. Nature 1993; 363:281–283.
43. Finkenzeller G, Marmé D, Weich HA, Hug H. Platelet-derived growth factor-induced transcription of the vascular endothelial growth factor gene is mediated by protein kinase C. Cancer Res 1992; 52:4821–4823.
44. Kieser A, Weich HA, Brandner G, Marmé D, Kolch W. Mutant p53 potentiates protein kinase C induction of vascular endothelial growth factor expression. Oncogene 1994; 9:963–969.
45. Fontanini G, Vignati S, Lucchi M, Mussi A, Calcinai A, Boldrini L, Chine S, Silvestri V, Angeletti CA, Basolo F, Bevilacqua G. Neoangiogenesis and p53 protein in lung cancer: Their prognostic role and their relation with vascular endothelial growth factor (VEGF) expression. Br J Cancer 1997; 75:1295–1301.
46. Fontanini G, Boldrini L, Calcinai A, Chine S, Lucchi M, Mussi A, Angeletti CA, Basolo F, Bevilacqua G. Thrombospondins I and II messenger RNA expression in lung carcinoma: Relationship with p53 alternations, angiogenic growth factors, and vascular density. Clin Cancer Res 1999; 5:155–161.
47. Giatromanolaki A, Koukourakis MI, Kakolyris S, Turley H, O'Byrne K, Scott PA, Pezzella F, Georgoulias V, Harris AL, Gatter KC. Vascular endothelial growth factor, wild-type p53, and angiogenesis in early operable non-small cell lung cancer. Clin Cancer Res 1998; 4:3017–3024.
48. Takahashi Y, Bucana CD, Cleary KR, Ellis LM. p53, Vessel count, and vascular endothelial growth factor expression in human colon cancer. Int J Cancer 1998; 79: 34–38.
49. Maeda K, Kang SM, Ogawa M, Onoda N, Sawada T, Nakata B, Kato Y, Chung YS, Sowa M. Combined analysis of vascular endothelial growth factor and platelet-derived endothelial cell growth factor expression in gastric carcinoma. Int J Cancer 1997; 74:545–550.
50. Kang SM, Maeda K, Onoda N, Chung YS, Nakata B, Nishiguchi Y, Sowa M. Combined analysis of p53 and vascular endothelial growth factor expression in colorectal carcinoma for determination of tumor vascularity and liver metastasis. Int J Cancer 1997; 74:502–507.
51. Bouvet M, Ellis LM, Nishizaki M, Fujiwara T, Liu W, Bucana CD, Fang B, Lee JJ, Roth JA. Adenovirus-mediated wild-type p53 gene transfer down-regulates vascular endothelial growth factor expression and inhibits angiogenesis in human colon cancer. Cancer Res 1998; 58:2288–2292.
52. Ueba T, Nosaka T, Takahashi JA, Shibata F, Florkiewicz RZ, Vogelstein B, Oda Y, Kikuchi H, Hatanaka M. Transcriptional regulation of basic fibroblast growth factor gene by p53 in human glioblastoma and hepatocellular carcinoma cells. Proc Natl Acad Sci U S A 1994; 91:9009–9013.
53. Bian J, Sun Y. Transcriptional activation by p53 of the human type IV collagenase (gelatinase A or matrix metalloproteinase 2) promoter. Mol Cell Biol 1997; 17: 6330–6338.

19

Regulation of Neoplastic Angiogenesis by the Organ Microenvironment

Rakesh Kumar and Isaiah J. Fidler
The University of Texas M. D. Anderson Cancer Center, Houston, Texas

I. INTRODUCTION

Most deaths from cancer result from metastases that are resistant to conventional therapies (1, 2). The design of better therapies depends on a thorough understanding of the metastatic process. The pathogenesis of cancer metastasis consists of a series of sequential, interrelated steps that include growth, invasion, circulation, survival, arrest in distant organs, extravasation, and proliferation (3). Each step in the pathogenesis of metastasis is rate limiting, and failure to complete any one prevents the malignant cells from producing a metastasis (2, 4, 5). One crucial step in the progressive growth of primary neoplasms and metastasis is vascularization of the tumor and its surroundings (6). Without angiogenesis, most tumors would not expand beyond 1 to 2 mm^3 (6, 7). The induction of angiogenesis is mediated by the positive and negative regulatory molecules released by both tumor and host cells (6–9). The extent of angiogenesis is determined by the balance of these mediators, which in the case of expanding neoplasms favors the positive mediators and the influence of the organ microenvironment (4, 5). In this regard, successful neoplastic metastatic cells subvert homeostatic mechanisms to their own gain (2). The host contributes to the angiogenesis of tumors, and hence their growth, by a mechanism that essentially subverts the normal process of wound healing. In other words, the body may treat cancers as wounds, albeit as

Dvorak (10) wrote, ''wounds that do not heal.'' This article will describe recent data regarding the regulation of the angiogenic phenotype and how the organ microenvironment modulates the extent of neoplastic angiogenesis.

II. THE PATHOGENESIS OF METASTASIS

During the last two decades, studies of the pathogenesis of cancer metastasis have established that the outcome of metastasis depends on the interactions of tumor cells with various host factors and that the pattern of metastasis is predictable, not random (11, 12). The metastatic patterns are determined by factors that are independent of vascular anatomy, rate of blood flow, and the number of tumor cells delivered to each organ (2). The search for factors that regulate the outcome of metastasis began in 1889, when Paget asked, ''What is it that decides what organs shall suffer in a case of disseminated cancer?'' (13). He analyzed postmortem data from a large number of women who died of breast or other cancers and noticed the high frequency of breast cancer metastasis to the ovaries and the different incidences of skeletal metastases produced by different primary tumors. Paget concluded that the organ distribution of secondary growths is not a matter of chance. The formation of metastases depends on both the ''seed'' (certain tumor cells with metastatic ability) and the ''soil'' (colonized organs providing growth advantage to the seeds); hence, a particular tumor cell (seed) would interact with the compatible organ environment (soil) (13). In recent years, Paget's hypothesis has received considerable experimental and clinical support (2, 4, 5, 14, 15). Site-specific metastasis occurs with many transplantable, experimental tumors and has been reported in autochthonous human tumors in patients with peritoneovenous shunts (16, 17).

A current definition of the ''seed and soil'' hypothesis consists of three principles: (a) neoplasms are biologically heterogeneous and contain subpopulations of cells with different angiogenic, invasive, and metastatic properties (2, 18); (b) metastasis represents a highly selective, nonrandom process favoring the survival and growth of a small subpopulation of cells that pre-exist in the parent neoplasm (11). The cells must succeed in invasion and embolization, survive in the circulation, arrest in a distant capillary bed, and extravasate into and multiply within the organ parenchyma (19). Thus, metastases can have a clonal origin, and different metastases can originate from the proliferation of different single cells (20, 21); (c) the outcome of metastasis depends on multiple interactions of metastatic cells (seed) with homeostatic mechanisms (soil). The contribution of host factors may vary in tumors arising from different tissues and in tumors of similar histologic origin in different patients.

III. TUMOR ANGIOGENESIS

It is now well established that angiogenesis is essential to the growth of both primary and metastatic tumors in that growth beyond 1 to 2 mm in diameter requires that a tumor develop an adequate blood supply (6–8). With few exceptions, benign tumors are sparsely vascularized and tend to grow slowly, whereas malignant neoplasms are highly vascular and fast growing (6–9, 22). The increase in vasculature also increases the probability that motile-invasive tumor cells will enter the circulation to disseminate to distant organs where they may give rise to a metastasis (23). The extent of vascularization in different malignancies correlates directly with their metastatic potential and hence inversely with the survival of the patient (24–26).

The process of angiogenesis consists of multiple, complex, interacting, and interdependent steps. It begins with local degradation of the basement membrane surrounding capillaries, followed by invasion of the surrounding stroma by the underlying endothelial cells in the direction of the angiogenic stimulus. Endothelial cell migration is accompanied by the proliferation of endothelial cells at the leading edge of the migrating column. Even as they move, the endothelial cells begin to organize into three-dimensional structures to form new capillary tubes (9, 27, 28) and R Kumar et al., unpublished data). Although most solid tumors are highly vascular, their vessels are not identical to the vessels of normal tissue. There are differences in cellular composition, vascular permeability, blood vessel stability, and growth regulation (28, 29).

IV. REGULATION OF ANGIOGENIC AND ANTIANGIOGENIC FACTORS

The onset of angiogenesis involves a change in the local equilibrium between positive and negative regulators (30). During the past decade, an increasing number of angiogenic molecules have been reported, including fibroblast growth factor (FGF) family members, vascular endothelial cell growth factor or vascular permeability factor (VEGF/VPF), interleukin-8 (IL-8), angiogenin, platelet-derived endothelial cell growth factor (PD-ECGF), platelet-derived growth factor (PDGF), hepatocyte growth factor (HGF), transforming growth factor-alpha and -beta (TGF-α and -β), and tumor necrosis factor-alpha (TNF-α) (7, 28, 31). Many different cytokines and growth factors that stimulate (e.g., basic FGF and VEGF) or inhibit (e.g., interferon-beta [IFN-β], thrombospondin, and tissue inhibitors of metalloproteinases) angiogenesis are present in different tissues (7, 32).

In many normal tissues, factors that inhibit angiogenesis predominate (7, 8). In rapidly dividing tissues, the balance of angiogenic molecules favors stimulation of the process. For example, in cultured fibroblasts, the loss of wild-type allele of the TP53 tumor suppressor gene coincides with the acquisition of the angiogenic phenotype and is the result of reduced production of thrombospondin-1 (TSP-1) (33). Moreover, experiments with different transgenic mouse models have shown that angiogenesis is activated through different pathways during the preneoplastic stages that precede the appearance of solid tumors, and that the mechanisms regulating the angiogenic switch may be tissue specific (34).

Our laboratory has investigated the role of cell density in the regulation of basic fibroblast growth factor (bFGF) expression in human renal cell carcinoma (HRCC) cells (35). Tumor cells expressed low levels of bFGF (both at mRNA and protein levels) under dense culture conditions compared with sparse cultures. Similar data were obtained in endothelial cells. In contrast to the inverse correlation of cell density and bFGF expression, expression of VEGF was directly correlated with cell density in human colon carcinoma cell lines (36).

Recent clinical observations noting an antiangiogenic effect of IFNs in tumors that express high levels of bFGF led us to investigate whether IFNs could modulate the expression of bFGF (7, 8, 37, 38). Interferon-α and IFN-β, but not IFN-γ, down-regulated the expression of bFGF mRNA and protein in HRCC (39). This effect was independent of the antiproliferative effect of IFNs. The down-regulation of bFGF required long exposure of the cells to a low concentration of IFNs. Moreover, once IFN was withdrawn, cells resumed production of bFGF. These observations are consistent with clinical experience indicating that IFN-α must be given for many months to induce a response (38). Incubation of human bladder, prostate, colon, and breast carcinoma cells with noncytostatic concentrations of IFN-α and IFN-β also inhibited bFGF production (39).

Constitutive expression of IL-8 directly correlates with the metastatic potential of human melanoma cells (40). Moreover, IL-8 has been shown to be angiogenic in vivo (41). Several organ-derived cytokines (produced by inflammatory cells) can up-regulate expression of IL-8 in normal and tumorigenic cells, indicating that specific organ microenvironments can influence the expression of IL-8 in melanoma cells (42). Further, IFN-α and IFN-β can down-regulate the expression of IL-8 induced by inflammatory cytokines such as IL-1β or TNF-α in melanoma cells (43).

Mechanisms regulating the angiogenic factor VEGF also have been investigated. Expression of VEGF is increased in necrotic areas of human tumors as shown by in situ hybridization (44, 45). In vitro studies have confirmed that VEGF is increased in response to hypoxia, probably because of increased transcription and mRNA stability (46–48). Numerous cytokines and growth factors that increase VEGF expression include IL-1, IL-6, IL-8, TGF-β, PDGF, HGF, and bFGF (49–53). Vascular endothelial growth factor expression is also regulated by certain oncogenes (*src* and *ras*) (54–56) and tumor suppressor genes like p53 (57).

V. HOST MICROENVIRONMENT-DEPENDENT EXPRESSION OF ANGIOGENESIS

Previous studies from our laboratory suggested that HRCC implanted into the different organ sites of nude mice have different metastatic phenotypes (58). We showed that expression of certain angiogenic factors depends on the implantation site of tumor cells (59). Human renal cell carcinoma grown in the kidney expressed tenfold to twentyfold the mRNA levels of subcutaneous HRCC, and the kidney tumors were more vascularized than tumors implanted in the subcutis. In sharp contrast, the expression of IFN-β was high in and around the subcutaneous tumors, whereas no IFN-β was found in the HRCC tumors growing in the kidney. The variation in bFGF level by the site of implantation was caused by adaptation to the organ microenvironment, inasmuch as cells that were taken from the implanted tumor and re-established in culture returned to the levels found in vitro after 4 weeks in culture (59).

The organ-specific expression of IL-8 was examined in two human melanoma cell lines (42). The A375P (parental) and A375SM (metastatic clone) lines were implanted into the subcutis, spleen (producing liver metastasis), and tail vein (producing lung metastasis). By Northern blot and immunohistochemical analyses, subcutaneous tumors expressed the greatest amounts of IL-8, followed by lung lesions, and lastly liver lesions. This differential expression was not the result of the selection of a subpopulation of cells. The cross-over experiment suggested that the IL-8 mRNA level was always high in skin and low in liver tumors, regardless of whether the melanoma cell had first been harvested from subcutaneous or liver tumors (42). Cells cocultured with keratinocytes or well-differentiated human hepatoma cells produced similar relative amounts of IL-8 as found in in vivo tumor extracts. These observations suggest that organ microenvironments modulate the expression of IL-8 in human melanoma cells.

Takahashi and colleagues (60) investigated the role of tumor implantation site on VEGF expression, tumor angiogenesis, tumor cell proliferation, and metastasis in the gastric cancer cell line KKLS. The tumor cells were implanted in orthotopic (stomach) and ectopic (subcutaneous) locations in nude mice. Tumors in the stomach demonstrated more vascularization, higher levels of VEGF expression, and greater proliferation than the subcutaneous tumors (60). In addition, metastasis occurred only from the tumors implanted in the stomach. These data suggest that the expression of VEGF, vascularization, metastasis, and proliferation of human gastric cancer cells are regulated, in part, by the organ microenvironment.

VI. LYMPHOID-MEDIATED ANGIOGENESIS

That cells of the immune system regulate angiogenesis is well established. Mast cells, T-lymphocytes, macrophages, and their cytokines all participate actively in neovascularization (61–70). Lymphoid-mediated angiogenesis has been recognized in cutaneous melanoma (71). A local inflammatory reaction consisting of T-lymphocytes and macrophages is often associated with invasive cutaneous melanoma, and an intense inflammatory reaction is often associated with increased risk of metastasis, suggesting that inflammatory-associated angiogenesis may contribute to melanoma metastasis (72, 73). Slower growth of tumors in senescent mice has been associated with decreased vascularization (74), which also may be caused by diminished immunological response with aging (75–77).

Immunological mechanisms are likewise involved in the physiological angiogenesis that occurs subsequent to wound healing (78–80). Systemic chemotherapy retards wound healing, possibly by decreasing the immune response; whether this is mediated by inhibition of angiogenesis is not clear (81, 82). We have investigated the role of tumor vascularization and its effect on tumor growth in immunosuppressed mice. The growth of weakly immunogenic B16 melanoma was retarded in myelosuppressed mice compared with control mice (83). Further evidence implicating myelosuppression in the retardation of tumor growth and vascularity was obtained from doxorubicin (DXR)-pretreated animals injected with normal spleen cells 1 day before tumor challenge. Tumor growth in these mice was comparable to that in control mice (83). Similar results were obtained in athymic mice, suggesting that the tumor vascularization observed in DXR-treated mice reconstituted with normal spleenocytes was not mediated solely by T-lymphocytes. Because reconstitution with spleen cells enhanced vascularization of the B16 tumors, the results suggest that myelosuppressive chemotherapeutic drugs, for example, DXR, can inhibit host-mediated vascularization and support the concept that developing tumors can usurp homeostatic mechanisms to their advantage (5).

The role of infiltrating cells in angiogenesis of human colon cancer has been reported by Takahashi and colleagues (61). They observed high expression of PD-ECGF in infiltrating cells, mostly macrophages and lymphocytes, and very little expression of PD-ECGF in the cancer epithelium. The intensity of staining for PD-ECGF in infiltrating cells correlated with vessel counts, suggesting the involvement of these cells in the angiogenesis of human colon cancer.

Macrophages have been recognized as important angiogenesis effector cells for several years (68, 69, 78, 84, 85). They may influence new capillary growth by several different mechanisms. First, macrophages produce factors that act directly to influence angiogenesis-linked endothelial cell functions. Studies have shown that macrophages produce more than 20 molecules that reportedly influence endothelial cell proliferation, migration, and differentiation in vitro (84, 85) and are potentially angiogenic in vivo. A second mechanism by which macrophages might modulate angiogenesis is by modifying extracellular matrix (ECM). The composition of the ECM influences endothelial cell shape and morphology dramatically and may profoundly influence new capillary growth (85–87). Macrophages can influence the composition of the ECM, either through the direct production of ECM components or through the production of proteases, which effectively alter the structure and composition of the ECM (69). A third mechanism is through production of substances that suppress angiogenesis. Macrophages have been shown to express the angiogenesis inhibitor thrombospondin-1 (TSP1) when treated with the chemopreventive agent retinoic acid (79, 85, 88, 89).

We have examined the mechanism for generation of angiostatin, an angiogenesis inhibitor isolated from plasma of mice bearing Lewis lung carcinoma (3LL) (90). Our results demonstrate that the generation of angiostatin by the subcutaneous tumors requires the presence of macrophages and is directly correlated with their metalloelastase activity (91). The addition of plasminogen to 3LL cells cultured in vitro did not result in generation of angiostatin, whereas the addition of plasminogen to cocultures of macrophages and 3LL cells did. Elastase activity in macrophages was up-regulated by the cytokine granulocyte macrophage-colony-stimulating factor (GM-CSF) (92). The GM-CSF secreted by 3LL cells significantly enhanced the production of elastase by macrophages and, hence, the generation of angiostatin from plasminogen (91). These data suggest that elastase released from tumor-infiltrating macrophages is responsible for the angiostatin production in this tumor model and the angiogenesis-inhibiting role of macrophages.

VII. CONCLUSION

The complement of positive and negative regulators of angiogenesis may vary among different physiological and pathological settings. To better understand the process of angiogenesis and its significance in tumor progression and metastasis, an angiogenic profile consisting of both pro- and antiangiogenic molecules is important. The recent elucidation of the cooperative interaction among positive and negative regulatory molecules during normal physiology and the apparent disruption of this program in pathology suggests that future studies of pathological angiogenesis must focus on the interaction of both positive and negative regulators of this process.

The crosstalk between the tumor cells and stromal cells occurs mainly through a complex network of extracellular signals, including cytokines and growth factors, their antagonists/inhibitors, and soluble receptors, all of which are released by and act on cells within the tumor microenvironment. The net effect is to regulate the proliferation of metastatic cells, to suppress the activity of infiltrating host cells, and to enhance the establishment of the stromal environment by inducing development of a new blood supply for the tumors.

Tumor cells express more than one angiogenic molecule, suggesting a redundant mechanism for regulation of new blood vessel growth. These factors may be regulated by different sets of host-derived cytokines. Understanding these events should allow the design of potent antiangiogenic therapies against cancer metastasis.

ACKNOWLEDGMENTS

This work was supported in part by Cancer Center Support Core grant CA16672 and grant R35-CA42107 (I.J.F.) from the National Cancer Institute, National Institutes of Health. The authors thank Walter Pagel for his editorial review and Lola López for excellent preparation of this manuscript.

REFERENCES

1. Sugarbaker EV. Cancer metastasis: a product of tumor-host interactions. Curr Probl Cancer 1979; 3:1–59
2. Fidler IJ. Critical factors in the biology of human cancer metastasis: twenty-eighth GHA Clowes Memorial Award Lecture. Cancer Res 1990; 50:6130–6138.
3. Weiss L. Principles of Metastasis. Orlando: Academic Press, 1985.
4. Fidler IJ. Experimental orthotopic models of organ-specific metastasis by human neoplasms. Adv Mol Cell Biol 1994; 9:191–215.
5. Fidler IJ. Modulation of the organ microenvironment for treatment of cancer metastasis. J Natl Cancer Inst 1995; 87:1588–1592.
6. Folkman J. The role of angiogenesis in tumor growth. Semin Cancer Biol 1992; 3: 65–71.
7. Folkman J. Angiogenesis in cancer, vascular, rheumatoid and other diseases. Nat Med 1995; 1:27–31.
8. Folkman J. Clinical applications of research on angiogenesis. N Engl J Med 1995; 333:1753–1763.
9. Auerbach W, Auerbach R. Angiogenesis inhibition: a review. Pharmacol Ther 1994; 63:265–311.
10. Dvorak HF. Tumors: wounds that do not heal. N Engl J Med 1986; 315:1650–1659.
11. Fidler IJ, Kripke ML. Metastasis results from preexisting variant cells within a malignant tumor. Science 1977; 197:893–895.
12. Poste G, Fidler IJ. The pathogenesis of cancer metastasis. Nature 1980; 283:139–146.
13. Paget S. The distribution of secondary growths in cancer of the breast. Lancet 1889; 1:571–573.

14. Price JE. Host-tumor interaction in progression of breast cancer metastasis. In Vivo 1994; 8:145–154.
15. Hart IR. ''Seed and soil'' revisited: mechanism of site-specific metastasis. Cancer Metastasis Rev 1982; 1:5–7.
16. Tarin D, Price JE, Kettlewell MGW, Souter RG, Vass ACR, Crossley B. Clinicopathological observations on metastasis in man studied in patients treated with peritoneovenous shunts. BMJ 1984; 288:749–751.
17. Tarin D, Price JE, Kettlewell MGW, Souter RG, Vass ACR. Mechanism of human tumor metastasis studied in patients with peritoneovenous shunts. Cancer Res 1984; 44:3584–3592.
18. Fidler IJ, Hart IR. Biological diversity in metastatic neoplasms: origin and implications. Science 1982; 217:998–1003.
19. Price JE, Aukerman SL, Fidler IJ. Evidence that the process of murine melanoma metastasis is sequential and selective and contains stochastic elements. Cancer Res 1986; 46:5172–5178.
20. Talmadge JE, Wolman SR, Fidler IJ. Evidence for the clonal origin of spontaneous metastasis. Science 1982; 217:361–363.
21. Fidler IJ, Talmadge JE. Evidence that intravenously derived murine pulmonary melanoma metastases can originate from the expansion of a single tumor cell. Cancer Res 1986; 46:5167–5171.
22. Ellis LM, Fidler IJ. Angiogenesis and metastasis. Eur J Cancer 1996; 32A:2451–2460.
23. Liotta LA, Kleinerman J, Saidel GM. Quantitative relationships of intravascular tumor cells, tumor vessels, and pulmonary metastases following tumor implantation. Cancer Res 1974; 34:997–1003.
24. Weidner N, Folkman J, Pozza F, Bevilacqua P, Allred EN, Moore DH, Meli S, Gaspanni G. Tumor angiogenesis: a new significant and independent prognostic indicator in early stage breast carcinoma. J Natl Cancer Inst 1992; 84:1875–1887.
25. Weidner N, Carroll PR, Flax J, Blumenfeld W, Folkman J. Tumor angiogenesis correlates with metastasis in invasive prostate carcinoma. Am J Pathol 1993; 143: 401–409.
26. Weidner N, Folkman J. Tumoral vascularity as a prognostic factor in cancer. In: DeVita VT, Hellman S, Rosenberg SA, eds. Important Advances in Oncology. Philadelphia: Lippincott-Raven, 1996:167–190.
27. Folkman J. How is blood vessel growth regulated in normal and neoplastic tissue? GHA Clowes Memorial Award Lecture. Cancer Res 1986; 46:467–473.
28. Folkman J, Klagsbrun M. Angiogenic factors. Science 1987; 235:442–447.
29. Gerlowski LE, Jain RK. Microvascular permeability of normal and neoplastic tissues. Microvasc Res 1986; 31:288–305.
30. Hanahan D, Folkman J. Patterns and emerging mechanisms of the angiogenic switch during tumorigenesis. Cell 1996; 86:353–364.
31. Bouck N, Stellmach V, Hsu SC. How tumors become angiogenic. Adv Cancer Res 1996; 69:135–174.
32. Fidler IJ, Ellis LM. The implication of angiogenesis to the biology and therapy of cancer metastasis. Cell 1994; 79:185–188.
33. Dameron KM, Volpert OV, Tanisky MA, Bouk N. Control of angiogenesis in fibroblasts by p53 regulation of thrombospondin-1. Science 1994; 265:1502–1504.

34. Hanahan D, Christofori G, Naik P, Arbeit J. Transgenic mouse models of tumor angiogenesis: the angiogenic switch, its molecular controls, and prospects for preclinical therapeutic models. Eur J Cancer 1996; 32A:2386–2393.
35. Singh RK, Llansa N, Bucana CD, Sanchez R, Koura A, Fidler IJ. Cell density-dependent regulation of basic fibroblast growth factor expression in human renal cell carcinoma cells. Cell Growth Differ 1996; 7:397–404.
36. Koura AN, Liu W, Kitadai Y, Radinsky R, Ellis LM. Regulation of vascular endothelial growth factor expression in human colon carcinoma cells by cell density. Cancer Res 1996; 56:3891–3894.
37. Takahashi K, Mulligan JB, Kozakewich HPW, Rogers RA, Folkman J, Ezekowitz RAB. Cellular markers that distinguish the phases of hemangioma during infancy and childhood. J Clin Invest 1994; 93:2357–2364.
38. Ezekowitz RAB, Mulliken JB, Folkman J. Interferon alfa-2a therapy for life-threatening hemangiomas of infancy. N Engl J Med 1992; 326:1456–1463.
39. Singh RK, Gutman M, Bucana CD, Sanchez R, Llansa N, Fidler IJ. Interferon-α and -β downregulate the expression of basic fibroblast growth factor in human carcinomas. Proc Natl Acad Sci U S A 1995; 92:4562–4566.
40. Singh RK, Gutman M, Radinsky R, Bucana CD, Fidler IJ. Expression of interleukin 8 correlates with the metastatic potential of human melanoma cells in nude mice. Cancer Res 1994; 54:3242–3247.
41. Koch AE, Polverini PJ, Kunkel SL, Harlow LA, DiPietro LA, Elner NM, Elner SG, Strieter RM. Interleukin-8 as a macrophage-derived mediator of angiogenesis. Science 1992; 258:1798–1801.
42. Gutman M, Singh RK, Xie K, Bucana CD, Fidler IJ. Regulation of interleukin-8 expression in human melanoma cells by the organ environment. Cancer Res 1995; 55:2470–2475.
43. Singh RK, Gutman M, Llansa N, Fidler IJ. Interferon-β prevents the upregulation of interleukin-8 expression in human melanoma cells. J Interferon Cytokine Res 1996; 16:577–584.
44. Brown LF, Berse B, Jackman RW, Tognazzi K, Manseau EJ, Dvorak HF, Senger DR. Expression of vascular permeability factor (vascular endothelial growth factor) and its receptors in adenocarcinomas of the gastrointestinal tract. Cancer Res 1993; 53:4727–4735.
45. Brown LF, Berse B, Jackman RW, Tognazzi K, Manseau EJ, Dvorak HF, Senger DR. Increased expression of vascular permeability factor (vascular endothelial growth factor) and its receptor in kidney and bladder carcinomas. Am J Pathol 1993; 143:1255–1262.
46. Shweiki D, Itin A, Stoffer D, Keshet E. Vascular endothelial growth factor induced by hypoxia may mediate hypoxia-initiated angiogenesis. Nature 1992; 359:843–845.
47. Ikeda E, Achen MG, Breier G, Risau W. Hypoxia-induced transcriptional activation and increased mRNA stability of vascular endothelial growth factor in C6 glioma cells. J Biol Chem 1995; 34:19761–19768.
48. Levy AP, Levy NS, Wegner S, Goldberg MA. Transcriptional regulation of the rat vascular endothelial growth factor gene by hypoxia. J Biol Chem 1995; 270:13333–13340.
49. Koochekpour S, Merzak A, Pilkington GJ. Vascular endothelial growth factor pro-

duction is stimulated in response to growth factors in human glioma cells. Oncol Rep 1995; 2:1059–1061.
50. Tsai JC, Goldman CK, Gillespie GY. Vascular endothelial growth factor in human glioma cell lines: induced secretion by EGF, PDGF-BB, and bFGF. J Neurosurg 1995; 358:311–315.
51. Cohen T, Nahari D, Cerem LW, Neufeld G, Levi BZ. Interleukin 6 induces the expression of vascular endothelial growth factor. J Biol Chem 1996; 271:736–741.
52. Li J, Perrella MA, Tsai JC, Yet SF, Hsieh CM, Yoshizumi M, Patterson C, Endego WO, Zhou F, Lee ME. Induction of vascular endothelial growth factor gene expression by interleukin-1β in rat aortic smooth muscle cells. J Biol Chem 1995; 270: 308–312.
53. Pertovaara L, Kaipainen A, Mustonen T, Orpana A, Ferrara N, Saksela O, Alitalo K. Vascular endothelial growth factor is induced in response to transforming growth factor-β in fibroblastic and epithelial cells. J Biol Chem 1994; 269:6271–6274.
54. Mukhopadhyay D, Tsiokas L, Zhou XM, Foster D, Brugge JS, Sukhatme VP. Hypoxic induction of human vascular endothelial growth factor expression through c-src activation. Nature 1995; 375:577–581.
55. Rak J, Mitsuhashi Y, Bayko L, Filmus J, Shirasawa S, Sasazuki T, Kerbel RS. Mutant *ras* oncogenes upregulate VEGF/VPF expression: implications for induction and inhibition of tumor angiogenesis. Cancer Res 1995; 55:4575–4580.
56. Rak J, Filmus J, Finkenzeller G, Grugel S, Marme D, Kerbel RS. Oncogenes as inducers of tumor angiogenesis. Cancer Metastasis Rev 1995; 14:263–277.
57. Mukhopadhyay D, Tsiokas L, Sukhatme VP. Wild-type p53 and v-src exert opposing influences on human vascular endothelial growth factor gene expression. Cancer Res 1995; 55:6161–6165.
58. Naito S, von Eschenbach AC, Giavazzi R, Fidler IJ. Growth and metastasis of tumor cells isolated from a human renal cell carcinoma implanted into different organs of nude mice. Cancer Res 1986; 46:4109–4115.
59. Singh RK, Bucana CD, Gutman M, Fan D, Wilson MR, Fidler IJ. Organ site-dependent expression of basic fibroblast growth factor in human renal cell carcinoma cells. Am J Pathol 1994; 145:365–374.
60. Takahashi Y, Mai M, Wilson MR, Kitadai Y, Bucana CD, Ellis LM. Site-dependent expression of vascular endothelial growth factor, angiogenesis, and proliferation in human gastric carcinoma. Int J Oncol 1996; 8:701–705.
61. Takahashi Y, Bucana CD, Liu W, Yoneda J, Kitadai Y, Cleary KR, Ellis LM. Platelet-derived endothelial cell growth factor in human colon cancer angiogenesis: role of infiltrating cells. J Natl Cancer Inst 1996; 88:1146–1151.
62. Sidky YA, Auerbach R. Lymphocyte-induced angiogenesis in tumor-bearing mice. Science 1976; 192:1237–1238.
63. Meininger CJ, Zetter BR. Mast cells and angiogenesis. Semin Cancer Biol 1992; 3: 73–79.
64. Fidler IJ. Lymphocytes are not only immunocytes (guest editorial). Biomedicine 1980; 32:1–3.
65. Fidler IJ, Gersten DM, Kripke ML. Influence of immune status on the metastasis of three murine fibrosarcomas of different immunogenicities. Cancer Res 1979; 39: 3816–3821.

66. Miguez M, Davel L, deLustig ES. Lymphocyte-induced angiogenesis: correlation with the metastatic incidence of two murine mammary adenocarcinomas. Invasion Metastasis 1986; 6:313–320.
67. Freeman MR, Schneck FX, Gagnon ML, Corless C, Soker S, Niknejad K, Peoples GE, Klagsbrun M. Peripheral blood T lymphocytes and lymphocytes infiltrating human cancers express vascular endothelial growth factor: a potential role for T cells in angiogenesis. Cancer Res 1995; 55:4140–4145.
68. Polverini P, Cotran R, Gimbrone N, Unanue E. Activated macrophages induce vascular proliferation. Nature 1977; 269:804–805.
69. Sunderkotter C, Steinbrink K, Goebeler M, Bhardwaj R, Sorg C. Macrophages and angiogenesis. J Leukoc Biol 1994; 55:410–422.
70. Leek RD, Harris AL, Lewis CE. Cytokine networks in solid human tumors: regulation of angiogenesis. J Leukoc Biol 1994; 56:423–435.
71. Srivastava A, Laidler P, Davies RP, Horgan K, Hughes LE. The prognostic significance of tumor vascularity in intermediate thickness (0.76–4.0 mm thick) skin melanoma: a quantitative histologic study. Am J Pathol 1988; 133:419–423.
72. Brocker EG, Rechenbeld C, Hamm H, Ruiter DJ, Sorg C. Macrophages in melanocytic naevi. Arch Dermatol Res 1992; 284:127–131.
73. Ruiter DJ, Bhan AK, Harris TJ, Sober AJ, Mihm MC Jr. Major histocompatibility antigens and the mononuclear inflammatory infiltrate in benign nevomelanocytic proliferation and malignant melanoma. J Immunol 1982; 129:2808–2815.
74. Kreisle RA, Stebler BA, Ershler WB. Effect of host age on tumor-associated angiogenesis in mice. J Natl Cancer Inst 1990; 82:44–47.
75. Ding A, Hwang S, Schwab R. Effect of aging on murine macrophages: diminished response to IFN-γ for enhanced oxidative metabolism. J Immunol 1994; 153:2146–2152.
76. Goidl E, ed. Aging and the Immune Response: Cellular and Humoral Aspects. New York: Marcel Dekker, 1987.
77. Weksler ME, Schwab R. The immunogenetics of immune senescence. Exp Clin Immunogenet 1992; 199:182–187.
78. Sunderkotter C, Goebeler M, Schultze-Osthoff K, Bhardwaj R, Sorg C. Macrophage-derived angiogenic factors. Pharmacol Ther 1991; 51:195–216.
79. DiPietro LA, Polverini PJ. Angiogenic macrophages produce the angiogenic inhibitor thrombospondin 1. Am J Pathol 1993; 143:678–684.
80. Rappolee DA, Mark D, Banda MJ, Werb Z. Wound macrophages express TGF-α and other growth factors in vivo: analysis by mRNA phenotyping. Science 1988; 241:708–712.
81. Fumagalli U, Trabucchi E, Soligo M, Rosati R, Rebuffat C, Tonelli C, Montorsi M. Effects of intraperitoneal chemotherapy on anastomotic healing in the rat. J Surg Res 1991; 50:82–87.
82. Noh R, Karp GI, Devereaux DF. The effect of doxorubicin and mitoxanthrone on wound healing. Cancer Chemother Pharmacol 1991; 29:141–144.
83. Gutman M, Singh RK, Yoon S, Xie K, Bucana CD, Fidler IJ. Leukocyte-induced angiogenesis and subcutaneous growth of B16 melanoma. Cancer Biother 1994; 9:163–170.
84. Polverini JJ, Leibovich SJ. Induction of neovascularization in vivo and endothelial

cell proliferation in vitro by tumor-associated macrophages. Lab Invest 1984; 51: 635–642.

85. Polverini PJ. How the extracellular matrix and macrophages contribute to angiogenesis-dependent diseases. Eur J Cancer 1996; 32A:2430–2437.
86. Ingber D. Extracellular matrix and cell shape: potential control points for inhibition of angiogenesis. J Cell Biochem 1991; 47:236–241.
87. Ingber DE, Folkman J. How does extracellular matrix control capillary morphogenesis. Cell 1989; 58:803–805.
88. Lingen MW, Polverini PJ, Bouck N. Inhibition of squamous cell carcinoma angiogenesis by direct interaction of retinoic acid with endothelial cells. Lab Invest 1996; 74:476–483.
89. Lingen MW, Polverini PJ, Bouck N. Retinoic acid induces cells cultured from oral squamous cell carcinomas to become antiangiogenic. Am J Pathol 1996; 149:247–258.
90. O'Reilly MS, Holmgren L, Shing Y, Chen C, Rosenthal RA, Moses M, Lane WS, Cao Y, Sage EH, Folkman J. Angiostatin: a novel angiogenesis inhibitor that mediates the suppression of metastases by a Lewis lung carcinoma. Cell 1994; 79:315–328.
91. Dong Z, Kumar R, Yang X, Fidler IJ. Macrophage-derived metalloelastase is responsible for the generation of angiostatin in Lewis lung carcinoma. Cell 1997; 88:801–810.
92. Kumar R, Dong Z, Fidler IJ. Differential regulation of metalloelastase activity in murine peritoneal macrophages by GM-CSF and M-CSF. J Immunol 1996; 157: 5104–5111.

20
Role of Macrophages in Tumor Angiogenesis

Peter J. Polverini
University of Minnesota School of Dentistry, Minneapolis, Minnesota

I. INTRODUCTION

The functional domain of the macrophage (Mø) extends far beyond its originally recognized role as a scavenger cell. Endowed with a rich array of secretory products, Mø are known to influence virtually every aspect of the immune response and inflammation as well as contribute to the etiology and pathogenesis of a number of diseases. Angiogenesis, the process that leads to the formation of new capillary blood vessels, is an essential feature of a number of important physiological processes. Furthermore, when angiogenesis occurs in excess or inappropriately, it can contribute to the etiology and pathogenesis of several inflammatory, degenerative, developmental, and neoplastic diseases. Macrophages are key angiogenesis effector cells that produce a number of growth stimulators and inhibitors, proteolytic enzymes, and cytokines that can influence one or more steps in the angiogenesis cascade. This chapter will include summaries of the evidence implicating Mø as important accessory cells in physiological angiogenic responses and a description of how disruption in the coordinate production of Mø-derived stimulators and inhibitors of angiogenesis contributes to tumor progression.

II. Mø ARE ANATOMICALLY AND FUNCTIONALLY DIVERSE

Cells belonging to the mononuclear phagocyte system are derived from myeloid precursors that originate from bone marrow stem cell populations. Macrophage progenitors, under the influence of colony-stimulating factors and differentiating-inducing signals, divide, differentiate, and migrate into the bloodstream as circulating monocytes (1–4). When called upon, as in inflammation or during immune responses, Mø undergo further differentiation and specialization whereby they become highly responsive to environmental signals that further modify their functional and morphological phenotype (5–8). Macrophages populate virtually every organ and tissue in which they perform several common as well as many specialized functions, depending on the tissues or organs in which they reside. Macrophages are capable of rapidly responding to changes in their environment by undergoing further differentiation and specialization. This process, termed "activation," is a tightly regulated biological process. When Mø are activated, they display properties such as increased phagocytic and microbiocidal activity, exhibit enhanced chemotactic activity, and secrete a wide spectrum of biologically active molecules, including a number of growth factors. Activation thus enables Mø to influence numerous biological processes in a precisely defined fashion.

Macrophages are among the most versatile cells in the mammalian organism. Recognized early on for their endocytic and phagocytic activity and their central role in host defense against infection and malignancy (1), Mø have gained considerable attention in recent years as potent secretory cells and have been shown to influence the growth and function of a diverse array of target cells (9). One of the first studies implicating Mø as promoting the growth of other mesenchymal cells was the work of Carrel (10), who recognized that leukocytes in inflammatory exudates could stimulate the growth of fibroblasts. In the early 70s, a number of studies reported that Mø culture fluids contained growth stimulatory and inhibitory activities for lymphoid and bone marrow-derived cells (11–15). The functional importance of the Mø in wound repair and fibroblast proliferation was first demonstrated when Leibovich and Ross (16) showed that guinea pigs depleted of monocytes and Mø exhibited significantly delayed wound repair. They later showed that Mø culture fluids contained growth promoting activity(s) for fibroblasts (17). The biochemical identity of this biological activity, termed "macrophage-derived growth factor (MDGF)," remained uncertain for several years. As the identity of many other growth-promoting activities and other secretory products became known, it became increasingly clear that a number of biochemically distinct molecules with a wide range of cell targets, including vascular endothelium, were responsible for the growth-promoting effects of Mø (18–20).

III. Mø ARE POTENT MEDIATORS OF ANGIOGENESIS

Shortly after Mø were reported to have growth-promoting activity for fibroblasts, they were shown to mediate angiogenesis. Early studies from several laboratories established a relationship between the presence of Mø and vascular proliferation

(19–23). The occurrence of endothelial cell proliferation during immunological reactions had been documented in several studies. Light microscopic and ultrastructural studies of hypersensitivity reactions in experimental animals and humans revealed the presence of activated and dividing endothelial cells (24, 25). Graham and Shannon (26) reported that endothelial mitoses were observed during lymphocyte migration through high endothelial venules in arthritic joints of rabbits. Anderson et al. (27) demonstrated extensive proliferation of postcapillary venular endothelium in lymph nodes draining skin allographs. Sidkey and Auerbach (28) showed that capillary proliferation occurred during local graft vs. host reactions in the skin of mice. It had been proposed that the accompanying dermal angiogenesis was induced by immunocompetent donor lymphocytes. Also, a number of in vitro studies indicated that Mø produced growth inhibitory and stimulatory factors for several mesenchymal cell types (12, 13, 16, 17, 29). Using a quantitative autoradiographic approach, Polverini et al. (21) demonstrated that incorporation of tritiated thymidine by microvascular endothelial cells in the skin of tuberculin-sensitized guinea pigs coincided with the onset and magnitude of mononuclear infiltration at the reaction site. The mechanisms responsible for endothelial proliferation were at the time conjectural: two explanations were proposed. First, endothelial replication was a reparative response to nonspecific injury and necrosis induced by humoral or cellular toxins. Alternatively, the proliferation was mediated by growth factors produced by one or more of the mononuclear cell types in the infiltrate. This possibility was addressed more directly by Clark et al. (30). These investigators showed that wound Mø, when introduced into the avascular corneas of rabbits, stimulated neovascularization in the wake of an acute inflammatory response. Polverini et al. (22) further showed that when Mø or their conditioned culture media were introduced into guinea pig corneas, they potently stimulated neovascularization. Peritoneal Mø obtained from Balb/c mice and Hartley albino guinea pigs by lavage or after injection of an inflammatory stimulant were processed by standard separation techniques to yield a preparation consisting of 85% to 90% Mø. Intracorneal injection of viable Mø or their conditioned culture media was potently angiogenic in more than 75% of corneas tested. In contrast, quiescent resident Mø were either weakly angiogenic or showed no activity at all. Similarly preparations of Mø from inbred strain II guinea pigs yielded essentially similar results, precluding the possibility that neovascularization occurred as a result of an immunologically mediated inflammatory response. The requirement that Mø be activated for expression of angiogenic activity was demonstrated with cultured cells. Brief exposure of quiescent resident peritoneal Mø to latex induced them to express angiogenic activity. Also, aliquots of cell-free, dialyzed, and concentrated culture media from Mø activated in vivo or in vitro induced angiogenesis when incorporated into Hydron polymer and implanted into corneas. These responses exhibited the same pattern of capillary growth as was observed with viable Mø. Collectively, these results indicated that activated Mø were able to induce angiogenesis in the absence of inflammation through an inducible secreted product. These studies were subsequently confirmed by Thakral et al. (31) and Hunt and coworkers (32) with wound-derived Mø and wound fluids rich in Mø, and by Moore and Sholley (33) with autologous rabbit peritoneal Mø.

Several environmental stimuli capable of inducing expression of the angiogenic phenotype by Mø have been identified. Knighton et al. (34) and Jensen et al. (35) showed that adherent Mø can be activated by low oxygen tension and high lactate concentration. Both of these agents are present in great abundance in organizing wound and are important stimuli for activating Mø at the wound site. Evidence exists that endothelial cell-derived cytokines and adhesion molecules may function to activate Mø (36). This may represent another mechanism of Mø activation at sites of inflammation. Before migrating into inflamed tissues, Mø and other leukocytes must adhere to endothelial cells (37). These cytokine-activated, postcapillary venular endothelial cells express a high number of adhesion molecules that are able to activate Mø, which in turn can participate in the generation of soluble adhesion molecules with proangiogenic activity (38).

Numerous substances have been reported to induce angiogenesis, and many of these mediators are produced by Mø (3, 19). These include polypeptide growth factors, cytokines, prostaglandins, and proteolytic enzymes (23, 39, 40). As a consequence, Mø can mediate new capillary growth by a several different mechanisms. First, the macrophage can produce factors that act directly to influence the angiogenic cascade. In vitro studies have shown that Mø produce more than 20 molecules that stimulate endothelial cell proliferation, migration, and differentiation (2), and many of them have been show to be potentially angiogenic in vivo. A second mechanism by which Mø might promote angiogenesis is by modifying the extracellular matrix (ECM). The composition of the ECM dramatically influences endothelial cell shape and morphology and may profoundly influence new capillary growth (41–43). Macrophages can influence the composition of the ECM, either through the direct production of ECM components or through the production of proteases that effectively alter the ECM.

IV. Mø PLAY A KEY ROLE IN WOUND NEOVASCULARIZATION

Wound healing is perhaps the most well studied and best example of a physiological process that is strictly dependent on the timely ingrowth of new capillary blood vessels. Wound healing is an essential biological process driven by the cooperative interaction of a variety of cell types and mediator systems. Normal tissue repair requires that the cells and mediators of the immune system, the connective tissue, and vascular endothelium function in a coordinated manner to effect the repair process in a timely and efficient manner. Although numerous cell types are involved, the monocyte-derived macrophage appears to play a central role in orchestrating the repair process. Macrophages migrating into healing wounds phagocytose wound debris, become activated, and secrete diffusable cytokines that modulate tissue repair (44, 45). In surgical models of wound healing, activated Mø are the predominant cell type approximately 5 days after injury when the proliferative phase of the repair process is most pronounced (16, 46). Several reports suggested that wound Mø function primarily to augment the repair response. The introduction of activated Mø into healing wounds results in enhanced wound repair (47), and activation of wound Mø, either by systemic or topical administration of the Mø stimulant, glucan, significantly increases wound-breaking strength (48).

Macrophages are believed to be responsible for coordinating much of the growth and tissue remodeling that occurs during the wound response. A key step in the repair process is the formation of inflammatory granulation tissue, a temporary tissue composed largely of new capillary blood vessels. It is now well established that Mø are key regulators of wound neovascularization. Activated Mø or their culture supernatants induce new capillary growth in vitro and angiogenesis in vivo (2, 3, 22, 30, 31, 32, 39, 49). During the proliferative phase, growing capillaries provide nutrient support for regenerating tissues, whereas during the resolution phase, many of the newly formed capillaries regress as tissue regeneration is complete. Recent evidence suggests that capillary regression may also be mediated by Mø, as they produce substances that are inhibitory to endothelial cell growth and some that are antiangiogenic in vivo (19, 50–53). Thus, a substantial body of evidence has implicated the Mø in both the stimulation and suppression of wound angiogenesis.

There has been much speculation regarding which of the known angiogenic substances produced by Mø might be key positive regulators of wound neovascularization. Using reverse transcriptase polymerase chain reaction (PCR) analysis, transcripts from a variety of potential angiogenic factors have been identified (54–56). However, among these mediators only tumor growth factor (TGF)-α and tumor necrosis factor (TNF)-β have been convincingly shown to mediate angiogenesis in vivo (57–59). Tumor necrosis factor α represents a likely candidate as an angiogenic regulator as it is (a) found in wound fluid; (b) transcribed in wounds, probably by Mø; and (c) described as a major angiogenic molecule produced by Mø (54, 58, 60). Strieter et al. (61) and Koch et al. (62, 63) demonstrated that interleukin 8 (IL-8), a major macrophage cytokine, is a potent mediator of angiogenesis in rodent corneas. Clearly, the induction and regulation of angiogenesis by Mø may involve redundancy so that any single factor may not be essential for adequate wound repair. To add to the complexity, wound Mø are capable of modulating other parameters of wound repair, such as the clearance of debris, and the growth and maturation of tissues (16, 17). Moreover, it is likely that some macrophage-derived factors may affect more than one aspect of wound repair. Although Mø influence many aspects of wound repair in vivo, the regeneration of the cellular and connective tissue components cannot proceed without the recruitment of new vasculature for nutrient support.

V. Mø PRODUCE INHIBITORS OF NEOVASCULARIZATION

One of the most important features distinguishing physiological from pathological angiogenesis is that in the former setting, angiogenesis is strictly delimited in both time and space (23, 64, 65). During wound neovascularization the rapid induction of new capillary vessels is tempered by inhibitors of neovascularization. One macrophage-derived mediator that has received considerable attention in recent years as a potent endogenous inhibitor of angiogenesis is thrombospondin-1 (TSP1) (66–68)

Thrombospondin-1 is a member of a family of five homologous proteins. It is a 450 kDa disulfide-linked trimer composed of three identical chains with a monomeric mass of about 140 kDa. Its modular structure in part enables it to interact with a variety of ECM proteins, cell-surface and serum protein, and cations. Thrombospondin-1 is present in great abundance in the platelet alpha granules and is secreted by a variety of epithelial and mesenchymal cells (66, 68–71). It participates in cell substrate interactions where many cells have been shown to attach, spread, and migrate on insoluble TSP1 (68, 72, 73). Thrombospondin-1 was first implicated as an inhibitor of neovascularization when an antiangiogenic hamster protein whose secretion was controlled by a tumor suppressor gene was found to have an amino acid sequence similar to human platelet TSP1 (74). Authentic TSP1 was then purified from platelets and shown to block neovascularization in vivo (72). A role for TSP1 in the inhibition of angiogenesis is supported by several observations. It is present adjacent to mature quiescent vessels and is absent from actively growing sprouts both in vivo (73) and in vitro (74). Hemangiomas that consist of rapidly proliferating endothelial cells fail to produce detectable TSP1 (75). Antibodies to TSP1 added to endothelial cell cultures enhance sprouting in vitro (76) and endothelial cells in which TSP1 production has been down-regulated by antisense TSP1 exhibit an accelerated rate of growth, enhanced chemotactic activity, and an increase in the number of capillary-like cords (76). DiPietro et al. (77) have shown that the addition of antisense TSP1 oligmers to wounds in the skin of mice results in delayed healing, suggesting that TSP1 is just as important in the initiation of the wound response as it is in the organization phase of wound repair. Also, Polverini et al. (78) reported that mice with a targeted disruption in TSP1 showed delayed wound organization and prolonged wound neovascularization.

Previous investigations have shown that both resting and activated Mø produce TSP1. DiPietro et al. (79) has reported an approximately sixfold increase in the steady-state levels of TSP1 mRNA expression in the murine monocyte line WEHI-3 when the cells were treated for 24 hours with the potent activating agent lipopolysaccharide (LPS) with peak secretion of TSP1 protein occurring by 8 hours. The finding that activated Mø produce the angiogenesis inhibitor TSP1 would seem paradoxical. There are several possible explanations for this apparent functional dichotomy. The angiogenic potential of Mø in vivo may be the result of the balanced production of both positive and negative regulators of angiogenesis. Alternatively macrophage-derived TSP1 may not exert significant effects on endothelial cells, particularly if TSP1 is rapidly degraded or sequestered into the ECM. In this instance the influence of activated Mø may be shifted toward diffusable mediators of angiogenesis rather than inhibitors such as TSP1. Several other functions of macrophage-derived TSP1 may influence wound repair and angiogenesis. The adhesive capacity of TSP1 may facilitate migration of activated Mø. Macrophages have surface receptors for TSP1 (80) and thus might lay TSP1 on the existing ECM as a scaffold upon which to migrate.

VI. Mø MEDIATE TUMOR NEOVASCULARIZATION

Mononuclear phagocytes are a frequent component of the stroma of neoplastic tissues (81). Interest in cells of the mononuclear phagocyte system in relation to the growth of neoplasms stem largely from the observation that these effector cells, when appropriately activated, are able to arrest the growth of or kill neoplastic and transformed target cells. Although there is substantial in vitro evidence supporting the antitumor activity of activated Mø, the in vivo relevance of these observations has not been unequivocally demonstrated even under conditions in which Mø are likely to have antitumor activity. Macrophages express diverse functions essential for tissue remodeling, inflammation, and immunity. Analysis of tumor-associated Mø (TAM) functions suggests that these multifunctional cells can affect diverse aspects of neoplastic development, including vascularization, growth rate and metastasis, stroma formation, and destruction. There is evidence that in some neoplasms, including human cancers, the protumor functions of Mø prevail. These observations emphasize the dual potential of TAM to influence neoplastic growth and progression in opposite directions, with protumor activity often prevailing in the absence of therapeutic interventions in many neoplasms.

The formation of new blood vessels is a crucial step in the growth of neoplastic tissues. Several lines of evidence suggested a relationship between the macrophage content of tumors, the rate of tumor growth, and the extent of their vascularization. In studies by Evans (82–84), it was reported that mice depleted of Mø by whole body X-irradiation of after the administration of azothioprine to tumor-bearing mice showed a delay in the appearance of tumors, suppression in the growth of established tumors, and a marked reduction in tumor neovascularization. Mostafa et al. (85, 86) and Stenzinger et al. (87) showed that neovascularization of several human tumors grown on the chick chorioallantoic membrane or subcutaneously in nude mice developed coincidental with mononuclear infiltration at the tumor site. This led these workers to speculate that tumor growth was partially dependent on the angiogenic activity of infiltrating macrophages. Polverini and Leibovich (38) reported that hamsters bearing chemical carcinogen-induced squamous cell carcinomas, when treated with low doses of steroid and antimacrophage serum, showed a significant reduction in thymidine incorporation of by endothelial cells and neovascularization of tumors. A more direct assessment of the role of TAM in tumor neovascularization was conducted, again by Polverini and Leibovich (39). They showed that TAM isolated from several transplantable chemical carcinogen-induced rat fibrosarcomas patently stimulated endothelial cell proliferation in vitro and neovascularization in vivo. Furthermore, they reported that tumors depleted of TAM grew more slowly when introduced into rat corneas. When TAM were added back to TAM-depleted tumors at concentrations equivalent to their original in situ concentration, tumor growth rate and the potency of neovascular responses were restored to levels observed in native tumors. The importance of a sustained influx of activated TAM to tumor neovascularization has been investigated by Lingen, Bouck and Polverini (unpublished observations). They found that human squamous carcinoma treated with the chemopreventive agent retinoic acid failed to activate Mø to express angiogenic activity and exhibited a diminished capacity to stimulate chemotaxis of Mø. These results suggest that the ability of retinoic acid to reduce the incidence of secondary tumor growths may induce the production of an inhibitor of angiogenesis by tumor cells and block the sustained infiltration of Mø into tumors and their subsequent activation for expression of angiogenic activity.

Another mechanism whereby tumors are able to subvert the defensive function of Mø is by suppressing the production of angioinhibitory substances (43). Kaposi's sarcoma (KS) is a complex neoplasm of suspected endothelial cell origin. Induction of angiogenesis is required for the progressive growth of KS tumors. Although much is known about the spectrum of proangiogenic cytokines produced by KS tumors cells, there is relatively little information on how other cells that populate KS tumors contribute to KS angiogenesis. Polverini et al. (43) have reported that human Mø, when grown in culture media conditioned by KS tumor cells, acquire potent angiogenic activity in association with significant suppression in the production of the angiogenesis inhibitor TSP1. These results suggest a mechanism by which KS tumor cells, and perhaps other tumors, can subvert the defensive properties of Mø and induce Mø to cooperate in sustaining a vigorous angiogenic response at the tumor site.

It is clear that Mø can influence angiogenesis in several physiological and pathological settings. Macrophages produce both stimulators and inhibitors of angiogenesis and thus have the ability to modulate angiogenesis either positively or negatively. In addition, tumor cells are able to recruit and modify the function of Mø to ensure expression of their protumor activities. Regardless of the setting in which angiogenesis is encountered and the great redundancy of mediator systems that participate in this process, the sorting of mechanisms that control the balanced production of positive and negative regulators of angiogenesis by accessory cell populations such as Mø is essential to develop novel approaches for the treatment of angiogenesis-dependent diseases such as neoplasia.

REFERENCES

1. Gordon S. The biology of the macrophage. J Cell Sci Suppl 1986; 4:267–286.
2. Sunderkotter C, Goebeler M, Schultze-Osthoff K, Bhardwaj R, Sorg C. Macrophage-derived angiogenesis factors. Pharmac Ther 1991; 51:195–216.
3. Sunderkotter C, Steinbrink K, Goebeler M, Bhardwaj R, Sorg C. Mø and angiogenesis. J Leukoc Biol 1994; 55:410–422.
4. Stein M, Keshav S. The versatility of Mø. Clin Exp Allergy 1992; 22:19–27.
5. Adams DO, Hamilton TA. The cell biology of the macrophage activation. Annu Rev Immunol 1984; 2:283–318.
6. Johnston RB Jr. Monocytes and Mø. New Engl J Med 1988; 318:747–752.
7. Van Furth R. Phagocytic cells: development and distribution of mononuclear phagocytes in normal steady state and in inflammation. In: Gallin JI, Goldstein IM, Snyderman R, eds. Inflammation: Basic Principles and Clinical Correlates. New York: Raven Press, 1988: 281–295.
8. Adams DO. Molecular interactions in macrophage activation. Immunol Today 1989; 10:33–35.
9. Nathan C. Secretory products of Mø. J Clin Invest 1987; 79:319–326.
10. Carrel A. Growth promoting functions of leukocytes. J Exp Med 1922; 36:385–391.
11. Gordon S, Unkeless JC, Cohn ZA. Induction of macrophage plasminogen activator by endotoxin stimulation and phagocytosis. J Exp Med 1974; 140:995–1010.
12. Calderon J, Kiely J-M, Lefko JL, Unanue ER. The modulation of lymphocyte functions by molecules secreted by Mø. I. Description and partial biochemical analysis. J Exp Med 1975; 142:151–164.
13. Calderon J, Unanue ER. Two biological activities regulating cell proliferation found in cultures of peritoneal exudate Mø. Nature 1975; 253:359–361.
14. Unanue ER. Secretory function of mononuclear phagocytes. Am J Pathol 1976; 83: 396–417.
15. Unanue ER, Kiely J-M, Calderon J. The modulation of lymphocyte functions of molecules secreted by Mø. II. Conditions leading to increased secretion. J Exp Med 1976; 144:155–166.

16. Leibovich SJ, Ross R. The role of the macrophage in wound repair: a study with hydrocortisone and antimacrophage serum. Am J Pathol 1975; 78:71–91.
17. Leibovich SJ, Ross R. A macrophage-dependent factor that stimulates the proliferation of fibroblasts in vitro. Am J Pathol 1976; 84:501–514.
18. Gillespie GY, Estes JE, Pledger WJ. Macrophage derived growth factors for mesenchymal cells. Lymphokines 1986; 2:213–242.
19. Polverini PJ. Macrophage-induced angiogenesis: a review. In: Sorg C, ed. Macrophage-Derived Regulatory Factors. Basel: S Karger, 1989; 54–73.
20. Polverini PJ. Role of the macrophage in angiogenesis-dependent diseases. ESX 1997; 79:11–28.
21. Polverini PJ, Cotran RS, Sholley MM. Endothelial proliferation in the delayed hypersensitivity reaction: an autoradiographic study. J Immunol 1977; 118:529–532.
22. Polverini PJ, Cotran RS, Gimbrone MA Jr, Unanue ER. Activated Mø induce vascular proliferation. Nature 1977; 269:804–806.
23. Polverini PJ. The pathophysiology of angiogenesis. Crit Rev Oral Biol Med 1995; 6:230–247.
24. Gell PGH. Cytological events in hypersensitivity reactions. In: Lawrence D, ed. Cellular and Humoral Aspects of the Hypersensitivity States. New York: Harper and Row, 1959:43–58.
25. Dvorak AM, Mim MC, Dvaork HF. Morphology of delayed-type hypersensitivity reactions in man. II. Ultrastructural alterations affecting the microvasculature and the tissue mast cell. Lab Invest 1976; 34:179–191.
26. Graham RC, Shannon S. Peroxidase arthritis. II. Lymphoid cell-endothelial interactions during developing immunologic inflammatory responses. Am J Pathol 1972; 69:7–14.
27. Anderson ND, Anderson AO, Wyllie RG. Microvascular changes in lymph nodes draining skin allographs. Am J Pathol 1975; 81:131–153.
28. Sidkey YA, Auerbach R. Lymphocyte-induced angiogenesis (LIA): a quantitative and sensitive assay of the graft vs. host reaction. J Exp Med 1975; 141:1084–1110.
29. Calderon J, Williams RT, Unanue ER. An inhibitor of cell proliferation released from cultures of Mø. Proc Natl Acad Sci U S A 1974; 71:4273–4277.
30. Clark RA, Stone RD, Leung DYK, Silver I, Hohn DD, Hunt TK. Role of Mø in wound healing. Surg Forum 1976; 27:16–18.
31. Thakral KK, Goodson W, Hunt TK. Stimulation of wound blood vessel growth by wound Mø. J Surg Res 1979; 26:430–436.
32. Hunt TK, Knighton DR, Thakral KK, Goodson WH, Andrews WS. Studies on inflammation and wound healing: angiogenesis and collagen synthesis stimulated in vivo by resident and activated wound Mø. Surgery 1984; 96:48–54.
33. Moore JW III, Sholley MM. Comparison of the neovascular effects of stimulated Mø and neutrophils in autologous rabbit corneas. Am J Pathol 1985; 120:87–98.
34. Knighton, DR, Hunt TK, Scheuenstuhl N, Halliday BT, Werb Z, Banda MJ. Oxygen tension regulates the expression of angiogenesis factor by macrophage. Science 1991; 221:1283–1285.
35. Jensen JA, Hunt TK, Scheuenstuhl H, Banda MJ. Effect of lactate, pyruvate, and pH on secretion of angiogenesis and mitogenesis factors by macrophages. Lab Invest 1986; 54:574–578.

36. Koch AE, Halloran MM, Haskell CJ, Shah MR, Polverini PJ. Angiogenesis mediated by soluble forms of E-selectin and vascular cell adhesion molecule-1. Nature 1995; 376:517–519.
37. Carlos TM, Harlan JM. Leukocyte-endothelial adhesion molecules. Blood 1994; 84: 2068–2101.
38. Szekanecz Z, Haines GK, Lin TR, Harlow LA, Goerdt S, Rayan G, Koch AE. Differential distribution of intercellular adhesion molecules (ICAM-1, ICAM-2, and ICAM-3) and the MS-1 antigen in normal and diseased human synovia. Their possible pathogenetic and clinical significance in rheumatoid arthritis. Arthritis Rheum 1994; 37:221–231.
39. Folkman J, Klagsbrun M. Angiogenic factors. Science 1987; 235:442–447.
40. Klagsbrun M, D'Amore PA. Regulators of angiogenesis. Annu Rev Physiol 1991; 53:217–239.
41. Ingber DE, Folkman J. Mechanochemical switching between growth and differentiation during fibroblast growth factor-stimulated angiogenesis in vitro. Role of the extracellular matrix. J Cell Biol 1989; 109:317–330.
42. Ingber DE. Extracellular matrix and cell shape: potential control points for the inhibition of angiogenesis. J Cell Biochem 1991; 47:236–241.
43. Polverini PJ. How the extracellular matrix and macrophages contribute to angiogenesis and vasoproliferative dependent diseases. Eur J Cancer 1996; 32A:2430–2437.
44. Leibovich SJ, Wiseman DM. Mø, wound repair and angiogenesis. Prog Clin Biol Res 1988; 266:131–145.
45. Riches DW. The multiple roles of Mø in wound healing. In: Clark RAF, Henson PM, eds. The Molecular and Cellular Biology of Wound Repair. New York: Plenum, 1988:23–36.
46. Ross R, Odland GF. Human wound repair. II. Inflammatory cells, epithelial-mesenchymal interrelations and fibrogenesis. J Cell Biol 1968; 39:152–168.
47. Danon D, Kowatch MA, Roth GS. Promotion of repair in old mice by local injection of Mø. Proc Natl Acad Sci U S A 1989; 86:2018–2020.
48. Browder W, Williams D, Lucore P, Pretus H, Jones E, McNamee R. Effect of enhanced macrophage function on early wound healing. Surgery 1988; 104:224–230.
49. Koch AE, Polverini PJ, Leibovich SJ. Stimulation of neovascularization by human rheumatoid synovial tissue Mø. Arthritis Rheum 1986; 29:471–479.
50. Jaffe EA, Ruggiero JT, Falcone DJ. Monocytes and Mø synthesize and secrete thrombospondin. Blood 1985; 65:79–84.
51. Vilette D, Setiadi H, Wautier M-P, Caen J, Wautier J-L. Identification of an endothelial cell growth inhibitory activity produced by human monocytes. Exp Cell Res 1990; 188:219–225.
52. Besner GE, Klagsbrun M. Mø secrete a heparin-binding inhibitor of endothelial cell growth. Microvasc Res 1991; 42:187–197.
53. DiPietro LA, Polverini PJ. Role of the macrophage in the positive and negative regulation of wound neovascularization. Behring Inst Mitt 1993; 92:238–247.
54. Ford H, Hoffman RA, Wing EJ, Magee M, McIntyre L, Simmons RL. Characterization of wound cytokines in the sponge matrix model. Arch Surg 1989; 124:1422–1428.

55. Grotendorst G, Grotendorst CA, Gilman T. Production of growth factors (PDGF and TGF-b) at the site of tissue repair. Prog Clin Biol Res 1988; 266:131–145.
56. Rappolee DA, Mark D, Banda MJ, Werb Z. Wound Mø express TGF-α and other growth factors in vivo: analysis by mRNA phenotyping. Science 1988; 241:708–712.
57. Schreiber AB, Winkler ME, Derynck R. Transforming growth factor-α: a more potent angiogenic mediator than epidermal growth factor. Science 1986; 232:1250–1253.
58. Leibovich SJ, Polverini PJ, Shepard HM, Wiseman DM, Shively V, Nusseir N. Macrophage-induced angiogenesis is mediated by tumor necrosis factor-alpha (TNF-α). Nature 1987; 329:630–632.
59. Fajardo LF, Kwan HH, Kowalski J, Prionas SD, Allison AC. Dual role of tumor necrosis factor-alpha in angiogenesis. Am J Pathol 1992; 140:539–544.
60. Fahey TJ, Sherry B, Tracey KJ, van Deventer S, Jones WG, Minei JP, Morgello S, Shires GT, Cerami A. Cytokine production in a model of wound healing: the appearance of MIP-1, MIP-2, cachetin/TNF, and IL-1. Cytokine 1991; 2:2–19.
61. Strieter RM, Kunkel SL, Elner VM, Martonyi CL, Koch AE, Polverini PJ, Elner SG. Interleukin-8: a corneal factor that induces neovascularization. Am J Pathol 1992; 141:1279–128.
62. Koch AE, Polverini PJ, Kunkel SL, Harlow LA, DiPietro LA, Elner VM, Elner SG, Strieter RM. Interleukin-8 (IL-8) is a potent macrophage-derived mediator of angiogenesis that is blocked by IL-8 antibody and antisense oligonucleotides. Science 1992; 258:179–1801.
63. Koch AE, Polverini PJ, Kunkel SL, Harlow LA, DiPietro LA, Elner VM, Elner SG, Strieter RM. Interleukin-8 (IL-8) is a potent macrophage-derived mediator of angiogenesis that is blocked by IL-8 antibody and antisense oligonucleotides. Science 1992; 258:179–1801.
64. Bouck N. Tumor angiogenesis: role of oncogenes and tumor suppressor genes. Cancer Cells 1990; 2:179–185.
65. Bouck N. Angiogenesis: a mechanism by which oncogenes and tumor suppressor genes regulate tumorigenesis. In: Benz CC, Liu ET, eds. Oncogenes and Tumor Suppressor Genes in Human Malignancy. Boston: Kluwer Academic, 1993:359–371.
66. Bornstein P. Diversity of function is inherent in matricellular proteins: an appraisal of thrombospondin 1. J Cell Biol 1995; 130:503–506.
67. Bornstein P. Thrombospondins: structure and regulation of expression. FASEB J 1992; 6:3290–3299.
68. Sage H, Bornstein P. Extracellular proteins that modulate cell-matrix interactions. J Biol Chem 1991; 266:14831–14834.
69. Lawler J. The structural and functional properties of thrombospondin. Blood 1986; 67:1197–1209.
70. Frazier WA. Thrombospondin: a modular adhesive glycoprotein of platelets and nucleated cells. J Cell Biol 1987; 105:625–632.
71. Frazier WA. Thrombospondin. Curr Opin Cell Biol 1991; 3:792–799.
72. Good DJ, Polverini PJ, Rastinejad F, Le Beau MM, Lemons RS, Frazier WA, Bouck NP. A tumor suppressor-dependent inhibitor of angiogenesis is immunologically and

functionally indistinguishable from a fragment of thrombospondin. Proc Natl Acad Sci U S A 1990; 87:6624–6628.

73. Bornstein P, Sage HE. Thrombospondins. Methods Enzymol 1994; 245:62–85.
74. Rastinejad F, Polverini PJ, Bouck NP. Regulation of the activity of a new inhibitor of angiogenesis by a cancer suppressor gene. Cell 1989; 56:345–355.
75. Sage H, Bornstein P. Endothelial cells from umbilical vein and a hemangioendothelioma secrete basement membrane largely to the exclusion of interstitial procollagens. Arteriosclerosis 1982; 2:27–36.
76. DiPietro LA, Nebgen DR, Polverini PJ. Downregulation of endothelial cell thrombospondin 1 enhances in vitro angiogenesis. J Vasc Res 1994; 31:178–185.
77. DiPietro LA, Nissen NN, Gamelli RL, Koch AE, Pyle JM, Polverini PJ. Thrombospondin 1 synthesis and function in wound repair. Am J Pathol 1996; 148:1851–1860.
78. Polverini PJ, DiPietro LA, Dixit VM, Hynes RO, Lawler J: Thrombospondin 1 knockout mice show delayed organization and neovascularization of skin wounds. FASEB J 1995; 9:272A.
79. DiPietro LA, Polverini PJ. Angiogenic Mø produce the angiogenesis inhibitor thrombospondin 1. Am J Pathol 1994; 143:678–684.
80. Silverstein RL, Nachman RL. Thrombospondin binds to monocytes and Mø and mediates platelet-monocyte adhesion. J Clin Invest 1987; 79:867–874.
81. Mantovani A. Biology of disease. Tumor-associated Mø in neoplastic progression: a paradigm for the in vivo function of chemokines. Lab Invest 1994; 71:5–16.
82. Evans R. Effect of x-irradiation on host cell infiltration and growth of murine fibrosarcoma. Br J Cancer 1977; 35:557–566.
83. Evans R. The effect of azothioprine on host-cell infiltration and growth of a murine fibrosarcoma. Int J Cancer 1977; 20:120–128.
84. Evans R. Macrophage requirement for growth of murine fibrosarcoma. Br J Cancer 1978; 37:1086–1095.
85. Mostafa LK, Jones DB, Wright DH. Mechanism of induction of angiogenesis by human neoplastic lymphoid tissue: studies on the chorioallantoic membrane (CAM) of the chick embryo. J Pathol 1980; 132:197–205.
86. Mostafa LK, Jones DB, Wright DH. Mechanism of induction of angiogenesis by human neoplastic lymphoid tissue: studies employing bovine aortic endothelial cells in vitro. J Pathol 1980; 132:207–216.
87. Stenzinger W, Bruggen J, Macher E, Sorg C. Tumor angiogenic activity (TAA) production in vivo and growth in the nude mouse by human malignant melanoma. Eur J Cancer Clin Oncol 1983; 19:649–656.
88. Polverini PJ, Leibovich SJ. Effect of macrophage depletion on growth and neovascularization of hamster buccal pouch carcinomas. J Oral Pathol 1987; 16:436–441.
89. Polverini PJ, Leibovich SJ. Induction of neovascularization in vivo and endothelial cell proliferation in vitro by tumor-associated Mø. Lab Invest 1984; 51:635–642.

21
Phenotypic Analysis of Endothelium from the Tumor Vasculature

Gerard Groenewegen
University Hospital Utrecht, Utrecht, The Netherlands

Arjan W. Griffioen
University Hospital Maastricht, Maastricht, The Netherlands

I. INTRODUCTION

Endothelial cells (EC) function as a barrier between bloodstream and tissue. There are probably similarities in function of endothelium in normal and tumor tissue; however, studies addressing this issue are limited. Those that have been done are hampered by a lack of techniques to analyze the phenotype of microvascular endothelium from the tumor vasculature. We recently developed a flow cytometry technique for this phenotypic analysis. It was used to study adhesion molecule expression in the tumor vasculature and other characteristics of tumor endothelial cells (TEC).

Endothelial cells play a role in the process of leukocyte extravasation during inflammatory responses. For this process, EC express a set of different adhesion molecules, allowing selective extravasation of subsets of leukocytes in selected sites of the vasculature. Different adhesion molecules participate in the adhesion cascade. The regulated expression of endothelial adhesion molecules allows a fine regulation of leukocyte extravasation. The most studied endothelial adhesion molecules are intercellular adhesion molecule (ICAM), vascular cell adhesion molecule (VCAM) and E-selectin. A brief description of the adhesion cascade allows that both VCAM and E-selection slow the velocity of the leukocytes in the blood vessel by brief interaction (rolling) with the respective ligands on the leukocytes (very late antigen-4 (VLA4) and E-selectin ligand). This interaction also causes activation of the leukocyte, with subsequent elevation in integrin expression. The reduced velocity allows tight binding of long duration to ICAM-1, necessary for transendothelial migration of the bound leukocyte. These processes have been reviewed extensively (1). However, this information was obtained in inflammation-based research. The situation in the tumor vasculature regarding endothelial expression of adhesion molecules has not been studied extensively, although available information has been reviewed (2). At this moment, the number of papers addressing endothelial adhesion molecule expression in many different tumor types is increasing. A complete overview cannot be presented yet. We will describe techniques used in our laboratory for analysis of adhesion molecule expression on tumor endothelium. These techniques also can be used to study other aspects of the phenotype of tumor EC.

II. IMMUNOHISTOCHEMISTRY

Standard immunohistochemistry can be used to obtain qualitative data on the expression of endothelial adhesion molecules (EAM) in the tumor vasculature.

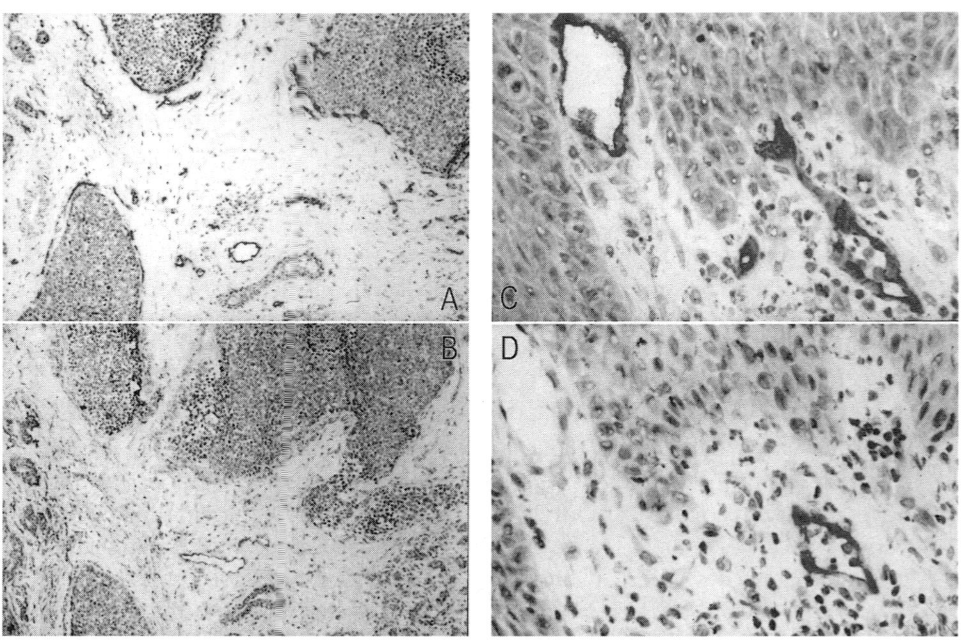

Figure 1 Immunohistochemistry for PAL-E (**A** and **C**), intercellular adhesion molecule (ICAM)-1 (**B**) and E-selectin (**D**) in representative cases of breast cancer (**A** and **B**) and head and neck squamous cell carcinoma (**C** and **D**).

Table 1 Expression of EAM by Capillaries and Postcapillary Venules

		ICAM-1				PECAM-1				VCAM-1				E-selectin			
EAM	n	0[b]	1	2	3	0	1	2	3	0	1	2	3	0	1	2	3
Tumor																	
Breast	18[a]	0/0[c]	0/2	16/16	2/0	0/1	0/2	3/5	15/10	17/17	1/1	0/0	0/0	18/18	0/0	0/0	0/0
RCC	12	0/0	0/1	4/10	8/1	0/0	0/0	0/0	12/12	2/8	3/3	5/1	2/0	12/12	0/0	0/0	0/0
Ovary	6	0/0	0/0	4/4	2/2	0/0	0/0	0/1	6/5	5/6	1/0	0/0	0/0	6/6	0/0	0/0	0/0
HNSCC	18	0/0	0/0	4/5	14/13	0/0	0/0	0/0	18/18	17/18	1/0	0/0	0/0	2/6	6/2	10/10	0/0

[a] Number of cases studied.

[b] Semiquantitative scoring: 0 = negative, 3 = all structures positive.

[c] Number of tumors with staining for capillaries/postcapillary venules.

Abbreviations: EAM, endothelial adhesion molecules; *ICAM-1*, intercellular adhesion molecule-1; *PECAM-1*, platelet endothelial cell adhesion molecule-1; *VCAM-1*, vascular cell adhesion molecule; *RCC*, renal cell carcinoma; *HNSCC*, squamous cell carcinoma of the head and neck.

Monoclonal antibodies against adhesion molecules are widely available. Markers of endothelium, such as CD34, CD31, EN4, and the antibody PAL-E (3), can be used in double-label staining techniques or by staining serial sections of a tumor. Figure 1 shows an example of the expression of ICAM-1 and E-selectin in breast cancer and squamous cell carcinoma of head and neck region (HNSCC) respectively; endothelium is identified with PAL-E-staining. Results from our laboratory regarding EAM expression in different human tumors are summarized in Table 1. Intercellular adhesion molecule-1 was detected in all tumors studied. Quantitative differences between different tumor types (breast, renal cell, ovarian adenocarcinoma, and HNSCC) were suggested by a difference in fraction of capillaries and postcapillary venules (PCV) stained; expression was lowest in breast cancer and highest in HNSCC. Additionally, in a series of 18 different HNSCC, E-selectin expression was noted in 16 cases—in 4 cases on capillaries only and in 12 cases on both capillaries and PCV. We did not observe E-selectin expression in the tumor vasculature in any of 36 cases of malignancies of different origin. E-selectin expression was reported by others, based on immunohistochemistry, to be present in dermal tumors (4,5), renal cell carcinoma (6), and colorectal cancer (7).

We noted VCAM-1 only in a subset of cases of renal cell carcinoma and to a very limited extent in the other tumors studied. Endothelial expression of this adhesion molecule has been reported in melanoma (8), albeit at a reduced level.

Although this technique yields topographical information on EAM-expression, immunohistochemistry is not suitable for quantifying expression. We, therefore, developed a technique for quantifying expression of endothelial adhesion molecules on a per-cell basis: flow cytometry of tumor EC.

III. FLOW CYTOMETRY

Flow cytometry allows the determination of expressed antigens on a per-cell basis. Cells must be examined in a single-cell suspension. Thus, the first issue addressed in the development of a technique for flow cytometry of TEC was the preparation of a single-cell suspension. We selected renal cell carcinoma as the tumor type to be studied because this tumor is known for its high degree of vascularization. When surgery is performed, normal tissue is also removed with the tumor nephrectomy. In this model, control nontransformed tissue can be obtained from the same donor, to allow comparison of TEC and normal tissue-derived endothelial cells (NEC). The local ethical review committee approved the use of fresh human tissue for in vitro research.

In our hands, the single-cell suspension was best obtained when fresh tumor tissue was first mechanically disrupted and then further enzymatically digested with collagenase and dispase. Comparison of 1- vs. 2-hour enzyme treatment showed that with a major increment in time, only a minimum 5% extra of TEC or NEC was obtained. Standard incubation time of 1 hour was chosen. After washing to remove enzymes, a brief adherence step was used to select viable cells and remove all nonvital material and nonadhering cells. Depending on the desired experiments, this preparation containing different cell types was released immediately or kept in culture.

A. Identification of EC

Because EC comprise only 10% to 50% (based on marker studies) of the prepared single-cell suspension, identification of the TEC and NEC is necessary. We selected two different markers for EC: uptake of DiI-LDL (9) and binding of the antibody EN4. DiI-LDL is an acetylated low density lipoprotein (LDL) conjugated to the red fluorochrome diI. It is taken up only by cells with an LDL receptor, such as monocytes/macrophages, EC, and hepatocytes. DiI-LDL can be analyzed by flow cytometry in the red part of the spectrum. Hepatocytes can be assumed to be absent from renal cell carcinomas and normal renal tissue. Monocytes/macrophages, likely to be present after the adherence step in the isolation, are not expected to be released by ethylenediaminetetraacetic acid (EDTA) or enzyme incubation from tissue culture plastic. Additionally, EC and peripheral blood mononuclear cells can be separated based on differences in forward/sideward scatter characteristics (Fig. 2). Therefore, EC will be the only cells present

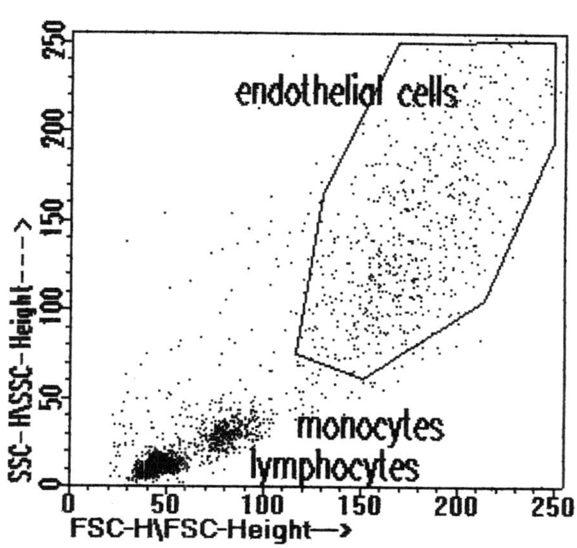

Figure 2 Flow cytometry forward/sideward characteristics after mixing human umbilical vein endothelial cells (HUVEC) and peripheral blood mononuclear cells in a 1:1 ratio. Populations have been labeled accordingly.

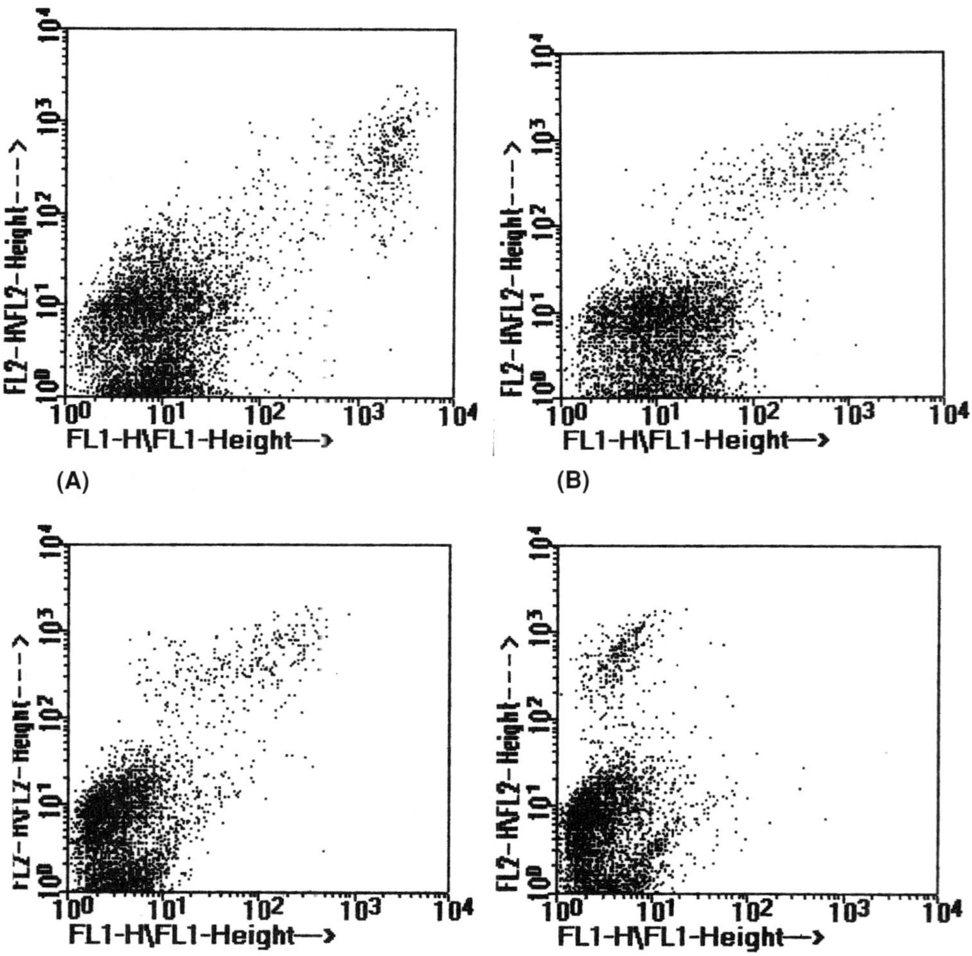

Figure 3 Fluorescence intensities of endothelial cells (EC) labeled with EN4 (vertical axis) and the EC markers CD105 (**A**), intercellular adhesion molecule (ICAM)-2 (**B**), and CD34 (**C**), all on the horizontal axis. In panel **D**, the conjugate control for these antibodies is shown.

in the flow cytometry sample that are stained by DiI-LDL. The EN4 monoclonal antibody recognizes a structure present on capillary, arteriolar, and venular endothelial cells, as reported from immunohistochemistry studies (3). Initial experiments in our laboratory with cultured human umbilical vein EC and dermis-derived microcapillary EC revealed that this marker is suitable for fluorescence-activated cell sorter (FACS) analysis.

Additional identification of EC can be obtained by staining TEC or NEC for expression of CD34, a structure present on EC and hematopoietic stem cells; of CD 105/endoglin (10), the transforming growth factor β receptor normally present on EC; or ICAM-2, an adhesion molecule present only on EC. Regarding the possible roles of these latter three molecules in control of phenotype of TEC, preference for EC identification was in the use of antibody EN4. This antibody was visualized by direct or indirect labeling with fluorescein isothiocyanate (FITC), a green fluorchrome, or phyco-erythrin (PE), a red fluorchrome. Phycoerythrin can be discriminated by FACS on both wavelength and intensity from DiI.

Double staining with EN4-FITC and the EC markers CD105, ICAM-2, and CD34 resulted in double-positive and double-negative population by FACS analysis, demonstrating identification of endothelium (Fig. 3). In addition, these double-positive cells have forward/sideward scatter characteristics similar to cultured EC. In summary, positive TEC identification is based on staining with EC-specific markers and forward/sideward scatter characteristics.

IV. APPLICATIONS OF FLOW CYTOMETRY TECHNIQUE

A. ICAM-1

We used the described FACS technique for the analysis of ICAM-1 expression in the TEC of renal cell carcinoma compared to the NEC removed at tumor nephrectomy (11). We observed that on all occasions, the expression of ICAM-1 by TEC was lower than by NEC from the same donor. These findings have been summarized in Figure 4, and one representative experiment of this series is shown in Figure 5.

We hypothesized that angiogenic factors are the causative agents for the down-regulation of ICAM-1 in the tumor vasculature. In vitro experiments with human umbilical vein EC (HUVEC) and dermis-derived capillary EC revealed that addition of basic fibroblast growth factor (bFGF) to these cells resulted in increased expression of ICAM-1 after 24 hours; longer incubation periods (72 hours) with bFGF resulted in near-total loss of ICAM-1 from the cell membrane. Similar results were obtained with exposure of HUVEC to vascular endothelial growth factor (VEGF). This down-regulated expression of ICAM-1 also was noted in adhesion assays with adhering cells using ICAM-1. Northern blot analy-

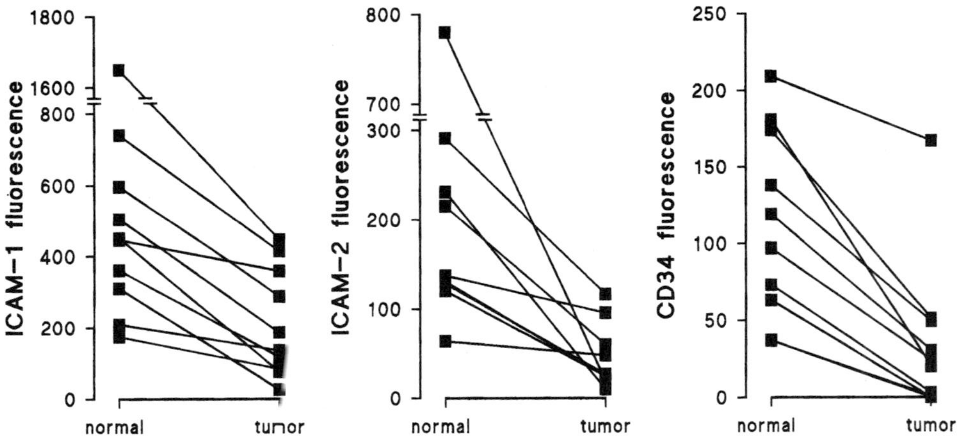

Figure 4 Comparison of fluorescence intensities for intercellular adhesion molecule (ICAM)-1, ICAM-2, and CD34 in tumor endothelial cells (EC) and normal tissue EC of different donors.

sis revealed that bFGF caused down-regulation of ICAM-1 expression by decreasing the number of copies of relevant mRNA (11).

Basic fibroblast growth factor not only induces down-regulation of expression of ICAM-1, this angiogenic factor also causes a state of EC anergy regarding the proinflammatory effect of tumor necrosis factor (TNF)α for increased expression of ICAM-1. Exposure of HUVEC to bFGF for 72 hours nearly completely prevented up-regulation by TNFα of ICAM-1 on EC, as observed in EC not exposed to bFGF. Also, incubation of TEC in TNFα had little influence on ICAM-1 expression, whereas incubation of NEC in TNFα resulted in significant up-regulation of ICAM-1 (12). We hypothesized that angiogenic factors play a role in the escape of tumors from inflammatory responses and infiltrating leukocytes by down-regulating expression of EAM in the tumor vasculature and by preventing up-regulation of endothelial adhesion molecules by proinflammaratory cytokines such as TNFα.

B. ICAM-2

As with ICAM-1 we also noted a decreased expression of ICAM-2 in the tumor vasculature (Figs. 4 and 5). The regulatory processes underlying ICAM-2 expression have not been studied for TEC. The contribution to the hypothesized immune escape needs further analysis.

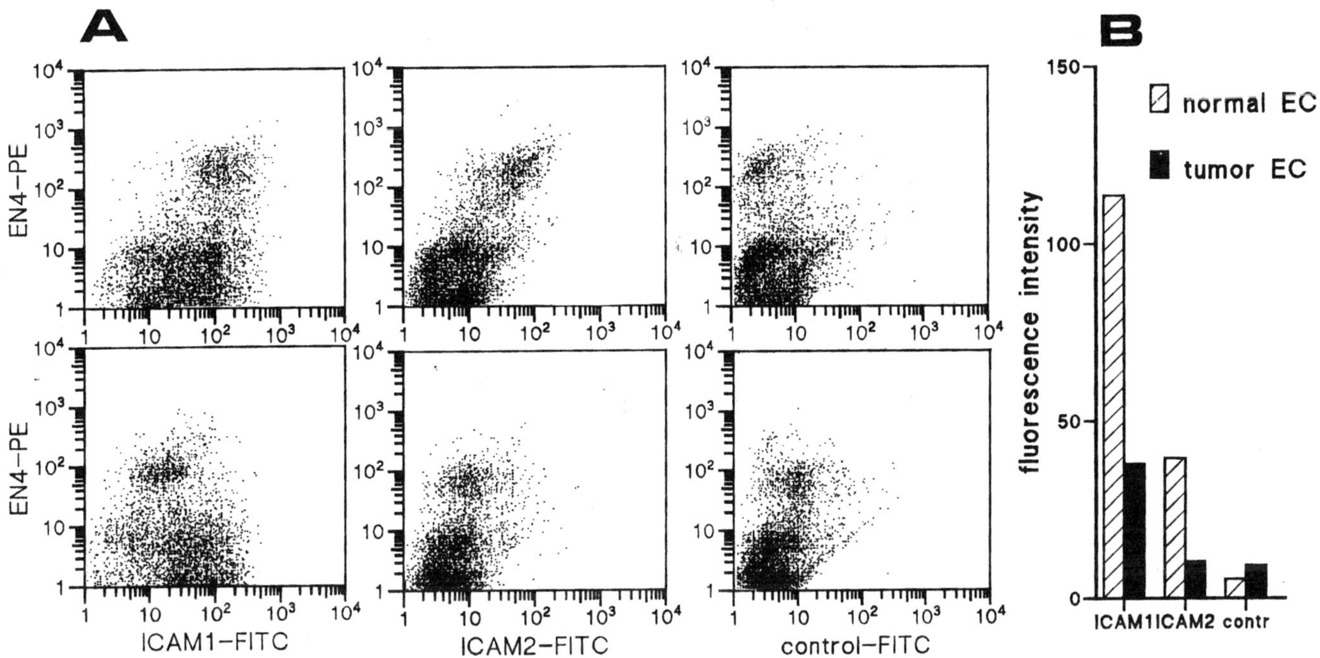

Figure 5 Suppressed endothelial intercellular adhesion molecule (ICAM)-1 and ICAM-2 expression in a representative case of renal cell carcinoma (*lower panels*), compared with normal renal tissue-derived endothelium (*upper panels*) is shown in **part A. Part B** shows a histogram of the mean fluorescence intensities of this experiment.

C. CD44

Because CD44 is a marker of activation on lymphocytes and other cell types, we also analyzed the expression of CD44 on EC of the tumor vasculature containing proliferating EC. It can be assumed that EC are somehow activated during angiogenesis. Therefore the expression of CD44 by these cells is of interest in analysis of TEC phenotype. We observed that CD44 is not present on HUVEC while they are still in the untreated umbilical cord, but that isolation of these cells results in the rapid appearance of CD44 on HUVEC. This expression is further increased by exposure to bFGF. Immunohistochemical localization of CD44 on renal cell carcinoma revealed a semiquantitative increase in expression in tumors compared with normal renal tissue. Flow cytometry demonstrated increased expression levels of CD44 on TEC compared with NEC (13).

D. CD34

We also analyzed the endothelial expression of CD34 in cell suspension of tumor tissue. The antigen is considered a marker for endothelium (3) and could be detected as expected on isolated EC. As shown in Figure 4, TEC express lower levels of CD34 than NEC. Further studies revealed that similar to ICAM-1, the expression of this antigen is affected by angiogenic factors (14). Recent observations have noted that the expression of CD34 is inversely related to other adhesion molecules (15) as well as the function of CD34 as an adhesion molecule (16). Further studies are needed to elucidate these issues.

E. Proliferation

Exposure of cells to 5-bromodeoxyuridine (BrdU) allows the detection of cells that were in S-phase of the cell cycle shortly before analysis. This technique also was applied to phenotype TEC in regard to proliferation. The permeabilization necessary for the demonstration of BrdU did not prevent the staining with the EN4-antibody to identify EC during flow cytometry. When both TEC and NEC were briefly exposed to BrdU during the isolation procedure and then stained with EN4 and anti-BrdU, a higher fraction of TEC-incorporated BrdU compared to the NEC was noted (data not shown).

This finding is in line with proliferation of EC during angiogenesis. Double- and triple-staining experiments will allow further discrimination between subsets of EC in areas of angiogenesis.

V. CONCLUDING REMARKS

The two techniques described here—immunohistochemistry and flow cytometry of EC from the tumor vasculature—can be used to analyze antigens present on tumor endothelium. Immunohistochemistry will give topographical information on distribution of the antigens. Flow cytometry will yield quantitative data on antigen expression on a per cell base. The isolation procedure used also allows the study of the effects of soluble mediators on this antigen expression. The technique can be used to sort EC from the tumor cell population, as a start for further experiments. Inclusion of normal tissue as comparison for tumor tissue as starting material allows the detection of in vitro artifacts during the experiments. We therefore consider the technique of flow cytometry of tumor vasculature derived endothelial cells a useful technique for the study of the phenotype of these cells.

We observed that there is a number of differences in the phenotype of EC derived from normal and from tumor tissue.

One of the general features of TEC is a decreased expression of EAM. However, activation markers like CD44 are expressed at a higher level. A role for angiogenetic factors is likely in the generation of these difference in phenotype between TEC and NEC, both for the down-regulated expression of ICAM-1 and the upregulated expression of CD44. Future studies will reveal whether the knowledge on phenotype and control of phenotype during angiogenesis of EC in the tumor vasculature can contribute to tumor therapy.

ACKNOWLEDGMENT

The authors are grateful to the local and regional urologists for supplying fresh tumor tissue. We appreciate the technical assistance of Cora Damen and the secretarial assistance of Marinella Bruinsma. Immunohistochemistry data were derived from the work of Karel Bos.

REFERENCES

1. Roitt IM, Brostof J, Male DK. Cell migration and inflammation. In: Immunology. London: Mosby, 1996.
2. Jain RK, Koenig GC, Dellian M, Fukumura D, Munn LL, Melder RJ. Leukocyte-endothelial adhesion and angiogenesis in tumors. Cancer Metastasis Rev 1996; 15: 195–204.
3. Schlingemann RO, Rietveld FJR, Kwaspen F, van de Kerkhof PCM, de Waal RMW, Ruiter DJ. Differential expression of markers of endothelial cells, pericytes and basal lamina in the vasculature of tumors and granulation tissue. Am J Pathol 1991; 138: 1335–1347.
4. Groves RW, Allen MH, Ross EL, Ashan G, Barker JN, MacDonald DM. Expression

of selectin ligands by cutaneous squamous cell carcinoma. Am J Pathol 1993; 143: 1220–1225.

5. Schadendorf D, Heidel J, Gawlik C, Suter C, Czarnetzki BM. Association with clinical outcome of expression of VLA-4 in primary cutaneous malignant melanoma as well as P-selectin and E-selectin in intratumoral vessels. J Natl Cancer Inst 1995; 87:366–371.
6. Droz D, Patey N, Paraf F, Chretien Y, Gugosev J. Composition of extracellular matrix and distribution of cell adhesion molecules in renal cell tumors. Lab Invest 1994; 71:710–748.
7. Ye C, Kiriyama K, Mistuoka C, Kannagi R, Watanabe T, Kondo K, Akiyama S, Takagi H. Expression of E-selectin on endothelial cells of small veins in human colorectal cancer. Int J Cancer 1995; 61:455–460.
8. Piali L, Fichtel A, Terpe HJ, Imhof BA, Gisler RH. Endothelial vascular cell adhesion molecule 1 expression is suppressed by melanoma and carcinoma. J Exp Med 1995; 181:811–816.
9. Netland PA, Zetter B, Via DP, Voyta JC. In situ labeling of vascular endothelium with fluorescent acetylated low density lipoprotein. Histochem J 1985; 17:1309–1320.
10. Griffioen AW, Damen CA, Blijham GH, Groenewegen G. Endoglin/CD105 expression on tumor endothelial cells. Breast Cancer Res Treat 1996; 39:239–40.
11. Griffioen AW, Damen CA, Martinotti S, Blijham GH, Groenewegen G. Endothelial ICAM-1 expression is suppressed in human malignancies: role of angiogenic factors. Cancer Res 1996; 56:1111–1117.
12. Griffioen AW, Damen CA, Blijham GH, Groenewegen G. Tumor angiogenesis is accompanied by a decreased inflammatory response of tumor associated endothelium. Blood 1996; 88:667–673.
13. Griffioen AW, Coenen MJH, Damen CA, Hellwig SMM, van Weering DHJ, Vooys W, Blijham GH, Groenewegen G. CD44 is involved in tumor angiogenesis: an activation antigen on human endothelial cells. Blood 1997; 90:1150–1159.
14. Hellwig SMM, Damen CA, van Adrichem NPH, Blijham GH, Groenewegen G, Griffioen AW. Endothelial CD34 is suppressed in human malignancies: role of angiogenic factors. Cancer Letters 1997; 120:203–211.
15. Delia D, Lampugnani MG, Resnati M, Dejana E, Aiello A, Fontanella E, Soligo D, Pierotti MA, Greaves MF. CD34 expression is regulated reciprocally with adhesion molecules in vascular endothelial cells in vitro. Blood 1993; 81:1001–1008.
16. Baumhueter S, Singer MS, Henzel W, Hemmerich S, Renz M, Rosen SD, Lasky LA. Binding of L-selectin to the vascular sialomucin CD34. Science 1993; 262:436–438.

22

Drug Delivery and Angiogenesis Inhibition in the Treatment of Brain Tumors

Laurence D. Rhines
The University of Texas M.D. Anderson Cancer Center, Houston, Texas

Matthew G. Ewend
University of North Carolina, Chapel Hill, North Carolina

Henry Brem
Johns Hopkins University School of Medicine, Baltimore, Maryland

I. BACKGROUND

The growth of solid tumors depends on the development of new blood vessels. In the absence of a blood supply, the three-dimensional growth of solid tumors is restricted by the limits of simple diffusion for delivery of nutrients and removal of wastes (1). In this avascular state, tumors grow slowly until an equilibrium is reached between the rate of cell proliferation at the periphery and the rate of cell death at the center (2). These tumors may remain viable for a prolonged period; however, they are considered dormant from the perspective of growth and metastatic potential.

Neoplastic cells are able to induce the activation of endothelial cells within the host microvasculature. This begins a cascade of endothelial cell proliferation, production of proteolytic enzymes leading to matrix degradation, migration, and invasion, which results in the formation of new blood vessels (3–6). This process, known as tumor angiogenesis, enables a dormant, avascular tumor to become vascularized. Once in this vascular phase of growth, the tumor is maintained by direct perfusion as opposed to diffusion from the periphery. Growth becomes rapid and tumor volume increases exponentially (1, 7). For neoplasms prone to metastasis, it is during this phase that metastatic colonies are most often detected (3, 8).

When Folkman initially described this phenomenon of tumor angiogenesis and demonstrated the existence of a tumor-angiogenesis factor, he introduced a new perspective into the treatment of malignant neoplasms (7, 9). If the induction of the vascular phase of tumor growth could be blocked, perhaps disease progression could be slowed or even halted.

Cartilage was the first tissue extensively examined for antiangiogenic properties. Because cartilage is vascularized in the embryo and avascular in the adult and had been observed to remain avascularized after implantation on the chorioallantoic membrane, it was selected as a possible source of inhibitors of angiogenesis. Initial studies showed that a diffusible material from cartilage inhibits capillary proliferation induced by tumors (10). Further extraction and purification yielded a cartilage fraction, the major component of which was a 16,000-dalton protein, with potent inhibitory effects on tumor-induced vascular proliferation (11). This discovery was significant in that it represented the first description of an antiangiogenesis factor. It is also noteworthy because the issues of bioavailability raised by the discovery of this new class of compounds provided an impetus for major advances in the field of drug delivery, some of which are currently in clinical use.

II. POLYMERIC DRUG DELIVERY

The fact that the antiangiogenic cartilage fraction contained large-molecular-weight proteins and that local, sustained exposure to safe doses of these compounds might be necessary to prevent angiogenesis, presented a challenging problem of drug delivery. In addition to being able to incorporate large molecules and release them locally in a sustained fashion, the delivery vehicle also needed to be biologically inert.

The development of biocompatible, controlled-release polymers provided a solution to many of these drug delivery issues. The first of these polymers were nonbiodegradable. An example of such a nonbiodegradable polymer is the ethyl-vinyl acetate copolymer (EVAc), which is biologically inert. It releases incorporated drugs by diffusion. In 1976, Langer and Folkman used EVAc polymers to achieve controlled release of biologically active molecules (12). These polymers also were used to release cartilage-derived angiogenesis inhibitors in the rabbit cornea model (11) This delivery system has been studied extensively and has been critical for establishing proof of the principle that controlled-release polymers provide a feasible, effective, and well-tolerated means of interstitial drug delivery. The major limitation of EVAc and other nonbiodegradable polymers, however, is that they remain as foreign bodies long after the drug has been completely released. This has limited the clinical use of these polymers.

Biodegradable polymers, as typified by the polyanhydrides, do not have this limitation. They release drug by erosion, or a combination of diffusion and erosion. These polymers degrade completely in water and release their incorporated drugs in the process. Thus, no foreign body remains after completion of drug release. Furthermore, the breakdown products are nontoxic and nonmutagenic (13). Two polyanhydride controlled-release systems have been studied most extensively. The first of these is poly (bis[p-carboxyphenoxy] propane-sebacic acid) (p[CPP-SA]). This polymer can be produced in a variety of forms including wafers, sheets, rods, microspheres, or nanospheres (14). Incorporation of the drug is a simple process that can be performed at room temperature. Modification of the CPP:SA ratio allows the time course of degradation to be optimized for the desired period of drug release. The p(CPP-SA) polymers are particularly well suited for delivery of hydrophobic compounds such as the nitrosoureas. The second polyanhydride polymer is fatty acid dimer-sebacic acid (FAD-SA). As with p(CPP-SA), drugs can be incorporated at room temperature and the polymer can be produced in a variety of forms. Fatty acid dimer-sebacic acid polymers, however, may be better suited for the delivery of hydrophilic and hydrolytically unstable compounds like carboplatin or methotrexate (15).

III. POLYMER-BASED LOCAL THERAPY FOR MALIGNANT BRAIN TUMORS

Despite advances in surgical technique, radiotherapy, and chemotherapy, the prognosis for patients with malignant gliomas remains dismal. Even with the most aggressive therapy, these tumors almost invariably recur, and 90% of them recur locally within 2 cm of the original resection site (16).

Chemotherapy for brain tumors has been limited, primarily by the lack of effective methods of drug delivery. The unique properties of tumor microvascular architecture and the presence of the blood-brain barrier make it difficult for efficacious levels of systemically delivered agents to reach brain tumor parenchyma. Tumor microvessels tend to be dilated and tortuous. Their organization is highly variable from one area of the tumor to another. In addition, their microvascular pressures tend to be low, particularly in relation to the high local interstitial pressures. These factors result in diminished blood flow within tumor vessels, and this limits the ability of agents within the bloodstream to reach tumor tissue. The presence of the blood-brain barrier further inhibits the movement of molecules from the blood to the brain. Anatomically, it is the tight junctions between the endothelial cells of the cerebral capillaries that form this barrier. Although it is essential for maintaining the biochemical milieu of the central nervous system, the blood-brain barrier significantly restricts the access of systemically delivered agents to the brain, particularly agents that are high in molecular weight, hydrophilic, or charged (17). Consequently, systemic administration of chemotherapeutic compounds often fails to achieve therapeutic concentrations within tumor despite toxic systemic levels.

The ability of polymeric delivery systems to locally release large molecules of varied hydrophobicity and charge in a controlled, biologically compatible fashion made the application of these systems to brain tumor therapy a natural choice. Not only could polymer-mediated interstitial therapy allow a variety of chemotherapeutic agents to be delivered in high concentrations directly at the site of the tumor, and a probable future recurrence, but the major impediments of access across the blood-brain barrier and systemic toxicity could be minimized.

IV. PRECLINICAL STUDIES

Before any specific agents could be tested in the polymers, the biocompatibility and biodistribution of the polymer itself needed to be rigorously tested. The p(CPP-SA) polymers were tested in vivo in the rabbit cornea, and rabbit, rat, and monkey brains. In the rabbit cornea assay, the polymers did not provoke a visible inflammatory response, nor was there any histological evidence of corneal neovascularization, edema, or inflammatory infiltrates during a 6-week implantation period (13). In the rat and rabbit brains, polymer implantation was similarly well tolerated. No animals displayed evidence of systemic or neurological toxicity. Histologically, the inflammatory response was minimal and transient, comparable to that provoked by commonly used biodegradable hemostatic implants such as Surgicel and Gelfoam (18, 19). Finally, implantation in the monkey brain confirmed the safety of the polymer (20).

The biodistribution of the p(CPP-SA) polymer was also examined. Two polymer types, one with [^{14}C]-radiolabeled SA and unlabeled CPP and the other with [^{14}C]-labeled CPP and unlabeled SA, were used to study the distribution and elimination of each monomer after polymer degradation in the rat brain. [^{14}C] Sebacic acid was released from the polymer in approximately 7 days. Eliminated radioactivity was found primarily in expired CO_2, as well as in the urine and feces. Unlike the SA monomer, the CPP monomer has very limited solubility in water. Thus, its elimination from the site of polymer implantation is slow and is probably dependent on the action of macrophages and other inflammatory cells once the polymer has disintegrated into smaller fragments (21, 22).

Once the biocompatibility and biodistribution of the p(CPP-SA) polymer were established, drug release and clinical efficacy could then be addressed. The drug chosen was the chemotherapeutic agent, carmustine, 1,3-bis(2-chloroethyl)-1-nitrosourea (BCNU). Nitrosoureas are a class of alkylating agents that are non-ionized and highly lipid soluble. This allows them some degree of penetration across the blood-brain barrier. BCNU was selected because it has been the most commonly used and most effective chemotherapeutic agent for brain tumors. Systemic administration of this drug has resulted in modest increases in patient survival, although its efficacy has been limited by side effects including myelosuppression, liver toxicity, and pulmonary fibrosis (23). It was hoped that polymer-based interstitial delivery of BCNU could result in higher local concentration, thereby increasing efficacy while avoiding systemic toxicity.

The in vivo biodistribution of BCNU delivered from intracranially implanted p(CPP-SA) (20:80 formulation) polymers was assessed in the rabbit brain by quantitative autoradiography. The intracerebral distribution of tritium-labeled BCNU released from polymers was compared to that of BCNU delivered through direct stereotactic injection. Three days after polymer implantation, radioactivity associated with BCNU was dispersed throughout the ipsilateral hemisphere. Three weeks after implantation, the brain tissue surrounding the degrading implant still showed drug concentrations two standard deviations above background. By contrast, such drug levels were no longer detectable 48 hours after direct injection (24). This study established that polymeric delivery could achieve a high, sustained, local concentration of BCNU in the brain. Subsequently, Fung and colleagues explored the pharmacokinetics and biodistribution of polymer-released BCNU, taxol, and 4-hydroperoxycyclophosphamide (4-HC) in the monkey brain. Using quantitative autoradiography, thin-layer chromatography, and scintillation counting, they have shown that BCNU levels achieved throughout the ipsilateral hemisphere 24 hours after polymer implantation are at least an order of magnitude higher than those achieved with maximal intravenous carmustine administration. Furthermore, significant levels of BCNU were detected 4 cm from the polymer implantation site 1 day after surgery, 2 cm from the implant at 7 days postoperatively, and 1.3 cm from the implantation site 30 days after surgery. This has confirmed that in the primate, polymers can be used to deliver high local drug levels in a sustained fashion (25).

Once the in vivo distribution of polymerically delivered BCNU had been established, the next step was to evaluate the efficacy of the BCNU polymers in an experimental tumor model. Polymeric local delivery of BCNU was compared to systemic (intraperitoneal) delivery in controlling the growth of the 9L gliosarcoma implanted in either the flank or the brain of Fisher 344 rats. For flank tumors, BCNU delivered by polymer was superior to systemic BCNU in limiting tumor growth. Similarly, when 9L gliosarcoma was implanted in the brains of the rats, local polymeric delivery was significantly more effective than systemic delivery at extending survival. The median survival was 11.6 days for the untreated controls, 27.3 days for the group receiving intraperitoneal BCNU, and 62.3 days for the group receiving intracranial BCNU-loaded polymer. Moreover, all of the control animals died by day 19 and all of the systemically treated animals by day 59 after tumor implantation. By contrast, approximately 17% of the BCNU polymer-treated animals were still alive 120 days after tumor challenge (26).

The final preclinical step was to demonstrate the safety and biocompatibility of BCNU-loaded p(CPP-SA) polymers in the primate brain. Macaca fascicularis monkeys receiving BCNU-impregnated polymers showed no physical signs of neurological or systemic toxicity after implantation. Blood tests were normal and radiological studies of the brain revealed degrading polymer with minimal brain reaction and edema. Autopsy and subsequent histologic evaluation were normal, except for some transient, local inflammation in the area of the implant (20).

In summary, the aforementioned preclinical studies demonstrate that BCNU-loaded p(CPP-SA) (20:80) polymers are biocompatible and safe in the brain, provide local delivery of active drug, and inhibit growth of tumor in animal models more effectively than maximal systemic dosages of the same chemotherapeutic agent. These findings were the basis for subsequent human clinical trials.

V. CLINICAL STUDIES

Two phase I-II clinical trials examining the safety of BCNU-loaded p(CPP-SA) polymers in human patients have been conducted. The first of these trials enrolled 21 patients with recurrent malignant gliomas. In these patients, polymer wafers containing BCNU were implanted in the surgical resection cavity at the time of tumor debulking. Three different polymer loading doses of BCNU (1.93%, 3.85%, and 6.37% weight of BCNU) were used. All were safe in the brain and well tolerated by the patients, and none caused any systemic toxicity (27).

A second, separate trial included 22 patients who received BCNU-impregnated p(CPP-SA) polymers at the time of initial craniotomy and tumor resection. Of these patients, 21 had glioblastoma multiforme, and 1 had anaplastic astrocytoma. All patients underwent subsequent standard radiation therapy averaging approximately 5600 cGy. Again, the polymers were well tolerated with no evidence of toxicity. In addition to establishing the safety of the BCNU polymers as the initial therapy for gliomas, the combination of the interstitial chemotherapy and standard radiation therapy also appeared to be safe (28).

The success of these studies led to a large, prospective, randomized, placebo-controlled phase III clinical trial examining the efficacy of p(CPP-SA) polymers containing 3.8% BCNU by weight in treating patients with recurrent malignant gliomas. Two hundred and twenty-two patients were treated at 27 medical centers (of these patients, 110 received polymers containing BCNU and 112 received placebo polymers). In this study, BCNU-loaded polymers significantly prolonged patient survival compared with placebo controls. Median survival was 31 weeks in the group receiving carmustine polymers and 23 weeks in the group receiving the placebo polymers. Furthermore, among patients with glioblastoma multiforme, 6-month survival was 50% greater in the patients treated with BCNU-loaded polymers compared with placebo controls. No clinically significant adverse effects were associated with the implants (29).

A subsequent study in Europe was carried out by Valtonen et al. (30). They performed a prospective, randomized, placebo-controlled study examining the efficacy of the BCNU polymers in treating patients with malignant gliomas when

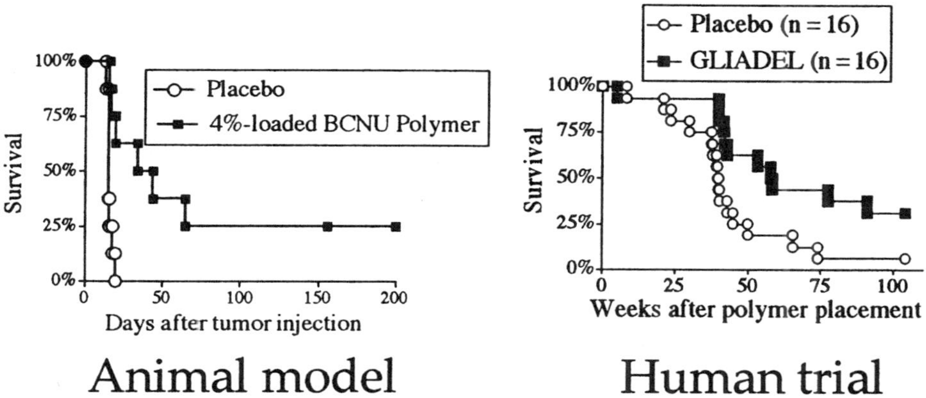

Figure 1 **Left**, survival of rats with intracranial 9L gliosarcoma treated with either BCNU-loaded polymer or empty placebo polymer (50). **Right**, survival of human patients with malignant gliomas treated at the time of initial surgery with Gliadel vs empty placebo polymer (30). The data show that the animal models successfully predict the results achieved in clinical trials.

implanted at the time of the initial surgery. Thirty-two patients from five institutions were randomized into two groups. One group received polymer containing 3.8% BCNU by weight and the other received empty polymer. All patients received standard postoperative radiotherapy. The median survival in the BCNU group was 58 weeks compared with 40 weeks in the control group. Two years after surgery, 33% of the patients who received BCNU were alive compared with 6% in the control group. Finally, 3 years after surgery, 25% of the patients in the BCNU polymer group were alive compared with 6% in the control group (30). Not only do these results demonstrate the efficacy of the BCNU-loaded polymers, but they clearly validate the findings seen in experimental animal brain tumor models (Fig. 1).

On the basis of these studies, the FDA approved the use of 3.8% BCNU-loaded polyanhydride polymers (Gliadel®) for the treatment of patients with recurrent glioblastoma multiforme. This was the first time in 23 years that the FDA had approved a new treatment for gliomas. These studies serve as "proof of principle" that controlled local delivery of therapeutic agents for brain tumors may play a significant role in their treatment.

VI. NEW DIRECTIONS

The preclinical and clinical studies with BCNU-impregnated polyanhydride polymers have served as a model for the evaluation of other potentially promising therapeutic agents aimed at treating brain tumors and other central nervous system diseases. To date, a variety of chemotherapeutic agents have been incorporated into polymers and tested in animal tumor models. 4-Hydroxyperoxycyclophosphamide (4-HC), a hydrophilic derivative of cyclophosphamide that does not require hepatic activation, has been incorporated into FAD-SA polymers and successfully used to treat animals with intracranial F98 gliomas (31). Similarly, carboplatin, a cisplatin derivative, has been incorporated into FAD-SA and p(CPP-SA) polymers and been shown to increase survival in rats bearing F98 intracranial gliomas (32). Camptothecin, a naturally occurring inhibitor of the DNA-replicating enzyme topoisomerase I, has been incorporated into EVAc polymers and, when delivered locally, has been shown to extend survival significantly in rats bearing intracranial 9L gliosarcoma (33). Finally, taxol, a microtubule-binding agent, has been incorporated into polyanhydride polymers and used successfully to extend survival in the rat intracranial 9L gliosarcoma model (34). Recent clinical experience has shown that even though taxol is effective against glioma cells in culture, it is relatively ineffective in patients with gliomas when given intravenously (35). Thus, it is an example of a potent drug that cannot be given systemically, but may offer significant benefit if delivered locally through a polymer implant. Other drugs currently under investigation include camptothecin analogues, taxotere (a taxol derivative), adriamycin, cytokines, and radiosensitizers.

The use of polymers to deliver therapy to the brain is not limited to chemotherapeutic agents. Dilantin, a commonly used anticonvulsant, has a number of systemic side effects, and proper plasma levels can be difficult to maintain. This prompted investigation into the efficacy of local delivery. Controlled, sustained release of dilantin from EVAc polymers effectively reduced the incidence of seizures in the rat model of cobalt-induced epileptic activity (36). In addition, dexamethasone, a corticosteroid used to treat vasogenic edema associated with brain tumors, can have serious adverse effects as a result of long-term systemic administration. When delivered locally by EVAc polymer in the rat 9L intracranial tumor model, dexamethasone was found to be as effective in controlling edema as when given systemically; however, only a fraction of the plasma steroid concentration was attained (37).

VII. POLYMERIC DELIVERY OF ANTIANGIOGENIC DRUGS

In concluding with a discussion of polymer-based local delivery of antiangiogenic drugs, this review has come full circle. Initially used as a vehicle for the sustained release of high-molecular-weight, possibly charged, putative inhibitors of angiogenesis in simple in vivo assays, polymeric delivery systems are now being used to deliver angiogenesis inhibitors directly to brain tumors in animal models as a prelude to potential human clinical trials.

Much experimental evidence supports the strategy of using antiangiogenesis compounds in the treatment of brain tumors. Angiogenic activity has been shown to be a marker of brain tumor malignancy. A grading system for the angiogenic response induced by human neoplasms was developed; it demonstrated that malignant gliomas were the most angiogenic of tumors (38). Moreover, among malignant gliomas, increasing angiogenesis score was associated with increasing degree of anaplasia (39). Biopsy specimens from human brain tumors transplanted to the rabbit cornea induced angiogenesis in proportion to their degree of malignancy (40). Pathologically, high-grade gliomas frequently show florid microvascular proliferation, suggesting that these neoplasms may be highly dependent on induction of new blood vessels for sustained growth. It is likely that other less infiltrative brain tumors (such as meningiomas and hemangiopericytomas) that grow as solid expanding masses also may rely heavily on angiogenesis for growth (41). Cerebrospinal fluid (CSF) from patients with brain tumor induced endothelial cell migration up to 10 times as actively as CSF from patients without tumors (42). In a study of 26 children with brain tumors, basic fibroblast growth factor, a highly angiogenic endothelial cell mitogen, was detected in the CSF of 62% of the patients, and this CSF stimulated mitogenic activity in endothelial cell cultures (43). These findings suggest that brain tumors may be a particularly susceptible target for inhibitors of angiogenesis.

As described at the beginning of this chapter, one early use of the controlled-release polymers was to test the activity of novel putative angiogenesis inhibitors in simple in vivo experimental assays (11). This continues to be an important application. To date, a number of different angiogenesis inhibitors representing several classes of compounds have been incorporated into polymers and shown to inhibit tumor-induced neovascularization in the rabbit corneal micropocket assay. These include cartilage-derived inhibitor, a high-molecular-weight protein extracted from calf cartilage; cortisone and other corticosteroids, the so-called angiostatic steroids; cortisone and heparin combined and released from a single polymer; minocycline, a semisynthetic tetracycline with antimicrobial and anticollagenase activity; and squalamine, a novel aminosterol derived from the dogfish shark (11, 44–47).

Given the performance of these agents when released from polymer in the rabbit cornea assay and the mounting success of polymeric, local delivery of traditional chemotherapeutic agents in treating brain tumors, several of these antiangiogenesis compounds have since been interstitially delivered in experimental brain tumor models. Tamargo et al. have shown that the localized, controlled release of the combination of heparin and cortisone, as well as of cortisone alone, inhibited the growth of a brain tumor, the 9L gliosarcoma, in the rat flank (45).

More recently, the efficacy of polymeric delivery of minocycline has been examined. When implanted adjacent to 9L gliosarcomas in the rat flank, the minocycline-loaded polymers significantly inhibited tumor growth (48). For

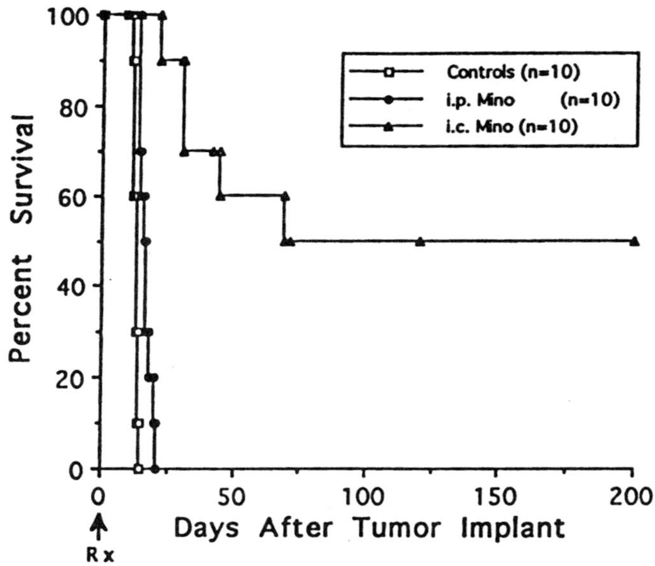

Figure 2 Survival of rats implanted with intracranial 9L gliosarcoma and treated at the time of implantation with minocycline-loaded polymer (i.c. Mino), systemic minocycline (i.p. Mino), or empty polymer (controls). Locally delivered minocycline significantly prolonged survival, whereas systemic minocycline was ineffective.

intracranial 9L tumors controlled-release minocycline polymers significantly extended survival when implanted at the time of tumor implantation or after tumor resection. When polymer treatment was begun 5 days after tumor implantation, no effect on survival was noted unless the polymer implantation was accompanied by a systemic dose of BCNU. In this case, median survival was extended significantly compared with the same systemic dose of BCNU without locally delivered minocycline. In summary, interstitial delivery of minocycline from polymers can prolong survival in rats with malignant brain tumors; however, this efficacy seems to depend on the timing of treatment, the state of the tumor, and concurrent adjuvant therapy (Fig. 2) (49).

VIII. CONCLUSION

The development of safe and effective drug delivery from biodegradable polymers has been a major advance in the treatment of malignant brain tumors. The ability to deliver a variety of different agents at high local concentrations while avoiding systemic toxicity has greatly broadened the range of drugs available to treat this devastating disease and its manifestations. One class of drugs that appears to be of potential importance are the inhibitors of angiogenesis. The role of these antiangiogenic compounds in cancer therapy is evolving as more is learned about their mechanisms of activity. Malignant brain tumors are among the most angiogenic of all malignancies. This suggests that these neoplasms may be a particularly attractive target for antiangiogenic therapy. As we continue to investigate these antiangiogenic agents and combine them with other emerging therapies, optimization of drug delivery will remain a critical issue. Laboratory and clinical experience suggests that local, polymer-based delivery may provide a safe and effective means of administering these therapies to patients, allowing us to continue to offer new hope to individuals with malignant brain tumors.

ACKNOWLEDGMENTS

We wish to thank Drs. Robert Langer, Pamela Talalay, and Rafael Tamargo for help in preparing the manuscript. The preclinical experiments described here were funded in part by the National Cooperative Drug Discovery Group grant U01-CA52857 and by the P20-NS31081 grant from the National Institutes of Health (NIH).

Dr. Brem is a consultant to Guilford Pharmaceuticals, Inc. and to Aventis Pharmaceuticals. The Johns Hopkins University and Dr. Brem own Guilford stock, the sale of which is subject to certain restrictions under University policy. The terms of this arrangement are being managed by the University in accordance with its conflict of interest policies.

Dr. Rhines is a recipient of the NIH National Research Service Award CA-09574.

REFERENCES

1. Knighton D, Ausprunk D, Tapper D, Folkman J. Avascular and vascular phases of tumour growth in the chick embryo. Br J Cancer 1977; 35:347–356.
2. Gimbrone M, Leapman S, Cotran R, Folkman J. Tumor dormancy in vivo by prevention of neovascularization. J Exp Med 1972; 136:261–276.
3. Blood CH, Zetter BR. Tumor interactions with the vasculature: angiogenesis and tumor metastasis. Biochim Biophys Acta 1990; 1032:89–118.
4. Furcht LT. Critical factors controlling angiogenesis: cell products, cell matrix and growth factors. Lab Invest 1986; 55:505–509.
5. D'Amore PA, Thompson RW. Mechanisms of angiogenesis. Annu Rev Physiol 1987; 49:453–464.
6. Folkman J, Brem H. Angiogenesis and inflammation. In: Gallin JI, Goldstein IM,

Snyderman R, eds. Inflammation: Basic Principles and Clinical Correlates. New York: Raven Press, Ltd., 1992:821–839.
7. Folkman J. Tumor angiogenesis: therapeutic implications. N Engl J Med 1971; 285: 1182–1186.
8. Sills AK, Sipos EP, Laterra J, Brem H. Angiogenesis inhibition in the treatment of central nervous system tumors. In: Kornblith PL, Walker MD, eds. Advances in Neuro-Oncology II. Armonk, NY: Futura Publishing Company, Inc., 1997:81–96.
9. Folkman J. Clinical application of research on angiogenesis. N Engl J Med 1996; 334:920–921.
10. Brem H, Folkman J. Inhibition of tumor angiogenesis mediated by cartilage. J Exp Med 1975; 141:427–439.
11. Langer R, Brem H, Falterman K, Klein M, Folkman J. Isolation of a cartilage factor that inhibits tumor neovascularization. Science 1976; 193:70–72.
12. Langer R, Folkman J. Polymers for the sustained release of proteins and other macromolecules. Nature 1976; 263:797–800.
13. Leong KW, D'Amore P, Marletta M, Langer R. Bioerodible polyanhydrides as drug-carrier matrices II: biocompatibility and chemical reactivity. J Biomed Mater Res 1986; 20:51–64.
14. Tamada J, Langer R. The development of polyanhydrides for drug delivery applications. J Biomat Sci Polymer Edition 1992; 3:315–353.
15. Domb A, Bogdansky S, Olivi A, Judy K, Dureza C, Lenartz D, Pinn ML, Colvin OM, Brem H. Controlled delivery of water soluble and hydrolytically unstable anticancer drugs from polymeric implants. Polymer Preprints 1991; 32:219–220.
16. Hochberg FH, Pruitt A. Assumptions in the radiotherapy of glioblastoma. Neurology 1980; 30:907–911.
17. Sipos EP, Brem H. New delivery systems for brain tumor therapy. Neurol Clin 1995; 13:813–825.
18. Tamargo RJ, Epstein JI, Reinhard CS, Chasin M, Brem H. Brain biocompatibility of a biodegradable controlled release polymer in rats. J Biomed Mater Res 1989; 23:253.
19. Brem H, Kader A, Epstein JI, Tamargo RJ, Domb A, Langer R, Leong K. Biocompatibility of biodegradable, controlled release polymer in the rabbit brain. Selective Cancer Therapeutics 1989; 5:55–65.
20. Brem H, Tamargo RJ, Olivi A, Pinn M, Weingart JD, Wharam M, Epstein JI. Biodegradable polymers for controlled delivery of chemotherapy with and without radiation therapy in the monkey brain. J Neurosurg 1994; 80:283–290.
21. Domb AJ, Rock M, Schwartz J, Perkin C, Yipchuk G, Broxup B, Villemure JG. Metabolic disposition and elimination studies of a radiolabelled biodegradable polymeric implant in the rat brain. Biomaterials 1994; 15:681–688.
22. Storm PB, Brem H. The treatment of brain tumors with drug-impregnated biodegradable polymers. In: Kornblith PL, Walker MD, eds. Advances in Neuro-Oncology II. Armonk, NY: Futura Publishing Company, Inc., 1997:435–446.
23. Kornblith P, Walker M. Chemotherapy for malignant gliomas. J Neurosurg 1988; 68:1–17.
24. Grossman SA, Reinhard C, Colvin OM, Chasin M, Brundrett R, Tamargo RJ, Brem

H. The intracerebral distribution of 1,3-bis(2-chloroethyl)-1-nitrosourea (BCNU) delivered by surgically implanted biodegradable polymers. J Neurosurg 1992; 76:640–647.

25. Fung LK, Ewend M, Sills A, Sipos EP, Thompson R, Watts M, Colvin OM, Brem H, Saltzman WM. Pharmacokinetics of interstitial delivery of carmustine, 4-hydroperoxycyclophosphamide and paclitaxel from a biodegradable polymer implant in the monkey brain. Cancer Res 1998. In press.
26. Tamargo RJ, Myseros JS, Epstein JI, Yang MB, Chasin M, Brem H. Interstitial chemotherapy of the 9L gliosarcoma: controlled release polymers for drug delivery to the brain. Cancer Res 1993; 53:329–333.
27. Brem H, Mahaley MSJ, Vick NA, Black K, Schold SC, Burger PC, Friedman AH, Ciric IS, Eller TW, Cozzens JW, Kenealy JN. Interstitial chemotherapy with drug polymer implants for the treatment of recurrent gliomas. J Neurosurg 1991; 74:441–446.
28. Brem H, Ewend MG, Piantadosi S, Greenhoot J, Burger PC, Sisti M. The safety of interstitial chemotherapy with BCNU-loaded polymer followed by radiation therapy in the treatment of newly diagnosed malignant gliomas: phase I trial. J Neurooncol 1995; 26:111–123.
29. Brem H, Piantadosi S, Burger PC, Walker M, Selker R, Vick NA, Black K, Sisti M, Brem S, Mohr G, Muller P, Morawetz R, Schold SC, and the Polymer-Brain Tumor Group. Placebo-controlled trial of safety and efficacy of intraoperative controlled delivery by biodegradable polymers of chemotherapy for recurrent gliomas. Lancet 1995; 345:1008–1012.
30. Valtonen S, Timonen U, Toivanen P, Kalimo H, Kivipelto L, Heiskanen O, Unsgaard G, Kuurne T. Interstitial chemotherapy with carmustine-loaded polymers for high grade gliomas: a randomized double-blind study. Neurosurgery 1997; 41:44–48.
31. Judy K, Olivi A, Buahin KG, Domb A, Epstein JI, Colvin OM, Brem H. Effectiveness of controlled release of a cyclophosphamide derivative with polymers against rat gliomas. J Neurosurg 1995; 82:481–486.
32. Olivi A, Ewend MG, Utsuki T, Tyler B, Domb AJ, Brat DJ, Brem H. Interstitial delivery of carboplatin via biodegradable polymers is effective against experimental glioma in the rat. Cancer Chemother Pharmacol 1996; 39:90–96.
33. Weingart JD, Thompson RC, Tyler B, Colvin OM, Brem H. Local delivery of the topoisomerase I inhibitor camptothecin sodium prolongs survival in the rat intracranial 9L gliosarcoma model. Int J Cancer 1995; 62:605–609.
34. Walter KA, Cahan MA, Gur A, Tyler B, Hilton J, Colvin OM, Burger PC, Domb A, Brem H. Interstitial taxol delivered from a biodegradable polymer implant against experimental malignant glioma. Cancer Res 1994; 54:2207–2212.
35. Fetell MR, Grossman SA, Fisher JD, Erlanger B, Rowinsky E, Stockel J, Piantadosi S. Preirradiation paclitaxel in glioblastoma multiforme: efficacy, pharmacology, and drug interactions. J Clin Oncol 1997; 15:3121–3128.
36. Tamargo RJ, Rossell LA, Tyler BM, Aryanpur J. Interstitial delivery of diphenylhydantoin in the brain for the treatment of seizures in a rat model. J Neurosurg 1994; 80:372.
37. Tamargo RJ, Sills AK Jr, Reinhard CS, Pinn ML, Long DM, Brem H. Interstitial

delivery of dexamethasone in the brain for the reduction of peritumoral edema. J Neurosurg 1991; 74:956–961.

38. Brem S, Cotran R, Folkman J. Tumor angiogenesis: a quantitative method for histologic grading. J Natl Cancer Inst 1972; 48:347–356.
39. Brem S. The role of vascular proliferation in the growth of brain tumors. Clin Neurosurg 1976; 23:440–453.
40. Brem H, Thompson D, Long DM, Patz A. Human brain tumors: differences in ability to stimulate angiogenesis. Surg Forum 1980; 31:471–473.
41. Wesseling P, Ruiter DJ, Burger PC. Angiogenesis in brain tumors: pathobiological and clinical aspects. J Neurooncol 1997; 32:253–265.
42. Brem H, Patz A, Tapper D. Detection of human central nervous system tumors: use of migration-stimulating activity of the cerebrospinal fluid. Surg Forum 1983; 34: 532–534.
43. Li VW, Folkerth RD, Watanabe H, Yu C, Barnes P, Scott RM, Black PM, Sallan SE, Folkman J. Microvessel count and cerebrospinal fluid basic fibroblast growth factor in children with brain tumors. Lancet 1994; 344:82–86.
44. Gross J, Azizkhan RG, Biswas C, Bruns RR, Hsieh DST, Folkman J. Inhibition of tumor growth, vascularization, and collagenolysis in the rabbit cornea by medroxyprogesterone. Proc Natl Acad Sci U S A 1981; 78:1176–1180.
45. Tamargo RJ, Leong KW, Brem H. Growth inhibition of the 9L glioma using polymers to release heparin and cortisone acetate. J Neurooncol 1990; 9:131–138.
46. Tamargo RJ, Bok RA, Brem H. Angiogenesis inhibition by minocycline. Cancer Res 1991; 51:672–675.
47. Sills AK, Williams JI, Tyler BM, Epstein DS, Sipos EP, Davis JD, McLane MP, Pitchford S, Chesire K, Gannon FH, Kinney WA, Chao TL, Donowitz M, Laterra J, Zasloff M, Brem H. Squalamine inhibits angiogenesis and tumor growth in vivo and perturbs embryonic vasculature. Cancer Research 1998; 58:2784–2792.
48. Tamargo RJ, Olivi A, Bok RA, Brem H. Angiogenesis inhibition by minocycline. Cancer Research 1991; 51:672–675.
49. Weingart JD, Sipos EP, Brem H. The role of minocycline in the treatment of intracranial 9L glioma. J Neurosurg 1995; 82:635–640.
50. Sipos EP, Tyler B, Piantadosi S, Burger PC, Brem H. Optimizing interstitial delivery of BCNU from controlled release polymers for the treatment of brain tumors. Cancer Chemother Pharmacol 1997; 39:383–389.

23

Matrix-Associated Endogenous Inhibitors of Angiogenesis

Raghu Kalluri and Vikas P. Sukhatme
Harvard Medical School and Beth Israel Deaconess Medical Center, Boston, Massachusetts

I. INTRODUCTION

It is now well established that growth of tumors beyond a few mm^3 requires angiogenesis—the formation of new capillaries from pre-existing blood vessels (1, 2). In adults, angiogenesis is associated with normal physiological processes such as wound healing and endometrial remodeling (3, 4). Angiogenesis involves a series of complex and sequential events that can be broadly divided into two phases: the inductive phase and the resolution phase (4). The inductive phase comprises the release of angiogenic factors such as basic fibroblast growth factor (bFGF) and vascular endothelial growth factor (VEGF) by the tumor cells, detachment of pericytes, degradation of vascular basement membrane (VBM), and activation of endothelial cells. The latter involves proliferation and migration toward the increasing concentration gradient of bFGF and VEGF under the influence of transitional matrix molecules (4). The resolution phase of angiogenesis is associated with inhibition of proliferation and migration of endothelial cells, reformation of vascular basement membrane, and reattachment of pericytes.

Induction and resolution of angiogenesis is a self-contained process in the human body (5). Induction of angiogenesis is presumably prevented because of the existence of an angiogenic barrier. When new blood capillaries are required, this barrier is overcome and angiogenesis ensues (6, 7). Several investigators have proposed various endogenous factors that help the human body maintain an angiogenically quiescent state (7–9). A balance between the progressive and regressive phases of angiogenesis is pivotal for homeostasis. Tumors themselves provide this balance to regulate new capillary formation (10). What constitutes the angiogenic barrier in the human body is currently an active area of investigation because of the promise of discovery of endogenous inhibitors of angiogenesis (11). In this regard, several endogenous inhibitors of angiogenesis have been discovered recently and some of these—endostatin, restin, and canstatin—are fragments of extracellular matrix molecules (12–14). In this chapter, we will review the discovery, activity, and therapeutic potential of these newly discovered inhibitors.

II. BACKGROUND AND SIGNIFICANCE

Specialized extracellular matrix exists as thin layers called basement membranes that provide supporting structure on which epithelial and endothelial cells grow and surround muscle, fat, etc. (15). Basement membranes are associated with cells and provide mechanical support as well as influence cellular behavior such as differentiation, proliferation, and migration. The major macromolecular constituents of basement membranes are type IV collagen, laminin, heparan sulfate proteoglycans, fibronectin, and entactin (13, 16). Vascular basement membrane constitutes the rigid structural wall of newly established capillaries and is speculated to play an important role in regulating proangiogenic and antiangiogenic events (17–19). In the last 2 decades, studies have illustrated the antiangiogenic properties of inhibitors of collagen metabolism, supporting the notion that VBM collagen synthesis and deposition is crucial for blood vessel formation and survival (18, 20–22). A more detailed role for extracellular matrix in angiogenesis process is provided by Dr. Joseph Madri (Chapter 2) in this book.

III. ENDOSTATIN

A. Discovery, Antiangiogenic Action, and Production

In 1996, O'Reilly et al. (12) isolated endostatin, an angiogenesis inhibitor from a murine hemangioendothelioma cell line (EOMA). Endostatin is a 20 kDa C-terminal fragment of type XVIII collagen, a VBM-associated matrix protein (12, 23–26). Endostatin specifically inhibits endothelial proliferation and potently inhibits tumor growth (12, 27). In the first two reports from the Folkman group, *Escherichia coli*-derived endostatin was administered as a suspension and by a hypothesized sustained release method. This molecule was shown to regress primary tumors in syngeneic and xenograft mouse models to dormant microscopic foci (12, 28, 29). Moreover, no drug resistance was noted in three of the tumor types studied: Lewis lung carcinoma, T241 fibrosarcoma, and B16 melanoma cells (28). Interestingly, repeated cycles of administration with endostatin resulted in tumor dormancy, that is, there was no tumor regrowth after cessation of drug administration (28). Immunohistochemical evaluation revealed that tumor regression in these studies was caused by blocked angiogenesis associated with increased proliferation and apoptosis of tumor cells, with proliferation dominated by apoptosis (12, 28). Notably, in these studies dosages less than 10 mg/kg (i.e., 2.5 mg/kg) were only partially effective in retarding tumor growth (12).

Results from these initial studies opened new avenues for potential treatment of cancer and provided a promising route for overcoming the drug resistance often seen during chemotherapy. However, in all these investigations, a presumably nonrefolded precipitated type of endostatin was administered in the form of a suspension to tumor-bearing animals. In addition, large amounts of protein were required to cause tumor regression and to lead to tumor dormancy. To obtain soluble endostatin for both in vitro and in vivo studies, Dhanabal et al. expressed mouse endostatin in the *Pichia pastoris* system (27). The yeast expression system was selected because of its ability to express heterologous proteins in large amounts with posttranslational modifications. These studies showed for the first time that it is possible to express biologically active mouse endostatin with a yield of 15 to 20 mg/l (27). Biological activity was demonstrated in vitro by effects on endothelial proliferation and migration and in the chick chorioallantoic membrane (CAM) assay, along with growth inhibition in a renal cell carcinoma tumor xenograft model (27). In the same report, two mutants of the endostatin protein were created, with one showing loss of function in vivo (27).

While O'Reilly and Dhanabal performed their in vivo studies with endostatin using syngeneic and xenograft mouse models, Bergers et al. used a transgenic model of pancreatic islet cell carcinogenesis (RIP1-Tag2). In this model, an angiogenic switch is known to occur in premalignant lesions, and angiogenesis continues during the progression to large and invasive solid carcinomas (12, 27, 30). These investigators showed that endostatin induced regressions of large end-stage tumors and targeted a specific stage in tumor growth (30). Recently, Chen et al. showed that liposomes complexed to plasmid-encoding endostatin reduced orthotopic breast cancer tumors in nude mice by 40% (31). These studies provide hope that nonviral delivery of endostatin to the tumor site may be particularly efficacious and may eliminate concerns that a contaminant in the endostatin preparations used in previous work was responsible for the observed antitumor activity (31).

Subsequent to this study, Boehm et al. showed that disruption of the KEX1 gene in *P. pastoris* was necessary for the recombinant expression of full-length endostatin (32). Dhanabal et al. showed that both mouse and human endostatin can be generated without the disruption of the KEX1 gene. They also showed that human endostatin specifically inhibited the proliferation (by G, arrest) and migration of human endothelial cells and caused apoptosis of these cells (33). Taddei et al. showed that full-length human endostatin is a potent inhibitor of bFGF- and VEGF-165-induced proliferation and migration of endothelial cells, and not of nonendothelial cells (34). In recent studies, Entremed scientists have shown that human endostatin is tenfold to twentyfold less potent in vivo on mouse vasculature than mouse endostatin (35).

B. Structure, Origin, Localization, and Mechanism of Action

Endostatin is a 185 amino acid molecule with a molecular mass of 20 kDa in reducing conditions and 18 kDa in nonreducing conditions (12). Secondary structure analysis estimated about 10% α-helix and about 70% β-structure (36). This protein fragment contains two disulfide bonds (36). The crystal structure of mouse endostatin at 1.5 A resolution revealed a compact folding pattern that is related to the C-type lectin carbohydrate recognition domain and the hyaluron-binding link module (36). Heparin binding was localized to a basic stretch formed by 11 arginine residues (36, 37). The intact NC10 domain of collagen XVIII was not an inhibitor of angiogenesis. It has been postulated that the NC10 domain potentially contributes to the steric blocking of angiogenic regions of the smaller endostatin through the N-terminal portion of the molecule (24). Sasaki et al. showed that mouse endostatin binds to heparin with a Kd of 0.3 μM (24, 37). They suggested that this interaction is crucial for its antiangiogenesis activity (however, see below). Alanine mutagenesis demonstrated that a cluster of arginine at positions 155, 158, 184, 270, 193, and 194 are important for this interaction (24, 36, 37). This same region also was shown to bind heparan sulfate proteoglycans (37).

Although the crystal structure suggests that endostatin may bind to heparan sulfate proteoglycans, Chang et al. showed that endostatin binds to blood vessels, and that this binding is not mediated by heparan sulfate proteoglycans (38). These investigators also showed that bFGF and heparin do not compete for endostatin binding (38). Another interesting feature of endostatin is the compact folding at the neutral pH, as also demonstrated by X-ray crystallography (36). Sasaki et al. showed that endostatin is very resistant to proteolysis by plasmin, trypsin, α-chymotrypsin, pancreatic elastase, or endoproteinase GLU-C at neutral pH. However, at pH 3, plasmin caused complete digestion of endostatin (24). These findings suggest that endostatin, and not the entire NC10 domain of collagen XVIII (which contains endostatin), is designed to be resistant to degradation by common proteases (24). These investigators also showed that tissue extracts from mouse brain, skeletal muscle, heart, kidney, testis, and liver contain endostatin in the range of 0.3 to 2 μg/ml (24). These amounts exceeded that of serum endostatin by at least a factor of 10, indicating that endostatin is generated specifically in tissues and not derived from serum (24).

The crystal structure of human endostatin also reveals a zinc binding site (39). The human endostatin zinc site is formed by three histidines at the N-terminus and an aspartic acid in the center of the molecule (36, 39). Dimerization of human endostatin is mediated by zinc. The location of the zinc site adjacent to the endostatin cleavage site suggests the possibility that zinc may play an important role in the activation of antiangiogenic activity after cleavage from the inactive type XVIII collagen molecule (39). Additionally, it was shown that for the bacterially produced protein in suspension form, the presence of zinc is crucial for the biological activity of endostatin (however, see below) (39, 40).

At present, how endostatin is generated in vivo is not known. Collagen XVIII, as a member of a family of collagen-like proteins, is localized mainly in the perivascular portion of blood vessels (24, 41, 42). Immunogold double-staining of elastic fibers of the aorta and other large arteries revealed a close colocalization of endostatin with fibulin-1, fibulin-2, and nidogen-2 (43). Collagen XVIII by itself was not inhibitory to endothelial cells; however, when processed by as yet unknown mechanisms, it may lead to the release of the carboxyl terminal portion (12). Sasaki et al. speculate that proteolytic release of endostatin can occur by a break in the central protease-sensitive hinge region (24). The protease(s) involved in the generation of endostatin are not defined, and how this process may be regulated also is not known. In this regard, Wen et al. showed that elastase can liberate endostatin from the recombinant NC10 domain of type XVIII collagen (44), although these studies do not address the in vivo generation of endostatin from type XVIII collagen when present as a large structural protein complex in the vascular basement membrane.

Dhanabal et al. showed that endostatin specifically caused endothelial cell apoptosis and this action is associated with reduction in Bcl-2 and Bcl-X_L anti-apoptotic protein without significant change in the Bax levels (12). These effects were not seen in several nonendothelial cells (12a). Angiogenesis induced by bFGF, but not VEGF, in a CAM assay could be inhibited by endostatin in a dose-dependent manner (37). In a different study by Yamaguchi et al., endostatin inhibited VEGF-induced endothelial cell migration and tumor growth in a zinc-independent fashion (45).

The mechanism of endostatin-mediated tumor regression is largely unknown. Whether inhibition of cell proliferation (perhaps by G, arrest, as shown in vitro) or apoptosis, or inhibition of cell migration is the relevant physiological action in vivo must be elucidated. A putative cell surface receptor and intracellular signaling events remain to be defined. It is conceivable that endostatin may compete with binding of angiogenic stimulators such as bFGF and VEGF to its appropriate receptors. Alternatively, it is possible that proliferating endothelial cells up-regulate $\alpha v\beta_3$, an endothelial integrin, and endostatin may act by disrupting the interaction of proliferating endothelial cells to matrix protein, thus driving endothelial cells to undergo apoptosis, as it has been well documented that lack of attachment of endothelial cells to matrix proteins such as vitronectin may result in programmed cell death (46).

C. Clinical Implications

Circulating levels of a fragment of human endostatin have been detected in patients with chronic renal insufficiency with no detectable tumor (30). These fragments were not active in vitro in endothelial cell assays, although no positive control was shown. It is likely that circulating levels many-fold higher will be required to affect tumor growth (based on doses used in mice in vivo and on in vitro data). A phase I clinical trial has recently begun at several hospitals. The expectation is that minimal or no toxicity will be found with this agent. Short-term use of this single drug is unlikely to lead to significant tumor growth inhibition, based on experience with other antiangiogenic therapies, such as interferon. Phase II trials, perhaps in conjunction with radiation or chemotherapy, will be eagerly awaited.

IV. RESTIN

Databank searches with mouse endostatin protein sequence yielded a high score hit for the human collagen XV protein, a homology significant in the 185 amino acid residues of the C-terminal region and present throughout this sequence. Thus Ramchandran et al. asked whether the C-terminal NC10 domain of human type XV collagen had antiangiogenic function (14). This 20 kDa fragment was cloned, expressed in *E. coli*, and named ''Restin'' (*re*lated to endo*s*ta*tin*) (14). It is found to inhibit migration, but not proliferation, of endothelial cells in vitro, in contrast to endostatin. Systemic administration of the refolded, bacterially expressed protein (20 mg/kg) caused suppression of tumor growth in a renal cell carcinoma xenograft nude mouse model. Because human protein was used in these studies, the potency was extrapolated to be similar to that of human endostatin used in similar mouse models (14).

Studies are in progress to determine the structure-function relationship of this protein, its effects on other tumors, and its mechanism of action. Interestingly, as with endostatin, a subfragment of restin has recently been isolated from human blood (47).

V. CANSTATIN

A. Discovery and In Vitro Antiangiogenic Activity

Type IV collagen in the human body is composed of six distinct α-chains, namely, α1–α6 (11). It is assembled into triple helices and forms a network to provide an interacting scaffold for other macromolecules in basement membranes (48–50). These α-chains are composed of three domains: N-terminal 7S domain, the middle triple helical domain, and C-terminal globular noncollagenous domain (NC1) (16, 50, 51). The α1 and α2 chains are ubiquitous in all human basement membranes (52). The other four chains exhibit more organ and tissue-specific distribution (52). Type IV collagen promotes cell adhesion, migration, differentiation, and growth (18, 19, 53). It also is thought to play a crucial role in endothelial cell proliferation and behavior during the angiogenic process (19, 53, 54). Based on these observations, it was postulated that collagen type IV could influence tumor angiogenesis and growth. Furthermore, the NC1 domain of type IV collagen is thought to play a crucial role in the assembly of type IV collagen to form trimers and thus influence basement membrane organization and associated endothelial cell behavior (9, 16). Recently, Kamphaus et al. demonstrated the ability of the NC1 domain of the α2 chain of type IV collagen, which was named canstatin, to inhibit angiogenesis in vitro and in vivo (13).

Human canstatin was produced in *E. coli* as a fusion protein with a C-terminal six histidine tag and as a secreted soluble protein in 293 embryonic kidney cells. In addition, human canstatin (24 kDa) was isolated from human placenta by gel filtration, high-performance liquid chromatography (HPLC), and affinity chromatography techniques. Canstatin selectively inhibits tube formation, proliferation, and migration of mouse and human endothelial cells, with no effect on tumor cells or primary epithelial cell lines (13).

B. In Vivo Antiangiogenic Activity

Canstatin inhibits the growth of small and large renal cell carcinoma (786-0) tumors by fourfold and threefold with respect to placebo-treated mice. Established human prostate (PC-3) tumors in severe combined immunodeficient mice or athymic mice exhibited fractional tumor volumes of 2.4-fold less than placebo-treated mice when treated with 3 mg/kg canstatin. A comparable dose of mouse endostatin revealed only partial tumor inhibitory effect. This decrease in tumor size was consistent with a decrease in CD31-positive vasculature (13).

C. Mechanism of Action

To further understand the molecular mechanisms involved in canstatin's antiproliferative and antimigratory activities, Kamphaus et al. assessed the effect of canstatin on ERK activation induced by 20% fetal bovine serum and endothelial mitogens (13). These results show that canstatin does not work primarily by inhibiting proximal events activated by VEGF or bFGF receptors (13). Alternatively, canstatin specifically induced apoptosis of endothelial cells, with no significant effect observed on nonendothelial cell lines. These results suggested that canstatin may act by driving the endothelial cells to apoptosis. Kamphaus et al. further confirmed this notion by showing that canstatin can induce a steady decrease in FLIP protein (an antiapoptotic protein associated with FAS-mediated apoptosis pathway) levels in the presence of both 20% serum and bFGF and VEGF. Interestingly, canstatin did not effect FLIP levels in the absence of growth factors. From these experiments, it was suggested that FLIP decrease may sensitize endothelial cells to an apoptotic signal. Importantly, canstatin's lack of effect on endothelial cells in the absence of growth factors may indicate that only angiogenic, not preformed endothelium is targeted (13).

VI. FUTURE DIRECTION

Because large doses and long-term use of antiangiogenic proteins will be needed to affect tumor growth, gene therapy approaches might be particularly useful. Alternatively, methods to enhance endogenous production of these agents through administration of suitable proteases also may prove efficacious. However, the latter may have to be used with care because deleterious effects could result.

Identification of the mechanism of action of these drugs, through delineation of signaling pathways, will allow for rational combinations within the antiangiogenic group, perhaps in conjunction with radiation or chemotherapy. In addition, receptor identification will facilitate the search for small molecule mimetics. Structure-function analysis of these proteins may reveal smaller fragments that are just as potent, or perhaps even have increased potency. Moreover, these smaller peptides also may be easier to produce in bulk.

REFERENCES

1. Folkman J, D'Amore PA. Blood vessel formation: what is its molecular basis? Cell 1996; 87:1153–1155.
2. Hanahan D, Weinberg R. Hallmarks of cancer. Cell 2000; 100:57–70.
3. Folkman J. Tumor angiogenesis and tissue factor. Nat Med 1996; 2:167–168.
4. Folkman J, Shing Y. Angiogenesis. J Biol Chem 1992; 267:10931–10934.
5. Folkman J. Angiogenesis—retrospect and outlook. EXS 1992; 61:4–13.

6. Hanahan D, Folkman J. Patterns and emerging mechanisms of the angiogenic switch during tumorigenesis. Cell 1996; 86:353–364.
7. Bouck N, Stellmach V, Hsu SC. How tumors become angiogenic. Adv Cancer Res 1996; 69:135–174.
8. Cheresh DA. Death to a blood vessel, death to a tumor. Nat Med 1998; 4:395–396.
9. Bouck N, Campbell S. Anti-cancer dividends from captopril and other inhibitors of angiogenesis. J Nephrol 1998; 11:3–4.
10. Folkman J. Angiogenesis inhibitors generated by tumors. Mol Med 1995; 1:120–122.
11. Folkman J. Angiogenesis and angiogenesis inhibition: an overview. EXS 1997; 79: 1–8.
12. O'Reilly MS, Boehm T, Shing Y, Fukai N, Vasios G, Lane WS, Flynn E, Birkhead JR, Olsen BR, Folkman J. Endostatin: an endogenous inhibitor of angiogenesis and tumor growth. Cell 1997; 88:277–285.
12a. Dhanabal M, Ramchandran R, Waterman MJF, Lu H, Knebelmann B, Segal M, Sukhatme VP. Endostatin induces endothelial cell apoptosis. J Biol Chem 1999; 274:11721–11726.
13. Kamphaus GD, Colorado PC, Panka DJ, Hopfer H, Ramchandran R, Torre A, Maeshima Y, Mier JW, Sukhatme VP, Kalluri R. Canstatin, a novel matrix-derived inhibitor of angiogenesis and tumor growth. J Biol Chem 2000; 275:1209–1215.
14. Ramchandran R, Dhanabal M, Volk R, Waterman MJ, Segal M, Lu H, Knebelmann B, Sukhatme VP. Antiangiogenic activity of restin, NC10 domain of human collagen XV: comparison to endostatin. Biochem Biophys Res Commun 1999; 255:735–739.
15. Paulsson M. Basement membrane proteins: structure, assembly, and cellular interaction. Crit Rev Biochem Mol Biol 1992; 27:93–127.
16. Timpl R. Structure and biological activities of basement membrane proteins. Eur J Biochem 1989; 180:487–502.
17. Madri JA, Pratt BM, Yurchenco PD, Furthmayr H. The ultrastructural organization and architecture of basement membranes. Ciba Foundation Symposium 1984; 108: 6–24.
18. Madri JA, Pratt BM. Endothelial cell-matrix interactions: in vitro models of angiogenesis. J Histochem Cytochem 1986; 34:85–91.
19. Form DM, Pratt BM, Madri JA. Endothelial cell proliferation during angiogenesis. In vitro modulation by basement membrane components. Lab Invest 1986; 55:521–530.
20. Ingber D, Folkman J. Inhibition of angiogenesis through modulation of collagen metabolism. Lab Invest 1988; 59:44–51.
21. Nicosia RF, Madri JA. The microvascular extracellular matrix. Developmental changes during angiogenesis in the aortic ring-plasma clot model. Am J Pathol 1987; 128:78–90.
22. Maragoudakis ME, Missirlis E, Karakiulakis GD, Sarmonica M, Bastakis M, Tsopanoglou N. Basement membrane biosynthesis as a target for developing inhibitors of angiogenesis with anti-tumor properties. Kidney Int 1993; 43:147–150.
23. Oh SP, Warman ML, Seldin MF, Cheng SD, Knoll JH, Timmons S, Olsen BR. Cloning of cDNA and genomic DNA encoding human type XVIII collagen and

localization of the alpha 1(XVIII) collagen gene to mouse chromosome 10 and human chromosome 21. Genomics 1994; 19:494–499.
24. Sasaki T, Fukai N, Mann K, Gohring W, Olsen BR, Timpl R. Structure, function and tissue forms of the C-terminal globular domain of collagen XVIII containing the angiogenesis inhibitor endostatin. Embo J 1998; 17:4249–4256.
25. Rehn M, Hintikka E, Pihlajaniemi T. Primary structure of the alpha 1 chain of mouse type XVIII collagen, partial structure of the corresponding gene, and comparison of the alpha 1(XVIII) chain with its homologue, the alpha 1(XV) collagen chain. J Biol Chem 1994; 269:13929–13935.
26. Rehn M, Hintikka E, Pihlajaniemi T. Characterization of the mouse gene for the alpha 1 chain of type XVIII collagen (Col18a1) reveals that the three variant N-terminal polypeptide forms are transcribed from two widely separated promoters. Genomics 1996; 32:436–446.
27. Dhanabal M, Ramchandran R, Volk R, Stillman IE, Lombardo M, Iruela-Arispe ML, Simons M, Sukhatme VP. Endostatin: yeast production, mutants, and antitumor effect in renal cell carcinoma. Cancer Res 1999; 59:189–197.
28. Boehm T, Folkman J, Browder T, O'Reilly MS. Antiangiogenic therapy of experimental cancer does not induce acquired drug resistance. Nature 1997; 390:404–407.
29. Black WR, Agner RC. Tumour regression after endostatin therapy. Nature 1998; 391:450.
30. Bergers G, Javaherian K, Lo KM, Folkman J, Hanahan D. Effects of angiogenesis inhibitors on multistage carcinogenesis in mice. Science 1999; 284:808–812.
31. Chen QR, Kumar D, Stass SA, Mixson AJ. Liposomes complexed to plasmids encoding angiostatin and endostatin inhibit breast cancer in nude mice. Cancer Res 1999; 59:3308–3312.
32. Boehm T, Pirie-Shepherd S, Trinh LB, Shiloach J, Folkman J. Disruption of the KEX1 gene in *Pichia pastoris* allows expression of full-length murine and human endostatin. Yeast 1999; 15:563–572.
33. Dhanabal M, Volk R, Ramchandran R, Simons M, Sukhatme VP. Cloning, expression, and in vitro activity of human endostatin. Biochem Biophys Res Commun 1999; 258:345–352.
34. Taddei L, Chiarugi P, Brogelli L, Cirri P, Magnelli L, Raugei G, Ziche M, Granger HJ, Chiarugi V, Ramponi G. Inhibitory effect of full-length human endostatin on in vitro angiogenesis. Biochem Biophys Res Commun 1999; 263:340–345.
35. Sim BKLF, Zhou XH, Liang H, Madsen JW, O'Reilley MS, Pranigrahy D, Fortier AH. Potent inhibition of experimental metastases and primary tumors by recombinant human endostatin that is suitable for human use. Proc Am Assoc Cancer Res 1999; 40:620.
36. Hohenester E, Sasaki T, Olsen BR, Timpl R. Crystal structure of the angiogenesis inhibitor endostatin at 1.5 A resolution. Embo J 1998; 17:1656–1664.
37. Sasaki T, Larsson H, Kreuger J, Salmivirta M, Claesson-Welsh L, Lindahl U, Hohenester E, Timpl R. Structural basis and potential role of heparin/heparan sulfate binding to the angiogenesis inhibitor endostatin [in process citation]. Embo J 1999; 18: 6240–6248.
38. Chang Z, Choon A, Friedl A. Endostatin binds to blood vessels in situ independent of heparan sulfate and does not compete for fibroblast growth factor-2 binding. Am J Pathol 1999; 155:71–76.

39. Ding YH, Javaherian K, Lo KM, Chopra R, Boehm T, Lanciotti J, Harris BA, Li Y, Shapiro R, Hohenester E, Timpl R, Folkman J, Wiley DC. Zinc-dependent dimers observed in crystals of human endostatin. Proc Natl Acad Sci U S A 1998; 95: 10443–10448.
40. Boehm T, O'Reilly MS, Keough K, Shiloach J, Shapiro R, Folkman J. Zinc-binding of endostatin is essential for its antiangiogenic activity. Biochem Biophys Res Commun 1998; 252:190–194.
41. Muragaki Y, Timmons S, Griffith CM, Oh SP, Fadel B, Quertermous T, Olsen BR. Mouse Col18a1 is expressed in a tissue-specific manner as three alternative variants and is localized in basement membrane zones. Proc Natl Acad Sci U S A 1995; 92: 8763–8767.
42. Saarela J, Ylikarppa R, Rehn M, Purmonen S, Pihlajaniemi T. Complete primary structure of two variant forms of human type XVIII collagen and tissue-specific differences in the expression of the corresponding transcripts. Matrix Biol 1998; 16: 319–328.
43. Miosge N, Sasaki T, Timpl R. Angiogenesis inhibitor endostatin is a distinct component of elastic fibers in vessel walls. Faseb J 1999; 13:1743–1750.
44. Wen W, Moses MA, Wiederschain D, Arbiser JL, Folkman J. The generation of endostatin is mediated by elastase [in process citation]. Cancer Res 1999; 59:6052–6056.
45. Yamaguchi N, Anand-Apte B, Lee M, Sasaki T, Fukai N, Shapiro R, Que I, Lowik C, Timpl R, Olsen BR. Endostatin inhibits VEGF-induced endothelial cell migration and tumor growth independently of zinc binding. Embo J 1999; 18:4414–4423.
46. Isik FF, Gibran NS, Jang YC, Sandell L, Schwartz SM. Vitronectin decreases microvascular endothelial cell apoptosis. J Cell Physiol 1998; 175:149–155.
47. John H, Preissner KT, Forssmann WG, Standker L. Novel glycosylated forms of human plasma endostatin and circulating endostatin-related fragments of collagen XV. Biochemistry 1999; 38:10217–10224.
48. Timpl R, Wiedemann H, Van Veldon V, Furthmayr H, Kuhn K. A network model for the organization of type IV collagen molecules in basement membranes. Eur J Biochem 1981; 120:203–211.
49. Yurchenco PD, Tsilibary EC, Charonis AS, Furthmayr H. Models for the self-assembly of basement membrane. J Histochem Cytochem 1986; 34:93–102.
50. Yurchenco PD, Ruben GC. Basement membrane structure in situ: evidence for lateral associations in the type IV collagen network. J Cell Biol 1987; 105:2559–2568.
51. Prockop DJ, Kivirikko KI. Collagens: molecular biology, diseases, and potentials for therapy. Annu Rev Biochem 1995; 64:403–434.
52. Hudson BG, Reeders ST, Tryggvason K. Type IV collagen: structure, gene organization, and role in human diseases. Molecular basis of Goodpasture and Alport syndromes and diffuse leiomyomatosis. J Biol Chem 1993; 268:26033–26036.
53. Madri JA, Williams SK. Capillary endothelial cell cultures: phenotypic modulation by matrix components. J Cell Biol 1983; 97:153–165.
54. Haas TL, Madri JA. Extracellular matrix-driven matrix metalloproteinase production in endothelial cells: implications for angiogenesis. Trends Cardiovasc Med 1999; 9: 70–77.

24

$\alpha v\beta 3$ and Its Antagonists in the Control of Angiogenesis

Brian P. Eliceiri and David A. Cheresh
The Scripps Research Institute, La Jolla, California

I. MECHANISM OF ANGIOGENESIS

Angiogenesis or vascular remodeling depends on both growth factor stimulation and cell adhesion events. Angiogenesis and vascular remodeling contribute to development and wound repair and facilitate inflammatory disease, retinopathy, and cancer. For example, growth of solid tumors requires angiogenesis to supply oxygen, nutrients, and growth factors. The process of tumor-induced angiogenesis can be divided generally into three phases: initiation, proliferation/invasion, and maturation. First, angiogenic cytokines or growth factors such as vascular endothelial growth factor (VEGF), basic fibroblast growth factor (bFGF), or transforming growth factor-alpha (TGFα) are released from tumors and inflammatory cells. Second, these factors stimulate vascular cell proliferation and invasive behavior, promoting blood vessel growth and invasion of tumors. Growth factors and other angiogenic inducers bound to the extracellular matrix (ECM) also can be released upon matrix proteolysis, facilitating the vascular cell invasion phase. Third, the invasive vascular sprouts deposit a basement membrane that facilitates differentiation and lumen formation. These basement membrane components maintain endothelial cells in a differentiated and quiescent state that is facilitated by cell-cell adhesive contacts. The newly formed vasculature provides nourishment for the tumor and acts as a conduit for metastatic cells to leave the primary site and metastasize to other locations (Fig. 1).

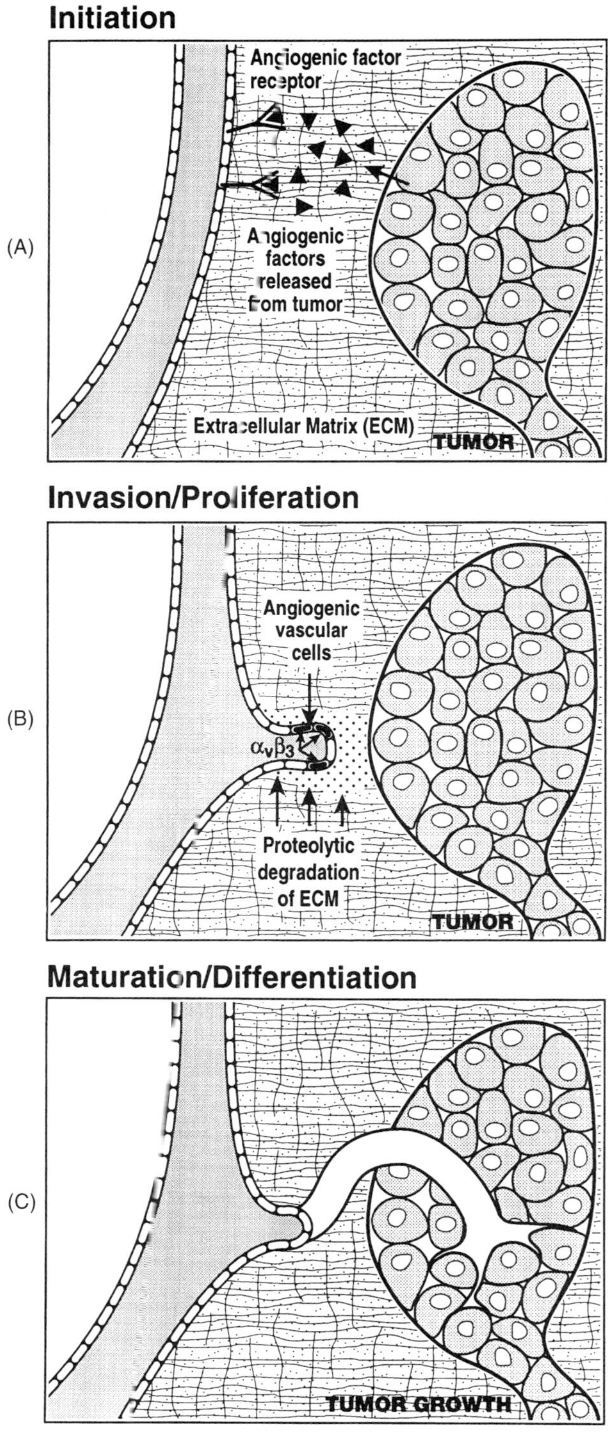
Initiation
(A)
Angiogenic factor receptor
Angiogenic factors released from tumor
Extracellular Matrix (ECM)
TUMOR
Invasion/Proliferation
(B)
Angiogenic vascular cells
$\alpha_v\beta_3$
Proteolytic degradation of ECM
TUMOR
Maturation/Differentiation
(C)
TUMOR GROWTH

II. CELL ADHESION MOLECULES IN ANGIOGENESIS

Angiogenesis depends on growth factors. It also is influenced by specific cell-cell and cell-ECM contacts. For example, antibodies to E-selectin, a transmembrane cell-adhesion glycoprotein, or sialyl-Lewis X or A, a cell-surface sialylated glycan, interfere with lumen formation in in vitro assays of blood vessel tube formation (Bischoff, 1995). Although E-selectin induces endothelial cell migration and angiogenesis in the rat cornea, E-selectin is not a mitogen nor does it influence endothelial cell mitogen production. In addition, a combined knockout of P- and E-selectin in mice does not result in blood vessel deformations (Frenette et al., 1996).

Immunoglobulin-like molecules such as intercellular adhesion molecule 1 and vascular adhesion molecule 1 (VCAM-1) expression levels are induced in endothelial cells after stimulation with inflammatory cytokines (interferon [IFN]-γ, interleukin [IL]-1, tumor necrosis factor [TNF]α, or lipopolysaccharides). Vascular adhesion molecule 1 induces angiogenesis in vivo and integrin $\alpha 4\beta 1$-dependent migration of endothelial cells in vitro. Vascular adhesion molecule 1 may act as an angiogenic stimulator through its interaction with $\alpha 4\beta 1$; however, VCAM-1 does not affect endothelial cell proliferation.

Cell adhesion to the ECM is mediated by integrins, heterodimeric transmembrane proteins that mediate cell-ECM interactions and comprise a diverse family of more than 15 α and 8 β subunits. Integrin subunits can heterodimerize in at least 20 different combinations. Different integrin combinations may recognize a single ECM ligand, and other integrins may bind several different ECM proteins. Integrins are known to mediate both the specificity of cell adhesion to a variety of matrix proteins and the regulation of the cell cycle (Guadagno et al., 1993; Varner et al., 1995; Dike and Farmer, 1988) and cell migration (Hynes, 1992; Cheresh, 1993). Integrin ligation is known to induce a wide range of intracellular signaling events, including tyrosine phosphorylation of focal adhesion kinase and other focal contact-associated proteins (Juliano and Haskill, 1993), elevated intracellular pH and Ca^{2+} levels, inositol lipid synthesis, cyclin synthesis, and the expression of immediate early genes (Kornberg et al., 1992; Guan and

Figure 1 Tumor-induced angiogenesis. Angiogenesis, the formation of new blood vessels from preexisting blood vessels, can be divided into three phases during tumor-induced angiogenesis. Angiogenic growth factors such as basic fibroblast growth factor or vascular endothelial growth factor are secreted from tumor cells (**A**). Tumor-secreted growth factors induce cell proliferation, cell invasion, expression of integrin $\alpha v\beta 3$ on vascular cells, and matrix degradation of surrounding extracellular matrix (**B**). The proteolytic degradation of the surrounding matrix microenvironment is a crucial step leading the remodeling of events that give rise to new blood vessel growth and the maturation of the newly sprouted blood vessels (**C**).

Shalloway, 1992; Schwartz and Lechene, 1992; Schwartz, 1993; McNamee et al., 1993; Guadagno et al., 1993; Varner et al., 1995). Prevention of integrin interactions suppresses cellular growth or induces apoptotic cell death (Varner et al., 1995; Meredith et al., 1993; Montgomery et al., 1994; Brooks et al., 1994b). Multiple integrins are expressed on endothelial cells, mediating adhesion to a wide variety of ECM proteins including fibronectin, vitronectin, laminin, collagen types I and IV, von Willebrand factor, fibrinogen, and denatured collagen (Cheng and Kramer, 1989).

III. CELL-ECM INTERACTIONS DURING ANGIOGENESIS

Angiogenesis involves multiple interactions between the ECM and vascular cells. Dynamic remodeling of the ECM surrounding blood vessels facilitates several steps during angiogenesis, including matrix degradation and deposition of new ECM components. Laminin, a major component of basement membranes, is important during capillary tube formation (Kubota et al., 1988; Grant et al., 1989). Various forms of collagen (types I, III, IV, and V) also are deposited during endothelial tube formation in vitro (Nicosia and Madri, 1987; Iruela-Arispe et al., 1991). The proteolysis of collagen also can influence endothelial tube formation because inhibition of matrix metalloproteinases (MMPs) block this process (Montesano and Orci, 1985; Mignatti et al., 1989; Fisher et al., 1994).

In vivo, ECM proteins are deposited during vasculogenesis and angiogenesis. For example, fibronectin is deposited, followed by laminin during wound healing in the skin and in retinal and intraembryonal vasculogenesis (Clark et al., 1982; Risau and Lemmon, 1988; Jiang et al., 1994). The role of collagens has been strongly implicated in angiogenesis based on studies by Ingber and Folkman who demonstrated that inhibition of collagen deposition and triple-helix formation, as well as inhibition of collagen crosslinking prevented angiogenesis (Ingber, 1991). De novo synthesis of collagen also has been shown to be important during angiogenesis (Haralabopoulos et al., 1994; Hanemaaijer et al., 1993). Genetic evidence for the role of collagen during angiogenesis is provided by a targeted gene knock-out of collagen type I $\alpha 1$-chain resulted in the rupture of blood vessels, indicating that collagen is essential for early blood vessel development (Lohler et al., 1984).

In addition to collagen deposition, collagen degradation by MMPs has been implicated as an important step during the invasive stage of angiogenesis. For example, angiogenic inducers such as bFGF, phorbal-12-myristate-13-acetate (PMA), and TNFα, stimulate the expression of MMPs in endothelial cells (Brooks et al., 1996; Takigawa et al., 1990). Tissue inhibitors of metalloproteinases (TIMPs), which regulate MMP activity on the cell surface, inhibit angiogenesis in the chick embryo yolk-sac, chick chorioallantoic membrane (CAM), and rat cornea (Takigawa et al., 1990; Moses et al., 1990; Johnson et al., 1994). The temporal and spatial coordination of collagen synthesis and collagen proteolysis in the ECM surrounding vascular cells is essential during angiogenesis. During the early phase of angiogenesis, local matrix degradation by MMPs may be required for invasion of preexisting vascular cells through the basement membrane and surrounding stroma followed by vascular cell migration and proliferation, which may depend on nascent expression and deposition of collagen. The proteolytic degradation of collagen may expose cryptic adhesive sites that are crucial for the invasive—and perhaps later the migration—phases of angiogenesis. For example, proteolysis of the intact collagen triple helix (types I and VI) can expose cryptic Arginine-Glycine-Aspartic Acid (RGD)-binding sites that are recognized by the integrin $\alpha v\beta 3$ (Davis, 1992; Pfaff et al., 1993; Montgomery et al., 1994). Integrin $\alpha v\beta 3$ is expressed preferentially on the surface of vascular cells undergoing angiogenesis in the chick CAM (Brooks et al., 1994a; Brooks et al., 1994b). Endothelial cells may use the cryptic RGD sites as a provisional matrix during the invasive and proliferative phases, providing a mechanism for how adhesive and proteolytic mechanisms may be coordinated during angiogenesis. Expression of collagen type IV and laminin during the deposition of new basement membrane may then facilitate differentiation and lumen formation during the later stages of angiogenesis (Ingber, 1991).

IV. INTEGRIN $\alpha v\beta 3$ AND ANGIOGENESIS

Of the wide spectrum of integrin subunit combinations expressed on the surface of cells, the $\alpha v\beta 3$ integrin has been identified as having an especially interesting expression pattern and distinct functional properties in vascular cells during angiogenesis. Integrin $\alpha v\beta 3$ is a receptor for a variety of ECM ligands with an exposed RGD moiety, including vitronectin, fibronectin, fibrinogen, laminin, collagen, von Willebrand factor, osteopontin, and adenovirus penton base (Cheresh, 1987; Leavesley et al , 1992; Cheresh 1993).

Integrin $\alpha v\beta 3$ has a very limited tissue distribution, as it is not typically expressed on epithelial cells and only at low levels on intestinal, vascular, and uterine smooth muscle cells (Brem et al., 1994; unpublished observations). This receptor is also expressed on some activated leukocytes, macrophages, and osteoclasts, where it may function during bone resorption (Sato et al., 1990; Horton et al., 1991; Ross et al., 1993). Some invasive tumors such as metastatic melanoma (Albelda et al., 1990) and late-stage glioblastoma (Gladson and Cheresh, 1991) also express $\alpha v\beta 3$. Some of the most prominent $\alpha v\beta 3$ expression levels have been identified in cytokine-activated endothelial or smooth muscle cells, especially on blood vessels in granulation tissue and tumors (Enenstein et al., 1994; Sepp et al., 1994; Brooks et al., 1994a; Brooks et al., 1994b). The expression of $\alpha v\beta 3$ on blood vessels suggests that it may be important for vascular cell proliferation and migration events associated with restenosis and angioplasty. The vascular smooth muscle cell migration that occurs during restenosis is dependent on αvβ3 ligation and is accompanied by increased expression levels of osteopontin, an αvβ3 ligand (Liaw et al., 1995). A function-blocking and β3 antibody has been shown to be beneficial in high-risk angioplasty patients (Topol et al., 1994). In addition to the role of αvβ3 during restenosis, there has been a significant advance in the understanding of the role of integrin αvβ3 during angiogenesis and vascular remodeling in recent years.

Integrin αvβ3 is expressed at low levels in quiescent or normal blood vessels, but is induced after exposure to cytokines, growth factors, or tumors (Brooks et al., 1994a). Basic FGF induces β3 mRNA and surface expression on cultured human dermal microvascular endothelial cells (Sepp et al., 1994; Enenstein et al., 1992). The bFGF-induced increase in αvβ3 mRNA depends on the nascent expression of the Hox D3 homeobox gene followed by αvβ3 expression (Boudreau et al., 1997). Furthermore, αvβ3 protein expression is induced by bFGF on blood vessels in the chick CAM (Brooks et al., 1994a) and on the rabbit cornea (Freidlander et al., 1995). αvβ3 Expression in vascular cells is also induced by human tumor cells cultured on the CAM (Brooks et al., 1994a,b) during wound healing (Brooks et al., 1994a), macular degeneration, diabetic retinopathy, and other neovascular diseases of the eye (unpublished observations).

The up-regulation of αvβ3 during angiogenesis suggests that integrins may have an important function during angiogenesis. In fact, disruption of integrin αvβ3 ligation with antibody (LM609) or cyclic peptide antagonists of αvβ3 prevent blood vessel formation in the chick CAM, quail embryo, rabbit cornea, mouse retina, and in human skin transplanted onto SCID mice (Drake et al., 1995; Brooks et al., 1995; Brooks et al., 1994a; Friedlander et al., 1995; Hammes et al., 1996). Angiogenesis induced by αvβ3-negative human tumor cells was also blocked with αvβ3 antagonists (Fig. 2). These antagonists prevented the growth of new blood vessels without detectably influencing the preexisting blood vessels. Furthermore, the inhibition of blood vessels supporting tumors not only blocked tumor growth but induced tumor regression (Brooks et al., 1994b). Histological examination of tumors treated with the αvβ3 antagonists revealed few if any viable tumor cells or detectable blood vessels (Brooks et al., 1994b). Cytokine or tumor cell-stimulated blood vessels treated with the αvβ3 antagonists undergo programmed cell death (apoptosis) in response to administration of the antagonists (Brooks et al., 1994a). These findings suggest that integrin αvβ3 can provide specific cell survival signals that facilitate vascular cell proliferation during angiogenesis.

A genetic approach to examining the role of the αv and the β3 integrin subunits has provided some insight into the role of these molecules during vasculogenesis and angiogenesis. In patients with Glanzmann thrombobastemia who lack functional β3 integrin protein (Coller et al., 1991; Djaffar and Rosa, 1993), there appears to be normal development of blood vessels, although the wound-healing response is impaired. This suggests that although functional β3 levels are diminished, perhaps the expression of integrin αvβ5, another RGD-specific

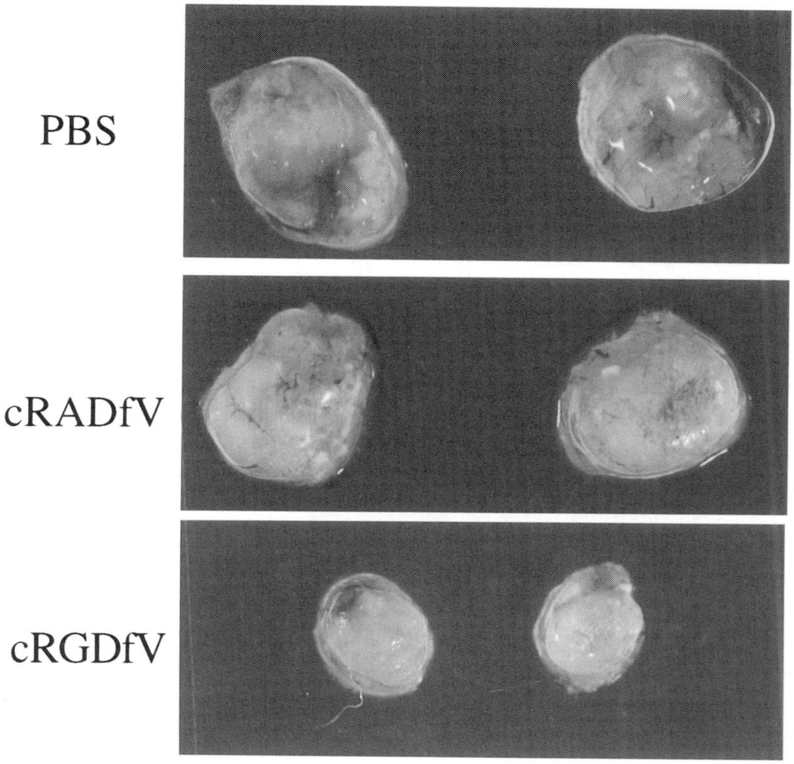

Figure 2 Tumor-induced angiogenesis blocked by integrin αvβ3 antagonists in the chick chorioallantoic membrane (CAM) angiogenesis model. M21L human tumor cells lacking αvβ3 or αvβ5 were inoculated onto the surface of the CAM of a 10-day old chick embryo. Intravenous injections of the embryo on day 11 with either phosphate buffered saline (PBS) (**top panel**), control cyclic RADfV peptide (**middle**), or cyclic RGDfV peptide (**bottom**) were administered. Tumors were excised 6 days later and analyzed for vascularization and tumor weight. Note that the αvβ3 antagonists acted on the CAM vessels, decreasing the tumor weight and vascularization, because the tumor cells do not express αvβ3 or αvβ5 (Felding-Habermann et al., 1992).

integrin, may compensate for the absence of functional αvβ3. In fact, integrin αvβ5 can potentiate a distinct pathway of VEGF-induced angiogenesis (Friedlander et al., 1995).

Genetic knock-out experiments of the αv gene in mice have shown that some mice survive to term but die shortly after birth (B. Bader and R. Hynes, personal communication). These αv-null mice have extensive brain and intestinal hemorrhaging, indicating a defect in blood vessel integrity, demonstrating the requirement for the expression of αv integrin in blood vessel formation and maturation. Other organs apparently have normal vascularization (B. Bader and R. Hynes, personal communication), suggesting that animals lacking αv integrins can compensate to some degree, perhaps by using other integrin-dependent adhesion pathways. However, until αv integrins are conditionally knocked out or crossed with other integrin knock-out mice, we will not understand why animals lacking αv integrins develop blood vessels at all.

V. INTEGRIN αvβ3 AND VASCULAR CELL SURVIVAL

Systemic administration of αvβ3 antagonists have been shown to induce apoptosis in cytokine or tumor cell-activated blood vessels (Brooks et al., 1994b). In fact, primary endothelial cells are known to be anchorage-dependent for growth and can undergo apoptosis when treated with anti-integrin function-blocking antibodies (Meredith et al., 1993; Re et al., 1994). These results suggest that ligation of αvβ3 on vascular cells may mediate a signaling event that is essential for the survival and differentiation of vascular cells undergoing angiogenesis in vivo. Using DNA laddering and measurements of free 3′OH groups from fragmented DNA as markers of apoptosis in endothelial cells, αvβ3 antagonists induced apoptosis after 48 hours of treatment (Brooks et al., 1994b). The αvβ3 antagonists administered during angiogenesis in the chick CAM also induced endothelial cell p53-dependent DNA-binding activity, which regulates the cell-cycle inhibitor $p21^{WAF1/CIP1}$ (Stromblad et al., 1996). In cultured endothelial cells, ligation of αvβ3 with immobilized antibody reduced the p53 activity and subsequent $p21^{WAF1/CIP1}$ protein levels. Ligation of αvβ3 was also shown to increase the expression of Bcl-2 and decrease Bax levels in primary endothelial cells, resulting in an increase in the Bcl-2: Bax ratio (Stromblad et al., 1996), a signal known to promote cell survival (White, 1996). Therefore, ligand binding by endothelial cell αvβ3 may suppress apoptosis and conflicting growth-arrest signals, facilitating the proliferation and differentiation of new blood vessels. It is important to point out that mice clearly survive without p53, indicating that alternative or compensatory apoptotic mechanisms can allow normal development. The fact that αv integrin antagonists activate a p53-dependent cell death pathway suggests that mice lacking p53 also may not depend on αv integrins for vascular development. This in turn may account for the presence of blood vessels in mice lacking αv integrins.

VI. REGULATION OF MITOGEN-ACTIVATED PROTEIN KINASE (MAPK) ACTIVITY IN ANGIOGENESIS

Angiogenesis is initiated by growth factors and depends on cell adhesion events to mediate the signaling events that lead to vascular cell proliferation, migration, and differentiation. Integrins and growth factor receptors have been colocalized on the cell surface and appear to cooperate in their capacity to activate the *ras*/ MAP kinase pathway (Miyamoto, 1996; Schwartz et al., 1995). Although growth factors can initiate MAP kinase activity and vascular cell proliferation, it is not clear how these signals ultimately lead to vascular remodeling events involving endothelial cell invasion and lumen formation of angiogenic sprouts in vivo. We recently have identified two bFGF-induced ERK activation signals in vascular cells required for angiogenesis (Eliceiri et al., unpublished observations). One is immediate and not influenced by integrin antagonists, and a second sustained signal is $\alpha v\beta 3$ dependent. Both the immediate and the sustained activated ERK were localized to vascular cells in the chick CAM model of angiogenesis. Using a synthetic inhibitor of the MAP kinase pathway, we demonstrated that active MAP kinase is required during angiogenesis in vivo. Previous studies have suggested that the duration of intracellular signaling events profoundly influences whether a cell undergoes proliferation and differentiation (reviewed in Marshall, 1995). For example, exposure of PC12 cells to epidermal growth factor induces a rapid and transient MAP kinase activity leading to cell proliferation, whereas nerve growth factor induces cell differentiation due to a sustained MAP kinase activation (Traverse et al., 1992).

We propose that during angiogenesis, ligation of $\alpha v\beta 3$ through appropriate matrix contacts may provide the positional or molecular cues necessary for sustained ERK activity. This may allow prolonged cell survival and differentiation of only those cells that are in the appropriate matrix microenvironment. In fact, antagonists of $\alpha v\beta 3$ caused apoptosis of proliferating vascular cells undergoing angiogenesis in the chick CAM, and this was associated with increased endothelial cell p53 activity. Interestingly, MAP kinase activity can regulate both p53 activity (Milne et al., 1994) and cell survival (Stromblad et al., 1996) in vitro. These observations indicate that sustained activation of ERK by $\alpha v\beta 3$ ligation during angiogenesis may suppress p53 activity, thereby promoting vascular cell survival and the maturation of newly sprouting blood vessels (Fig. 3).

VII. FUTURE PERSPECTIVES

The elucidation of the molecular basis of angiogenesis remains a challenge because of the complex interactions between the ECM and vascular cells that must be temporally and spatially coordinated. Further examination of the signaling events transduced by cell adhesion molecules to the smooth muscle and endothelial cells will probably reveal mechanisms by which cells can process cytokine or growth factor stimuli to have an impact on changes in intracellular phosphorylation cascades, gene expression levels, and ECM-associated enzymatic activities.

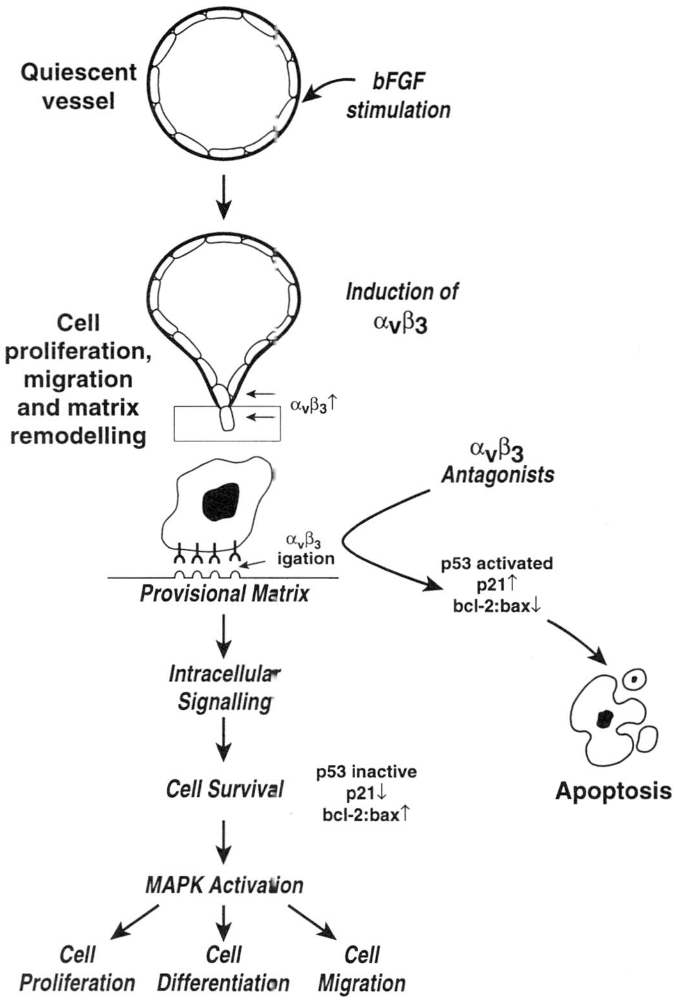

Figure 3 Hypothetical model for the role of integrin $\alpha v\beta 3$ in angiogenesis. Angiogenic stimulus by basic fibroblast growth factor (bFGF) induces expression of $\alpha v\beta 3$ and causes cells to invade the surrounding extracellular matrix and to enter the cell cycle. When ligation of integrin $\alpha v\beta 3$ is blocked, proliferating vascular cells undergo apoptosis, accompanied by an increase in p53 activity, $p21^{WAF1/CIP1}$ expression and a decrease in the Bcl2:Bax ratio. Basic FGF induces the activation of MAP kinase in vascular cells and leads to cell proliferation, differentiation, and migration.

The coordinated response to these inputs may direct the processes of vascular cell invasion, migration, proliferation, and differentiation during angiogenesis.

Clinical trials are now underway to examine the effects of a humanized form of the anti-αvβ3 antibody, LM609. This antibody is being administered to late-stage cancer patients in a dose-escalation study. If this or other αv integrin antagonists prove to be safe, it will be important to evaluate the clinical benefits of disrupting αv integrins on angiogenesis and the growth and malignant behavior of human cancer or other diseases associated with aberrant neovascularization.

REFERENCES

1. SM Abelda, SA Mette, DE Elder, R Stewart, L Damjanovich, M Herlyn, CA Buck. Canc Res 1990; 50:6757–6764.
2. J Bischoff. Trends Cell Biol 1995; 5:69–74.
3. N Boudreau, C Andrews, A Srebrow, A Ravanpay, DA Cheresh. J Cell Biol 1997; 139:257–264.
4. RB Brem, SG Robbins, DJ Wilson, LM O'Rourke, RN Mixon, JE Robertson, SR Planck, JT Rosenbaum. Invest Ophthalmol Vis Sci 1994; 35:3466–3474.
5. PC Brooks, RAF Clark, DA Cheresh. Science 1994; 264:569–571.
6. PC Brooks, AM Montgomery, M Rosenfeld, RA Reisfeld, T Hu, G Klier, DA Cheresh. Cell 1994; 79:1157–1164.
7. PC Brooks, S Stromblad, R Klemke, D Visscher, FH Sarkar, DA Cheresh. J Clin Invest 1995; 96:1815–1822.
8. PC Brooks, S Stromblad, LC Sanders, TL von Scholscha, RT Aimes, WG Stetler-Stevenson, JP Quigley, DA Cheresh. Cell 1996; 85:683–693.
9. Y-F Cheng, RH Kramer. J Cell Physiol 1989; 139:275–286.
10. DA Cheresh. Proc Natl Acad Sci 1987; 84:6471–6475.
11. DA Cheresh. Adv Molec Cell Biol 1993; 6:225–252.
12. RAF Clark, P DellaPelle, et al. J Invest Dermatol 1982; 79:269–276.
13. BS Coller, DA Cheresh, E Asch, U Seligsohn. Blood 1991; 77:75–83.
14. GE Davis. Biochem Biophys Res Commun 1992; 182:1025–1031.
15. LE Dike, SR Farmer. Proc Natl Acad Sci 1988; 85:6792–6796.
16. I Djaffar, JP Rosa. Hum Mol Genet 1993; 2:2179–2180.
17. CJ Drake, DA Cheresh, CD Little. J Cell Sci 1995; 108:2655–2661.
18. J Enenstein, RH Kramer. J Invest Dermat 1994; 103:381–386.
19. B Felding-Habermann, B Mueller, C Romerdahl, D Cheresh. J Clin Investig 1992; 89:2018–2022.
20. C Fisher, S Gilbertson-Beadling, et al. Dev Biol 1994; 162:499–510.
21. PS Frenette, TN Mayadas, H Rayburn, RO Hynes, DD Wagner. Cell 1996; 84:563–574.
22. M Friedlander, PC Brooks, et al. Science 1995; 270:1500–1502.
23. C Gladson, DA Cheresh. J Clin Invest 1991; 88:1924–1932.
24. DS Grant, K. Tashiro, et al. Cell 1989; 58:933–943.
25. TM Guadagno, M Ohtsubo, JM Roberts, RK Assoian. Science 1993; 262:1592–1675.

26. JL Guan, D Shalloway. Nature 1992; 358:690–692.
27. HP Hammes, M Brownlee, A Jonczyk, A Sutter, KT Preissner. Nat Med 1996; 2: 529–533.
28. R Hanemaajier, P Koolwijk, L Le Clercq, WJA De Wree, VWM van Hinsbergh. Biochem J 1993; 296:803–809.
29. GC Haralabopoulos, DS Grant, et al. Lab Invest 1994; 71:575–582.
30. MA Horton, ML Taylor, TR Arnett, MH Helfrich. Exp Cell Res 1991; 195:368–375.
31. RO Hynes. Cell 1992; 79:1157–1164.
32. D Ingber. J Cell Biochem 1991; 47:236–241.
33. ML Iruela-Arispe, P Hasselar, H Sage. Lab Invest 1991; 64:174–186.
34. B Jiang, GI Liuo, MA Behzadian, RB Caldwell. J Cell Sci 1994; 107:2499–2508.
35. MD Johnson, HR Kim, et al. J Cell Physiol 1994; 160:194–202.
36. RL Juliano, S Haskill. J Cell Biol 1993; 120:577–585.
37. L Kornberg, HS Earp, JT Parsons, M Schaler, RL Juliano. J Biol Chem 1992; 117: 1101–1107.
38. Y Kubota, HK Kleinman, GR Martin, TJ Lawley. J Cell Biol 1988; 107:1589–1598.
39. DI Leavesley, GD Ferguson, EA Wayner, DA Cheresh. J Cell Biol 1992; 117:1101–1107.
40. L Liaw, MP Skinner, et al. J Clin Invest 1995; 95:713–724.
41. J Lohler, R Timpl, R Jaenisch. Cell 1984; 38:597–607.
42. CJ Marshall. Cell 1995; 80:179–185.
43. HP McNamee, DE Ingber, MA Schwartz. J Cell Biol 1993; 121:673–678.
44. JE Meredith Jr, B Fazeli, MA Schwartz. Mol Biol Cell 1993; 4:953–961.
45. P Mignatti, R Tsuboi, E Robbins, DB Rifkin. J Cell Biol 1989; 108:671–682.
46. DM Milne, DG Campbell, FB Caudwell, DW Meek. J Biol Chem 1994; 269:9253.
47. S Miyamoto, JS Teramoto, JS Gutkind, K Yamada. J Cell Biol 1996; 135:1633.
48. R Montesano, L Orci. Cell 1985; 42:469–477.
49. AMP Montgomery, RA Reisfeld, DA Cheresh. Proc Natl Acad Sci 1994; 91:8856–8860.
50. MA Moses, J Sudhalter, R Langer. Science 1990; 248:1408–1410.
51. RF Nicosia, JA Madri. Am J Pathol 1987; 128:78–90.
52. M Pfaff, M Aumailley, et al. Exp Cell Res 1993; 206:167–176.
53. F Re, A Zanetti, M Sironi, et al. J Cell Biol 1994; 127:537–546.
54. W Risau, V Lemmon. Dev Biol 1988; 125:441–450.
55. FP Ross, J Chappel, et al. J Biol Chem 1993; 268:9901–9907.
56. M Sato, MK Sardana, et al. J Cell Biol 1990; 111:1713–1723.
57. M Schwartz, C Lechene. Proc Natl Acad Sci 1992; 89:6138–6141.
58. MA Schwartz, MD Schaller, MH Ginsberg. Annu Rev Cell Dev Biol 1995; 11:549–599.
59. M Schwartz. Cancer Res 1993; 51:1503–1505.
60. NT Sepp, LJ Li, et al. J Invest Dermatol 1994; 103:295–299.
61. S Stromblad, JC Becker, M Yebra, PC Brooks, DA Cheresh. J Clin Invest 1996; 98:426–433.
62. M Takigawa, Y Nishida, et al. Biochem Biophys Res Comm 1990; 171:1264–1271.
63. EJ Topol, RM Califf, et al. Lancet 1994; 343:881–886.
64. S Traverse, N Gomez, H Paterson, et al. Biochem J 1992; 288:351.
65. JA Varner, D Emerson, R Juliano. Mol Cell Biol 1995; 6:725–740.
66. E White. Genes Dev 1996; 10:1–15.

25
The Role of Vascular Endothelial Growth Factor in Angiogenesis

Napoleone Ferrara
Genentech, Inc., South San Francisco, California

I. INTRODUCTION

The development of a vascular supply is fundamental for organ development and differentiation during embryogenesis, as well as for wound healing and reproductive functions in the adult (1). Angiogenesis also is implicated in the pathogenesis of a variety of disorders: proliferative retinopathies, age-related macular degeneration, tumors, rheumatoid arthritis, and psoriasis (1, 2).

The search for positive regulators of angiogenesis has yielded several candidates, including aFGF, basic fibroblast growth factor (bFGF), tumor growth factor (TGF)-α, TGF-β, human growth factor (HGF), tumor necrosis factor (TNF)-α, angiogenin, interleukin (IL)-8, and, most recently, a TIE-2 receptor ligand called angiopoietin-1 (3, 4). The negative regulators so far identified include thrombospondin (5, 6), the 16-kD N-terminal fragment of prolactin (7), angiostatin (8), and endostatin (9).

This chapter discusses the molecular and biological properties of vascular endothelial growth factor (VEGF) proteins. Over the last few years, several members of the VEGF gene family have been identified, including VEGF-B, VEGF-C, placenta growth factor, and VEGF-D (10). This chapter focuses primarily on VEGF, also referred to as "VEGF-A." Work done by several laboratories over the last few years has elucidated the pivotal role of VEGF and its receptors in the regulation of normal and abnormal angiogenesis (10). The finding that the loss of even a single VEGF allele results in embryonic lethality points to the important role played by this factor in the development and differentiation of the vascular system (11, 12). Furthermore, VEGF-induced angiogenesis has been shown to result in a therapeutic effect in animal models of coronary (13) or limb (14) ischemia and, more recently, in humans as well (15).

At present, both the recombinant VEGF protein and a humanized anti-VEGF monoclonal antibody are in clinical trials, for the treatment of coronary ischemia and solid tumors, respectively.

II. BIOLOGICAL ACTIVITIES OF VEGF

Vascular endothelial growth factor is a mitogen for vascular endothelial cells derived from arteries, veins, and lymphatics, but it is devoid of consistent and appreciable mitogenic activity for other cell types (10). It promotes angiogenesis in tridimensional in vitro models, inducing confluent microvascular endothelial cells to invade collagen gels and form capillary-like structures (16). Also, VEGF induces sprouting from rat aortic rings embedded in a collagen gel (17). It also elicits a pronounced angiogenic response in a variety of in vivo models, including the chick chorioallantoic membrane (18).

Vascular endothelial growth factor induces expression of the serine proteases urokinase-type and tissue-type plasminogen activators (PA) and PA inhibitor 1 (PAI-1) in cultured bovine microvascular endothelial cells (19). Moreover, VEGF increases expression of the metalloproteinase interstitial collagenase in human umbilical vein endothelial cells but not in dermal fibroblasts (20). Other studies have shown that VEGF promotes expression of urokinase plasminogen activator receptor (uPAR) in vascular endothelial cells (21). Additionally, VEGF stimulates hexose transport in cultured vascular endothelial cells (22).

Vascular endothelial growth factor is known also as vascular permeability factor (VPF) based on its ability to induce vascular leakage in the guinea pig skin (23). Dvorak and colleagues proposed that an increase in microvascular permeability is a crucial step in angiogenesis associated with tumors and wounds (24). According to this hypothesis, a major function of VPF/VEGF in the angiogenic process is the induction of plasma protein leakage. This effect would result in the formation of an extravascular fibrin gel, a substrate for endothelial and tumor cell growth (25). Recent studies also have suggested that VEGF may induce fenestrations in endothelial cells (26, 27). Topical administration of VEGF resulted in the development of fenestrations in the endothelium of small venules and capillaries, even in regions where endothelial cells are not normally fenestrated, and was associated with increased vascular permeability (26, 27).

Melder et al. have shown that VEGF promotes expression of vascular cell adhesion molecule (VCAM)-1 and intercellular adhesion molecule (ICAM)-1 in endothelial cells (28). This induction results in the adhesion of activated natural killer (NK) cells to endothelial cells, mediated by specific interaction of endothelial VCAM-1 and ICAM-1 with CD18 and viruslike agent (VLA)-4 on the surface of NK cells.

Vascular endothelial growth factor has been reported to have regulatory effects on blood cells. Clauss et al. reported that VEGF may promote monocyte chemotaxis (29). Broxmeyer et al. have shown that VEGF induces colony formation by mature subsets of granulocyte-macrophage progenitor cells (30). These findings may be explained by the common origin of endothelial cells and hematopoietic cells and the presence of VEGF receptors in progenitor cells as early as hemangioblasts in blood islands in the yolk sac. Furthermore, Gabrilovich et al. have reported that VEGF may have an inhibitory effect on the maturation of host professional antigen-presenting cells such as dendritic cells (31). Vascular endothelial growth factor was found to inhibit immature dendritic cells without having a significant effect on the function of mature cells. These findings led to the suggestion that VEGF may facilitate tumor growth by allowing the tumor to avoid the induction of an immune response (31).

Vascular endothelial growth factor induces vasodilation in vitro in a dose-dependent fashion (32, 33) and produces transient tachycardia, hypotension, and a decrease in cardiac output when injected intravenously in conscious, instrumented rats (33). Such effects appear to be caused by a decrease in venous return, mediated primarily by endothelial cell-derived nitric oxide (NO), as assessed by the requirement for an intact endothelium and the prevention of the effects by N-methyl-arginine (33). Accordingly, VEGF has no direct effect on contractility or rate in isolated rat heart in vitro (33). These hemodynamic effects, however, are not unique to VEGF: other angiogenic factors such as aFGF and bFGF also have the ability to induce NO-mediated vasodilation and hypotension (34, 35).

III. ORGANIZATION OF THE VEGF GENE AND CHARACTERISTICS OF THE VEGF PROTEINS

The human VEGF gene is organized into eight exons, separated by seven introns. The coding region spans approximately 14 kilobases (kb) (36, 37). The human VEGF gene has been assigned to chromosome 6p21.3 (38). It is now well established that alternative exon splicing of a single VEGF gene results in the generation of four different molecular species, having respectively 121, 165, 189, and 206 amino acids following signal sequence cleavage ($VEGF_{121}$, $VEGF_{165}$, $VEGF_{189}$, $VEGF_{206}$). Vascular endothelial growth $factor_{165}$ lacks the residues encoded by exon 6, whereas $VEGF_{121}$ lacks the residues encoded by exons 6 and 7. Compared with $VEGF_{165}$, $VEGF_{121}$ lacks 44 amino acids; $VEGF_{189}$ has an insertion of 24 amino acids highly enriched in basic residues; and $VEGF_{206}$ has an additional insertion of 17 amino acids (36).

Vascular endothelial growth factor$_{165}$ is the predominant molecular species produced by a variety of normal and transformed cells. Transcripts encoding VEGF$_{121}$ and VEGF$_{189}$ are detected in the majority of cells and tissues expressing the VEGF gene (36). In contrast, VEGF$_{206}$ is a very rare form, so far identified only in a human fetal liver cDNA library (36). The genomic organization of the murine VEGF gene also has been described (39). Similarly to the human gene, the coding region of the murine VEGF gene encompasses approximately 14 kb and is composed of eight exons interrupted by seven introns. Analysis of exons suggests the generation of three isoforms: VEGF$_{120}$, VEGF$_{164}$, and VEGF$_{188}$. Therefore, murine VEGFs are shorter than human VEGF by one amino acid. However, a fourth isoform comparable to VEGF$_{206}$ is not predicted, because an in-frame stop codon is present in the region corresponding to the human VEGF$_{206}$ open reading frame. Analysis of the 3′ untranslated region of the rat VEGF mRNA has revealed the presence of four potential polyadenylation sites (40). A frequently used site is about 1.9 kb further downstream from the previously reported transcription termination codon (41). The sequence within this 3′ untranslated region reveals a number of sequence motifs known to be involved in the regulation of mRNA stability (40).

Native VEGF is a basic, heparin-binding, homodimeric glycoprotein of 45,000 daltons (42). These properties correspond to those of VEGF$_{165}$, the major isoform (43). Vascular endothelial growth factor$_{121}$ is a weakly acidic polypeptide that fails to bind to heparin (43); VEGF$_{189}$ and VEGF$_{206}$ are more basic and bind to heparin with greater affinity than VEGF$_{165}$ (43). Such differences in the isoelectric point and in affinity for heparin may profoundly affect the bioavailability of the VEGF. Vascular endothelial growth factor$_{121}$ is a freely diffusible protein; VEGF$_{165}$ is also secreted, although a significant fraction remains bound to the cell surface and the extracellular matrix (ECM). In contrast, VEGF$_{189}$ and VEGF$_{206}$ are almost completely sequestered in the ECM (44). However, these isoforms may be released in a soluble form by heparin or heparinase, suggesting that their binding site is represented by proteoglycans containing heparinlike moieties. The long forms also may be released by plasmin after cleavage at the COOH terminus. This action generates a bioactive proteolytic fragment having molecular weight of ~34,000 daltons (43). Plasminogen activation and generation of plasmin play an important role in the angiogenesis cascade. Thus, proteolysis of VEGF is likely to occur also in vivo. Keyt et al. have shown that the bioactive product of plasmin action comprises the first 110 NH_2-terminal amino acids of VEGF (45). These findings suggest that the VEGF proteins may become available to endothelial cells by at least two different mechanisms: as freely diffusible proteins (VEGF$_{121}$, VEGF$_{165}$) or after protease activation and cleavage of the longer isoforms. However, loss of heparin binding, whether it is caused by alternative splicing of RNA or plasmin cleavage, results in a substantial loss of mitogenic activity for vascular endothelial cells: compared to VEGF$_{165}$, VEGF$_{121}$ or VEGF$_{110}$ demonstrates 50-

to 100-fold reduced potency when tested in endothelial cell growth assay (45). It has been suggested that the stability of VEGF-heparan sulfate-receptor complexes contributes to effective signal transduction and stimulation of endothelial cell proliferation (45). Thus, VEGF has the potential to express structural and functional heterogeneity to yield a graded and controlled biological response. Recently, Poltcrak et al. have provided evidence for the existence of an additional alternatively spliced molecular species of VEGF (46). A VEGF isoform containing exons 1–6 and 8 of the VEGF gene was found to be expressed as a major VEGF mRNA form in several cell lines derived from carcinomas of the female reproductive system. This mRNA is predicted to encode a VEGF form of 145 amino acids ($VEGF_{145}$). Recombinant $VEGF_{145}$ induced the proliferation of vascular endothelial cells, albeit at much lower potency than $VEGF_{165}$. Vascular endothelial growth $factor_{145}$ binds to the KDR receptor on the surface of endothelial cells. It also binds to heparin with an affinity similar to that of $VEGF_{165}$.

Recently, Muller et al. (47) determined the crystal structure of VEGF at a resolution of 2.5 A. Overall, the VEGF monomer resembles that of platelet-derived growth factor (PDGF), but its N-terminal segment is helical rather than extended. The dimerization mode of VEGF is similar to that of PDGF and very different from that of TGF-β.

IV. REGULATION OF VEGF GENE EXPRESSION

A. Oxygen Tension

Among the mechanisms thought to participate in the regulation of VEGF gene expression, oxygen tension plays a major role, both in vitro and in vivo. Vascular endothelial growth factor mRNA expression is rapidly and reversibly induced by exposure to low partial pressure of oxygen (pO_2) in a variety of normal and transformed cultured cell types (48, 49). Also, ischemia caused by occlusion of the left anterior descending coronary artery results in a dramatic increase in VEGF mRNA levels in the pig and rat myocardium, suggesting the possibility that VEGF may mediate the spontaneous revascularization that follows myocardial ischemia (50, 51). Furthermore, hypoxic up-regulation of VEGF mRNA in neuroglial cells, secondary to the onset of neuronal activity, is thought to play an important physiological role in the development of the retinal vasculature (52).

Similarities exist between the mechanisms leading to hypoxic regulation of VEGF and erythropoietin (Epo) (53). Hypoxia inducibility is conferred on both genes by homologous sequences. By deletion and mutation analysis, a 28-base sequence has been identified in the 5′ promoter of the rat and human VEGF gene that mediated hypoxia-induced transcription (54, 55). Such a sequence reveals a high degree of homology and similar protein-binding characteristics as the hypoxia-inducible factor 1-(HIF-1) binding site within the Epo gene (56).

Hypoxia-inducible factor-1 has been identified as a mediator of transcriptional responses to hypoxia and is a basic, heterodimeric, helix-loop-helix protein (57). When reporter constructs containing the VEGF sequences that mediate hypoxia-inducibility were cotransfected with expression vectors encoding HIF-1 subunits, reporter gene transcription was much greater than that observed in cells transfected with the reporter alone, both in hypoxic and normoxic conditions (58).

Transcriptional activation is not the only mechanism leading to VEGF up-regulation in response to hypoxia (40, 59). Increased mRNA stability has been identified as a significant posttranscriptional component. Sequences that mediate increased stability were identified in the 3′ untranslated region of the VEGF mRNA.

B. Cytokines

Various cytokines or growth factors may up-regulate VEGF mRNA expression. Epidermal growth factor (EGF), TGF-β, or KGF results in a significant induction of VEGF mRNA expression (60). Epidermal growth factor also stimulates VEGF release by cultured glioblastoma cells (61). In addition, treatment of quiescent cultures of epithelial and fibroblastic cell lines with TGF-β resulted in induction of VEGF mRNA and release of VEGF protein in the medium (62). Based on these findings, it has been proposed that VEGF may function as a paracrine mediator for indirect-acting angiogenic agents such as TGF-β (62). Furthermore, IL-1-β induces VEGF expression in aortic smooth muscle cells (63). Both IL-1-α and PGE_2 induce expression of VEGF in cultured synovial fibroblasts, suggesting the participation of such inductive mechanisms in inflammatory angiogenesis (64). Interleukin-6 significantly induces VEGF expression in several cell lines (65). Insulinlike growth factor (IGF)-1, a mitogen implicated in the growth of several malignancies, induces VEGF mRNA and protein in cultured colorectal carcinoma cells (66).

C. Differentiation and Transformation

Cell differentiation plays an important role in the regulation of VEGF gene expression (67). The VEGF mRNA is up-regulated during the conversion of 3T3 preadipocytes into adipocytes or during the myogenic differentiation of C2C12 cells. Conversely, VEGF gene expression is repressed during the differentiation of the pheochromocytoma cell line PC12 into nonmalignant, neuronlike cells.

Specific transforming events also result in induction of VEGF gene expression. A mutated form of the murine p53 tumor suppressor gene results in induction of VEGF mRNA expression in NIH 3T3 cells in transient transfection assays (68). Likewise, oncogenic mutations or amplification of *ras* lead to VEGF up-regulation (69, 70). Interestingly, expression of oncogenic *ras*, either constitutive or transient, potentiated the induction of VEGF by hypoxia (71). Moreover, the von Hippel-Lindau (VHL) tumor suppressor gene has been implicated in the regulation of VEGF gene expression (72–74). The VHL tumor suppressor gene is inactivated in patients with VHL disease and in most sporadic clear-cell renal carcinomas. Although the function of the VHL protein has not been fully elucidated, it is known that such protein interacts with the elongin BC subunits in vivo and regulates RNA polymerase II elongation activity in vitro by inhibiting formation of the elongin ABC complex. Human renal cell carcinoma cells either lacking as endogenous wild-type VHL gene or expressing an inactive mutant demonstrated altered regulation of VEGF gene expression, which was corrected by introduction of the wild-type VHL gene. Most of the endothelial cells' mitogenic activity released by tumor cells expressing mutant VHL gene was neutralized by anti-VEGF antibodies (72). These findings suggest that VEGF is a key mediator of the abnormal vascular proliferations and solid tumors characteristics of VHL syndrome. Iliopulos et al. (73) have shown that a function of the VHL protein is to provide a negative regulation of a series of hypoxia-inducible genes, including the VEGF, PDGF B chain, and the glucose transporter GLUT1 genes. In the presence of a mutant VHL, mRNAs for such genes were produced under both normoxic and hypoxic conditions. Reintroduction of wild-type VHL resulted in inhibition of mRNA production under normoxic conditions and restored the characteristic hypoxia-inducibility of those genes (73). In addition, Gnarra et al. (74) have shown that VHL regulates VEGF expression at a posttranscriptional level and that VHL inactivation in target cells causes a loss of VEGF suppression, leading to formation of a vascular stroma. Interestingly, despite fivefold differences in VEGF mRNA levels, VHL overexpression did not affect VEGF transcription initiation.

V. THE VEGF RECEPTORS

Two classes of high-affinity VEGF binding sites were initially described in the surface of bovine endothelial cells, with K_d values of 10 pM and 100 pM, respectively (75, 76). Lower affinity binding sites on mononuclear phagocytes were subsequently described (77). Such binding sites may be involved in mediating chemotactic effects for monocytes by VEGF (29).

Ligand autoradiography studies on fetal and adult rat tissue sections demonstrated that high-affinity VEGF binding sites are localized to the vascular endothelium of large or small vessels in situ (78, 79). Vascular endothelial growth factor binding was apparent on both proliferating and quiescent endothelial cells (78, 79). Also, the earliest developmental identification of high-affinity VEGF binding was in the hemangioblasts in the blood islands in the yolk sac (79).

A. The Flt-1 and Flk-1/KDR Tyrosine Kinases

1. Binding Characteristics and Structure Function Analysis

Two VEGF receptor tyrosine kinases (RTKs) have been identified. The Flt-1 (FMS-like tyrosine kinase) (80) and KDR (kinase domain region) (81) receptors bind VEGF with high affinity. The murine homologue of KDR, Flk-1 (fetal liver kinase-1), shares 85% sequence identity with human KDR (82). Both Flt-1 and KDR/Flk-1 have seven immunoglobulin (Ig)-like domains in the extracellular domain (ECD), a single transmembrane region and a consensus tyrosine kinase sequence that is interrupted by a kinase-insert domain (82–84). FMS-like tyrosine kinase-1 has the highest affinity for $rhVEGF_{165}$, with a K_d of approximately 10–20 pM (80). The KDR has a somewhat lower affinity for VEGF: the K_d has been estimated to be approximately 75–125 pM (81).

A cDNA coding an alternatively spliced soluble form of Flt-1 (sFlt-1), lacking the seventh Ig-like domain, transmembrane sequence, and the cytoplasmic domain, has been identified in human umbilical vein endothelial cells (85). This sFlt-1 receptor binds VEGF with high affinity (K_d 10–20 pM). It is able to inhibit VEGF-induced mitogenesis and may be a physiological negative regulator of VEGF action (85).

An additional member of the family of RTKs with seven Ig-like domains in the ECD is Flt-4 (86–88). However, it is not a receptor for VEGF but rather binds a newly identified ligand called VEGF-C or VEGF-related peptide (VRP) (89, 90). Interestingly, VEGF-C/VRP is a regulator of lymphatic angiogenesis (91).

Recent studies have mapped the binding site for VEGF to the second immunoglobulinlike domain of Flt-1 and KDR. Deletion of the second domain of Flt-1 completely abolished the binding of VEGF. Introduction of the second domain of KDR into an Flt-1 mutant lacking the homologous domain restored VEGF binding. However, the ligand specificity was characteristic of the KDR receptor. To further test this hypothesis, chimeric receptors in which the first three or just the second Ig-like domains of Flt-1 replaced the corresponding domains in Flt-4 were created. Both swaps conferred on Flt-4 the ability to bind VEGF with an affinity nearly identical to that of wild-type Flt-1. Furthermore, transfected cells expressing these chimeric Flt-4 receptors exhibited increased DNA synthesis in response to VEGF or placenta growth factor (PlGF) (92).

An application of these structure-function studies is the generation of inhibitors of VEGF activity. The first three Ig-like domains of Flt-1 fused to a heavy chain Fc potently inhibits VEGF bioactivity across species. The Fc may confer sufficient half-life and stability when injected systemically (93). Therefore, this agent may be useful in determining the role of endogenous VEGF in several in vivo models.

Very recently, the crystal structure of VEGF in complex with the second Ig-like domain of Flt-1 has been solved (94). These studies show that the interaction between VEGF and Flt-1 is predominantly hydrophobic. Other studies have shown that several charged residues within the second Ig-like domain, especially Asp^{187}, are important to maintain appropriate structural stability and integrity, even though they are not directly involved in ligand binding (95).

2. Signal Transduction

Vascular endothelial growth factor induces the phosphorylation of at least 11 proteins in bovine aortic endothelial cells (96). PLC-γ, and two proteins that associate with PLC-γ, were phosphorylated in response to VEGF. Furthermore, immunoblot analysis for mediators of signal transduction that contain SH2 domains demonstrated that VEGF induces phosphorylation of phosphatidylinositol 3-kinase, *ras* GTPase activating protein (GAP), and several others. These findings suggest that VEGF promotes the formation of multimeric aggregates of VEGF receptors with proteins that contain SH2 domains. These studies, however, did not identify which VEGF receptor(s) are involved in these events. It has been suggested that NO mediates, at least in part, the mitogenic effect of VEGF on cultured microvascular endothelium isolated from coronary venules (97). The proliferative effect of VEGF was reduced by pretreatment of the cells with NO synthase inhibitors. Exposure of the cells to VEGF induced a significant increment in cGMP levels. These findings suggest that VEGF stimulates proliferation of postcapillary endothelial cells through the production of NO and cGMP accumulation.

Several studies have indicated that Flt-1 and KDR have different signal transduction properties (98, 99). Porcine aortic endothelial cells lacking endogenous VEGF receptors display chemotaxis and mitogenesis in response to VEGF when transfected with a plasmid coding for KDR (98). In contrast, transfected cells expressing Flt-1 lack such responses (98, 99). Fetal liver kinase-1/KDR undergoes strong ligand-dependent tyrosine phosphorylation in intact cells, whereas Flt-1 reveals a weak or undetectable response (98, 99). Also, VEGF stimulation results in weak tyrosine phosphorylation that does not generate any mitogenic signal in transfected NIH 3T3 cells expressing Flt-1 (99). These findings agree with other studies that PlGF, which binds with high affinity to Flt-1 but not to Flk-1/KDR, lacks direct mitogenic or permeability-enhancing properties or the ability to stimulate effectively tyrosine phosphorylation in endothelial cells (100). Therefore, interaction with Flk-1/KDR is a critical requirement to induce the full spectrum of VEGF biological responses. In further support of this conclusion, VEGF mutants that bind selectively to Flk-1/KDR are fully active endothelial cell mitogens (101). These findings cast doubt on the role of Flt-1 as a truly signaling receptor. However, more recent evidence indicates that Flt-1 indeed signals, although our understanding of these events is fragmentary. Cunningham et al. have demonstrated an interaction between Flt-1 and the p85 subunit of phosphatidylinositol 3-kinase (102), suggesting that p85 couples Flt-1 to intracellular signal transduction systems and implicating elevated levels of PtdIns(3,4,5)P3 levels in this process (102). Also, members of the Src family, such as Fyn and Yes, show an increased level of phosphorylation after VEGF stimulation in transfected cells expressing Flt-1 but not KDR (98). Furthermore, a specific biological response, the migration of monocytes in response to VEGF (or PlGF), is mediated by Flt-1 (103).

3. Regulation

The expression of Flt-1 and Flk-1/KDR genes is largely restricted to the vascular endothelium. The promoter region of Flt-1 has been cloned and characterized and a 1-kb fragment of the 5′ flanking region essential for endothelial-specific expression was identified (104). Likewise, a 4-kb 5′ flanking sequence has been identified in the promoter of KDR that confers endothelial cell-specific activation (105).

Similarly to VEGF, hypoxia has been thought to play an important role in the regulation of VEGF receptor gene expression. Exposure of rats to acute or chronic hypoxia led to pronounced up-regulation of both Flt-1 and Flk-1/KDR genes in the lung vasculature (106). Also, Flk-1/KDR and Flt-1 mRNAs were substantially up-regulated throughout the heart after myocardial infarction in the rat (107). However, in vitro studies have yielded unexpected results. Hypoxia increases VEGF receptor number by 50% in cultured bovine retinal capillary endothelial cells. The expression of KDR, however, is not induced but paradoxically shows an initial down-regulation (108). Brogi et al. proposed that the hypoxic up-regulation of KDR observed in vivo is not direct but requires the release of an unidentified paracrine mediator from ischemic tissues (109). Recent studies have provided evidence for a differential transcriptional regulation of the Flt-1 and KDR genes by hypoxia (110). When human umbilical vein endothelial cells (HUVEC) were exposed to hypoxic conditions in vitro, increased levels of Flt-1 expression were observed. In contrast, Flk-1/KDR mRNA levels were unchanged or slightly repressed. Promoter deletion analysis demonstrated a 430-bp region of the Flt-1 promoter to be required for transcriptional activation in response to hypoxia. This region includes a heptamer sequence matching the HIF-1 consensus-binding site previously found in other hypoxia-inducible genes. The element mediating the hypoxia response was further defined as a 40 bp sequence including the putative HIF-1 binding site. Such an element was not found in the Flk-1/KDR promoter. These findings indicate that, unlike the KDR/Flk-1 gene, the Flt-1 receptor gene is directly up-regulated by hypoxia through a hypoxia-inducible enhancer element located at position -976 to -937 of the Flt-1 promoter (110). Also, recent studies have shown that both TNF-α (111) and TGF-β (112) have the ability to inhibit the expression of the KDR gene in cultured endothelial cells.

VI. ROLE OF VEGF AND ITS RECEPTORS IN PHYSIOLOGICAL ANGIOGENESIS

A. Distribution of VEGF, Flk-1/KDR, and Flt-1 mRNA

The proliferation of blood vessels is crucial for a wide variety of physiological processes such as embryonic development, normal growth and differentiation, wound healing, and reproductive functions.

During embryonic development, VEGF expression is first detected within the first few days after implantation in the giant cells of the trophoblast (79, 113). At later developmental stages in the mouse or rat embryos, the VEGF mRNA is expressed in several organs, including heart, vertebral column, kidney, and along the surface of the spinal cord and brain. In the developing mouse brain, the highest levels of mRNA expression are associated with the choroid plexus and the ventricular epithelium (113). In the human fetus (16–22 weeks), VEGF mRNA expression is detectable in virtually all tissues and is most abundant in lung, kidney, and spleen (114).

In situ hybridization studies have shown that the Flk-1 mRNA is expressed in the yolk sac and intraembryonic mesoderm, and later in angioblasts, endocardium, and small and large vessel endothelium (115, 116). These findings strongly suggested a role for Flk-1 in the regulation of vasculogenesis and angiogenesis. Other studies have demonstrated that expression of Flk-1 mRNA is first detected in the proximal-lateral embryonic mesoderm, which gives rise to the heart (117). Fetal liver kinase-1 is then detectable in the endocardial cells of heart primordia and subsequently in the major embryonic and extraembryonic vessels (117). These studies indicated that Flk-1 may be the earliest marker of endothelial cells precursors. The Flt-1 mRNA is selectively expressed in vascular endothelial cells, both in fetal and adult mouse tissues (118). Similarly to the high affinity VEGF binding, the Flt-1 mRNA is expressed in both proliferating and quiescent endothelial cells, suggesting a role for Flt-1 in the maintenance of endothelial cells (118).

Vascular endothelial growth factor expression is also detectable around microvessels in areas where endothelial cells are normally quiescent, such as kidney glomerulus, pituitary, heart, lung, and brain (119, 120). These findings raised the possibility that VEGF may be required to induce active vascular proliferation and, at least in some circumstances, for the maintenance of the differentiated state of blood vessels (119). In agreement with this hypothesis, Alon et al. have shown that VEGF acts as a survival factor, at least for the developing retinal vessels (121). They proposed that hyperoxia-induced vascular regression in the retina of neonatal animals is a consequence of inhibition of VEGF production by glial cells.

B. The Flk-1/KDR, Flt-1, and VEGF Gene Knock-Outs in Mice

Recent studies have demonstrated that both Flt-1 and Flk-1/KDR are essential for normal development of embryonic vasculature. However, their roles in endothelial cell proliferation and differentiation appear to be distinct (122, 123). Mouse embryos homozygous for a targeted mutation in the Flt-1 locus died in utero between days 8.5 and 9.5 (122). Endothelial cells developed in both embryonic and extra-embryonic sites but failed to organize in normal vascular channels. Mice in which the Flk-1 gene had been inactivated lacked vasculogenesis and failed to develop blood islands. Hematopoietic precursors were severely disrupted, and organized blood vessels failed to develop throughout the embryo or the yolk sac, resulting in death in utero between days 8.5 and 9.5 (123).

These findings do not necessarily mean that VEGF is equally essential, as other ligands might potentially activate the Flt-1 and Flk-1 receptors and thus substitute VEGF action. Very recent studies (11, 12) have generated direct evidence for the role played by VEGF in embryonic vasculogenesis and angiogenesis. Inactivation of the VEGF gene in mice resulted in embryonic lethality in heterozygous embryos, between days 11 and 12. The VEGF+/− embryos were growth retarded and exhibited a number of developmental anomalies. The forebrain region appeared significantly underdeveloped. In the heart region, the outflow region was grossly malformed; the dorsal aortae were rudimentary, and the thickness of the ventricular wall was significantly decreased. The yolk sac revealed a very reduced number of nucleated red blood cells within the blood islands. Also, the vitelline veins failed to fuse with the vascular plexus of the yolk sac. Significant defects in the vasculature of other tissues and organs, including placenta and nervous system, were observed. In situ hybridization confirmed expression of VEGF mRNA in heterozygous embryos. Thus, the VEGF+/− phenotype appears to be the result of gene dosage, not maternal imprinting.

Although several heterozygous phenotypes have been described (124), this may be the first example of embryonic lethality after the loss of a single allele of a gene that is not maternally imprinted. Therefore, VEGF and its receptors are essential for blood island formation and angiogenesis, so that even reduced concentrations of VEGF are inadequate to support a normal pattern of development. Interestingly, inactivation of the PlGF gene does not result in embryonic lethality, even in the homozygous state (125). Placenta growth factor−/− mice are viable and fertile, although they may have some impairment of wound healing. These findings suggest that other members of the VEGF gene family may not be equally critical for vascular development.

C. Role of VEGF in Corpus Luteum Angiogenesis

The development and endocrine function of the ovarian corpus luteum (CL) depend on the growth of new capillary vessels (126). Previous studies have shown that the VEGF mRNA is temporally and spatially related to the proliferation of blood vessels in the rat, mouse, and primate ovary and in the rat uterus, suggesting that VEGF is a mediator of the cyclical growth of blood vessels that occurs in the female reproductive tract (127–130). Very recently, the hypothesis that VEGF may be has been examined in a rat model of gonadotropin-induced ovulation (131). Treatment with Flt (1-3)-IgG resulted in virtually complete suppression of CL angiogenesis. This effect was associated with inhibition of CL development and progesterone release. Failure of maturation of the endometrium was also observed. Areas of ischemic necrosis were demonstrated in the CL of treated animals. However, no effect on the pre-existing ovarian vasculature was observed. These findings demonstrate that, in spite of the redundancy of potential mediators, VEGF is essential for CL angiogenesis. Furthermore, they have implications for the control of fertility and the treatment of ovarian disorders characterized by hypervascularity and hyperplasia, such as policystic ovary syndrome.

VII. ROLE OF VEGF IN PATHOLOGIC ANGIOGENESIS

A. Tumor Angiogenesis

Many tumor cell lines secrete VEGF in vitro (119). In situ hybridization studies demonstrated that the VEGF mRNA is significantly up-regulated in the vast majority of human tumors thus far examined. These include lung (132, 133), breast (134, 135), gastrointestinal tract (136, 137), kidney (138), bladder (138), ovary (139), endometrium (140), and uterine cervix (141) carcinomas; angiosarcoma (142), germ cell tumors (143), and several intracranial tumors including glioblastoma multiforme (144–146) and sporadic, as well as VHL syndrome-associated, capillary hemangioblastoma (147, 148). In glioblastoma multiforme and other tumors with significant necrosis, the expression of VEGF mRNA is highest in hypoxic tumor cells adjacent to necrotic areas (144–146). A correlation exists between the degree of vascularization of the malignancy and VEGF mRNA expression (141, 147, 148). In virtually all specimens examined, the VEGF mRNA was expressed in tumor cells but not in endothelial cells. In contrast, the mRNAs for Flt-1 and KDR were up-regulated in the endothelial cells associated with the tumor (136, 149). These findings are consistent with the hypothesis that VEGF is primarily a paracrine mediator (150). Immunohistochemical studies have localized the VEGF protein to both the tumor cells and the vasculature (136, 145). This indicates that tumor-secreted VEGF accumulates in the target cells (151). Interestingly, studies have suggested that the angiogenesis mediated by the HIV-1 Tat protein (152) requires activation of the KDR receptor (153). Tat induces growth of Kaposi's sarcoma (KS) spindle cells and has been implicated in the vascularity of the KS lesions (153).

Elevations in VEGF levels have been detected in the serum of some cancer patients (154). Also, a correlation has been noted between VEGF expression and microvessel density in primary breast cancer sections (155). Postoperative surveys indicated that the relapse-free survival rate of patients with VEGF-rich tumors was significantly worse than those with VEGF-poor tumors, suggesting that expression of VEGF is associated with stimulation of angiogenesis and with early relapse in primary breast cancer (156). A similar correlation has been described in gastric carcinoma patients (157). Vascular endothelial growth factor positivity in tumor sections was correlated with vessel involvement, lymph node metastasis, and liver metastasis. Furthermore, patients with VEGF-positive tumors had a worse prognosis than those with VEGF-negative tumors (157).

The availability of specific monoclonal antibodies capable of inhibiting VEGF-induced angiogenesis in vivo and in vitro (158) made it possible to generate direct evidence for a role of VEGF in tumorigenesis. In a study published by Kim et al. in 1993, such antibodies were found to exert a potent inhibitory effect on the growth of three human tumor cell lines injected subcutaneously in nude mice: the SK-LMS-1 leiomyosarcoma, the G55 glioblastoma multiforme, and the A673 rhabdomyosarcoma (159). The growth inhibition ranged from 70% to more than 95%. Subsequently, other tumor cell lines were found to be inhibited in vivo by this treatment (160–162).

In agreement with the hypothesis that inhibition of neovascularization is the mechanism of tumor suppression, the density of blood vessels was significantly lower in sections of tumors from antibody-treated animals as compared with controls. Furthermore, neither the antibodies nor VEGF had any effect on the in vitro growth of the tumor cells (159). Intravital videomicroscopy techniques have allowed a more direct verification of the hypothesis that anti-VEGF antibodies block tumor angiogenesis (163). Noninvasive imaging of the vasculature revealed a nearly complete suppression of tumor angiogenesis in anti–VEGF-treated animals as compared with controls, at all time points examined (163).

Vascular endothelial growth factor is a mediator of the in vivo growth of human colon carcinoma HM7 cells in a nude mouse model of liver metastasis (160). Treatment with anti-VEGF monoclonal antibodies resulted in a dramatic decrease in the number and size of metastases. Similarly, administration of anti-VEGF neutralizing antibodies inhibited primary tumor growth and metastasis of A431 human epidermoid carcinoma cells in Scid mice (161) or HT-1080 fibrosarcoma cells implanted in BALB/c nude mice (162). Recent studies have shown that VEGF is also a mediator of stromal-induced enhancement of human prostate cancer LNCaP cell growth in vivo (164).

Borgström et al. (165) have shown that a combination treatment that includes anti-VEGF monoclonal antibody and doxorubicin significantly enhances either agent alone and, in some cases, led to complete regression of tumors derived from MCF-7 breast carcinoma cells in nude mice.

Intravital fluorescence microscopy and video imaging analysis also have been applied to address the important issue of the effects of VEGF on permeability and other properties of tumor vessels (166). Treatment with anti-VEGF monoclonal antibodies was initiated when tumor xenografts were already established and vascularized and resulted in time-dependent reductions in vascular permeability (166). These effects were accompanied by striking changes in the morphology of vessels, with dramatic reduction in diameter and tortuosity. This reduction in diameter is expected to block the passage of blood elements and eventually stop the flow in the tumor vascular network. A regression of blood vessels was observed after repeated administrations of anti-VEGF antibody. These findings suggest that tumor vessels require constant stimulation with VEGF to maintain their proliferative properties as well as some key morphological features (166).

An independent verification of the hypothesis that the VEGF action is required for tumor angiogenesis has been provided by the finding that retrovirus-mediated expression of a dominant negative Flk-1 mutant, which inhibits signal transduction through wild-type Flk-1 receptor, suppresses the growth of glioblastoma multiforme as well as other tumor cell lines in vivo (167, 168).

Further evidence that VEGF action is necessary for effective tumor angiogenesis has been obtained in an in vivo model of embryonic stem (ES) cell tumorigenesis (11). Vascular endothelial growth factor null ES cells were dramatically impaired in their ability to form tumors in nude mice. The number of vessels in the VEGF−/− group was substantially reduced and showed a much less complex branching pattern than was observed in controls. These findings indicate that, even in a pluripotent system such as the ES cells, VEGF is required for effective in vivo growth.

B. Angiogenesis Associated with Other Pathological Conditions

Diabetes mellitus, occlusion of central retinal vein, or prematurity with subsequent exposure to oxygen can all be associated with intraocular neovascularization (2). The new blood vessels may lead to vitreous hemorrhage, retinal detachment, neovascular glaucoma, and eventual blindness (2). Diabetic retinopathy is the leading cause of blindness in the working population (169). All of these conditions are known to be associated with retinal ischemia (170). In 1948, Michaelson proposed that a key event in the pathogenesis of these conditions is the release by the ischemic retina into the vitreous diffusible angiogenic factor(s) (''factor X'') responsible for retinal and iris neovascularization (171). Vascular endothelial growth factor, by virtue of its diffusible nature and hypoxia inducibility, was an attractive candidate as a mediator of intraocular neovascularization. Accordingly, elevations of VEGF levels in the aqueous and vitreous of eyes with proliferative retinopathy have been described (172–174). In a large series, a strong correlation was found between levels of immunoreactive VEGF in the aqueous and vitreous humors, and active proliferative retinopathy VEGF levels were undetectable or very low (< 0.5 ng/ml) in the eyes of patients affected by nonneovascular disorders or diabetes without proliferative retinopathy (172). In contrast, the VEGF levels were in the range of 3 to 10 ng/ml in the presence of active proliferative retinopathy associated with diabetes, occlusion of central retinal vein, or prematurity.

More direct evidence of a role for VEGF as a mediator of intraocular neovascularization has been generated in a primate model of iris neovascularization and in a murine model of retinopathy of prematurity (175, 176). In the former, intraocular administration of anti-VEGF antibodies dramatically inhibits the neovascularization that follows occlusion of central retinal veins (177). Likewise, soluble Flt-1 or Flk-1 fused to an IgG suppresses retinal angiogenesis in the mouse model (178).

Neovascularization is a major cause of visual loss in age-related macular degeneration (AMD), the overall leading cause of blindness (2). Most AMD patients have atrophy of the retinal pigment epithelial and characteristic formations called ''drusen.'' A significant percentage of AMD patients (about 20%) manifest the neovascular (exudative) form of the disease. In this condition, the new vessels stem from the extraretinal choriocapillary (2). Leakage and bleeding from these vessels may lead to damage to the macula and ultimately to loss of central vision. Because of the proximity of the lesions to the macula, laser photocoagulation or surgical therapy are of very limited value. Studies have documented the immunohistochemical localization of VEGF in surgically resected choroidal neovascular membranes from AMD patients (179, 180). These findings suggest a role for VEGF in the progression of AMD-related choroidal neovascularization, raising the possibility that a pharmacological treatment with monoclonal antibodies or other VEGF inhibitors may constitute a therapy for this condition.

Two independent studies have suggested that VEGF is involved in the pathogenesis of rheumatoid arthritis (RA), an inflammatory disease in which angiogenesis plays a significant role (181, 182). The RA synovium is characterized by the formation of pannus, an extensively vascularized tissue that invades and destroys the articular cartilage (183). Levels of immunoreactive VEGF were found to be high in the synovial fluid of RA patients, but very low or undetectable in the synovial fluid of patients affected by other forms of arthritis or by degenerative joint disease (181, 182). Furthermore, anti-VEGF antibodies significantly reduced the endothelial cell chemotactic activity of the RA synovial fluid (181).

Vascular endothelial growth factor expression is increased in psoriatic skin (184). Increased vascularity and permeability are characteristic of psoriasis. Also, VEGF mRNA expression has been examined in three bullous disorders with subepidermal blister formation: bullous pemphigoid, erythema multiforme, and dermatitis herpetiformis (185).

Angiogenesis is also important in the pathogenesis of endometriosis, a condition characterized by ectopic endometrium implants in the peritoneal cavity. Elevation of VEGF in the peritoneal fluid of patients with endometriosis has been reported (186, 187). Immunohistochemistry indicated that activated peritoneal fluid macrophages as well as tissue macrophages within the ectopic endometrium are the main source of VEGF in this condition (186, 187). Vascular endothelial growth factor up-regulation also has been implicated in the hypervascularity of the ovarian stroma that characterizes Stein-Leventhal syndrome (188).

Moreover, Sato et al. proposed that VEGF may be responsible for the characteristic hypervascularity of Graves' disease (189). Thyroid-stimulating hormone (TSH), insulin phorbol ester, dibutiryl cyclic adenosine monophosphate (cAMP) and Graves' IgG were found to stimulate VEGF mRNA expression in cultured human thyroid follicles (189).

VIII. CONCLUSIONS

The demonstration that heterozygous mutations inactivating the VEGF gene result in profound deficits in vasculogenesis and blood island formation that lead to early intrauterine death emphasizes the pivotal role played by this molecule in the development of the vascular system. Further studies, using inducible gene knock-out technology (190) should help determine when the embryo is most vulnerable to VEGF deficiency.

The elucidation of the signal transduction properties of the Flt-1 and KDR receptors may help dissect the pathways leading to such fundamental biological events as endothelial cell differentiation, morphogenesis, and angiogenesis. Furthermore, a more complete understanding of the signaling events involving other endothelial cell-specific tyrosine kinases, as well as cell adhesion molecules and their interrelation with the VEGF/VEGF receptor system, should provide a more integrated view of the biology of the endothelial cell, in both normal and abnormal circumstances. In this context, studies have shown that VEGF-mediated angiogenesis requires a specific vascular integrin pathway, mediated by $\alpha v\beta 5$ (191). Furthermore, a ligand selective for the endothelial cell-specific tyrosine kinase Tie-2 has been identified and named angiopoietin (Ang)-1 (192). Gene knock-out studies have shown that Ang-1 is required for the correct assembly of the vessel wall (193). Angiopoietin-1 seems to play a crucial role in mediating reciprocal interactions between the endothelium and surrounding matrix and mesenchyme, and has a later role than VEGF in angiogenesis. Also, unlike VEGF, Ang-1 does not directly stimulate endothelial cell growth. Interestingly, very recent studies provide evidence for the existence of Ang-2, a natural antagonist for Tie-2 receptor (194). Transgenic expression of Ang-2 disrupted blood vessel formation. The interrelation between the VEGF and Ang systems is likely to be an area of intense investigation in vascular biology.

An attractive possibility is that recombinant VEGF or gene therapy with VEGF gene may be used to promote endothelial cell growth and collateral vessel formation. This would represent a novel therapeutic modality for conditions that frequently are refractory to conservative measures and unresponsive to pharmacological therapy. rhVEGF$_{165}$ is already in clinical trials for the treatment of myocardial ischemia associated with coronary artery disease.

The high expression of VEGF mRNA in human tumors, the presence of the VEGF protein in ocular fluids of individuals with proliferative retinopathies and in the synovial fluid of RA patients, as well as the localization of VEGF in AMD lesions strongly support the hypothesis that VEGF is a key mediator of angiogenesis associated with various disorders. Therefore, anti-VEGF antibodies or other inhibitors of VEGF may be of therapeutic value for a variety of malignancies and other disorders, whether used alone or in combination with other agents. A humanized version of a high-affinity anti-VEGF monoclonal antibody, which retains the same affinity and efficacy as the original murine antibody, has been generated (195) and is being tested in humans as a treatment for solid tumors, alone or in combination with chemotherapy.

In conclusion, in spite of the many factors potentially involved in angiogenesis, one specific factor, VEGF, plays an irreplaceable role in a variety of physiological and pathological circumstances.

REFERENCES

1. Folkman J. Angiogenesis in cancer, vascular, rheumatoid and other disease. Nat Med 1995; 1:27–31.
2. Garner A. Vascular Disease. 2d ed. New York: Marcel Dekker, 1994.
3. Folkman J, Shing Y. Angiogenesis. J Biol Chem 1992; 267:10931–10934.
4. Risau W. Mechanisms of angiogenesis. Nature 1997; 386:671–4.
5. Good D, Polverini P, Rastinejad F, Beau M, Lemons R, Frazier W, Bouck N. Proc Natl Acad Sci U S A 1990; 87:6624–6628.
6. DiPietro LA. Thrombospondin as a regulator of angiogenesis. In: Goldberg I, Rosen E, eds. Regulation of Angiogenesis. Springer Verlag, 79:295–314.

7. Ferrara N, Clapp C, Weiner R. The 16K fragment of prolactin specifically inhibits basal or fibroblast growth factor stimulated growth of capillary endothelial cells. Endocrinology 1991; 129:896–900.
8. O'Reilly MS, Holmgren L, Shing Y, Chen C, Rosenthal RA, Moses M, Lane WS, Cao Y, Sage EH, Folkman J. Angiostatin: a novel angiogenesis inhibitor that mediates the suppression of metastases by a Lewis lung carcinoma. Cell 1994; 79:315–328.
9. O'Reilly MS, Boehm T, Shing Y, Fukai N, Vasios G, Lane WS, Flynn E, Birkhead JR, Olsen BR, Folkman J. Endostatin: an endogenous inhibitor of angiogenesis and tumor growth. Cell 1997; 88:277–285.
10. Ferrara N, Davis-Smyth T. The biology of vascular endothelial growth factor. Endocr Rev 1997; 18:4–25.
11. Ferrara N, Carver Moore K, Chen H, Dowd M, Lu L, O'Shea KS, Powell Braxton L, Hillan KJ, Moore MW. Heterozygous embryonic lethality induced by targeted inactivation of the VEGF gene. Nature 1996; 380:439–442.
12. Carmeliet P, Ferreira V, Breier G, Pollefeyt S, Kieckens L, Gertsenstein M, Fahrig M, Vandenhoeck A, Harpal K, Eberhardt C, Declercq C, Pawling J, Moons L, Collen D, Risau W, Nagy A. Abnormal blood vessel development and lethality in embryos lacking a single VEGF allele. Nature 1996; 380:435–439.
13. Pearlman JD, Hibberd MG, Chuang ML, Harada K, Lopez JJ, Gladstone SR, Friedman M, Sellke FW, Simons M. Magnetic resonance mapping demonstrates benefits of VEGF-induced myocardial angiogenesis. Nat Med 1995; 1:1085–1089.
14. Takeshita S, Zhung L, Brogi E, Kearney M, Pu L-Q, Bunting S, Ferrara N, Symes JF, Isner JM. Therapeutic angiogenesis: a single intra-arterial bolus of vascular endothelial growth factor augments collateral vessel formation in a rabbit ischemic hind-limb model. J Clin Invest 1994; 93:662–670.
15. Isner JM, Pieczek A, Schainfeld R, Blair R, Haley L, Asahara T, Rosenfield K, Razvi S, Walsh K, Symes JF. Clinical evidence of angiogenesis after arterial gene transfer of phVEGF165 in patient with ischaemic limb. Lancet 1996; 348:370–374.
16. Pepper MS, Ferrara N, Orci L, Montesano R. Potent synergism between vascular endothelial growth factor and basic fibroblast growth factor in the induction of angiogenesis in vitro. Biochem Biophys Res Commun 1992; 189:824–831.
17. Nicosia R, Nicosia SV, Smith M. Vascular endothelial growth factor, platelet-derived growth factor and insulin-like growth factor stimulate angiogenesis in vitro. Am J Pathol 1994; 145:1023–1029.
18. Leung DW, Cachianes G, Kuang WJ, Goeddel DV, Ferrara N. Vascular endothelial growth factor is a secreted angiogenic mitogen. Science 1989; 246:1306–1309.
19. Pepper MS, Ferrara N, Orci L, Montesano R. Vascular endothelial growth factor (VEGF) induces plasminogen activators and plasminogen activator inhibitor-1 in microvascular endothelial cells. Biochem Biophys Res Commun 1991; 181:902–906.
20. Unemori EN, Ferrara N, Bauer EA, Amento EP. Vascular endothelial growth factor induces interstitial collagenase expression in human endothelial cells. J Cell Physiol 1992; 153:557–562.
21. Mandriota SJ, Seghezzi G, Vassalli JD, Ferrara N, Wasi S, Mazzieri R, Mignatti

P, Pepper MS. Vascular endothelial growth factor increases urokinase receptor expression in vascular endothelial cells. J Biol Chem 1995; 270:9709–9716.
22. Pekala P, Marlow M, Heuvelman D, Connolly D. Regulation of hexose transport in aortic endothelial cells by vascular permeability factor and tumor necrosis factor-alpha, but not by insulin. J Biol Chem 1990; 265:18051–18054.
23. Dvorak HF, Brown LF, Detmar M, Dvorak AM. Vascular permeability factor/vascular endothelial growth factor, microvascular hyperpermeability, and angiogenesis. Am J Pathol 1995; 146:1029–1039.
24. Dvorak HF. Tumors: wounds that do not heal. Similarities between tumor stroma generation and wound healing. N Engl J Med 1986; 315:1650–1659.
25. Dvorak HF, Harvey VS, Estrella P, Brown LF, McDonagh J, Dvorak AM. Fibrin containing gels induce angiogenesis. Implications for tumor stroma generation and wound healing. Lab Invest 1987; 57:673–686.
26. Roberts WG, Palade GE. Increased microvascular permeability and endothelial fenestration induced by vascular endothelial growth factor. J Cell Sci 1995; 108:2369–2379.
27. Roberts WG, Palade GE. Neovasculature induced by vascular endothelial growth factor is fenestrated. Cancer Res 1997; 57:765–772.
28. Melder RJ, Koenig GC, Witwer BP, Safabakhsh N, Munn LL, Jain RK. During angiogenesis, vascular endothelial growth factor and basic fibroblast growth factor regulate natural killer cell adhesion to tumor endothelium. Nat Med 1996; 2:992–997.
29. Clauss M, Gerlach M, Gerlach H, Brett J, Wang F, Familletti PC, Pan YC, Olander JV, Connolly DT, Stern D. Vascular permeability factor: a tumor-derived polypeptide that induces endothelial cell and monocyte procoagulant activity, and promotes monocyte migration. J Exp Med 1990; 172:1535–1545.
30. Broxmeyer HE, Cooper S, Li ZH, Lu L, Song HY, Kwon BS, Warren RE, Donner DB. Myeloid progenitor cell regulatory effects of vascular endothelial cell growth factor. Int J Hematol 1995; 62:203–215.
31. Gabrilovich DI, Chen HL, Girgis KR, Cunningham HT, Meny GM, Nadaf S, Kavanaugh D, Carbone DP. Production of vascular endothelial growth factor by human tumors inhibits the functional maturation of dendritic cells. Nat Med 1996; 2:1096–103.
32. Ku DD, Zaleski JK, Liu S, Brock TA. Vascular endothelial growth factor induces EDRF-dependent relaxation in coronary arteries. Am J Physiol 1993; 265:H586–592.
33. Yang R, Thomas GR, Bunting S, Ko A, Ferrara N, Keyt B, Ross J, Jin H. Effects of vascular endothelial growth factor on hemodynamics and cardiac performance. J Cardiovasc Pharmacol 1996; 27:838–844.
34. Cuevas P, Carceller F, Ortega S, Zazo M, Nieto I, Gimenez-Gallego G. Hypotensive activity of fibroblast growth factor. Science 1991; 254:1208–1210.
35. Cuevas P, Garcia-Calvo M, Carceller F, Reimers D, Zazo M, Cuevas B, Munoz-Willery I, Martinez-Coso V, Lamas S, Gimenez-Gallego G. Correction of hypertension by normalization of endothelial levels of fibroblast growth factor and nitric oxide synthase in spontaneously hypertensive rats. Proc Natl Acad Sci U S A 1996; 93:11996–2001

36. Houck KA, Ferrara N, Winer J, Cachianes G, Li B, Leung DW. The vascular endothelial growth factor family: identification of a fourth molecular species and characterization of alternative splicing of RNA. Mol Endocrinol 1991; 5:1806–1814.
37. Tischer E, Mitchell R, Hartman T, Silva M, Gospodarowicz D, Fiddes JC, Abraham JA. The human gene for vascular endothelial growth factor. Multiple protein forms are encoded through alternative exon splicing. J Biol Chem 1991; 266:11947–11954.
38. Vincenti V, Cassano C, Rocchi M, Persico G. Assignment of the vascular endothelial growth factor gene to human chromosome 6p21.3. Circulation 1996; 93:1493–1495.
39. Shima DT, Kuroki M, Deutsch U, Ng YS, Adamis AP, D'Amore PA. The mouse gene for vascular endothelial growth factor. Genomic structure, definition of the transcriptional unit, and characterization of transcriptional and post-transcriptional regulatory sequences. J Biol Chem 1996; 271:3877–3883.
40. Levy AP, Levy NS, Goldberg MA. Post-transcriptional regulation of vascular endothelial growth factor by hypoxia. J Biol Chem 1996; 271:2746–2753.
41. Conn G, Bayne ML, Soderman DD, Kwok PW, Sullivan KA, Palisi TM, Hope DA, Thomas KA. Amino acid and cDNA sequences of a vascular endothelial cell mitogen that is homologous to platelet-derived growth factor. Proc Natl Acad Sci U S A 1990; 87:2628–2632.
42. Ferrara N, Henzel WJ. Pituitary follicular cells secrete a novel heparin-binding growth factor specific for vascular endothelial cells. Biochem Biophys Res Commun 1989; 161:851–858.
43. Houck KA, Leung DW, Rowland AM, Winer J, Ferrara N. Dual regulation of vascular endothelial growth factor bioavailability by genetic and proteolytic mechanisms. J Biol Chem 1992; 267:26031–26037.
44. Park JE, Keller H-A, Ferrara N. The vascular endothelial growth factor isoforms (VEGF): differential deposition into the subepithelial extracellular matrix and bioactivity of extracellular matrix-bound VEGF. Mol Biol Cell 1993; 4:1317–1326.
45. Keyt BA, Berleau LT, Nguyen HV, Chen H, Heinsohn H, Vandlen R, Ferrara N. The carboxyl-terminal domain (111–165) of vascular endothelial growth factor is critical for its mitogenic potency. J Biol Chem 1996; 271:7788–7795.
46. Poltorak Z, Cohen T, Sivan R, Kandelis Y, Spira G, Vlodavsky I, Keshet E, Neufeld G. VEGF145, a secreted vascular endothelial growth factor isoform that binds to extracellular matrix. J Biol Chem 1997; 272:7151–7158.
47. Muller YA, Li B, Christinger HW, Wells JA, Cunningham BC, de Vos AM. Vascular endothelial growth factor: crystal structure and functional mapping of the kinase domain receptor binding site. Proc Natl Acad Sci U S A 1997; 94:7192–7197.
48. Minchenko A, Bauer T, Salceda S, Caro J. Hypoxic stimulation of vascular endothelial growth factor expression in vivo and in vitro. Lab Invest 1994; 71:374–379.
49. Shima DT, Adamis AP, Ferrara N, Yeo KT, Yeo TK, Allende R, Folkman J, D'Amore PA. Hypoxic induction of endothelial cell growth factors in retinal cells: identification and characterization of vascular endothelial growth factor (VEGF) as the mitogen. Mol Med 1995; 1:182–193.
50. Banai S, Shweiki D, Pinson A, Chandra M, Lazarovich G, Keshet E. Upregulation of vascular endothelial growth factor expression induced by myocardial ischemia: implications for coronary angiogenesis. Cardiovasc Res 1994; 28:1176–1179.

51. Hashimoto E, Ogita T, Nakaoka T, Matsuoka R, Takao A, Kira Y. Rapid induction of vascular endothelial growth factor expression by transient ischemia in rat heart. Am J Physiol 1994; 267:H1948–H1954.
52. Stone J, Itin A, Alon T, Pe'er J, Gnessin H, Chan Ling T, Keshet E. Development of retinal vasculature is mediated by hypoxia-induced vascular endothelial growth factor (VEGF) expression by neuroglia. J Neurosci 1995; 15:4738–4747.
53. Goldberg MA, Schneider TJ. Similarities between the oxygen-sensing mechanisms regulating the expression of vascular endothelial growth factor and erythropoietin. J Biol Chem 1994; 269:4355–4361.
54. Levy AP, Levy NS, Wegner S, Goldberg MA. Transcriptional regulation of the rat vascular endothelial growth factor gene by hypoxia. J Biol Chem 1995; 270:13333–13340.
55. Liu Y, Cox SR, Morita T, Kourembanas S. Hypoxia regulates vascular endothelial growth factor gene expression in endothelial cells. Identification of a 5′ enhancer. Circ Res 1995; 77:638–643.
56. Madan A, Curtin PT. A 24-base-pair sequence 3′ to the human erythropoietin gene contains a hypoxia-responsive transcriptional enhancer. Proc Natl Acad Sci U S A 1993; 90:3928–3932.
57. Wang GL, Semenza GL. Purification and characterization of hypoxia-inducible factor 1. J Biol Chem 1995; 270:1230–1237.
58. Forsythe JA, Jiang BH, Iyer NV, Agani F, Leung SW, Koos RD, Semenza GL. Activation of vascular endothelial growth factor gene transcription by hypoxia-inducible factor 1. Mol Cell Biol 1996; 16:4604–4613.
59. Ikeda E, Achen MG, Breier G, Risau W. Hypoxia-induced transcriptional activation and increased mRNA stability of vascular endothelial growth factor in C6 glioma cells. J Biol Chem 1995; 270:19761–19766.
60. Frank S, Hubner G, Breier G, Longaker MT, Greenhalg DG, Werner S. Regulation of VEGF expression in cultured keratinocytes. Implications for normal and impaired wound healing. J Biol Chem 1995; 270:12607–12613.
61. Goldman C, Kim J, Wonf W-L, King V, Brock T, Gillespie Y. Epidermal growth factor stimulates vascular endothelial growth factor production by malignant glioma cells. A model of glioblastoma multiforme pathophysiology. Mol Biol Cell 1993; 4:121–133.
62. Pertovaara L, Kaipainen A, Mustonen T, Orpana A, Ferrara N, Saksela O, Alitalo K. Vascular endothelial growth factor is induced in response to transforming growth factor-beta in fibroblastic and epithelial cells. J Biol Chem 1994; 269:6271–6274.
63. Li J, Perrella MA, Tsai JC, Yet SF, Hsieh CM, Yoshizumi M, Patterson C, Endego WO, Zhou F, Lee M. Induction of vascular endothelial growth factor gene expression by interleukin-1 beta in rat aortic smooth muscle cells. J Biol Chem 1995; 270:308–312.
64. Ben-Av P, Crofford LJ, Wilder RL, Hla T. Induction of vascular endothelial growth factor expression in synovial fibroblasts. FEBS Lett 1995; 372:83–87.
65. Cohen T, Nahari D, Cerem LW, Neufeld G, Levi BZ. Interleukin 6 induces the expression of vascular endothelial growth factor. J Biol Chem 1996; 271:736–741.
66. Warren RS, Yuan H, Matli MR, Ferrara N, Donner DB. Induction of vascular endo-

thelial growth factor by insulin-like growth factor 1 in colorectal carcinoma. J Biol Chem 1996; 271:29483–29488.
67. Claffey KP, Wilkison WO, Spiegelman BM. Vascular endothelial growth factor. Regulation by cell differentiation and activated second messenger pathways. J Biol Chem 1992; 267:16317–16322.
68. Kieser A, Weich H, Brandner G, Marme D, Kolch W. Mutant p53 potentiates protein kinase C induction of vascular endothelial growth factor expression. Oncogene 1994; 9:963–969.
69. Rak J, Mitsuhashi Y, Bayko L, Filmus J, Shirasawa S, Sasazuki T, Kerbel RS. Mutant ras oncogenes upregulate VEGF/VPF expression: implications for induction and inhibition of tumor angiogenesis. Cancer Res 1995; 55:4575–4580.
70. Grugel S, Finkenzeller G, Weindel K, Barleon B, Marme D. Both v-Ha-Ras and v-Raf stimulate expression of the vascular endothelial growth factor in NIH 3T3 cells. J Biol Chem 1995; 270:25915–25919.
71. Mazure NM, Chen EY, Yeh P, Laderoute KR, Giaccia AJ. Oncogenic transformation and hypoxia synergistically act to modulate vascular endothelial growth factor expression. Cancer Res 1996; 56:3436–3440.
72. Siemeister G, Weindel K, Mohrs K, Barleon B, Martiny Baron G, Marme D. Reversion of deregulated expression of vascular endothelial growth factor in human renal carcinoma cells by von Hippel-Lindau tumor suppressor protein. Cancer Res 1996; 56:2299–2301.
73. Iliopoulos O, Levy AP, Jiang C, Kaelin WG Jr, Goldberg MA. Negative regulation of hypoxia-inducible genes by the von Hippel-Lindau protein, Proc Natl Acad Sci U S A 1996; 93:10595–10599.
74. Gnarra JR, Zhou S, Merrill MJ, Wagner JR, Krumm A, Papavassiliou E, Oldfield EH, Klausner RD, Linehan WM. Post-transcriptional regulation of vascular endothelial growth factor mRNA by the product of the VHL tumor suppressor gene. Proc Natl Acad Sci U S A 1996; 93:10589–10594.
75. Vaisman N, Gospodarowicz D, Neufeld G. Characterization of the receptors for vascular endothelial growth factor. J Biol Chem 1990; 265:19461–19466.
76. Plouet J, Moukadiri HJ. Characterization of the receptors for vasculotropin on bovine adrenal cortex-derived capillary endothelial cells. J Biol Chem 1990; 265: 22071–22075.
77. Shen H, Clauss M, Ryan J, Schmidt AM, Tijburg P, Borden L, Connolly D, Stern D, Kao J. Characterization of vascular permeability factor/vascular endothelial growth factor receptors on mononuclear phagocytes. Blood 1993; 81:2767–2773.
78. Jakeman LB, Winer J, Bennett GL, Altar CA, Ferrara N. Binding sites for vascular endothelial growth factor are localized on endothelial cells in adult rat tissues. J Clin Invest 1992; 89:244–253.
79. Jakeman LB, Armanini M, Philips HS, Ferrara N. Developmental expression of binding sites and mRNA for vascular endothelial growth factor suggests a role for this protein in vasculogenesis and angiogenesis. Endocrinology 1993; 133:848–859.
80. de Vries C, Escobedo JA, Ueno H, Houck K, Ferrara N, Williams LT. The fms-like tyrosine kinase, a receptor for vascular endothelial growth factor. Science 1992; 255:989–991.

81. Terman BI, Dougher Vermazen M, Carrion ME, Dimitrov D, Armellino DC, Gospodarowicz D, Bohlen P. Identification of the KDR tyrosine kinase as a receptor for vascular endothelial cell growth factor. Biochem Biophys Res Commun 1992; 187:1579–1586.
82. Matthews W, Jordan CT, Gavin M, Jenkins NA, Copeland NG, Lemischka IR. A receptor tyrosine kinase cDNA isolated from a population of enriched primitive hematopoietic cells and exhibiting close genetic linkage to c-kit. Proc Natl Acad Sci U S A 1991; 88:9026–9030.
83. Shibuya M, Yamaguchi S, Yamane A, Ikeda T, Tojo A, Matsushime H, Sato M. Nucleotide sequence and expression of a novel human receptor-type tyrosine kinase (flt) closely related to the fms family. Oncogene 1990; 8:519–527.
84. Terman BI, Carrion ME, Kovacs E, Rasmussen BA, Eddy RL, Shows TB. Identification of a new endothelial cell growth factor receptor tyrosine kinase. Oncogene 1991; 6:1677–1683.
85. Kendall RL, Wang G, Thomas KA. Identification of a natural soluble form of the vascular endothelial growth factor receptor, FLT-1, and its heterodimerization with KDR. Biochem Biophys Res Comm 1996; 226:324–328.
86. Pajusola K, Aprelikova O, Korhonen J, Kaipainen A, Pertovaara L, Alitalo R, Alitalo K. FLT4 receptor tyrosine kinase contains seven immunoglobulin-like loops and is expressed in multiple human tissues and cell lines. Cancer Res 1992; 52: 5738–5743.
87. Galland F, Karamysheva A, Mattei MG, Rosnet O, Marchetto S, Birnbaum D. Chromosomal localization of FLT4, a novel receptor-type tyrosine kinase gene. Genomics 1992; 13:475–478.
88. Finnerty H, Kelleher K, Morris GE, Bean K, Merberg DM, Kriz R, Morris JC, Sookdeo H, Turner KJ, Wood CR. Molecular cloning of murine FLT and FLT4. Oncogene 1993; 8:2293–2298.
89. Joukov V, Pajusola K, Kaipainen A, Chilov D, Lahtinen I, Kukk E, Saksela O, Kalkkinen N, Alitalo K. A novel vascular endothelial growth factor, VEGF-C, is a ligand for the Flt4 (VEGFR-3) and KDR (VEGFR-2) receptor tyrosine kinases. EMBO J 1996; 15:1751.
90. Lee J, Gray A, Yuan J, Luoh SM, Avraham H, Wood WI. Vascular endothelial growth factor-related protein: a ligand and specific activator of the tyrosine kinase receptor Flt4. Proc Natl Acad Sci U S A 1996; 93:1988–1992.
91. Jeltsch M, Kaipainen A, Joukov V, Meng X, Lakso M, Rauvala H, Awartz M, Fukumura D, Jain RK, Alitalo K. Hyperplasia of lymphatic vessels in VEGF-C transgenic mice. Science 1997; 276:1423–1425.
92. Davis-Smyth T, Chen H, Park J, Presta LG, Ferrara N. The second immunoglobulin-like domain of the VEGF tyrosine kinase receptor Flt-1 determines ligand binding and may initiate a signal transduction cascade. EMBO J 1996; 15:4919–4927.
93. Chamow SM, Ashkenazi A. Immunoadhesions: principles and applications. Trends Biotechnol 1996; 14:52–60.
94. Weissmann C, Fuh G, Christinger H, Eigenbrot C, Wells JA, de Vos AM. Crystal structure at 1.7: a resolution of VEGF in complex with domain 2 of the Flt-1 receptor. Cell 1997; 91:695–704.
95. Davis-Smyth T, Presta LG, Ferrara N. Mapping the charged residues in the second

immunoglobulin-like domain of the vascular endothelial growth factor/placenta growth factor receptor Flt-1 required for binding and structural stability. J Biol Chem 273: 1998; 273:3216–3222.

96. Guo D, Jia Q, Song HY, Warren RS, Donner DB. Vascular endothelial cell growth factor promotes tyrosine phosphorylation of mediators of signal transduction that contain SH2 domains. Association with endothelial cell proliferation. J Biol Chem 1995; 270:6729–6733.
97. Morbidelli L, Chang CH, Douglas JG, Granger HJ, Ledda F, Ziche M. Nitric oxide mediates mitogenic effect of VEGF on coronary venular endothelium. Am J Physiol 1996; 270:H411–H415.
98. Waltenberger J, Claesson Welsh L, Siegbahn A, Shibuya M, Heldin CH. Different signal transduction properties of KDR and Flt1, two receptors for vascular endothelial growth factor. J Biol Chem 1994; 269:26988–26995.
99. Seetharam L, Gotoh N, Maru Y, Neufeld G, Yamaguchi S, Shibuya M. A unique signal transduction from FLT tyrosine kinase, a receptor for vascular endothelial growth factor VEGF. Oncogene 1995; 10:135–147.
100. Park JE, Chen HH, Winer J, Houck KA, Ferrara N. Placenta growth factor. Potentiation of vascular endothelial growth factor bioactivity, in vitro and in vivo, and high affinity binding to Flt-1 but not to Flk-1/KDR. J Biol Chem 1994; 269:25646–25654.
101. Keyt BA, Nguyen HV, Berleau LT, Duarte CM, Park J, Chen H, Ferrara N. Identification of vascular endothelial growth factor determinants for binding KDR and FLT-1 receptors. Generation of receptor-selective VEGF variants by site-directed mutagenesis. J Biol Chem 1996; 271:5638–5646.
102. Cunningham SA, Waxham MN, Arrate PM, Brock TA. Interaction of the Flt-1 tyrosine kinase receptor with the p85 subunit of phosphatidylinositol 3-kinase. Mapping of a novel site involved in binding. J Biol Chem 1995; 270:20254–20257.
103. Barleon B, Sozzani S, Zhou D, Weich HA, Mantovani A, Marme D. Migration of human monocytes in response to vascular endothelial growth factor (VEGF) is mediated via the VEGF receptor flt-1. Blood 1996; 87:3336–3343.
104. Morishita K, Johnson DE, Williams LT. A novel promoter for vascular endothelial growth factor receptor (flt-1) that confers endothelial-specific gene expression. J Biol Chem 1995; 270:27948–27953.
105. Patterson C, Perrella MA, Hsieh CM, Yoshizumi M, Lee ME, Haber E. Cloning and functional analysis of the promoter for KDR/flk-1, a receptor for vascular endothelial growth factor. J Biol Chem 1995; 270:23111–23118.
106. Tuder RM, Flook BE, Voelkel NF. Increased gene expression for VEGF and the VEGF receptors KDR/Flk and Flt in lungs exposed to acute or to chronic hypoxia. Modulation of gene expression by nitric oxide. J Clin Invest 1995; 95:1798–1807.
107. Li J, Brown LF, Hibberd MG, Grossman JD, Morgan JP, Simons M. VEGF, flk-1, and flt-1 expression in a rat myocardial infarction model of angiogenesis. Am J Physiol 1996; 270:H1803–H1811.
108. Takagi H, King GL, Ferrara N, Aiello LP. Hypoxia regulates vascular endothelial growth factor receptor KDR/Flk gene expression through adenosine A2 receptors in retinal capillary endothelial cells. Invest Ophthalmol Vis Sci 1996; 37:1311–1316.

109. Brogi E, Schatteman G, Wu T, Kim EA, Varticovski L, Keyt B, Isner JM. Hypoxia-induced paracrine regulation of vascular endothelial growth factor receptor expression. J Clin Invest 1996; 97:469–476.
110. Gerber HP, Condorelli F, Park J, Ferrara N. Differential transcriptional regulation of the two VEGF receptor genes. Flt-1, but not Flk-1/KDR, is up-regulated by hypoxia. J Biol Chem 1997; 272:23659–23667.
111. Patterson C, Perrella MA, Endege WO, Yoshizumi M, Lee ME, Haber E. Downregulation of vascular endothelial growth factor receptors by tumor necrosis factor-alpha in cultured human vascular endothelial cells. J Clin Invest 1996; 98:490–496.
112. Mandriota SJ, Menoud PA, Pepper MS. Transforming growth factor beta 1 down-regulates vascular endothelial growth factor receptor 2/flk-1 expression in vascular endothelial cells. J Biol Chem 1996; 271:11500–11505.
113. Breier G, Albrecht U, Sterrer S, Risau W. Expression of vascular endothelial growth factor during embryonic angiogenesis and endothelial cell differentiation. Development 1992; 114:521–532.
114. Shifren JL, Doldi N, Ferrara N, Mesiano S, Jaffe RB. In the human fetus, vascular endothelial growth factor is expressed in epithelial cells and myocytes, but not vascular endothelium: implications for mode of action. J Clin Endocrinol Metab 1994; 79:316–322.
115. Quinn TP, Peters KG, De Vries C, Ferrara N, Williams LT. Fetal liver kinase 1 is a receptor for vascular endothelial growth factor and is selectively expressed in vascular endothelium. Proc Natl Acad Sci U S A 1993; 90:7533–7537.
116. Millauer B, Wizigmann Voos S, Schnurch H, Martinez R, Moller NP, Risau W, Ullrich A. High affinity VEGF binding and developmental expression suggest Flk-1 as a major regulator of vasculogenesis and angiogenesis. Cell 1993; 72:835–846.
117. Yamaguchi TP, Dumont DJ, Conlon RA, Breitman ML, Rossant J. Flk-1, an flt-related receptor tyrosine kinase is an early marker for endothelial cell precursors. Development 1993; 118:489–498.
118. Peters KG, De Vries C, Williams LT. Vascular endothelial growth factor receptor expression during embryogenesis and tissue repair suggests a role in endothelial differentiation and blood vessel growth. Proc Natl Acad Sci U S A 1993; 90:8915–8919.
119. Ferrara N, Houck K, Jakeman L, Leung DW. Molecular and biological properties of the vascular endothelial growth family of proteins. Endocr Rev 1992:18–32.
120. Monacci WT, Merrill MJ, Oldfield EH. Expression of vascular permeability factor/vascular endothelial growth factor in normal rat tissues. Am J Physiol 1993; 264: C995–1002.
121. Alon T, Hemo I, Itin A, Pe'er J, Stone J, Keshet E. Vascular endothelial growth factor acts as a survival factor for newly formed retinal vessels and has implications for retinopathy of prematurity. Nat Med 1995; 1:1024–1028.
122. Fong GH, Rossant J, Gertsenstein M, Breitman ML. Role of the Flt-1 receptor tyrosine kinase in regulating the assembly of vascular endothelium. Nature 1995; 376:66–70.
123. Shalaby F, Rossant J, Yamaguchi TP, Gertsenstein M, Wu XF, Breitman ML,

Schuh AC. Failure of blood-island formation and vasculogenesis in Flk-1-deficient mice. Nature 1995; 376:62–66.

124. Brandon EP, Idzerda RL, McKnight GS. Targeting the mouse genome: a compendium of knockouts (part III). Curr Biol 1995; 5:873–881.
125. Carmeliet P, Collen D. Genetic analysis of blood vessel formation: role of endothelial versus smooth muscle cells. Trends Cardiovasc Med 1997; 8:271–281.
126. Bassett DL. The changes in the vascular pattern of the ovary of the albino rat during the estrous cycle. Am J Anat 1943; 73:251.
127. Phillips HS, Hains J, Leung DW, Ferrara N. Vascular endothelial growth factor is expressed in rat corpus luteum. Endocrinology 1990; 127:965–967.
128. Ravindranath N, Little-Ihrig L, Phillips HS, Ferrara N, Zeleznik AJ. Vascular endothelial growth factor messenger ribonucleic acid expression in the primate ovary. Endocrinology 1992; 131:254–260.
129. Shweiki D, Itin A, Neufeld G, Gitay-Goren H, Keshet E. Patterns of expression of vascular endothelial growth factor (VEGF) and VEGF receptors in mice suggest a role in hormonally mediated angiogenesis. J Clin Invest 1993; 91:2235–2243.
130. Cullinan-Bove K, Koos RD. Vascular endothelial growth factor/vascular permeability factor expression in the rat uterus: rapid stimulation by estrogen correlates with estrogen-induced increases in uterine capillary permeability and growth. Endocrinology 1993; 133:829–837.
131. Ferrara N, Chen H, Davis-Smyth T, Gerber H-P, Nguyen T-N, Peers D, Chisholm V, Hillan KJ, Schwall RH. Vascular endothelial growth factor is essential for corpus luteum angiogenesis. Nat Med 1998; 4:336–340.
132. Volm M, Koomagi R, Mattern J, Stammler G. Angiogenic growth factors and their receptors in non-small cell lung carcinomas and their relationships to drug response in vitro. Anticancer Res 1997; 17:99–103.
133. Volm M, Koomagi R, Mattern J. Prognostic value of vascular endothelial growth factor and its receptor Flt-1 in squamous cell lung cancer. Int J Cancer 1997; 74: 64–68.
134. Brown LF, Berse B, Jackman RW, Tognazzi K, Guidi AJ, Dvorak HF, Senger DR, Connolly JL, Schnitt SJ. Expression of vascular permeability factor (vascular endothelial growth factor) and its receptors in breast cancer. Hum Pathol 1995; 26: 86–91.
135. Yoshiji H, Gomez DE, Shibuya M, Thorgeirsson UP. Expression of vascular endothelial growth factor, its receptor, and other angiogenic factors in human breast cancer. Cancer Res 1996; 56:2013–2016.
136. Brown LF, Berse B, Jackman RW, Tognazzi K, Manseau EJ, Senger DR, Dvorak HF. Expression of vascular permeability factor (vascular endothelial growth factor) and its receptors in adenocarcinomas of the gastrointestinal tract. Cancer Res 1993; 53:4727–4735.
137. Suzuki K, Hayashi N, Miyamoto Y, Yamamoto M, Ohkawa K, Ito Y, Sasaki Y, Yamaguchi Y, Nakase H, Noda K, Enomoto N, Arai K, Yamada Y, Yoshihara H, Tujimura T, Kawano K, Yoshikawa K, Kamada T. Expression of vascular permeability factor/vascular endothelial growth factor in human hepatocellular carcinoma. Cancer Res 1996; 56:3004–3009.
138. Brown LF, Berse B, Jackman RW, Tognazzi K, Manseau EJ, Dvorak HF, Senger

DR. Increased expression of vascular permeability factor (vascular endothelial growth factor) and its receptors in kidney and bladder carcinomas. Am J Pathol 1993; 143:1255–1262.
139. Olson TA, Mohanraj D, Carson LF, Ramakrishnan S. Vascular permeability factor gene expression in normal and neoplastic human ovaries. Cancer Res 1994; 54: 276–280.
140. Guidi AJ, Abu Jawdeh G, Tognazzi K, Dvorak HF, Brown LF. Expression of vascular permeability factor (vascular endothelial growth factor) and its receptors in endometrial carcinoma. Cancer 1996; 78:454–460.
141. Guidi AJ, Abu-Jawdeh G, Berse B, Jackman RW, Tognazzi K, Dvorak HF, Brown LF. Vascular permeability factor (vascular endothelial growth factor) expression and angiogenesis in cervical neoplasia. J Natl Cancer Inst 1995; 87:1237–1245.
142. Hashimoto M, Ohsawa M, Ohnishi A, Naka N, Hirota S, Kitamura Y, Aozasa K. Expression of vascular endothelial growth factor and its receptor mRNA in angiosarcoma. Lab Invest 1995; 73:859–863.
143. Viglietto G, Romano A, Maglione D, Rambaldi M, Paoletti I, Lago CT, Califano D, Monaco C, Mineo A, Santelli G, Manzo G, Botti G, Chiappetta G, Persico MG. Neovascularization in human germ cell tumors correlates with a marked increase in the expression of the vascular endothelial growth factor but not the placenta-derived growth factor. Oncogene 1996; 13:577–587.
144. Shweiki D, Itin A, Soffer D, Keshet E. Vascular endothelial growth factor induced by hypoxia may mediate hypoxia-initiated angiogenesis. Nature 1992; 359:843–845.
145. Plate KH, Breier G, Weich HA, Risau W. Vascular endothelial growth factor is a potential tumour angiogenesis factor in human gliomas in vivo. Nature 1992; 359: 845–848.
146. Phillips HS, Armanini M, Stavrou D, Ferrara N, Westphal M. Intense focal expression of vascular endothelial growth factor mRNA in human intracranial neoplasms: association with regions of necrosis. Int J Oncol 1993; 2:913–919.
147. Berkman RA, Merrill MJ, Reinhold WC, Monacci WT, Saxena A, Clark WC, Robertson JT, Ali IU, Oldfield EH. Expression of the vascular permeability factor/vascular endothelial growth factor gene in central nervous system neoplasms. J Clin Invest 1993; 91:153–159.
148. Wizigmann Voos S, Breier G, Risau W, Plate KH. Up-regulation of vascular endothelial growth factor and its receptors in von Hippel-Lindau disease-associated and sporadic hemangioblastomas. Cancer Res 1995; 55:1358–1364.
149. Plate KH, Breier G, Millauer B, Ullrich A, Risau W. Up-regulation of vascular endothelial growth factor and its cognate receptors in a rat glioma model of tumor angiogenesis. Cancer Res 1993; 53:5822–5827.
150. Ferrara N, Winer J, Burton T, Rowland A, Siegel M, Phillips HS, Terrell T, Keller GA, Levinson AD. Expression of vascular endothelial growth factor does not promote transformation but confers a growth advantage in vivo to Chinese hamster ovary cells. J Clin Invest 1993; 91:160–170.
151. Qu H, Nagy JA, Senger DR, Dvorak HF, Dvorak AM. Ultrastructural localization of vascular permeability factor/vascular endothelial growth factor (VPF/VEGF) to

the abluminal plasma membrane and vesiculovacuolar organelles of tumor microvascular endothelium. J Histochem Cytochem 1995; 43:381–389.

152. Albini A, Benelli R, Presta M, Rusnati M, Ziche M, Rubartelli A, Paglialunga G, Bussolino F, Noonan D. HIV-tat protein is a heparin-binding angiogenic growth factor. Oncogene 1996; 12:289–297.
153. Albini A, Soldi R, Giunciuglio D, Giraudo E, Benelli R, Primo L, Noonan D, Salio M, Camussi G, Rockl W, Bussolino F. The angiogenesis induced by HIV-1 tat protein is mediated by the Flk-1/KDR receptor on vascular endothelial cells. Nat Med 1996; 2:1371–1375.
154. Kondo S, Asano M, Matsuo K, Ohmori I, Suzuki H. Vascular endothelial growth factor/vascular permeability factor is detectable in the sera of tumor-bearing mice and cancer patients. Biochim Biophys Acta 1994; 1221:211–214.
155. Toi M, Kondo S, Suzuki H, Yamamoto Y, Inada K, Imazawa T, Taniguchi T, Tominaga T. Quantitative analysis of vascular endothelial growth factor in primary breast cancer. Cancer 1996; 77:1101–1106.
156. Gasparini G, Toi M, Gion M, Verderio P, Dittadi R, Hanatani M, Matsubara I, Vinante O, Bonoldi E, Boracchi P, Gatti C, Suzuki H, Tominaga T. Prognostic significance of vascular endothelial growth factor protein in node-negative breast carcinoma. J Natl Cancer Inst 1997; 89:139–147.
157. Maeda K, Chung YS, Ogawa Y, Takatsuka S, Kang SM, Ogawa M, Sawada T, Sowa M. Prognostic value of vascular endothelial growth factor expression in gastric carcinoma. Cancer 1996; 77:858–863.
158. Kim KJ, Li B, Houck K, Winer J, Ferrara N. The vascular endothelial growth factor proteins: identification of biologically relevant regions by neutralizing monoclonal antibodies. Growth Factors 1992; 7:53–64.
159. Kim KJ, Li B, Winer J, Armanini M, Gillett N, Phillips HS, Ferrara N. Inhibition of vascular endothelial growth factor-induced angiogenesis suppresses tumor growth in vivo. Nature 1993; 362:841–844.
160. Warren RS, Yuan H, Matli MR, Gillett NA, Ferrara N. Regulation by vascular endothelial growth factor of human colon cancer tumorigenesis in a mouse model of experimental liver metastasis. J Clin Invest 1995; 95:1789–1797.
161. Melnyk O, Shuman MA, Kim KJ. Vascular endothelial growth factor promotes tumor dissemination by a mechanism distinct from its effect on primary tumor growth. Cancer Res 1996; 56:921–924.
162. Asano M, Yukita A, Matsumoto T, Kondo S, Suzuki H. Inhibition of tumor growth and metastasis by an immunoneutralizing monoclonal antibody to human vascular endothelial growth factor/vascular permeability factor 121. Cancer Res 1995; 55: 5296–5301.
163. Borgstrom P, Hillan KJ, Sriramarao P, Ferrara N. Complete inhibition of angiogenesis and growth of microtumors by anti-vascular endothelial growth factor neutralizing antibody: novel concepts of angiostatic therapy from intravital videomicroscopy. Cancer Res 1996; 56:4032–4039.
164. Kirshembaum A, Wang J-P, Ren M, Schiff JD, Aaronson SA, Droller MJ, Ferrara N, Holland J, Levine A. Inhibition of vascular endothelial growth factor suppresses the in vivo growth of human prostate tumors. Urol Oncol 3:1997.

165. Borgström P, Hillan KJ, Sriraramao P, Ferrara N. Combination treatment with anti-vascular endothelial growth factor antibody and doxorubicin suppresses growth of breast carcinoma cells, submitted.
166. Yuan F, Chen Y, Dellian M, Safabakhsh N, Ferrara N, Jain RK. Time-dependent vascular regression and permeability changes in established human tumor xenografts induced by an anti-vascular endothelial growth factor/vascular permeability factor antibody. Proc Natl Acad Sci U S A 1996; 93:14765–14770.
167. Millauer B, Shawver LK, Plate KH, Risau W, Ullrich A. Glioblastoma growth inhibited in vivo by a dominant-negative Flk-1 mutant. Nature 1994; 367:576–579.
168. Millauer B, Longhi MP, Plate KH, Shawver LK, Risau W, Ullrich A, Strawn LM. Dominant-negative inhibition of Flk-1 suppresses the growth of many tumor types in vivo. Cancer Res 1996; 56:1615–1620.
169. Olk RJ, Lee CM. Diabetic Retinopathy: Practical Management. Philadelphia: Lippincott, 1993.
170. Patz A. Studies on retinal neovascularization. Invest Ophthalmol Vis Sci 1980; 19: 1133–1138.
171. Michaelson IC. The mode of development of the vascular system of the retina with some observations on its significance for certain retinal disorders. Trans Ophthalmol Soc UK. 1948; 68:137–180.
172. Aiello LP, Avery RL, Arrigg PG, Keyt BA, Jampel HD, Shah ST, Pasquale LR, Thieme H, Iwamoto MA, Park JE, Nguyen H, Aiello LM, Ferrara N, King GL. Vascular endothelial growth factor in ocular fluid of patients with diabetic retinopathy and other retinal disorders. N Engl J Med 1994; 331:1480–1487.
173. Adamis AP, Miller JW, Bernal MT, D'Amico DJ, Folkman J, Yeo TK, Yeo KT. Increased vascular endothelial growth factor levels in the vitreous of eyes with proliferative diabetic retinopathy. Am J Ophthalmol 1994; 118:445–450.
174. Malecaze F, Clemens S, Simorer-Pinotel V, Mathis A, Chollet P, Favard P, Bayard F, Plouet J. Detection of vascular endothelial growth factor mRNA and vascular endothelial growth factor-like activity in proliferative diabetic retinopathy. Arch Ophthalmol 1994; 112:1476–1482.
175. Miller JW, Adamis AP, Shima DT, D'Amore PA, Moulton RS, O'Reilly MS, Folkman J, Dvorak HF, Brown LF, Berse B. Vascular endothelial growth factor/vascular permeability factor is temporally and spatially correlated with ocular angiogenesis in a primate model. Am J Pathol 1994; 145:574–584.
176. Pierce EA, Avery RL, Foley ED, Aiello LP, Smith LE. Vascular endothelial growth factor/vascular permeability factor expression in a mouse model of retinal neovascularization. Proc Natl Acad Sci U S A 1995; 92:905–909.
177. Adamis AP, Shima DT, Tolentino MJ, Gragoudas ES, Ferrara N, Folkman J, D'Amore PA, Miller JW. Inhibition of vascular endothelial growth factor prevents retinal ischemia-associated iris neovascularization in a nonhuman primate. Arch Ophthalmol 1996; 114:66–71.
178. Aiello LP, Pierce EA, Foley ED, Takagi H, Chen H, Riddle L, Ferrara N, King GL, Smith LE. Suppression of retinal neovascularization in vivo by inhibition of vascular endothelial growth factor (VEGF) using soluble VEGF-receptor chimeric proteins. Proc Natl Acad Sci U S A 1995; 92:10457–10461.

179. Lopez PF, Sippy BD, Lambert HM, Thach AB, Hinton DR. Transdifferentiated retinal pigment epithelial cells are immunoreactive for vascular endothelial growth factor in surgically excised age-related macular degeneration-related choroidal neovascular membranes. Invest Ophthalmol Vis Sci 1996; 37:855–862.
180. Kvanta A, Algvere PV, Berglin L, Seregard S. Subfoveal fibrovascular membranes in age-related macular degeneration express vascular endothelial growth factor. Invest Ophthalmol Vis Sci 1996; 37:1929–1934.
181. Koch AE, Harlow L, Haines GK, Amento EP, Unemori EN, Wong W-L, Pope RM, Ferrara N. Vascular endothelial growth factor: a cytokine modulating endothelial function in rheumatoid arthritis. J Immunol 1994; 152:4149–4156.
182. Fava RA, Olsen NJ, Spencer-Green G, Yeo KT, Yeo TK, Berse B, Jackman RW, Senger DR, Dvorak HF, Brown LF. Vascular permeability factor/endothelial growth factor (VPF/VEGF): accumulation and expression in human synovial fluids and rheumatoid synovial tissue. J Exp Med 1994; 180:341–346.
183. Fassbender HJ, Simling-Annenfeld M. The potential aggressiveness of synovial tissue in rheumatoid arthritis. J Pathol 1983; 10:845–851.
184. Detmar M, Brown LF, Claffey KP, Yeo KT, Kocher O, Jackman RW, Berse B, Dvorak HF. Overexpression of vascular permeability factor/vascular endothelial growth factor and its receptors in psoriasis. J Exp Med 1994; 180:1141–1146.
185. Brown LF, Harrist TJ, Yeo KT, Stahle-Backdahl M, Jackman RW, Berse B, Tognazzi K, Dvorak HF, Detmar M. Increased expression of vascular permeability factor (vascular endothelial growth factor) in bullous pemphigoid, dermatitis herpetiformis, and erythema multiforme. J Invest Dermatol 1995; 104:744–749.
186. McLaren J, Prentice A, Charnock-Jones DS, Smith SK. Vascular endothelial growth factor (VEGF) concentrations are elevated in peritoneal fluid of women with endometriosis. Hum Reprod 1996; 11:220–223.
187. Shifren JL, Tseng JF, Zaloudek CJ, Ryan IP, Meng YG, Ferrara N, Jaffe RB, Taylor RN. Ovarian steroid regulation of vascular endothelial growth factor in the human endometrium: implications for angiogenesis during the menstrual cycle and in the pathogenesis of endometriosis. J Clin Endocrinol Metab 1996; 81:3112–3118.
188. Kamat BR, Brown LF, Manseau EJ, Senger DR, Dvorak HF. Expression of vascular permeability factor/vascular endothelial growth factor by human granulosa and theca lutein cells. Role in corpus luteum development. Am J Pathol 1995; 146: 157–165.
189. Sato K, Yamazaki K, Shizume K, Kanaji Y, Obara T, Ohsumi K, Demura H, Yamaguchi S, Shibuya M. Stimulation by thyroid-stimulating hormone and Grave's immunoglobulin G of vascular endothelial growth factor mRNA expression in human thyroid follicles in vitro and flt mRNA expression in the rat thyroid in vivo. J Clin Invest 1995; 96:1295–1302.
190. Kuhn R, Schwenk F, Aguet M, Rajewsky K. Inducible gene targeting in mice. Science 1995; 269:1427–1429.
191. Friedlander M, Brooks PC, Shaffer RW, Kincaid CM, Varner JA, Cheresh DA. Definition of two angiogenic pathways by distinct alpha v integrins. Science 1995; 270:1500–1502.
192. Davis S, Aldrich TH, Jones PF, Acheson A, Compton DL, Jain V, Ryan TE, Bruno J, Radziejewski C, Maisonpierre PC, Yancopoulos GD. Isolation of angiopoietin-

1, a ligand for the TIE2 receptor, by secretion-trap expression cloning. Cell 1996; 87:1161–1169.
193. Suri C, Jones PF, Patan S, Bartunkova S, Maisonpierre PC, Davis S, Sato TN, Yancopoulos GD. Requisite role of angiopoietin-1, a ligand for the TIE2 receptor, during embryonic angiogenesis. Cell 1996; 87:1171–1180.
194. Maisonpierre PC, Suri C, Jones PF, Bartunkova S, Wiegend SJ, Radziejewski C, Compton D, McClain J, Aldrich TH, Papadopulos N, Daly TJ, Davis S, Sato TN, Yancopoulos GD. Angiopoietin-2, a natural antagonist for Tie-2 that disrupts in vivo angiogenesis. Science 1997; 277:55–60.
195. Presta LG, Chen H, O'Connor SJ, Chisholm V, Meng YG, Krummen L, Winkler M, Ferrara N. Humanization of an anti-VEGF monoclonal antibody for the therapy of solid tumors and other disorders. Cancer Res 1997; 57:4593–4599.

26

TNP-470

Preclinical and Clinical Development

Deborah M. Milkowski and Rachelle A. Weiss
TAP Pharmaceutical Products Inc., Lake Forest, Illinois

I. INTRODUCTION

Preclinical and clinical aspects of the development of TNP-470, an angiogenesis inhibitor, as a potential therapeutic modality for cancer, are presented in this chapter. Preclinical pharmacology studies of the compound's efficacy in a variety of animal models are discussed first. A summary of observations emanating from phase I clinical trials follows.

II. HISTORICAL PERSPECTIVE

TNP-470 is a synthetic analogue of fumagillin, a natural product secreted by the fungus *Aspergillus fumigatus fresenius* (1). Studies demonstrating fumagillin's angioinhibitory activity were initiated in the laboratory of Judah Folkman, M.D. after observations of morphological changes in endothelial cell cultures inadvertently contaminated by this fungus. The results of these studies confirmed that fumagillin inhibited endothelial cell proliferation in vitro as well as angiogenesis and tumor growth in vivo. However, severe weight loss in laboratory animals after prolonged administration of fumagillin precluded its further development. A collaborative agreement between Harvard University and Takeda Chemical Industries, Ltd. resulted in the synthesis by Takeda scientists of a series of less

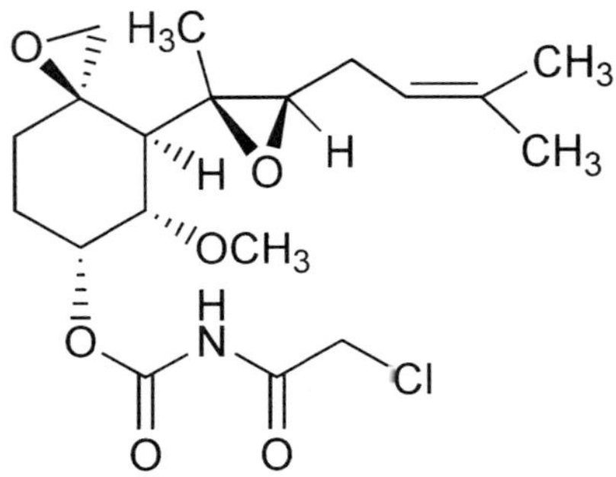

TNP-470

Figure 1 Chemical structure of TNP-470. The chemical formula and molecular weight are $C_{19}H_{28}ClNO_6$ and 401.89.

toxic analogues, termed angioinhibins. Of these, *O*-(chloroacetyl carbamoyl) fumagillol or AGM-1470, now referred to as TNP-470, was among the most potent identified (1). The chemical structure of TNP-470 is depicted in Figure 1.

III. IN VITRO CELL BIOLOGY STUDIES

The endothelial cell response to growth factors such as basic fibroblast growth factor (bFGF) includes proliferation, migration, and capillary-like tube formation. TNP reversibly inhibits the mitogen-induced proliferation of a variety of endothelial cells (bovine capillary, human umbilical vein [HUVEC]) with an IC_{50} in the pg/mL range (1–4). Cytotoxicity is not observed until μg/mL concentrations are reached. These concentrations correlate with the observation that DNA synthesis and RNA and protein synthesis in HUVECs are inhibited by pg/mL and μg/mL concentrations, respectively (3). In a rat blood vessel organ culture assay consisting of a mixed cell population, TNP specifically inhibited the proliferation of and capillary-like tube formation by endothelial cells (2). TNP does not have a cytostatic effect on transformed endothelial cells (5).

The effect of TNP-470 on the endothelial cell cycle has been examined. Time course studies suggest that TNP affects processes that occur late in G_1, but prior to the transition to S phase (5–7). The results of these studies are dependent on the source of the cultured endothelial cells, the actual length of exposure to TNP, and the time of addition of TNP relative to that of growth factor. The effects of TNP within G_1 of HUVECs include inhibition or attenuation of several cyclins, attenuation of bFGF-induced activation of cyclin-dependent kinases cdc2 and cdk2, and inhibition of the phosphorylation of the RB protein (7). Again, the results of these experiments depend on the time of TNP addition relative to that of bFGF. Additional in vitro experiments indicate that TNP does not interact directly with DNA (8). Further work will be required before the exact mechanism of action of TNP-470 can be determined.

The effect of TNP-470 on the proliferation of a wide variety of rodent and human, transformed or tumor-derived cell lines also has been examined. In general, IC_{50} values for these cell types are several orders of magnitude higher than those that have been reported for normal endothelial cells, that is, in the ng/mL to μg/mL range, and cytostatic and cytotoxic concentrations are comparable. Notable exceptions include human fibroblasts and two of six tested human glioblastoma lines that have IC_{50} values in the pg/mL range (9). It also appears that TNP enhances the proliferation of normal human, but not tumor-derived, lymphocytes (10, 11). These data clearly indicate that the effects of TNP-470 are cell specific.

IV. IN VIVO TUMOR STUDIES

TNP-470 inhibits growth factor-induced angiogenesis in a dose-dependent manner in several model systems including embryonic chick chorioallantoic membrane (2), rat and rabbit corneal micropocket assays (8, 12), and surgically implanted sponges (2). In a mouse sarcoma model, TNP specifically decreased the proliferation index of tumor-associated endothelial cells (13).

The rate of wound healing is not affected by treatment with TNP-470 if the drug is administered before wounding, but wound healing is delayed if the drug is given immediately after injury (12).

TNP-470 is effective in decreasing the overall growth of primary tumor and the growth and incidence of pulmonary and hepatic metastases in a wide variety of rodent homograft and xenograft models using a variety of dosing schedules and routes of administration. In most instances, antitumor effects were dose dependent. Rodent tumor models included hemangioendothelioma (14), melanoma (15–17), osteosarcoma (18, 19), reticulum cell sarcoma (16), glioma (20, 21) hepatoma (22), and mammary (23, 24), lung (16), and pancreatic carcinomas (25). Human xenograft models included glioblastoma (9), meningioma (26), fibrosarcoma (4), neurofibrosarcoma (27), and colon (28) and prostate (29) carcinomas. In some instances, the antitumor effect was accompanied by an increase in tumor necrosis and an increase in mean survival (16, 20). Studies with Lewis lung carcinoma suggest that repeated exposure to TNP by sequential passage does not result in the development of resistance (i.e., no change in the Treated/Control (T/C) ratio). No efficacy against primary tumor was seen in three cases: a rat astrocytoma (20), a human endometrioid carcinoma (30), and a human gastric carcinoma (30). With few exceptions, weight loss or failure to gain weight was observed in animals receiving high doses of TNP.

Routes of administration included subcutaneous (s.c.), intravenous (i.v.), intraperitoneal (i.p.), and intra-arterial (i.a.), with s.c. being the most frequently used. Dosing schedules ranged from 10 to 60 mg/kg every other day (q.o.d.) to 50 to 200 mg/kg once per week, with 30 mg/kg q.o.d. being the most common. Encapsulation of TNP-470 into microspheres or dissolved in either a lipid-based contrast medium or medium chain triglycerides provides the opportunity for i.a. administration, resulting in prolonged antitumor effects from even a single dose (31, 32).

V. COMBINATION THERAPY STUDIES

Potentiation of tumor response is observed when TNP-470 is coadministered with hyperthermia, other antiangiogenic agents, or cytotoxic drugs in a number of rodent homograft and xenograft models. This is the case when TNP is used in combination with tamoxifen (23) or 5′-deoxy-5-fluorouridine (24) in a rat mammary carcinoma model; with mitomycin C (33) or α/β interferon (34) against murine melanoma and Lewis lung carcinoma; with adriamycin against murine renal cell carcinoma (35); with 5-fluorouracil against Lewis lung carcinoma (32); and with hyperthermia against murine squamous cell carcinoma (36). Xenograft models in which combination therapy resulted in an increase in efficacy include breast carcinoma with tamoxifen (37) and esophageal and gastric carcinomas with hyperthermia (38).

Several studies included TNP in a regimen of multiple therapeutic agents. In a drug-resistant murine mammary carcinoma model, TNP in combination with cisplatin, cyclophosphamide, or thiotepa with or without minocycline resulted in potentiation of cytotoxicity against the primary tumor as well as a decrease in the incidence of metastatic disease and an increase in long-term survival (39, 40).

Several experiments included attempts to elucidate the mechanism of these observed synergies. Using a transgenic mouse model of progressive pancreatic cancer, a combination of TNP with minocycline and α/β interferon resulted in growth inhibition of the primary tumor with a concomitant reduction in tumor capillary density and an increase in the apoptotic index of tumor cells (41). These observations suggest that, in addition to or as a consequence of its effect on the endothelium, TNP-470 is able to increase the effectiveness of biological therapy by shifting the equilibrium between cell proliferation and death.

A study using radiolabeled cyclophosphamide or tracing the platinum moiety of cisplatin demonstrated an increase in DNA cross-linking and an increase in both tissue and tumor uptake of cytotoxic drug when TNP was included in the regimen (42). This suggests that TNP, most likely through its effect on the vasculature, increases the relative availability of therapeutic agents. A study in a rat glioma model that used a microdialysis probe to collect tumor interstitial fluid samples indicated that when TNP was given in combination with temozolamide (TMZ), there was a 25% decrease in interstitial TMZ levels (43). This seems to be in conflict with the results of the cyclophosphamide/cisplatin study. However, the combination of TNP and TMZ did result in a 59% decrease in tumor volume. Further, in this study, neither the level of DNA alkylation nor survival time were determined.

A variety of dosing regimens was used in the combination therapy experiments. In general, it appears that although TNP-470 is effective as a single agent, it is also able to increase the effectiveness of both cytotoxic and biological therapies. This is most probably mediated through its effect on tumor vasculature. Studies are currently underway to optimize the combination dosing regimens and to further elucidate the basis of the observed synergies.

VI. OVERVIEW OF PHASE I EXPERIENCE

The development of TNP-470 began in September 1992 when the first of seven phase I clinical trials was initiated. The patient population in this and one other clinical trial consisted of individuals with AIDS-associated Kaposi's sarcoma. The last of the remaining five clinical trials was initiated in December 1994. These include four that enrolled adult cancer patients (two for adult solid tumors, one for prostate cancer, and one for cervical cancer) and one limited to pediatric cancer patients. Three phase I clinical trials have concluded (prostate cancer, cervical cancer, and AIDS-associated Kaposi's sarcoma), and two are approaching closure (adult solid tumor); only one trial in AIDS-associated Kaposi's sarcoma patients and the pediatric trial continue.

Admission criteria for all four adult patient phase I protocols were similar, including only patients with histological documentation of malignancy that was either metastatic or inoperable and for which there was no alternative, standard, curative, or palliative regimen. Patients' disease had to be either evaluable or measurable, and their performance status could be no greater than two on the Eastern Cooperative Oncology Group (ECOG) or Zubrod scale. Concurrent therapy with antineoplastic drugs was not permitted, and an interval of at least 3 weeks (depending on the prior treatment modality) between the end of a prior treatment regimen and initiation of TNP-470 treatment was required. The hematology and chemistry baseline values that were required were standard for oncology clinical trials. However, based on preclinical toxicology findings, more rigorous criteria were applied to coagulation parameters, and patients with certain conditions were excluded (e.g., history of bleeding diathesis, seizures, peripheral neuropathy, and primary or metastatic brain tumor). Also excluded were pregnant or lactating female patients. Finally, signed informed consent was to be obtained before initiation of treatment.

The observations included in this overview of clinical experience with TNP-470 derive primarily from the 4 adult (data for 101 patients) and 1 pediatric (data for 5 patients) phase I clinical trials in cancer patients. The databases for the two trials in patients with AIDS-associated Kaposi's sarcoma are held by their respective institutional sponsors, precluding detailed analysis at this time. Further, only the database for the phase I clinical trial in prostate cancer patients has been finalized. Although addition of patient information to the other databases is an ongoing process, these databases currently are representative of but a portion

Table 1 Dosing Schedules in Phase I Clinical Trials of TNP-470

Patient population	Infusion duration	Infusion frequency	Cycle definition
Prostate cancer, n = 32	1 hour	Every other day for 28 days	28 days plus 14-day rest period; restaging evaluations every 6 weeks
Cervical cancer, n = 21	1 hour	Every other day for 28 days	28 days plus 14-day rest period; restaging evaluations every 6 weeks
Adult solid tumor, n = 35 (schedule A)	1 hour	Every Monday, Wednesday, and Friday	6 weeks; no rest period; restaging evaluations every 6 weeks
Adult solid tumor, n = 31 (schedule B)	4 hour	Once weekly	Continuous; no rest period; restaging evaluations every 8 weeks
Pediatric, n = 15	1 hour	Every Monday, Wednesday, and Friday	Continuous; no rest period; restaging evaluations at the end of 8 weeks, 6 months, and 12 months
AIDS-associated Kaposi's sarcoma, n = 28	1 hour	Every other day	18 weeks; no rest period; restaging evaluations every 6 weeks
AIDS-associated Kaposi's sarcoma, n = 40	1 hour	Once weekly	12 weeks, followed by a 2-week rest period; sentinel lesion restaging at weeks 2, 4, 8, 12, 14, 18, 22, and 26

of patients treated in the clinical trials. Thus, more detailed analyses will be limited to observations made in the phase I prostate cancer clinical trial.

TNP-470 is administered as an intravenous infusion. Several different dosing schedules, ranging from once weekly to every other day, were used in the phase I clinical trials. Once-weekly schedules included administration over the course of either 1 or 4 hours, whereas the more frequent administration schedules (either every other day or every Monday, Wednesday, and Friday) used a 1-hour infusion. A priori definitions of treatment cycles differed between protocols as well, and some schedules incorporated rest periods before initiation of additional cycles. Table 1 describes the dosing schedules.

VII. PATIENT DEMOGRAPHICS

In the four phase I clinical trials enrolling adult patients (prostate cancer, cervical cancer, and two adult solid tumor), ages ranged from 22 to 82 years, with the prostate cancer population having the highest mean age (63 years). Eighty-five percent of the patients in the four adult and one pediatric phase I clinical trials

Table 2 Summary of Demographic Characteristics of Patients in Phase I Clinical Trials

Patient population distribution by sex (patients in database/total enrollment)	Mean age and range (years)	Mean height and range (cm)	Mean weight and range (kg)	Race White (W) Black (B) Other (O)
Prostate cancer, male = 32 (32/32)	63.0 38–82	178.4 162.6–198.1	87.0 67.0–119.0	W = 28 B = 2 O = 2
Cervical cancer, female = 18 (18/21)	46.1 25–55	161.7 150.0–174.0	60.3 44.4–76.0	W = 9 B = 2 O = 7
Adult solid tumor, (schedule A), male = 14, female = 11 (25/35)	50.4 22–75	168.8 155.0–183.0	74.9 45.4–114.1	W = 25 B = 0 O = 0
Adult solid tumor, (schedule B), male = 14, female = 12 (26/31)	54.8 22–73	171.4 152.4–190.0	73.9 43.1–107.2	W = 25 B = 1 O = 0
Pediatric, male = 4, female = 1 (5/15)	17.2 14–20	165.9 155.5–171.0	60.3 41.7–73.3	W = 3 B = 0 O = 2

were white, 5% were black, and 10% were categorized as belonging to other races. Table 2 contains detailed patient demographic information.

Sarcomas were the most common tumor types in the adult solid tumor phase I protocols, accounting for almost half of the 51 cases currently in the database. Representative tumor types in order of prevalence were: leiomyosarcoma, angiosarcoma, fibrous histiocytoma, chondrosarcoma, rhabdomyosarcoma, dermatofibrosarcoma, and hemangiopericytoma. Adenocarcinomas were documented for approximately 20 patients, and 5 patients had diagnoses of melanoma. With few exceptions, patients had metastatic disease.

VIII. OUTCOMES

The most common primary reason for discontinuation from the clinical trials was disease progression; in the four adult patient phase I clinical trials, this accounted

Table 3 Summary of Primary Reasons for Treatment Termination in Phase I Clinical Trials

Primary reason cited for termination from the trial	Prostate cancer n = 32	Cervical cancer n = 17	Adult solid tumor n = 25 schedule A	Adult solid tumor n = 25 schedule B	Pediatric (n = 5)
Disease progression	27 84.4%	12 70.6%	17 68.0%	15 60.0%	3 60.0%
Toxicity	3 9.4%	2 11.8%	4 16.0%	3 12.0%	1 20.0%
Intercurrent medical event	2 6.2%	1 5.9%	2 8.0%	4 16.0%	0
Death	0	1 5.9%	0	1 4.0%	0
Study completed	0	0	1 4.0%	0	0
Personal reasons	0	0	1 4.0%	0	0
Lost to follow-up	0	1 5.9%	0	0	0
Other	0	0	0	2 8.0%	1 20.0%
Median duration of participation (days, cycles)	69 days 2 cycles	27 days 1 cycle	40 days 1 cycle	50 days 1 cycle	50 days 1 cycle

n = number of patients for whom termination data are in the database. Several patients continue on treatment and are not reflected in Table 3.

for more than 70% of terminations. The next most common primary reason was toxicity, cited for about 12% of terminations. Intercurrent medical events accounted for almost 9% of the primary reasons for discontinuation, with other reasons (e.g., personal decision, lost to follow-up, etc.) individually being cited for no more than 2% of terminations. The median duration of participation ranged from 27 to 69 days, translating to 1 or 2 treatment cycles, depending on study design. Table 3 summarizes the primary reasons for all terminations for each study individually and indicates the median duration of participation.

The deaths reported in Table 3 each occurred 9 days after the last dose of TNP-470. The primary cause of death cited for the cervical cancer patient was pelvic hemorrhage; treatment duration was 27 days. The primary cause of death for the adult solid tumor patient was malignant melanoma, with superior vena cava syndrome constituting a secondary cause. Duration of treatment was 15 days.

The full range of treatment duration in the database for patients in the 4 adult and 1 pediatric phase I studies extended from 1 to 357 days. Several patients continue to receive treatment and the database does not reflect their entire experience. Three patients have received treatment for more than 1 year; of these, 2 have been treated for more than 18 months. In these cases, as well as others in which the duration of treatment was prolonged, disease stabilization was a common observation. Further details will be provided in the discussion of efficacy.

IX. DOSE-LIMITING TOXICITIES AND MAXIMAL TOLERATED DOSE DETERMINATIONS

The primary objectives of all seven phase I clinical trials included determination of dose-limiting toxicities (DLT) and the maximal tolerated dose (MTD), defined as the dose level at which no more than one third of patients experienced DLTs. In the four clinical trials that have either concluded or are reaching closure, the MTD and the DLTs contributing to its determination have been established. The two ongoing clinical trials have not yet reached the MTD, and one clinical trial in AIDS-associated Kaposi's sarcoma patients was discontinued before determination of the MTD because of accrual difficulties.

Ten DLTs, of which nine were neurological, were reported in the four adult phase I studies. The neurological DLTs involved aspects of cortical, cerebellar, mood, and vision function. Complaints included memory impairment, gait disturbance, incoordination, dizziness, nystagmus, increased anxiety, emotional lability, and blurred vision. The median duration of treatment before occurrence of DLTs in patients receiving TNP-470 either every other day or every Monday, Wednesday, and Friday was 27 days, with a range of 13 to 40 days. In contrast, DLTs were observed later, at 52 and 78 days, for the two patients on a once-weekly schedule. Hemoptysis (grade 1), the only nonneurological DLT, was reported for a patient with non–small-cell lung cancer (NSCLC) who had a history of similar occurrences.

At the time the neurological DLTs were observed, the patients' complaints were evaluated with a range of diagnostic modalities, including radiologic (CT scans and MRI) and neuropsychological assessments. Radiological findings were negative, whereas neuropsychological testing revealed decrements in cognitive function and affect. The DLTs were reversible, with resolution occurring within 3 weeks after discontinuation of TNP-470 in most cases.

The MTDs for administration as a 1-hour infusion every other day for 28 days followed by a 2-week rest period were 47.1 and 60.0 mg/m^2. Administration

Table 4 Dose-Limiting Toxicities/Maximal Tolerated Doses in Phase I Clinical Trials

Patient population	Dose-limiting toxicities and dose level	Maximal tolerated dose
Prostate cancer	*Neurological grade 3*: gait disturbance, impaired coordination, memory impairment, increased anxiety and emotional lability; occurred at the 70.6 (2 of 7 patients) and 105.9 (1 of 1 patient) mg/m^2 dose levels.	47.1 mg/m^2
Cervical cancer	*Neurological grade 3*: gait disturbance, dizziness, nystagmus; occurred in 2 of 4 patients at the 71 mg/m^2 dose level.	60.0 mg/m^2
Adult solid tumor (schedule A)	*Neurological grade 1*: unsteadiness; occurred in 1 of 6 patients at the 32.4 mg/m^2 dose level. *Neurological grade 3*: gait disturbance and nystagmus; occurred in 1 of 6 patients at the 76.5 mg/m^2 dose level. *Hemorrhage grade 1*: hemoptysis; occurred in 1 of 6 patients at the 76.5 mg/m^2 dose level.	57.4 mg/m^2
Adult solid tumor (schedule B)	*Neurological grades 1 and 2*: dizziness; occurred in 2 of 6 patients at the 235 mg/m^2 dose level.	177 mg/m^2
Pediatric	*Hemorrhage grade 1*: petechiae; occurred in 1 of 3 patients at the 23.2 mg/m^2 dose level.	To be determined

every Monday, Wednesday and Friday had an associated MTD of 57.4 mg/m^2. Extending the infusion time to 4 hours with once-weekly administration resulted in an MTD of 177 mg/m^2. Table 4 presents detailed information about DLTs.

X. ADVERSE EVENTS

In the four adult patient phase I clinical trials, at least one treatment-emergent adverse event (AE) was reported for 79 of 101 patients (78.2%) for whom such data have been collected. The most commonly reported AEs were: asthenia (41 patients or 40.6%); nausea (31 patients or 30.7%); anorexia (18 patients or 17.8%); and dizziness (16 patients or 15.8%). Pain and vomiting were each reported by 11 patients (10.9%), whereas the frequency of reports of all other AEs was less than 10% each. The majority of AEs were tolerable, with 69.8% either grade 1 or mild, 20.4% grade 2 or moderate, and only 8.8% grade 3 or 4 or severe. Excepting AEs involving the nervous system (where a dose-response relationship was observed in the prostate cancer population), the incidence of AEs was not related to the dose level of TNP-470. The complaints of anorexia were not reflected in the incidence of weight loss of 10% or greater, which was reported for fewer than 5% of patients.

XI. LABORATORY AND SPECIAL EVALUATIONS

Observations of multisystem microhemorrhage, laboratory abnormalities, and cataract development in preclinical toxicology studies suggested parameters that required careful monitoring in phase I clinical trials. Treatment-emergent low platelet counts ($< 100{,}000/\mu L$), attributed to the patient's underlying condition in most cases, were recorded for less than 7% of patients. Although the incidence of treatment-emergent lymphocyte counts less than $500/\mu L$ was almost 25%, the majority were sporadic, limited to one or two low values, and not considered to be clinically significant by the investigators. Only two patients had treatment-emergent abnormally high serum glutamic pyruvic transaminase (SGPT) values ($>$ 3 times the upper limit of normal), and in both cases this was attributed to the patient's cancer. Treatment-emergent coagulation abnormalities ($>$ 1.5 times the upper limit of normal) included one not clinically significant elevation in prothrombin time, and six patients with elevations in partial thromboplastin time, all attributable to anticoagulant treatment.

Development of cataracts was observed for two phase I patients. TNP-470 (47.1 mg/m^2) was administered to a 69-year-old patient with prostate cancer for 126 days before cataract development was noted. A 70-year-old female patient with metastatic colon cancer received TNP-470 (235 mg/m^2) for 85 days before mild cataract changes were documented. In both cases, ophthalmological examinations performed earlier during treatment were negative for these findings.

XII. PHARMACOKINETIC ANALYSES

TNP-470 is rapidly and extensively metabolized. Although numerous metabolites have been observed, only two have been characterized. Briefly, the proposed metabolic pathway involves an initial enzymatic degradation to a metabolite known as AGM-1883 (M-IV), which is further metabolized by hydrolysis of the epoxide rings to metabolite M-II. The stability of TNP-470 is pH-dependent, with a pH of 3 to 5 providing the greatest degree of stability. Hence, degradation of TNP-470 occurs rapidly in whole blood or plasma samples unless the pH of the sample is properly adjusted.

Preliminary results from a phase I study (n = three patients; dose level = 235 mg/m^2) suggested that the TNP-470 and AGM-1883 $t_{1/2}$ values were only several minutes (about 7 to 8 minutes), and the mean $t_{1/2}$ for M-II was 2.8 hours. Mean $AUC_{0-\infty}$ values for TNP-470, AGM-1883, and M-II were 1610, 32, and 3280 ng·hr/mL, respectively. Degradation of TNP-470 and AGM-1883 occurs rapidly. Further, M-II elimination appears to be consistent with a two-compartment model with a terminal $t_{1/2}$ of about 3 hours. Additional studies are necessary to confirm these preliminary results and conclusions.

XIII. EFFICACY

Preclinical pharmacology studies demonstrated that treatment with TNP-470 resulted primarily in growth inhibition of both the primary tumor and metastases rather than tumor regression. Such observations suggest that clinical outcomes of TNP-470 administration might include disease stabilization, and indeed, observations in phase I clinical trials have supported this. Table 5 presents information about patients who experienced either a period of disease stabilization or response while treated with TNP-470 in the three adult phase I protocols that did not impose a treatment duration limit (44–46). Although there were some patients with disease stabilization in the fourth adult phase I protocol, treatment was limited to only 18 weeks, and these patients are excluded from Table 5.

XIV. FUTURE DIRECTIONS

In addition to these phase I studies, TNP-470 is also being tested in phase II clinical trials. Patient populations in the latter setting include glioblastoma multi-

Table 5 Patients in Phase I Clinical Trials with Disease Stabilization/Response

Patient population	Dose level (mg/m^2)	Disease status	Treatment duration
Prostate cancer[a]	9.3	Prostate cancer with bone metastases	9 months prior to disease progression
Cervical cancer[a]	14 → 47.5	Cervical cancer with lung metastases	6.5 months prior to disease progression
	31.5 → 47.5 47.5 → 71	Cervical cancer with lymph node involvement	5 months prior to disease progression
	71	Cervical cancer with lung metastases	Complete response treated from 02/95 until 01/97
	60	Cervical cancer with lung metastases	Stable disease; ongoing treatment for 21 months
Adult solid tumor[b]	25	Metastatic melanoma	6 months prior to disease progression
	50	Fibrous histiocytoma	Stable disease treated 05/95 until 03/97
	235 → 177	Colon cancer with lung metastases	Stable disease treated from 12/95 until 01/97

TNP-470 administered as a: [a]1-hour infusion every other day, 28 days plus 14-day rest period; [b]4-hour infusion once weekly.

forme, pancreatic cancer, breast cancer, cervical cancer, and renal cell carcinoma. The majority of these clinical trials began enrollment during 1996 and it is too early to know whether treatment with TNP-470 is beneficial for these patient populations. Future studies will depend, in large part, on observations in the current phase II programs, but will certainly include evaluations of combination treatment modalities.

Clinical investigators working in the field of angiogenesis inhibition as applied to oncology face a great challenge. The standard response criteria on which oncology clinical trial design is based are not entirely applicable to outcomes predicted for angiogenesis inhibitors. If tumor regression is not an a priori expectation for angiogenesis inhibitors, and if disease stabilization is, then it is very difficult to establish efficacy because disease stabilization is traditionally viewed as treatment failure. Further, clinical endpoints appropriate for this treatment modality are neither readily available nor attainable in the short term. Surrogate endpoints have been much discussed and debated, but they must be validated before they will be accepted by the regulatory and medical communities. Validation will require studies that track the time to disease progression and survival, endpoints that may not occur for many years in certain cancers. In addition, the literature is based in large part on standard response criteria and derived endpoints, such as response rate. This makes it increasingly difficult to conduct single-arm phase II clinical trials with angiogenesis inhibitors because an historical control database for parameters such as time to progression and survival is often nonexistent. Thus, phase II clinical trial design must approach that of traditional phase III studies, requiring the presence of a concurrent control arm to assess the efficacy of an angiogenesis inhibitor. It is important to note that the above definitions of phase II and phase III clinical trial design as open-label and controlled, respectively, are used in oncology and are not generally applicable to clinical research in other disease indications. In contrast, phase II clinical trials provide the first opportunity to assess the efficacy of an investigational drug under controlled circumstances in a carefully defined patient population. To maximize the future applicability of information obtained in phase II clinical trials, the design incorporates control treatment arms, and the most common control used is the placebo control. Although these challenges in protocol design and implementation are well known to investigators working in this area, there is a critical need to educate the larger medical community about the need to adopt new paradigms—for both clinical trial design and goals for cancer treatment.

ACKNOWLEDGMENTS

The authors wish to acknowledge the contributions of their colleagues in preclinical and clinical disciplines at TAP Holdings Inc., Takeda Chemical Industries, Ltd., and Abbott Laboratories. In addition, the efforts of the clinical investigators and respective staff in conducting the clinical trials are appreciated. Most important, the authors are indebted to the patients, who by virtue of their participation in these and future clinical trials, make invaluable contributions to the advancement of medical knowledge.

REFERENCES

1. Ingber D, Fujita T, Kishimoto S, Sudo K, Kanamaru T, Brem H, Folkman J. Synthetic analogues of fumagillin that inhibit angiogenesis and suppress tumor growth. Nature 1990; 348:555–557.
2. Kusaka M, Sudo K, Fujita T, Marui S, Itoh F, Ingber D, Folkman J. Potent antiangiogenic action of AGM-1470: comparison of the fumagillin parent. Biochem Biophys Res Commun 1991; 174:1070–1076.

3. Kusaka M, Sudo K, Matsutani E, Kozai Y, Marui S, Fujita T, Ingber D, Folkman J. Cytostatic inhibition of endothelial cell growth by the angiogenesis inhibitor TNP-470 (AGM-1470). Br J Cancer 1994; 69:212–216.
4. Ito Y, Iwamoto Y, Oshima N, Sugioka Y. Quantitative evaluation of the effects of an angiogenesis inhibitor, TNP-470, by an in vivo tumor angiogenesis assay using basement membrane extracts. Cancer J (France) 1996; 9:95–100.
5. Antoine N, Greimers R, De Roanne C, Kusaka M, Heinen E, Simar LJ, Castronovo V. AGM-1470, a potent angiogenesis inhibitor, prevents the entry of normal but not transformed endothelial cells into the G_1 phase of the cell cycle. Cancer Res 1994; 54:2073–2076.
6. Dike L, Ingber D. Inhibition of cell cycle progression in capillary endothelial cells by TNP-470. Takeda Report N-5-112; March 1992.
7. Abe J, Zhou W, Takuwa N, Taguchi J, Kurokawa K, Kumada M, Takuwa Y. A fumagillin derivative angiogenesis inhibitor, AGM-1470, inhibits activation of cyclin-dependent kinases and phosphorylation of retinoblastoma gene product but not protein tyrosyl phosphorylation or protooncogene expression in vascular endothelial cells. Cancer Res 1994; 54(13):3407–3412.
8. Kito G. Summary of pharmacological studies of TNP-470. Takeda Report N-5-111; March 1992.
9. Takamiya Y, Brem H, Ojeifo J, Mineta T, Martuza RL. AGM-1470 inhibits the growth of human glioblastoma cells in vitro and in vivo. Neurosurgery 1994; 34(5): 869–875.
10. Antoine N, Daukandt M, Locigno R, Heinen E, Simar LJ, Castronovo V. The potent angioinhibin AGM-1470 stimulates normal but not tumor lymphocytes. Tumor (Italy) 1996; 82:27–30.
11. Schoof DD, Obando JA, Cusack JC Jr, Goedegeburre PS, Brem H, Eberlein TJ. The influence of angiogenesis inhibitor AGM-1470 on immune system status and tumor growth in vitro. Int J Cancer 1993; 55:630–635.
12. Brem H, Ingber D, Gonzalez E, Goto F, Blood C, Budson A, Tsakayannis D, Takamiya Y, Martuza R, Adamis A, Folkman J. Takeda Report N-5-113; 1992.
13. Yamamoto T, Sudo K, Fujita T. Significant inhibition of endothelial cell growth in tumor vasculature by an angiogenesis inhibitor, TNP-470 (AGM-1470). Anti-cancer Res 1994; 14:1–3.
14. O'Reilly MS, Brem H, Folkman J. Treatment of murine hemangioendotheliomas with the angiogenesis inhibitor AGM-1470. J Pediatr Surg 1995; 30:325–330.
15. Brem H, Ingber D, Blood CH, Bradley D, Urioste S, Folkman J. Suppression of tumor metastasis by angiogenesis inhibition. Am Coll Surg 1991 Surgical Forum Volume 1993; XLII:439–441.
16. Yamaoka M, Yamamoto T, Masaki T, Ikeyama S, Sudo K, Fujita T. Inhibition of tumor growth and metastasis of rodent tumors by the angiogenesis inhibitor *O*-(chloroacetyl-carbamoyl)fumagillol (TNP-470; AGM-1470). Cancer Res 1993; 53:4262–4267.
17. Tsujimoto H, Hagiwara H, Osaki K, Ohyama T, Sakakibara T, Sakuyama A, Ohgaki M, Imanishi T, Watanabe N, Yamazaki J, Shirasu M, Sakakura C, Shimotsuma M, Takahashi T. Therapeutic effects of the angiogenesis inhibitor TNP-470 against carcinomatous peritonitis in mice. Anticancer Drugs 1995; 6:438–442.

18. Mori S, Ueda T, Kuratsu S, Hosono N, Izawa K, Uchida A. Suppression of pulmonary metastasis by angiogenesis inhibitor TNP-470 in murine osteosarcoma. Int J Cancer 1995; 61:148–152.
19. Mortishita T, Mii Y, Miyauchi Y, Miura S, Honoki K, Aoki M, Kido A, Tamai S, Tsutsumi M, Konishi Y. Efficacy of the angiogenesis inhibitor *O*-(chloroacetyl-carbamoyl) fumagillol (AGM-1470) on osteosarcoma growth and lung metastasis in rats. Jpn J Clin Oncol 1995; 25:25–31.
20. Isobe N, Vozumi T, Kurisu K, Kawamoto K. Antitumor effect of TNP-470 on glial tumors transplanted in rats. Anticancer Res 1996; 16:71–76.
21. Wilson JT, Penar PL. The effect of AGM-1470 in an improved intracranial 9L gliosarcoma rat model. Neurol Res 1994; 16:121–124.
22. Ahmed MH, Konno H, Tanaka T, Matsuda I, Naitou Y, Baba S. Inhibition of metastasis of rat hepatoma (AH-130) by the angiogenesis inhibitor TNP-470. Proc Ann Meeting Jpn Cancer Assoc 1994; 6:324.
23. Toi M, Yamamoto Y, Imazawa T, Takayanagi T, Akutsu K, Tominaga T. Antitumor effect of the angiogenesis inhibitor AGM-1470 and its combination effect with tamoxifen in DMBA induced mammary tumors in rats. Int J Oncol 1993; 3:525–528.
24. Yamamoto Y, Toi M, Yamada R, Tominaga T. Combination effect of an angiogenesis inhibitor AGM-1470 with 5′deoxy-5-fluorouridine, and with hormonal drugs in DMBA-induced rat mammary tumors. Oncol Rep 1995; 2:793–798.
25. Egawa S-I, Tsutsumi M, Konishi Y, Kobari M, Matsumo S, Nagasaki K, Futami H, Yamaguchi K. The role of antiogenesis in the tumor growth of Syrian hamster pancreatic cell line HPD-NR. Gastroenterology 1995; 108:1526–1533.
26. Yazaki T, Takamiya Y, Costello PC, Mineta T, Menon A, Rabkin SD, Martuza RL. Inhibition of angiogenesis and growth of human non-malignant and malignant meningiomas by TNP-470. J Neurooncol 1995; 23:23–29.
27. Takamiya Y, Friedlander RM, Brem H, Malick A, Martuza RL. Inhibition of angiogenesis and growth of human nerve-sheath tumors by AGM-1470. J Neurosurg 1993; 78:470–476.
28. Konno H, Tanaka T, Kanai T, Maruyama K, Nakamura S, Baba S. Efficacy of an angiogenesis inhibitor TNP-470, in xenotransplanted human colorectal cancer with high metastatic potential. Cancer (supp) 1996; 77:1736–1740.
29. Yamaoka M, Yamamoto T, Ikeyama S, Sudo K, Fujita T. Angiogenesis inhibitor TNP-470 (AGM-1470) potently inhibits the tumor growth of hormone-independent human breast and prostate carcinoma cell lines. Cancer Res 1993; 53:5233–5236.
30. Yanase T, Tamura M, Fujita K, Kodama S, Tanaka K. Inhibitory effect of angiogenesis inhibitor TNP-470 on tumor growth and metastasis of human cell lines in vitro and in vivo. Cancer Res 1993; 53:2566–2570.
31. Kamei S, Okada H, Inoue Y, Yoshioka T, Ogawa Y, Toguchi H. Antitumor effects of angiogenesis inhibitor TNP-470 in rabbits bearing VX-2 carcinoma by arterial administration of microspheres and oil solution. J Pharmacol Exp Ther 1993; 264(1): 469–474.
32. Yanai S, Okada H, Misaki M, Saito K, Kuge Y, Ogawa Y, Toguchi H. Antitumor activity of a medium-chain triglyceride solution of the angiogenesis inhibitor TNP-470 (AGM-1470) when administered via the hepatic artery to rats bearing Walker 256 carcinosarcoma in the liver. J Pharmacol Exp Ther 1994; 271(3):1267–1273.

33. Kato T, Sato K, Kakinuma H, Matsuda Y. Enhanced suppression of tumor growth by combination of angiogenesis inhibitor *O*-(chloroacetyl-carbamoyl) fumagillol (TNP-470) and cytotoxic agents in mice. Cancer Res 1994; 54(19):5143–5147.
34. Brem H, Gresser I, Grosfeld J, Folkman J. The combination of antiangiogenic agents to inhibit primary tumor growth and metastasis. J Pediatr Surg 1993; 28:1253–1257.
35. Sato M, Fujiuka T, Hasegawa M, Ogiu K, Matsushita Y, Ishikura K, Tanji S, Nomura K, Okamoto T, Kubo T. Enhanced antitumor effects by combination of angiogenesis inhibitor TNP-470 and Adriamycin on murine renal cell carcinoma. Biotherapy (Japan) 1995; 9:1411–1416.
36. Nishimura N, Murata R, Hiraoka M. Combined effects of an angiogenesis inhibitor (TNP-470) and hyperthermia. Br J Cancer 1996; 73:270–274.
37. McLesky SE, Zhang L, Trock BJ, Kharbanda S, Liu Y, Gottardis MM, Lippman ME, Kern EG. Effects of AGM-1470 and pentosan polysulfate on tumorigenicity and metastasis of FGF-transfected MCF-7 cells. Br J Cancer 1996; 73:1053–1062.
38. Yano T, Tanase M, Watanabe A, Sawada H, Yamada Y, Shino Y, Nakano H, Ohnishi T. Enhancement effect of an anti-angiogenic agent, TNP-470, on hyperthermia-induced growth suppression of human esophageal and gastric cancers transplantable to nude mice. Anticancer Res 1995; 15:1355–1358.
39. Teicher BA, Holden SA, Dupuis NP, Kakeji Y, Ikebe M, Emi Y, Goff D. Potentiation of cytotoxic therapies by TNP-470 and minocycline in mice bearing EMT-6 mammary carcinoma. Breast Cancer Res Treat 1995; 36:227–236.
40. Teicher BA, Holden SA, Ara G, Alvarez Sotomayor E, Huang ZD, Chen Y-N, Brem H. Potentiation of cytotoxic cancer therapies by TNP-470 alone and with other anti-angiogenic agents. Int J Cancer 1994; 57(6):920–925.
41. Parangi S, O'Reilly M, Christofori G, Holmgren L, Grosfeld J, Folkman J, Hanahan D. Antiangiogenic therapy of transgenic mice impairs de novo tumor growth. Proc Nat Acad Sci U S A 1996; 93:2002–2007.
42. Teicher BA, Dupuis NP, Robinson MF, Emi Y, Goff DA. Anti-angiogenic treatment (TNP-470/minocycline) increases tissue levels of anticancer drugs in mice bearing Lewis lung carcinoma. Oncol Res 1995; 7:237–243.
43. Devineni D, Klein-Szanto A, Gallo J. Uptake of temozolamide in a rat glioma model in the presence and absence of the angiogenesis inhibitor TNP-470. Cancer Res 1996; 56:1983–1987.
44. Levy T, Kudelka A, Vershraegen CF, Edwards CL, Freedman RS, Kaplan A, Kieback D, Steger M, Mante R, Gutterman J, Piamsomboon S, Termrungruanglert W, Kavanagh JJ. A Phase I study of TNP-470 administered to patients with advanced squamous cell cancer of the cervix (abstr). Proc Am Assoc Cancer Res 1996; 37: 166.
45. Kudelka AP, Levy T, Verschraegen CF, Edwards CL, Piamsomboon S, Termrungruanglert W, Freedman RS, Kaplan AL, Kieback DG, Meyers CA, Jaeckle KA, Loyer E, Steger M, Mante R, Mavligit G, Killian A, Tang RA, Gutterman JU, Kavanagh JJ. A Phase I study of TNP-470 administered to patients with advanced squamous cell cancer of the cervix. Clin Cancer Res 1997; 3:1501–1505.
46. Bhargava P, Marshall J, Rizvi N, Dahut W, Yoe J, Figuera M, Phipps K, Ong VS, Kato A, Hawkins MI. A Phase I and pharmacokinetic study of TNP-470 administered weekly to patients with advanced cancer. Clin Cancer Res 1999; 5:1989–1995.

27
Matrix Metalloproteinase Inhibitors

Peter D. Brown
British Biotech Pharmaceuticals Ltd., Oxford, England

I. INTRODUCTION

Matrix metalloproteinases, and the roles played by these enzymes in angiogenesis, have been described in Part I of this book. This chapter will focus on the development of synthetic inhibitors of matrix metalloproteinases and the therapeutic applications of these compounds. Excessive matrix metalloproteinase activity is thought to be involved in the pathogenesis of several diseases including cancer (1), rheumatoid arthritis (2), osteoarthritis (3), inflammatory bowel disease (4), neurodegenerative diseases (5), and cerebral hemorrhage (6). Matrix metalloproteinase inhibitors have been considered as treatments for each of these conditions, and the first clinical trials in patients with cancer have started.

Although pharmaceutical research on matrix metalloproteinase inhibitors was originally directed toward arthritis, much of the development work has focused on the treatment of cancer. This disease provides a useful framework within which to discuss these novel drugs. Research into the matrix metalloproteinase family dates back to the late 1960s when the first mammalian enzyme activities were isolated and characterized (7, 8). The practical significance of this work was recognized very early when, writing in 1972, Strauch noted that ". . . it suggests an idea which may open new possibilities for the treatment of cancer. By reducing the rate of collagen degradation and simultaneously stimulating collagen biosynthesis, the body may be able to encapsulate the invading tumour in collagen structures and isolate it from adjoining tissue not yet affected. The invasion and metastases would thus be limited and the surgical removal or destruction of the primary tumour would stand a better chance of successful outcome (9)." These words provide a succinct summary of the intended therapeutic action of matrix metalloproteinase inhibitors in the treatment of cancer and today, 25 years later, we have the compounds to be able to test the hypothesis.

II. DEVELOPMENT OF MATRIX METALLOPROTEINASE INHIBITORS

Both endogenous and synthetic inhibitors have been considered as potential therapies for the treatment of cancer. Tissue inhibitor of metalloproteinases-1 (TIMP-1) and TIMP-2 were cloned and sequenced in 1985 and 1989, respectively (10, 11), and both have shown activity in models of tumor invasion, metastasis, and angiogenesis (12–16). Unfortunately, the therapeutic use of these molecules has been limited by the fact that they are proteins (M_r 20,000–28,000), which makes long-term systemic administration particularly difficult. It is likely that interest in the use of TIMPs or TIMP-derived peptides will continue because of the observation that these endogenous inhibitors can modulate the proliferation of human endothelial cells—and thereby angiogenesis—in an apparently protease-independent fashion. Studies with a cartilage-derived matrix metalloproteinase inhibitor have demonstrated the ability of this TIMP-related protein to block both capillary endothelial cell proliferation and migration, as well as in vivo angiogenesis in the chick chorioallantoic membrane assay (17). Similarly, TIMP-2 was shown to inhibit the proliferation of human microvascular endothelial cells in conditions in which neither batimastat, a synthetic matrix metalloproteinase inhibitor (BB-94, British Biotech), nor anti-gelatinase A antibodies were effective (18).

The first synthetic matrix metalloproteinase inhibitors were developed in the early 1980s. These molecules were pseudopeptide derivatives based on the structure of the collagen molecule at the site of cleavage by interstitial collagenase. Compounds designed from the Ile-Ala-Gly and Leu-Leu-Ala sequences on the right-hand side of the cleavage site have emerged as the most promising drugs. The structure of one such compound, marimastat (BB-2516, British Biotech) is shown in Figure 1. The inhibitor binds reversibly at the active site of the matrix metalloproteinase in a stereospecific manner. The zinc-binding group, in this case hydroxamic acid (-CONHOH), is then positioned to chelate the active site zinc ion. Modification of the stereochemistry of the molecule results in loss of inhibitory activity. Several zinc-binding groups have been tested, including carboxylates, aminocarboxylates, sulfhydryls, and derivatives of phosphorus acids (19), but hydroxamates have proved to be the most useful and the majority of inhibitors currently in clinical testing contain this group.

Highly potent compounds with K_i values in the low nanomolar range were developed early without the assistance of X-ray crystal structures. These compounds, typified by the hydroxamate batimastat (Fig. 2), showed broad specificity for members of the matrix metalloproteinase family but displayed little detectable

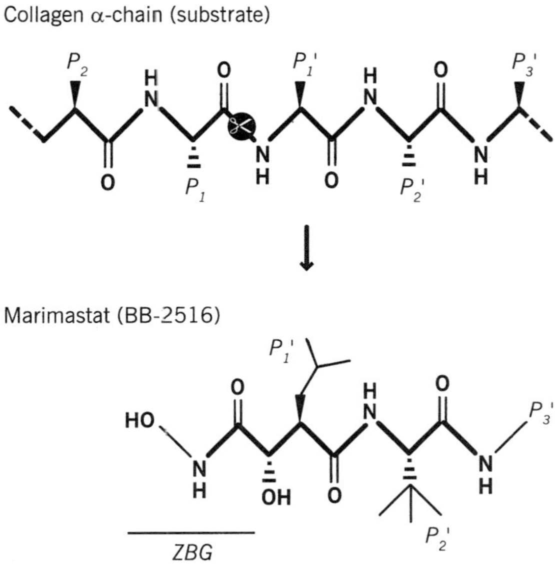

Figure 1 Structure of marimastat. Many of the inhibitors currently being studied are derived from the peptide structure of the α-chain of type I collagen at the point at which collagenase first cleaves the molecule. Marimastat is based on the right hand side of this cleavage site, although the chemical groups at the P1′, P2′, and P3′ positions are different from the original amino acid residues. The zinc binding group (ZBG), in this case a hydroxamate (-CONHOH), binds the zinc atom in the active site of the matrix metalloproteinase enzyme.

activity against other classes of metalloproteinase such as angiotensin-converting enzyme and enkephalinase (20). Unfortunately, these early compounds showed poor oral bioavailability and, therefore, offered little advantage over the endogenous TIMPs.

The design of synthetic matrix metalloproteinase inhibitors then proceeded with two goals: the development of compounds with good oral bioavailability and the development of compounds with selective inhibitory activity against individual matrix metalloproteinases. In both cases, the design of new compounds was assisted by X-ray crystallography data on the three-dimensional structure of the collagenase active site (21). Marimastat (Fig. 1) was one of the first inhibitors to show good oral bioavailability in both animals and man, differing from its predecessor batimastat in the group adjacent to the hydroxamate and the group at the P2′ position. In both positions a small substituent, -hydroxyl and -t-butyl, respectively, replaces a larger cyclic group.

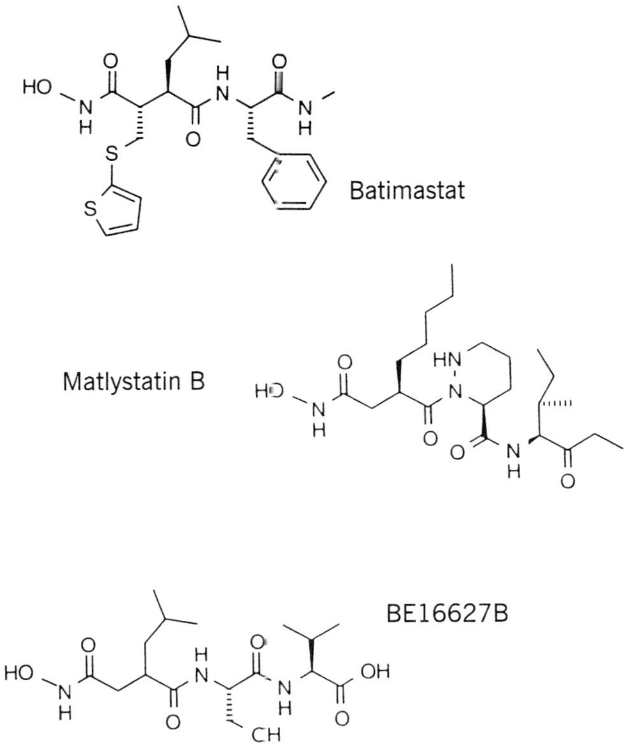

Figure 2 Structure of three matrix metalloproteinase inhibitors showing the similarity between inhibitors derived by rational drug design (batimastat) and those that are natural products identified through conventional screening: BE16627B from *Streptomyces* and matlystatin B from *Actinomadura atramentaria*.

More selective compounds also have been developed. In practice these compounds are not selective for one particular matrix metalloproteinase, but instead show a selective loss of activity against one or more of the enzymes. A series of compounds described by Morphy et al. take advantage of differences in the active site of gelatinase A and B that allow larger hydrophobic groups at the P1′ position (22). These compounds show more than 1000-fold selectivity for gelatinases over interstitial collagenase, but are also potent inhibitors of stromelysin-1. Unfortunately, these early selective inhibitors have not shown good bioavailability when given orally and CDP-845 (Celltech), a potent selective gelatinase inhibitor, has been withdrawn from clinical development partly for this reason. Ro32-3555 (Roche) is a hydroxamate-based inhibitor with relatively weak activity against gelatinase A and stromelysin-1, but good activity against interstitial collagenase. This compound shows good activity when given orally in animal models of arthritis and is currently in clinical development as a treatment for rheumatoid arthritis (23). It is expected that other orally bioavailable selective matrix metalloproteinase inhibitors will follow Ro32-3555 into the clinic.

Low-molecular-weight matrix metalloproteinase inhibitors also have been developed from natural products such as the tetracyclines. Chemical modification of this group of molecules has led to the separation of antibiotic and protease inhibitory activity (24). Interestingly, the more potent natural products such as BE16627B (Banyu) (25) and matlystatin B (Sankyo) (26) are naturally occurring hydroxamates and are structurally very similar to the right-hand side pseudopeptide inhibitors obtained by rational substrate-based design (Fig. 2).

III. PRECLINICAL STUDIES

Studies of the effects of matrix metalloproteinase inhibitors in experimental models of disease are an important part of the preclinical development of potential drugs and provide some indication of what might be expected in the way of therapeutic effect in the subsequent clinical trials. Early studies with synthetic matrix metalloproteinase inhibitors, such as the hydroxamate SC44463 (G.D. Searle), and recombinant TIMPs demonstrated that these inhibitors could block tumor cell invasion through matrix barriers in vitro and inhibit organ colonization by tumor cells (experimental metastasis) in vivo (13, 27). At this time matrix metalloproteinase inhibitors were primarily thought of as antimetastatic drugs; that is drugs to block the passage of metastatic cells ''into'' and ''out of'' lymphatic and vascular channels. However, as further studies were carried out, these inhibitors were thought to have the potential to inhibit the growth of established tumors, at either their primary or secondary site.

Mechanistically, it was proposed that matrix metalloproteinase inhibitors could inhibit tumor growth either by encouraging ''stromal encapsulation'' of the tumor, thereby preventing invasive growth, or by inhibiting angiogenesis. In a model of rat mammary carcinoma, batimastat was shown to reduce both the spread of metastatic cells and the growth of established metastases (28). Batimastat was also shown to inhibit locoregional regrowth and metastasis of a human breast carcinoma, MDA-MB-435, after resection in athymic nude mice (29). In another series of experiments, increased expression of TIMP-2, in clones of rTIMP-2 transfected metastatic 4R cells, was associated with marked suppression of tumor growth and local invasion after subcutaneous implantation. Clones showing suppressed growth were surrounded by a capsule of dense connective tissue (16).

One interesting feature of certain experimental tumors treated with matrix metalloproteinase inhibitors is the development of an enlarged necrotic core. This was reported for C170HM$_2$ human colon tumors grown in the intraperitoneal cavity of nude mice (30) These tumors grow rapidly by invading the liver. In addition to reducing the number and size of the liver tumors, batimastat treatment was associated with a significant increase in the size of necrotic core. An increase in the proportion of necrotic tumor was also observed in the treatment of Mat Ly Lu rat prostate tumors with the synthetic matrix metalloproteinase inhibitors, GI168 and GI173 (Glaxo Inc.) (31). This increase in necrosis may be the result of antiangiogenic activity. Alternatively, it is possible that in certain tumors, constriction of invasive growth by matrix metalloproteinase inhibitors results in increased interstitial pressure. This in turn leads to compression of blood vessels in the center of the tumor causing ischemia and subsequent necrosis (32, 33).

Anti-angiogenic activity has been demonstrated directly for synthetic matrix metalloproteinase inhibitors. Batimastat was shown to reduce the angiogenic response in vivo to heparin-Matrigel implants to levels comparable to controls without added heparin (34). In the same study it was shown that batimastat inhibited the invasion of human umbilical vein endothelial cells through Matrigel in vitro, but did not significantly alter endothelial cell proliferation, haptotaxis, or chemotaxis. The related compound, ilomastat (GM6001, Glycomed) inhibited angiogenesis in the chick chorioallantoic membrane assay and a rat corneal model (35, 36). As discussed earlier, the antiangiogenic activity of the synthetic matrix metalloproteinase inhibitors appears to be mediated through inhibition of endothelial cell invasion rather than the sort of effects shown by TIMPs on endothelial cell proliferation (17, 18). It is also clear that serine proteinase inhibitors can inhibit endothelial cell invasion and angiogenesis (37, 38). This suggests an interdependence of the different proteinase systems that presumably act in concert during the processes of endothelial cell migration, invasion, and vessel formation. However, the recent observation of normal development in plasminogen activator-deficient mice indicates the existence of compensatory mechanisms, at least in nonpathological angiogenesis (39).

Of particular relevance to the therapeutic application of matrix metalloproteinase inhibitors is the recent finding that these inhibitors may be combined effectively with established cytoreductive cancer treatments. In a study of the synthetic inhibitor CT1746 (Celltech) and cyclophosphamide, the two compounds combined were significantly more effective in inhibiting the growth and metastasis of the murine Lewis lung carcinoma than either agent used alone (40).

Similarly, in a model of human ovarian carcinoma, batimastat and cisplatin were shown to be significantly more effective in prolonging survival than either single agent and, as in the study with CT1746, the additive therapeutic effects did not appear to be accompanied by additive toxicity (R. Giavazzi, personal communication). Although the mechanisms underlying these changes are not well understood, these results have already led to clinical studies of the combined use of matrix metalloproteinase inhibitors and cytotoxic agents.

Collectively, these preclinical studies show that in addition to inhibiting metastatic spread of tumors, matrix metalloproteinase inhibitors can directly inhibit the growth of solid tumors. The means by which they do this will probably vary with tumor type. Figure 3 shows a diagrammatic representation of a tumor divided into quarters with each quarter showing a different facet of the possible treatment effect. Section A shows an untreated tumor with a high proportion of viable tumor cells and no detectable stromal tissue. The boundary of the tumor is characterized by motile tumor cells moving into adjacent tissue. The effects of batimastat on the C170HM$_2$ colorectal tumors is shown in Section B. In these tumors, there was no clear evidence of fibrotic tissue development, but the tumors were smaller than control tumors and the enlarged necrotic core may have re-

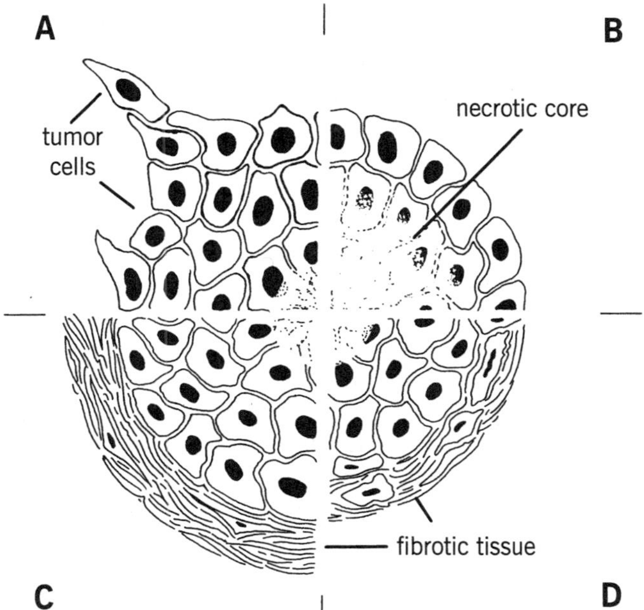

Figure 3 A diagrammatic representation of the possible effects of matrix metalloproteinase inhibition on a solid tumor. Section **A** shows an untreated tumor with tumor cells moving into adjacent tissue. Section **B** shows an enlarged necrotic core seen in some treated experimental tumors. Section **C** shows a capsule of dense stromal tissue surrounding the tumor. Section **D** shows fibrotic replacement of tumor with tumor cells showing signs of damage.

sulted from increased interstitial pressure as the invasive growth was constricted (30, 33). Section C shows the development of fibrotic tissue around the tumor mass, as originally envisioned by Strauch (9). This has been seen experimentally in tumors transfected with TIMP-2 (16) and with tumours treated with batimastat (unpublished observations). Section D shows a third possible treatment effect in which part of the cellular mass has been replaced by fibrotic tissue. Tumor cells entrapped in this region show pyknotic nuclei and signs of necrosis. Again this has been observed experimentally with batimastat (unpublished observations) and, as will be discussed later, has been seen in the tumor of a patient treated with marimastat (41). It is also clear, from a recent study of the effects of CT1746 (Celltech), that tumor growth may simply be slowed by matrix metalloproteinase inhibitors without any of these visible features being present (42). The different treatment effects probably reflect fundamental differences in the biology of the tumors treated.

Some of these features may be hallmarks of the effect of matrix metalloproteinase inhibitors on solid tumors. In this regard, they may provide useful ways of demonstrating the activity of these inhibitors in early clinical trials in which effects on metastasis and clinical outcome would require too long and too large a study to be practical in dose-finding designs.

IV. EARLY CLINICAL TRIALS

The first matrix metalloproteinase inhibitors to be tested in patients were characterized by their poor oral bioavailability. Consequently, alternative routes of administration were explored. Ilomastat was administered in eyedrops to normal volunteers and subsequently to patients with corneal ulcers (35). Batimastat was administered directly into the peritoneum or pleural space of patients with malignant effusions. A phase I study of intraperitoneal batimastat was conducted in patients with symptomatic malignant ascites. Patients with any form of malignancy who required paracentesis for symptomatic relief were eligible for the study. Patients received a single intraperitoneal dose of batimastat in 500 ml of 5% dextrose (150–1350 mg/m^2) after paracentesis. In this study, batimastat was generally well tolerated and there were early signs of efficacy, with several patients requiring no further paracentesis for more than 3 months. The intraperitoneal administration of batimastat also gave rise to unexpectedly high and sustained plasma concentrations of the drug with 100 to 200 ng/ml batimastat still detectable 28 days after a single administration (43). Further development of batimastat for this indication was hindered by peritoneal irritation and poor tolerability.

A second phase I study of similar design was conducted in patients with malignant pleural effusion. Patients with symptomatic malignant pleural effusion received lower doses of batimastat (15–135 mg/m^2), given intrapleurally in 50 ml of 5% dextrose after aspiration of the effusion. Batimastat was well tolerated, and again, there were early signs that the drug might be effective in palliation of this condition. In patients receiving batimastat at 60 to 135 mg/m^2, there was a significant reduction in the number of aspirations, with an average of 2.33 ± 0.15 in the month before treatment and only 0.22 ± 0.15 in the month after ($P < 0.01$) (44).

Another series of early clinical trials involved the use of tetracycline derivatives with anticollagenase activity. In a placebo-controlled study, lymecycline in combination with conventional nonsteroidal anti-inflammatory treatment resulted in a decrease in the severity and duration of reactive arthritis triggered by *Chlamydia trachomatis* (45). Low-dose doxycycline (20 mg twice daily) was also reported to decrease urinary pyridinoline collagen cross-link excretion in patients with rheumatoid arthritis (46). In a randomized study of patients with periodontal disease, tetracycline and minocycline gels were shown to reduce significantly the concentration of stromelysin in gingival crevicular fluid. This effect was not observed with metronidazole antimicrobial treatment (47). The relative importance of the antimicrobial and antimetalloproteinase properties in mediating these different effects will become clearer with the development and testing of non–antimicrobial tetracycline derivatives.

V. CLINICAL TRIALS OF SECOND GENERATION INHIBITORS

The development of low-molecular-weight matrix metalloproteinase inhibitors with good oral bioavailability represents an important milestone in this area of research. The great majority of clinical settings for the potential use of these inhibitors involve chronic conditions requiring long-term treatments for months and years. As in many cases of drug design, the early phase of engineering site recognition and potency must give way to the need to overcome a purely practical problem: the ability to deliver the drug. Many of the early peptide-based inhibitors were poorly absorbed. Enzymatic degradation and high first-pass metabolism also may have contributed to the disappointing plasma concentrations achieved with these compounds (19). Replacement of specific groups with the intention of shielding the peptide backbone and of increasing hydrogen bonding has led to the development of inhibitors with good oral bioavailability, without loss of inhibitory potency.

Currently, at least six matrix metalloproteinase inhibitors are believed to be in clinical trial as oral treatments in patients. AG3340 (Agouron), CGS-27023A (Novartis), BAY12-9566 (Bayer), and marimastat (British Biotech) in cancer patients; D5410 (Chiroscience) in patients with inflammatory bowel disease; and Ro32-3555 (Roche) in patients with rheumatoid arthritis. Preliminary results have been presented for marimastat, Ro32-3555, and AG3340. Marimastat displays limited oral bioavailability in rodents; however, preliminary results from healthy volunteer studies showed high blood concentrations after oral administration with pharmacokinetic parameters indicating once or twice daily administration (48). Results from a phase I study of AG3340 in healthy volunteers indicate that this compound shows a similar pharmacokinetic profile to marimastat, although the terminal elimination half-life appears shorter (49). Both compounds were well tolerated in these phase I settings. Ro32-3555 also has been studied in healthy volunteers, and good oral bioavailability has been reported (23).

Marimastat is currently being tested in a series of trials in cancer patients. Results from the first of these trials were presented at a European Society for Medical Oncology meeting and provide the first indications that the therapeutic potential seen in animal cancer models may be realized in the clinic. A series of studies in patients with advanced malignancy examined the effect of different doses of marimastat on the serum cancer antigens CA125, carcino embryonic antigen (CEA), prostate specific antigen (PSA), and CA19-9. Serum concentrations of these antigens are followed clinically as surrogate markers of disease progression (50–53). There was a dose-related reduction in the rate of rise of these markers, with a proportion of patients showing a fall in the absolute cancer antigen serum concentration over the 28-day study period (54–56).

In a separate study in patients with advanced gastric cancer, treatment with marimastat was associated with changes in the macroscopic and histological appearance of the tumors consistent with an increase in the quantity of fibrotic stromal tissue. The changes were very similar to those seen in various cancer models, and several of the patients appeared to benefit from these alterations in tumor/stroma ratio (41).

Preliminary indications are that marimastat is generally well tolerated when given for periods of 3 to 6 months. The nature of trials in patients with advanced malignancy complicates the analysis of potential side effects and a clearer picture must await randomized, placebo-controlled trials. Musculoskeletal pain has emerged as the principal treatment-related side effect with marimastat. The severity and rate of onset of symptoms were found to be dose related and the effects were considered manageable at the dose range selected for future studies. The condition generally resolved rapidly on discontinuation of marimastat, and several patients restarted treatment after an interruption of 2 to 4 weeks (54–56). The mechanism responsible for the musculoskeletal pain has not been established, but it seems likely that it is related to inhibition of metalloproteinase activity in the normal physiological remodeling of the connective tissue of tendons and joints.

VI. PROMISE AND EXPECTATIONS

The therapeutic potential of matrix metalloproteinase inhibitors can now be studied in a range of diseases in which extracellular matrix degradation or angiogenesis is part of the pathogenic mechanism. Trials in arthritis and cancer patients have already begun and trials in other diseases will follow. As more selective orally bioavailable inhibitors become available for clinical testing, we might expect different inhibitors to be used in different diseases, possibly with an improved side effect profile.

In the particular case of cancer, the use of matrix metalloproteinase inhibitors represents a fundamentally different approach from conventional treatments. A malignant tumor shows a remarkable ability to adapt to the various cytotoxic agents directed toward it, driven both by its genetic instability and high proliferative rate. Matrix metalloproteinase inhibitors, and other antiangiogenic compounds, differ from cytoreductive treatments in that they are essentially targeting the other component of malignancy, the stroma. The tumor stroma, including the vasculature, plays a vital role in the growth, invasion, and spread of malignant disease. Perhaps this target will be less able than the tumor to evade treatment. In blocking the ability of the tumor to utilize the adjacent tissue for its own purposes, these new treatments may reveal an ''Achilles' heel'' in the malignant phenotype, namely its reliance on the ''collaboration'' of nonmalignant tissue.

If significant inhibition of tumor growth and spread can be achieved, it will alter the way both surgeons and oncologists view their respective means of intervention. Resection of more widespread disease might become worthwhile if it is known that the residual tumor can be held in check. Equally, the use of radiotherapy and chemotherapy in patients in whom the responses are short-lived should become more worthwhile if the time-to-relapse can be significantly extended. The near future is likely to reveal whether matrix metalloproteinase inhibitors will achieve their potential as new therapies for some of the most common and poorly treated diseases.

REFERENCES

1. Liotta LA, Stetler-Stevenson WG. Metalloproteinases and cancer invasion. Sem Cancer Biol 1990; 1:99–106.
2. Gordon JL, Drummond AH, Galloway WA. Metalloproteinase inhibitors as therapeutics. Clin Exp Rheum 1993; 11:S91–S94.

3. O'Byrne EM, Parker DT, Roberts ED, Goldberg RL, MacPherson LJ, Blancuzzi V, Wilson D, Singh HN, Ludewig R, Ganu VS. Oral administration of a matrix metalloproteinase inhibitor, CGS 27023A, protects the cartilage proteoglycan matrix in a partial meniscectomy model of osteoarthritis in rabbits. Inflamm Res (suppl) 1995; 44:S117–S118.
4. Saarialho-Kere UK, Vaalamo M, Puolakkainen P, Airola K, Parks WC, Karjalainen-Lindsberg ML. Enhanced expression of matrilysin, collagenase and stromelysin-1 in gastrointestinal ulcers. Am J Pathol 1996; 148:519–526.
5. Gijbels K, Masure S, Carton H, Opdenakker G. Gelatinase in cerebrospinal fluid of patients with multiple sclerosis and other inflammatory neurological disorders. J Neuroimmunol 1992; 41:29–34.
6. Rosenberg GA. Matrix metalloproteinases in brain injury. J Neurotrauma 1995; 12: 833–842.
7. Jeffrey JJ, Gross J. Isolation and characterization of a mammalian collagenolytic enzyme. Fed Proc 1967; 26:670.
8. Taylor AC, Levy BM, Simpson JW. Collagenolytic activity of sarcoma tissues in culture. Nature 1970; 228:366–367.
9. Strauch L. The role of collagenases in tumour invasion. In: Tarin D, ed. Tissue Interactions in Carcinogenesis. New York: Academic Press, 1972:399–434.
10. Docherty AJP, Lyons A, Smith BJ, Wright EM, Stephens PE, Harris TJR. Sequence of human tissue inhibitor of metalloproteinases and its identity to erythroid-potentiating activity. Nature 1985; 318:66–69.
11. Stetler-Stevenson WG, Krutzsch HC, Liotta LA. Tissue inhibitor of metalloproteinase (TIMP-2). A new member of the metalloproteinase inhibitor family. J Biol Chem 1989; 264:17374–17378.
12. Johnson MD, Kim HR, Chesler L, Tsao-Wu G, Bouck N, Polverini PJ. Inhibition of angiogenesis by tissue inhibitor of metalloproteinase. J Cell Physiol 1994; 160: 194–202.
13. Schultz RM, Silberman S, Persky B, Bajkowski AS, Carmichael DF. Inhibition by human recombinant tissue inhibitor of metalloproteinases of human amnion invasion and lung colonization by murine B16-F10 melanoma cells. Cancer Res 1988; 48: 5539–5545.
14. Albini A, Melchiori A, Santi L, Liotta LA, Brown PD, Stetler-Stevenson WG. Tumour cell invasion inhibited by TIMP-2. J Natl Cancer Inst 1991; 83:775–779.
15. DeClerck YA, Yean T-D, Chan D, Shimada H, Langley KE. Inhibition of tumour invasion of smooth muscle cell layers by recombinant human metalloproteinase inhibitor. Cancer Res 1991; 51:2151–2157.
16. DeClerck YA, Perez N, Shimada H, Boone TC, Langley KE, Taylor SM. Inhibition of invasion and metastasis in cells transfected with an inhibitor of metalloproteinases. Cancer Res 1992; 52:701–708.
17. Moses MA, Sudhalter J, Langer R. Identification of an inhibitor of neovascularization from cartilage. Science 1990; 248:1408–1410.
18. Murphy AN, Unsworth EJ, Stetler-Stevenson WG. Tissue inhibitor of metalloproteinases-2 inhibits bFGF-induced human microvascular endothelial cell proliferation. J Cell Physiol 1993; 157:351–358.
19. Beckett RP, Davidson AH, Drummond AH, Huxley P, Whittaker M. Recent ad-

vances in matrix metalloproteinase inhibitor research. Drug Dev Today 1996; 1:16–26.

20. Brown PD, Giavazzi R. Matrix metalloproteinase inhibition: a review of anti-tumour activity. Ann Oncol 1995; 6:967–974.
21. Grams F, Crimmin M, Hinnes L, Huxley P, Pieper M, Tschesche H, Bode W. Structure determination and analysis of human neutrophil collagenase complexed with a hydoxamate inhibitor. Biochemistry 1995; 34:14012–14020.
22. Morphy JR, Beeley NRA, Boyce BA. Potent and selective inhibitors of gelatinase A. 2. Carboxylic acids and phosphonic acid derivatives. Bioorg Med Chem Lett 1994; 4:2747–2752.
23. Lewis EJ, Bishop J, Bottomley KMK, Bradshaw D, Brewster M, Broadhurst MJ, Brown PA, Budd JM, Elliott L, Greenham AK, Johnson WH, Nixon JS, Rose F, Sutton B, Wilson K. Ro32-3555, an orally active collagenase inhibitor, prevents cartilage breakdown in vitro and in vivo. Br J Pharmacol 1997; 121:540–546.
24. Golub LM, McNamara TF, D'Angelo G, Greenwald RA, Ramamurthy NS. A non-antibacterial chemically-modified tetracycline inhibits mammalian collagenase activity. J Dental Res 1987; 66:1310–1314.
25. Naito K, Nakajima S, Kanbayashi N, Okuyama A, Goto M. Inhibition of metalloproteinase activity of rheumatoid arthritis synovial cells by a new inhibitor [BE16627B; L-N-(N-hydroxy-2-isobutylsuccinamoyl)-seryl-L-valine]. Agents Actions 1993; 39: 182–186.
26. Tamaki K, Tanzawa K, Kurihara S, Oikawa T, Monma S, Shimada K, Sugimura Y. Synthesis and structure-activity relationships of gelatinase inhibitors derived from matlystatins. Chem Pharm Bull 1995; 43:1883–1893.
27. Reich R, Thompson EW, Iwamoto Y, Martin GR, Deason JR, Fuller GC, Miskin R. Effects of inhibitors of plasminogen activator, serine proteinases, and collagenase IV on the invasion of basement membranes by metastatic cells. Cancer Res 1988; 48:3307–3312.
28. Eccles SA, Box GM, Court WJ, Bone EA, Thomas W, Brown PD. Control of lymphatic and hematogenous metastases of a rat mammary carcinoma by the matrix metalloproteinase inhibitor batimastat (BB-94). Cancer Res 1996; 56:2815–2822.
29. Sledge GW, Qulali M, Goulet R, Bone EA, Fife R. Effect of matrix metalloproteinase inhibitor batimastat on breast cancer regrowth and metastasis in athymic mice. J Natl Cancer Res 1995; 87:1546–1550.
30. Watson SA, Morris TM, Robinson G, Crimmin M, Brown PD, Hardcastle JD. Inhibition of organ invasion by metalloproteinase inhibitor, BB-94 (batimastat) in two human colon metastasis models. Cancer Res 1995; 55:3629–3633.
31. Conway JG, Trexler SJ, Wakefield JA, Marron BE, Emerson DL, Bickett DM, Deaton DN, Garrison D, Elder M, McElroy A, Willmott N, Docherty AJP, McGeehan GM. Effect of matrix metalloproteinase inhibitors on tumour growth and spontaneous metastasis. Clin Exp Metastasis 1996; 14:115–124.
32. Jain RK. Barriers to drug delivery in solid tumours. Sci Am 1994; 271:58–65.
33. Folkman J. New perspectives in clinical oncology from angiogenesis research. Eur J Cancer 1996; 32A:2535–2539.
34. Taraboletti G, Garofalo A, Belotti D, Drudis T, Borsotti P, Scanziani E, Brown P, Giavazzi R. Inhibition of angiogenesis and murine hemangioma growth by batima-

stat, a synthetic inhibitor of matrix metalloproteinases. J Natl Cancer Inst 1995; 87: 293–298.
35. Galardy RE, Cassabone ME, Giese C, et al. Low molecular weight inhibitors in corneal ulceration. Ann N Y Acad Sci 1994; 732:315–323.
36. Galardy RE, Grobelny D, Foellmer HG, Fernandez LA. Inhibition of angiogenesis by the matrix metalloproteinase inhibitor N-[2R-2-(hydroxyamidocarbonylmethyl)-4-(methylpentanoyl)]-L-tryptophan methylamide. Cancer Res 1994; 54:4715–4718.
37. Mignatti P, Tsuboi R, Robbins E, Rifkin DB. In vitro angiogenesis on the human amniotic membrane: requirements for basic fibroblast growth factor-induced proteinases. J Cell Biol 1989; 108:671–682.
38. Min HY, Doyle LV, Vitt CR, Zandonella CL, Stratton-Thomas JR, Shuman MA, Rosenberg S. Urokinase receptor antagonists inhibit angiogenesis and primary tumor growth in syngeneic mice. Cancer Res 1996; 56:2428–2433.
39. Carmeliet P, Schoonjans L, Kieckens L, Ream B, Degen J, Bronson R, De Vos R, van den Oord JJ, Collen D, Mulligan RC. Physiological consequences of loss of plasminogen activator gene function in mice. Nature 1994; 386:419–425.
40. Anderson IC, Shipp MA, Docherty AJP, Teicher BA. Combination therapy including a gelatinase inhibitor and cytotoxic agent reduces local invasion and metastasis of murine Lewis lung carcinoma. Cancer Res 1996; 56:715–710.
41. Parsons SL, Watson SA, Griffin NR, Steele RJC. An open phase I/II study of the oral matrix metalloproteinase inhibitor marimastat in patients with inoperable gastric cancer. Ann Oncol 1996; 7:47 (abstr).
42. An Z, Wang X, Willmott N, Chander SK, Tickle S, Docherty AJP, Mountain A, Millican AT, Morphy R, Porter JR, Epemolu RO, Kubota T, Moossa AR, Hoffman RM. Conversion of a highly malignant colon cancer from an aggressive to a controlled disease by oral administration of a metalloproteinase inhibitor. Clin Exp Metastasis 1997; 15:184–195.
43. Beattie GJ, Young HA, Smyth JF. Phase I study of intra-peritoneal metalloproteinase inhibitor BB-94 in patients with malignant ascites. Abstract presented at the 8th NCI-EORTC Symposium on New Drug Development, Amsterdam, The Netherlands, March 1994.
44. Macaulay VM, O'Byrne KJ, Saunders MP, Salisbury A, Long L, Gleeson F, Ganesan TS, Harris AL, Talbot DC. Phase I study of matrix metalloproteinase (MMP) inhibitor batimastat (BB-94) in patients with malignant pleural effusions. Br J Cancer 1995; 71:11 (abstr).
45. Lauhio A, Leirisalo-Repo M, Lahdevirta J, Saikku P, Repo H. Double-blind, placebo-controlled study of the three month treatment with lymecycline in reactive arthritis, with special reference to *Chlamydia* arthritis. Arthritis Rheum 1991; 24:6–14.
46. Greenwald RA, Moak SA, Golub LM. Low dose doxycycline inhibits pyridinoline excretion in selected patients with rheumatoid arthritis. Ann N Y Acad Sci 1994; 732:419–421.
47. Pourtaghi N, Radvar M, Mooney J, Kinane DF. The effect of subgingival antimicrobial therapy on the levels of stromelysin and tissue inhibitor of metalloproteinases in gingival crevicular fluid. J Periodontology 1996; 67:866–870.
48. Millar AW, Brown PD, Moore J, Galloway WA, Cornish AG, Lenehan TJ, Lynch

KP. Results of single and repeat dose studies of the oral matrix metalloproteinase inhibitor marimastat in healthy male volunteers. Br J Clin Pharm 1998; 45:21–26.

49. Collier MA, Yuen GJ, Bansal SK, Kolis S, Chew TG, Appelt K, Clendeninn NJ. A phase I study of the matrix metalloproteinase (MMP) inhibitor AG3340 given in single doses to healthy volunteers. Proc Am Assoc Cancer Res 1997; 38:13.
50. Rubin SC, Hoskins WJ, Hakes TB. CA125 levels and surgical findings in patients undergoing secondary operations for epithelial ovarian cancer. Am J Obstet Gynecol 1989; 160:667–671.
51. Goldenberg DM, Neville A, Carter A. CEA (carcinoembryonic antigen): its role as a marker in the management of cancer. J Cancer Res Clin Oncol 1981; 101:239–242.
52. Stamey TA, Kabalin JW, McNeal JE. Prostate-specific antigen in the diagnosis and treatment of adenocarcinoma of the prostate II radical prostatectomy treated patients. J Urol 1989; 141:1076–1083.
53. Steinberg W, Gelfand R, Anderson K. Comparison of the sensitivity and specificity of the CA19-9 and CEA assays in detecting cancer of the pancreas. Gastroenterology 1986; 90:343–349.
54. Primrose J, Bleiberg H, Daniel F, Johnson P, Mansi J, Neoptolemos J, Seymour M, van Belle S. A dose-finding study of marimastat, an oral matrix metalloproteinase inhibitor, in patients with advanced colorectal cancer. Ann Oncol 1996; 7:35 (abstr).
55. Poole C, Adams M, Barley V, Graham J, Kerr D, Louviaux I, Perren T, Piccart M, Thomas H. A dose-finding study of marimastat, an oral matrix metalloproteinase inhibitor, in patients with advanced ovarian cancer. Ann Oncol 1996; 7:68 (abstr).
56. Millar A, Brown P. 360 patient meta-analysis of studies of marimastat, a novel matrix metalloproteinase inhibitor. Ann Oncol 1996; 7:123 (abstr).

28

Tumoral Vascularity

What Does It Tell Us About the Growth and Spread of Cancer?

Noel Weidner
University of California, San Diego, San Diego, California

I. EVIDENCE THAT TUMOR GROWTH IS ANGIOGENESIS DEPENDENT

Without blood vessels, tumor cell clusters grow until passive diffusion can no longer provide adequate nutrients or allow waste products to exit into the adjacent medium (1–5). These avascular clusters grow as spheroids, reaching up to approximately 2 mm^3 in vivo (6–8), and further growth and metastases do not occur until they become vascularized (9, 7–17). Further indirect evidence that tumor angiogenesis is important in tumor growth is that intratumoral endothelial cells proliferate faster than endothelial cells in adjacent benign stroma on average 45-fold faster within breast carcinoma and 30-fold faster within prostate carcinoma) (18, 19), and the rate of tumor progression is associated with increased intratumoral vascularity (19–87). More direct evidence is that different methods of specifically inhibiting angiogenesis, which are not cytostatic to tumor cells in vitro, clearly inhibited tumor growth in vivo (88–99). For example, a synthetic analogue of fumagillin (also called AGM-1470 or TNP-470) inhibits endothelial proliferation in vitro and tumor-induced angiogenesis in vivo (90), and this substance will suppress tumor growth with few side effects. AGM-1470, as well as other angiogenesis inhibitors, are now in various phases of clinical trials as therapeutic agents for a variety of malignant solid tumors, leukemias, and infantile hemangiomas (1, 88, 89). Also, Kim et al. (92) showed that inhibition of vascular endothelial growth factor (VEGF)-induced angiogenesis suppresses tumor growth in vivo. These investigators injected human malignant cell lines into nude mice. They found that treatment of these mice with a monoclonal antibody specific for VEGF inhibited the growth of the tumors and reduced tumor vessel density, but had no effect on the growth rate of the tumor cells in vitro. Further, Millauer et al. (94) reported that tumor growth was significantly suppressed by the introduction of defective VEGF receptors into tumor endothelial cells. It has been reported that a single intravascular injection of antagonists of the alpha$_v$beta$_3$ integrin disrupts ongoing angiogenesis on the chick chorioallantoic membrane. This leads to the rapid regression of histologically distinct human tumors transplanted onto the chorioallantoic membrane (95). Also, induction of angiogenesis by a tumor or cytokine promotes vascular cell entry into the cell cycle and expression of alpha$_v$beta$_3$ integrin. After angiogenesis is initiated, antagonists of this integrin induce apoptosis (programmed cell death) of the proliferative angiogenic vascular cells, leaving preexisting quiescent blood vessels unaffected. Finally, very compelling evidence that tumor growth and metastases are angiogenesis dependent comes from experiments showing that angiostatin, which specifically inhibits proliferation of vascular endothelial cells, causes metastases to remain dormant and small (< 0.2 mm) (96). Also, angiostatin significantly inhibits growth of animal and human tumors (97).

II. MECHANISMS BY WHICH TUMOR GROWTH IS STIMULATED BY ANGIOGENESIS

Clearly, tumor neovascularization promotes growth because the new vessels allow exchange of nutrients, oxygen, and waste products by a crowded cell population for which simple diffusion is inadequate. Also, activated endothelial cells may release important paracrine growth factors for tumor cells (e.g., basic fibroblast growth factor [bFGF], insulin growth factors, platelet-derived growth factor, and colony stimulating factors) (98, 100–102). To allow ingrowth, those activated endothelial cells located at the tips of growing capillaries secrete collagenases, urokinases, and plasminogen activator (PA) (103–105). It is likely that these degradative enzymes facilitate spread of tumor cells into and through the adjacent fibrin-gel matrix and connective tissue stroma. In breast carcinoma patients, increased intratumoral levels of urokinase-type plasminogen activator (uPA) and PA inhibitor-1 (PA-1) are reported to be independent predictors of poor prognosis. Fox et al. (104) have showed a significant association of uPA and PA-1 with intratumoral microvessel density. These investigators concluded that the poor prognosis in breast carcinomas associated with elevated uPA and PA-1 might be the result of an interaction between endothelial and tumor cells using the uPA enzyme system. Thus, the additive impact of the perfusion and paracrine tumor effects, plus the endothelial cell-derived, invasion-associated enzymes, all likely contribute to a phase of rapid tumor growth and signal a switch to a potentially lethal angiogenic phenotype. These same effects may contribute to a much higher metastatic potential by facilitating entry of tumor cells into blood vessels and the lymphatic system.

III. MEDIATORS OF TUMOR ANGIOGENESIS

Tumor neovascularization is similar to normal wound healing (106), and it is likely mediated by similar and specific angiogenic molecules. These mediators are released by the tumor cells and/or host immune cells (i.e., macrophages) or are possibly mobilized from substances within the tumor stroma (1, 6, 107, 108). We reported that some breast ducts containing ductal carcinoma in situ (DCIS) have a cuff or ring of microvessels around the duct. The nearness of this cuff of neovascularization to the DCIS cells suggested that it formed in response to angiogenic factor(s) released by the DCIS cells. The cuff was limited to ducts containing DCIS and did not correlate with periductal inflammation, suggesting that the angiogenic stimulus was a diffusible factor coming from the DCIS cells and not from inflammatory cells. Guidi et al. (109) subsequently reported similar observations in 38% of DCIS cases. Likewise, Smith-McCune et al. (110) found that microvessels were increased immediately beneath cervical intraepithelial neoplasia (CIN) when compared to adjacent normal epithelium. Yet the neovascularization was not related to the number of macrophages within the CIN lesions, indicating that the production of the angiogenic factor(s) is likely a property of the dysplastic epithelial cells themselves (110).

The factor(s) or cell(s) causing tumor angiogenesis have not been determined. The leading candidates are bFGF (111, 112) and VEGF (113). Vascular endothelial growth factor and vascular permeability factor (VPF) are the same substance. Vascular permeability factor/VEGF is a potent vascular permeability factor, a selective endothelial cell growth factor, and likely an important tumor angiogenic factor (114, 115). Moreover, VPF/VEGF causes endothelial cells to express PA, PAI, interstitial collagenase, and procoagulant activity (113, 116). By increasing vascular permeability, VPF/VEGF promotes extravasation of plasma fibrinogen, leading to fibrin deposition within the tumor matrix. This matrix or scaffold promotes the ingrowth of macrophages, fibroblasts, and endothelial cells (113, 116). Possibly, molecules derived from the fibrin gel matrix have important angiogenic properties, and Thompson et al. (117) found that fibrin degradation products have angiogenic potential. Furthermore, the work of Kim et al. (92), Millauer et al. (94), and Warren et al. (99) strongly supports VPF/VEGF as an important tumor angiogenic factor. Toi et al. (118) found that VPF/VEGF expression was higher in breast tumors with higher intratumoral microvessel densities, and that relapse-free survival was shorter in patients with tumor showing relatively high VPF/VEGF expression. However, VPF/VEGF may not act alone, and

Goto et al. (119) have shown that VPF/VEGF and bFGF can act synergistically to cause angiogenesis. Finally, various low-molecular-weight, nonpeptide angiogenic factors are known (e.g., nitric oxide and 12(R)-hydroxy-eicosatrienoic acid) (6, 107, 120, 121); their significance remains unclear, yet likely important.

Angiogenic stimulators may be necessary but not sufficient for tumor angiogenesis. Bouck et al. (122, 123) suggest that tumor angiogenesis results from a net balance between positive and negative regulators of blood vessel growth. Zajchowski et al. (124) reported that somatic hybrid cells (i.e., MCF-7 human breast carcinoma cells fused with normal human mammary epithelial cells) did not form tumors in nude mice. The hybrids increased the expression of thrombospondin, an angiogenesis inhibitor, suggesting that angiogenic capability contributes to tumorigenicity in human breast carcinoma. Also, Dameron et al. (125) showed that the switch to the angiogenic phenotype by fibroblasts cultured from Li-Fraumeni patients coincided with loss of the wild-type allele of the p53 tumor suppressor gene and was the result of reduced expression of thrombospondin-1. Finally, O'Reilly et al. (96, 97) reported that a novel angiogenesis inhibitor, angiostatin, is produced by the primary tumor mass of a Lewis lung carcinoma. In this model, when the primary tumor is present, metastatic tumor growth is suppressed by angiostatin. After primary tumor removal, the metastases neovascularize and grow. This mechanism may explain one form of dormancy, but some metastatic deposits appear to remain dormant in spite of the fact that the primary tumor had been previously removed (126).

IV. ANGIOGENESIS IS NECESSARY FOR METASTASES TO FORM

To metastasize, a tumor cell must sequentially overcome a series of physical barriers and biochemical deficiencies. Usually, less than one cell in approximately 100,000 has all the properties necessary to produce a successful metastasis (127–129). Tumor cells must induce angiogenesis to gain access to the vasculature from the primary tumor, survive the circulation, escape immune surveillance, localize in the microvasculature of the target organ, escape from or grow from within the vasculature into the target organ, and induce tumor angiogenesis (127, 128). If the primary tumor is highly angiogenic, then its daughter metastases (clones) are likely to be highly angiogenic. Tumor growth and spread are amplified geometrically, when the newly established angiogenic metastasis sheds additional tumor cells to form even more metastases by following the same cascade of events (128).

Angiogenesis is necessary at the beginning of this journey because without it, tumor cells are only rarely shed into the circulation (130–132). Liotta et al. (131, 132), using a transplantable mouse fibrosarcoma model, showed that the number of tumor cells shed into the bloodstream increased dramatically with tumor growth, and this increase in circulating tumor cells correlated very closely with increasing intratumoral microvessel density. These studies showed that the number of lung metastases was directly related to the number of cells shed into the circulation (6, 131, 132). Obviously, these data suggested that intratumoral microvessel density might correlate with aggressive tumor behavior, a suggestion subsequently shown to be true (19–87).

New, proliferating capillaries have fragmented basement membranes and are leaky, making them more accessible to tumor cells than mature vessels (133). Furthermore, the invasive chemotactic behavior of endothelial cells at the tips of growing capillaries is facilitated by the secretion of collagenases, urokinases, and PA (105). These degradative enzymes may facilitate the escape of tumor cells into the tumor neovasculature. Indeed, the ''invading'' capillaries may actively participate in the metastatic process by engulfing, and thus facilitating the entry of tumor cells into vascular spaces, allowing systemic spread. Sugino et al. (134) observed, in a naturally occurring mouse mammary carcinoma model (C3H/He mice), that intravasating tumor cells and tumor emboli within blood vessel lumina retained their nested architecture within a continuous basement membrane and were invested by an endothelial cell layer. These investigators believed the findings indicated a ''passive'' mechanism of tumor cell intravasation, distinct from invasive properties of tumor cells, in which endothelial cells in sinusoidal vessels can envelop tumor cell nests, which then become detached into the blood. Arrest of such encapsulated emboli in pulmonary arterioles downstream could form new metastatic tumor foci.

Also, supporting the role of angiogenesis in the metastatic process is the observation that India ink injected into the rabbit cornea will stay at the injection site indefinitely as a tattoo, unless neovascularization is induced in the cornea (135, 136). As new capillaries approach the ink spot, the ink fragments and reappears in the ipsilateral lymph nodes. Tumor cells can invade adjacent lymphatics that form concomitantly with blood capillaries or, hypothetically, they can pass from the bloodstream into the lymphatics through lymphaticovenous junctions (6, 137). Also, tumor angiogenesis may facilitate this process by increasing tumor volume, thus enhancing tumor cell-lymphatic contact at the growing edge of the tumor.

V. ASSOCIATION OF INTRATUMORAL MICROVESSEL DENSITY WITH TUMOR AGGRESSIVENESS

Although Brem et al. (138) were among the first to suggest that the intensity of intratumoral angiogenesis may correlate with tumor grade and aggressiveness, the first clear-cut evidence that tumor angiogenesis in a human solid tumor could predict the probability of metastasis was reported for cutaneous melanoma. Srivastava et al. (63) studied the vascularity of 20 intermediate thickness skin melanomas. Vessels were highlighted and the stained histological sections analyzed with an image analysis system. The 10 cases that developed metastases had a vascular area at the tumor base that was more than twice that seen in the 10 cases without metastases ($P = 0.025$).

Next, in 1990, my colleagues and I asked if the extent of angiogenesis (i.e., measured by intratumoral microvessel density) in human breast carcinoma correlated with metastasis (20). If so, such information might prove valuable in selecting subsets of breast carcinoma patients for aggressive adjuvant therapies. To be true, it is important that a spectrum of intratumoral microvessel densities exist within the spectrum of invasive breast carcinomas. When the microvessel counts in a number of invasive breast carcinomas are sorted in ascending order on a log scale, the spectrum of low to high microvessel densities becomes apparent. The densities are an evenly distributed continuum, extending from about 10 to 200 microvessels per 0.74 mm^2 (200×) field.

My colleagues and I examined primary tumor specimens from randomly selected patients with invasive breast carcinoma (20). Hematoxylin and eosin (H&E)-stained sections of the breast tumor were used to choose one paraffin-embedded tissue block clearly representative of a generous cross-section of the invasive carcinoma, and one 5-micron thick section from this block was immunostained for factor VIII-related antigen/von Willebrand's factor (F8RA/vWF) to highlight the endothelial cells lining the blood vessels. Intratumoral microvessel density was assessed by light microscopic analysis for areas of the tumor that contained the most capillaries and small venules (microvessels). Finding these neovascular "hot spots" is critical to accurately assess a particular tumor's angiogenic potential. This is to be expected, as there is considerable evidence that, like tumor proliferation rate, tumor angiogenesis is heterogeneous within tumors (20, 102, 111, 139). The technique for identifying neovascular hot spots is very similar to that for finding mitotic hot spots for assessing mitotic figure content and is subject to the same kinds of inter- and intraobserver variability. In our study, sclerotic, hypocellular areas within tumors and immediately adjacent to benign breast tissue were not considered in intratumoral microvessel density determinations. Only tumors that produced a high quality and distinct microvessel immunoperoxidase staining pattern with low background staining were included in this or subsequent studies. This is very important, because the quality of immunoperoxidase staining can vary considerably among laboratories, and before measuring intratumoral microvessel density, high quality immunoperoxidase staining must be consistently achieved.

Areas of highest neovascularization were found by scanning the tumor sections at low power (40× and 100× total magnification) and selecting those areas of invasive carcinoma with the greatest density of distinct F8RA/vWF-staining microvessels. These highly neovascular areas could occur anywhere within the tumor but appeared most frequently at the tumor margins. After the area of highest neovascularization was identified, individual microvessel counts were made on a 200× field (20× objective and 10× ocular, Olympus BH-2 microscope, 0.74 mm^2 per field with the field size measured with an ocular micrometer). Any highlighted endothelial cell or endothelial-cell cluster clearly separate from adjacent microvessels, tumor cells, and other connective tissue elements was considered a single, countable microvessel. Even those distinct clusters of brown-staining endothelial cells, which might be from the same microvessel ''snaking'' its way in and out of the section, were considered distinct and countable as separate microvessels. Vessel lumens, although usually present, were not necessary for a structure to be defined as a microvessel, and red cells were not used to define a vessel lumen. Results were expressed as the highest number of microvessels in any single 200×field. An average of multiple fields was not performed.

Invasive breast carcinomas from patients with metastases (either lymph nodal or distant site) had a mean microvessel count of 101 per 200× field. For those carcinomas from patients without metastases, the corresponding value was 45 per 200× field ($P = 0.003$). We plotted the percent of patients with metastatic disease in whom a vessel count was carried out within progressive 33 vessel increments. The plot showed that the incidence of metastatic disease increased with the number of microvessels, reaching 100% for patients having invasive carcinomas with more than 100 microvessels per 200× field.

To further define the relationship of intratumoral microvessel density to overall and relapse-free survival and to other reported prognostic indicators in breast carcinoma, a blinded study of 165 consecutive carcinoma patients was performed using identical techniques to measure intratumoral microvessel density (23). The other prognostic indicators evaluated were metastasis to axillary lymph nodes, patient age, menopausal status, tumor size, histological grade (i.e., Scarff-Bloom-Richardson criteria), peritumoral lymphatic-vascular invasion (PLVI), flow DNA ploidy analysis, flow S-phase fraction, growth fraction by Ki-67 binding, c-erbB2 oncoprotein expression, pro-cathepsin-D content, estrogen-receptor content, progesterone-receptor content, and epidermal growth factor receptor (EGFR) expression. We found a highly significant association of intratumoral microvessel density with overall survival and relapse-free survival in all patients, including node-negative and node-positive subsets. All patients with breast carcinomas having more than 100 microvessels per 200× field experienced tumor recurrence within 33 months of diagnosis, compared with less than 5% of patients who had less than 33 microvessels per 200× field. Moreover, intratumoral microvessel density was the only significant predictor of overall and relapse-free survival among node-negative women. Weidner et al. (23) concluded that intratumoral microvessel density in the area of most intense neovascularization in invasive breast carcinoma is an independent, highly significant, and accurate prognostic indicator in predicting metastasis, as well as overall and relapse-free survival in patients with stage I to II breast carcinoma. Such an indicator would be useful in the selection of high-risk, node-negative patients with breast carcinoma for systemic adjuvant therapy.

Other studies performed on different patient databases by different investigators at different medical centers have observed this same association of increasing intratumoral vascularity with various measures of tumor aggressiveness, such as higher stage at presentation, greater incidence of metastases, or decreased patient survival. This has been shown in studies of patients with carcinoma of the breast (20–44) and in those with prostate carcinoma (45–50), head-and-neck squamous carcinoma (51–55), non–small-cell lung carcinoma (56–61), malignant melanoma (62–68), gastrointestinal carcinoma (69–72), testicular germ-cell malignancies (73), multiple myeloma (74), central nervous system tumors (75, 76), ovarian carcinoma (77, 78), cervical squamous carcinoma (79–81), endometrial carcinoma (82), and transitional cell carcinoma of the bladder (83–86). In many of these studies, intratumoral vascularity was found to have independent prognostic significance when compared with traditional prognostic markers by multivariate analysis.

Although assaying intratumoral microvessel density has been used most often to assay tumor vascularity, some investigators found similar associations with tumor aggressiveness using image analysis to measure vascular area or Doppler ultrasound to measure blood flow. The optimum technique for assaying intratumoral vascularity has not been completely defined. Finally, it is important that some studies have found that high intratumoral microvessel density can be significantly associated with a favorable outcome, apparently when specific forms of therapy are given in which therapeutic effectiveness depends directly on the extent of blood flow (86, 87). Kohno et al. (86) found that cervical carcinomas treated with hypertensive intra-arterial chemotherapy are more responsive when highly vascular, and Zatterstrom et al. (87) found that highly vascular squamous carcinomas of the head and neck are more responsive to radiation therapy when highly vascular.

VI. PITFALLS IN MEASURING INTRATUMORAL VASCULARITY

Many pathology laboratories can perform the standard immunohistochemical assays for highlighting microvessels for assessing intratumoral microvessel density. However, it is very important that previously published protocols for measuring intratumoral microvessel density be followed carefully. Also, considerable experience is needed at the senior staff pathologist level for assessing intratumoral microvessel density. It is necessary both for supervising the immunostaining of endothelial cells and for selecting generous sections of representative invasive tumor and for localizing the neovascular "hot spot." Counting microvessels is reproducible (140), especially following a period of training. Brawer et al. (48) compared manual intratumoral microvessel determinations with those determined by automated counting (i.e., Optimas Image Analysis) and found a very tight correlation ($r^2 = 0.98$, $P < 0.001$). Finally, accurate staging and adequate patient follow-up are needed to determine those patients who have metastases or will experience recurrent tumor, and proper technique must be supplemented with unbiased case selection and proper statistical analysis of data. These reasons may explain why some investigators have not found this association between intratumoral microvessel density and prognosis in some solid tumors, including breast and others (141–156). Why these reports are contradictory to other reports is not clear; however, Leedy et al. (146) noted that the tongue was already a highly vascular organ. They implied that tumor growth and spread may be facilitated by preexisting vessels in highly vascular organs, and it may be that intratumoral microvessel density will prove less useful in predicting outcome in patients with tumors developing in such highly vascular organs such as the tongue, liver, skin, kidney, or gastrointestinal tract. Clearly, it should not prove useful in solid tumor systems, wherein there is no spectrum from low to high intratumoral microvessel density (152). Paradoxically, Kainz et al. (156) found that patients with cervical cancers showing relatively low microvessel density had a significantly poorer recurrence-free survival than those with higher densities.

VII. TECHNIQUES FOR HIGHLIGHTING MICROVESSELS

No endothelial marker is trouble free. When applied properly, anti-F8RA/vWF remains the most specific endothelial marker, providing very good contrast between microvessels and other tissue components. Unfortunately, anti-F8RA/vWF may not highlight all intratumoral microvessels. Although apparently more sensitive, CD31 strongly cross-reacts with plasma cells (157, 158). This complication can greatly obscure the microvessels in those tumors with a prominent plasma cellular inflammatory background. CD34 is an acceptable alternative and the most reproducible endothelial-cell highlighter in many laboratories; however, it will highlight perivascular stromal cells and has been noted to stain a wide variety of stromal neoplasms (159, 160). Like antibodies to F8RA/vWF, antibodies to CD31, CD34, and PAL-E also do not immunostain all intratumoral microvessels (161). Ulex europeus lectin will stain many tumor cells, seriously decreasing its specificity; it is not recommended.

Wang et al. (162, 163) have developed a monoclonal antibody (Mab E9) that was raised against proliferating or "activated" endothelial cells of human umbilical vein origin and grown in tissue culture. Mab E9 strongly reacted with endothelial cells of all tumors, fetal organs, and in regenerating and inflamed tissues, but it only rarely and weakly immunostained endothelial cells of normal tissues. Unfortunately, Mab E9 immunoreacted only in frozen tissue sections, although whether microwave antigen-retrieval techniques were applied to formalin-fixed, paraffin-embedded tissues is unknown. Antibodies such as Mab E9 may provide the most sensitive staining of intratumoral microvessels and preferentially immunostain ''activated or proliferating'' endothelial cells such that the overall staining intensity may correlate best with the intensity of tumor angiogenesis and hence, tumor aggressiveness. Staining for the endothelial activation marker *alphavbeta3* may also yield very useful data for clinicopathological correlations (95). Automated (''machine'') immunostaining and application of computer-aided image analysis may help to standardize microvessel counts and help eliminate interobserver and even intraobserver variables, such as inexperience and ''hot spot'' selection biases (33). The latter approach may make determination of intratumoral microvessel density a simple, reliable, and reproducible prognostic factor in a variety of solid tumors, not just in breast carcinoma.

Actually, measuring intratumoral microvessel density may prove to be a relatively crude method for estimating a tumor's angiogenic capacity. Other methods may prove more reliable and reproducible, such as measuring levels of angiogenic molecules in serum or urine, or directly measuring angiogenic molecules or inhibitors from tumor extracts (i.e., in a manner similar to hormone receptor assays). Indeed, using an immunoassay, Watanabe et al. (164) and Nguyen et al. (165) reported elevated levels of bFGF in the serum and urine of patients with a wide variety of solid tumors, including breast carcinoma. Higher levels were found in patients with metastatic disease vs those of localized disease. Moreover, Li et al. (166) measured bFGF in the cerebral spinal fluids of children with various brain tumors and correlated increasing fluid levels with greater intratumoral microvessel density and increased likelihood of recurrence. As a final note in this section, it is important that immunohistochemistry of any given angiogenic factor (ie., bFGF or VPF/VEGF) in a tumor would not by itself be expected to correlate with microvessel count (or with patient outcome), because the microvessel count is the sum total of positive and negative angiogenic factors, and most likely more than one of each.

VIII. EXPLANATIONS FOR THE ASSOCIATION OF INTRATUMORAL MICROVESSEL DENSITY WITH TUMOR AGGRESSIVENESS

The association between intratumoral microvessel density and tumor aggressiveness could be explained in the following ways. First, a highly angiogenic primary tumor with a high intratumoral microvessel density is more likely to seed distant sites with highly angiogenic clones (1, 167). Second, solid tumors are composed of two discrete yet interdependent components (i.e., the malignant cells and the stroma they induce), and measuring intratumoral microvessel density could be a valid measure of the success that a particular tumor has in forming this very important stromal compartment. Also, the endothelial cells of this stromal component may be stimulating the growth of the tumor cells in a reverse paracrine fashion. If true, the more microvessels and, thus, more endothelial cells, the greater this paracrine growth stimulation. Third, the density of the microvessel bed within a tumor is likely a direct measure of the size of the vascular window through which tumor cells pass to spread to distant body sites. The larger that window, the greater the number of circulating tumor cells from which a metastasis could develop. Finally, if true that endothelial cells play a very active role in the metastatic process and that tumor cells are actually more ''passive'' than previously thought, then intratumoral microvessel density could be a measure of those endothelial-derived forces promoting metastases. I believe all of these factors are acting together to encourage tumor growth and metastasis. Indeed, it is no surprise that intratumoral microvessel density correlates with various measures of tumor aggressiveness.

IX. FINAL COMMENT

Finally, it should be emphasized that tumor angiogenesis alone is not sufficient to cause metastases. Tumor cells also must proliferate, penetrate host tissues and vessels, survive within the vasculature, escape the host's immune system, and then begin growth at a new body site. The behavior of typical bronchial carcinoids illustrates this point; they are highly vascular tumors, yet they uncommonly metastasize to distant sites. Also, it remains to be seen whether intratumor microvessel density, as reviewed here, will be universally reproducible and continue to hold up as a predictor of metastasis or patient outcome when used in a prospective manner by pathologists in many different centers. As tumor therapies become more effective in preventing tumor recurrence, the ability of a prognostic test to stratify patients into various prognostic categories becomes diminished. With a 100% cure rate (or death rate, for that matter), all prognostic tests for predicting patient survival become meaningless. In any event, the well-documented association of increasing intratumoral microvessel density with various measures of tumor aggressiveness has increased our understanding about the critical role of angiogenesis in human tumor growth and metastasis.

REFERENCES

1. Folkman J. Clinical applications of angiogenesis research. N Engl J Med 1995. In press.

2. Folkman J. Tumor angiogenesis: therapeutic implications. N Engl J Med 1971; 285:1182–1186.
3. Folkman J, Hochberg M, Knighton D. Self-regulation of growth in three dimensions: the role of surface area limitations. In: Clarkson B, Baserga R, eds. Control of Proliferation in Animal Cells. Cold Spring Harbor: Cold Spring Harbor Laboratory, 1974:833–842.
4. Sutherland RM. Cell and environment interactions in tumor microregions: the multicell spheroid model. Science 1988; 240:177–184.
5. Sutherland RM, McCredie JA, Inch WR. Growth of multicell spheroids in tissue culture as a model of nodular carcinomas. J Natl Cancer Inst 1971; 46:113–120.
6. Blood CH, Zetter BR. Tumor interactions with the vasculature: angiogenesis and tumor metastasis. Biochim Biophys Acta 1990; 1032:89–118.
7. Gimbrone MA, Leapman SB, Cotran RS, Folkman J. Tumor dormancy in vivo by prevention of neovascularization. J Exp Med 1972; 136:261–276.
8. Gimbrone MA, Cotran RS, Leapman SB, Folkman J. Tumor growth neovascularization: an experimental model using rabbit cornea. J Natl Cancer Inst 1974; 52: 413–427.
9. Folkman J. What is the evidence that tumors are angiogenesis-dependent? J Natl Cancer Inst 1990; 82:4–6.
10. Antonelli-Orlidge A, Saunders KB, Smith SR, D'Amore PA. An activated form of transforming growth factor-beta is produced by co-cultures of endothelial cells and pericytes. Proc Natl Acad Sci U S A 1989; 86:4544–4588.
11. Ausprunk DH, Folkman J. Migration and proliferation of endothelial cells in preformed and newly formed blood vessels during tumor angiogenesis. Microvasc Res 1977; 14:53–65.
12. Adam JA, Maggelakis AA. Diffusion of regulated growth characteristics of a spherical prevascular carcinoma. Bull Math Biol 1990; 52:549–582.
13. Roberts AB, Sporn MB, Assoian RK, Smith JM, Roche NS, Wakefield LM, Heine UI, Liotta LA, Falanga V, Kehrl JH, Fauci AS. Transforming growth factor type-beta: rapid induction of fibrosis and angiogenesis in vivo and stimulation of collagen formation in vitro. Proc Natl Aca Sci U S A 1986; 83:4167–4171.
14. Knighton D, Ausprunk D, Tapper D, Folkman J. Avascular and vascular phases of tumor growth in the chick embryo. Br J Cancer 1977; 35:347–356.
15. Lien W, Ackerman N. The blood supply of experimental liver metastases. II. A microcirculatory study of normal and tumor vessels of the liver with the use of perfused silicone rubber. Surgery 1970; 68:334–340.
16. Thompson WD, Shiach KJ, Fraser RA, McIntosh LC, Simpson JG. Tumors acquire their vasculature by vessel incorporation, not vessel ingrowth. J Pathol 1987; 151: 323–332.
17. Skinner SA, Tutton PJM, O'Brien PE. Microvascular architecture of experimental colon tumors in the rat. Cancer Res 1990; 50:2411–2417.
18. Vartanian R, Weidner N. Correlation of intratumoral endothelial-cell proliferation with microvessel density (tumor angiogenesis) and tumor-cell proliferation in breast carcinoma. Am J Pathol 1994; 144:1188–1194.
19. Vartanian RK, Weidner N. Endothelial cell proliferation in human prostatic carci-

noma and hyperplasia: correlation with microvessel density, epithelial cell proliferation, and Gleason's score. Lab Invest 1996. In press.
20. Weidner N, Semple JP, Welch WR, Folkman J. Tumor angiogenesis and metastasis—correlation in invasive breast carcinoma. N Engl J Med 1991; 324:1–8.
21. Bosari S, Lee AKC, DeLellis RA, et al. Microvessel quantitation and prognosis in invasive breast carcinoma. Hum Pathol 1992; 23:755–761.
22. Horak E, Leek R, Klenk N, LeJeune S, Smith K, Stuart N, Greenall M, Stepniewska K, Harris AL. Angiogenesis, assessed by platelet/endothelial cell adhesion molecule antibodies, as indicator of node metastases and survival in breast cancer. Lancet 1992; 340:1120–1124.
23. Weidner N, Folkman J, Pozza F, Bevilacqua P, Allred EN, Moore DH, Meli S, Gasparini G. Tumor angiogenesis: a new significant and independent prognostic indicator in early-stage breast carcinoma. J Natl Cancer Inst 1992; 84:1875–1887.
24. Visscher DW, Smilanetz S, Drozdowicz S, Wykes SM. Prognostic significance of image morphometric microvessel enumeration in breast carcinoma. Anal Quant Cytol Histol 1993; 15:88–92.
25. Toi M, Kashitani J, Tominaga T. Tumor angiogenesis is an independent prognostic indicator of primary breast carcinoma. Int J Cancer 1993; 55:371–374.
26. Gasparini G, Weidner N, Bevilacqua P, Maluta S, Dalla Palma P, Caffo O, Barbareschi M, Boracchi P, Marubini E, Pozza F. Tumor microvessel density, p53 expression, tumor size, and peritumoral lymphatic vessel invasion are relevant prognostic markers in node-negative breast carcinoma. J Clin Oncol 1994; 12:454–466.
27. Obermair A, Czerwenka K, Kurz C, Buxbaum P, Schemper M, Sevela P. Influence of tumoral microvessel density on the recurrence-free survival in human breast cancer: preliminary results. Onkologie 1994; 17:44–49.
28. Gasparini G, Bevilacqua P, Boracchi P, Maluta S, Pozza F, Barbareschi M, Dalla Palma P, Mezzetti M, Harris AL. Prognostic value of p53 expression in early-stage breast carcinoma compared with tumor angiogenesis, epidermal growth factor receptor, c-erbB2, cathepsin D, DNA ploidy, parameters of cell kinetics and conventional features. Int J Oncol 1994; 4:155–162.
29. Fox SB, Leek AK, DeLellis RA, et al. Tumor angiogenesis in node-negative breast carcinomas: relationship with epidermal growth factor receptor, estrogen receptor, and survival. Breast Can Res Treat 1994; 29:109–116.
30. Gasparini G, Barbareschi M, Boracchi P, Bevilacqua P, Verderio P, Dalla Palma P, Menard S. 67-kDa laminin-receptor expression adds prognostic information to intra-tumoral microvessel density in node-negative breast cancer. Int J Cancer 1995; 60:7604–7610.
31. Inada K, Toi M, Hoshina S, Hayashi K, Tominaga T. Significance of tumor angiogenesis as an independent prognostic factor in axillary node-negative breast cancer. Gan To Kagaku Ryoho 1995; 22(suppl 1):59–65.
32. Charpin C, Devictor B, Bergeret D, Andrac L, Boulat J, Horschowski N, Lavaut MN, Piana L. CD 31 quantitative immunocytochemical assays in breast carcinomas. Correlation with current prognostic factors. Am J Clin Pathol 1995; 103:443–448.
33. Barbareschi M, Gasparini G, Weidner N, Morelli L, Forti S, Eccher C, Fina P, Leonardi E, Mauri F, Bevilacqua P, Dalla Palma P. Microvessel density quantifica-

tion in breast carcinomas: assessment by manual vs. a computer-assisted image analysis system. Appl Immunohistochem 1995; 3:75–84.

34. Obermair A, Czerwenka K, Kurz C, Kaider A, Sevelda P. Tumor vascular density in breast tumors and their effect on recurrence free survival. Chirurg 1994; 65: 611–615.

35. Toi M, Hoshina S, Yamamoto Y, Ishii T, Hayashi K, Tominaga T. Tumor angiogenesis in breast carcinoma: significance of vessel density as a prognostic indicator. Gan To Kagaku Ryoho 1994; 21(suppl 2):178–182.

36. Gasparini G, Barbareschi M, Boracchi P, Verderio P, Caffo O, Meli S, Palma PD, Marubini E, Bevilacqua P. Tumor angiogenesis may predict clinical outcome of node-positive breast cancer patients treated either with adjuvant hormone therapy or chemotherapy. Cancer J Sci Am 1995; 1:131–141.

37. Ogawa Y, Chung Y-S, Nakata B, Takatsuka S, Maeda K, Sawada T, Kato Y, Yoshikawa K, Sakurai M, Sowa M. Microvessel quantitation in invasive breast cancer by staining for factor VIII-related antigen. Br J Cancer 1995; 71:1297–1301.

38. Obermair A, Kurz C, Czervenka K, Thoma M, Kaider A, Wagner T, Gitsch G, Sevelda P. Microvessel density and vessel invasion in lymph node negative breast cancer: effect on recurrence-free survival. Int J Cancer 1995; 62:126–130.

39. Bevilacqua P, Barbareschi M, Verderio P, Boracchi P, Caffo O, Dalla Palma P, Meli S, Weidner N, Gasparini G. Prognostic value of intratumoral microvessel density, a measure of tumor angiogenesis, in node-negative breast carcinoma—results of a multiparametric study. Breast Cancer Res Treat 1995; 36:205–217.

40. Toi M, Inada K, Suzuki H, Tominaga T. Tumor angiogenesis in breast cancer: its importance as a prognostic indicator and the association with vascular endothelial growth factor expression. Breast Cancer Res Treat 1995; 36:193–204.

41. Gasparini G, Barbareschi M, Boracchi P, Bevilacqua P, Verderio P, Calla Palma P, Menard S. 67-kDa laminin-receptor expression adds prognostic information to intratumoral microvessel density in node-negative breast cancer. Int J Cancer 1995; 60:604–610.

42. Fox SB, Turner GDH, Leek RD, Whitehouse RM, Gatter KC, Harris AL. The prognostic value of quantitative angiogenesis in breast cancer and role of adhesion molecule expression in tumor endothelium. Breast Cancer Res Treat 1995; 36:219–226.

43. Scopinaro F, Schillaci O, Scarpini M, Mingazzini PL, diMacio L, Banci M, Danieli R, Zerilli M, Limiti MR, Centi Colella A. Technetium-99m sestamibi: an indicator of breast cancer invasiveness. Eur J Nucl Med 1994; 21:984–987.

44. Lipponen P, Ji H, Aaltomaa S, Syrjanen K. Tumor vascularity and basement membrane structure in breast cancer as related to tumor histology and prognosis. J Cancer Res Clin Oncol 1994; 120:645–650.

45. Wakui S, Furusato M, Itoh T, Sasaki H, Akiyama A, Kinoshita I, Asano K, Tokuda T, Aizawa S, Ushigome S. Tumor angiogenesis in prostatic carcinoma with and without bone marrow metastasis: a morphometric study. J Pathol 1992; 168:257–262.

46. Weidner N, Carroll PR, Flax J, Blumenfeld W, Folkman J. Tumor angiogenesis correlates with metastasis in invasive prostate carcinoma. Am J Pathol 1993; 143: 401–409.

47. Fregene TA, Khanuja PS, Noto AC, Gehani SK, Van Egmont EM, Luz DA, Pienta KJ. Tumor-associated angiogenesis in prostate cancer. Anticancer Res 1993; 13: 2377–2381.
48. Brawer MK, Deering RE, Brown M, Preston SD, Bigler SA. Predictors of pathologic stage in prostate carcinoma. Cancer 1994; 73:678–687.
49. Vesalainen S, Lipponen P, Talja M, Alhava E, Syrjanen K. Tumor vascularity and basement membrane structure as prognostic factors in T1-2M0 prostatic adenocarcinoma. Anticancer Res 1994; 14:709–714.
50. Hall MC, Troncoso P, Pollack A, Zhau HY, Zagars GK, Chung LW, von Eschenbach AC. Significance of tumor angiogenesis in clinically localized prostate carcinoma treated with external beam radiotherapy. Urology 1994; 44:869–875.
51. Mikami Y, Tsukuda M, Mochimatsu I, Kokatsu T, Yago T, Sawaki S. Angiogenesis in head and neck tumors. Nippon Jibiinkoka Gakkai Kaiho 1991; 96:645–650.
52. Gasparini G, Weidner N, Bevilacqua P, Maluta S, Boracchi P, Testolin A, Pozza F, Folkman J. Intratumoral microvessel density and p53 protein: correlation with metastasis in head-and -neck squamous-cell carcinoma. Int J Cancer 1993; 55:739–744.
53. Albo D, Granick MS, Jhala N, Atkinson B, Solomon MP. The relationship of angiogenesis to biological activity in human squamous cell carcinomas of the head and neck. Ann Plast Surg 1994; 32:588–594.
54. Williams JK, Carlson GW, Cohen C, Derose PB, Hunter S, Jurkiewicz MJ. Tumor angiogenesis as a prognostic factor in oral cavity tumors. Am J Surg 1994; 168: 373–380.
55. Alcalde RE, Shintani S, Yoshihama Y, Matsumura T. Cell proliferation and tumor angiogenesis in oral squamous cell carcinomas. Anticancer Res 1995; 15:1417–1422.
56. Macchiarini P, Fontanini G, Hardin MJ, Hardin MJ, Squartini F, Angeletti CA. Relation of neovasculature to metastasis of non-small-cell lung cancer. Lancet 1992; 340:145–146.
57. Macchiarini P, Fontanini G, Dulmet E, de Montpreville V, Chapelier AR, Cerrin J, Le Roy Ladurie F, Dartevelle PG. Angiogenesis: an indicator of metastasis in non-small-cell lung cancer invading the thoracic inlet. Ann Thorac Surg 1994; 57: 1534–1539.
58. Yamazaki K, Abe S, Takekawa H, Sukoh N, Watanabe N, Ogura S, Nakajima I, Isobe H, Inoue K, Kawakami Y. Tumor angiogenesis in human lung adenocarcinoma. Cancer 1994; 74:2245–2250.
59. Yuan A, Yang P-C, Yu C-J, Yao Y-T, Lee Y-C, Kuo S-H, Luh K-T. Tumor angiogenesis correlates with histologic type and nodal metastasis in non-small cell lung carcinoma. Amer J Resp Critical Care Med. In press.
60. Fontanini G, Bigini D, Vignati S, Basolo F, Mussi A, Lucchi M, Chine S, Angeletti CA, Bevilacqua G. Recurrence and death in non small cell lung carcinomas: a prognostic model using pathological parameters, microvessel count, and gene protein products. J Pathol 1995; 177:57–63.
61. Fontanini G, Vignati S, Bigini D, Mussi A, Lucchi M, Chine S, Angeletti CA, Bevilacqua G. Recurrence and death in non small cell lung carcinomas: a prognostic

model using pathological parameters, microvessel count, and gene protein products. Clin Cancer Res 1996. In press.
62. Srivastava A, Laidler P, Hughes LE, Woodcock J, Shedden EJ. Neovascularization in human cutaneous melanoma: a quantitative morphological and Doppler ultrasound study. Eur J Cancer Clin Oncol 1986; 22:1205–1209.
63. Srivastava A, Laidler P, Davies R, Horgan K, Hughes LE. The prognostic significance of tumor vascularity in intermediate-thickness (0.76–4.0 mm thick) skin melanoma. Am J Pathol 1988; 133:419–423.
64. Smolle J, Soyer H-P, Hofmann-Wellenhof R, Smolle-Juettner FM, Kerl H. Vascular architecture of melanocytic skin tumors. A quantitative immunohistochemical study using automated image analysis. Pathol Res Pract 1989; 185:740–745.
65. Fallowfield ME, Cook MG. The vascularity of primary cutaneous melanoma. J Pathol 1991; 164:241–244.
66. Barnhill RL, Levy MA. Regressing thin cutaneous malignant melanomas (< 1.0 mm) are associated with angiogenesis. Am J Pathol 1993; 43:99–104.
67. Vacca A, Ribatti D, Roncali L, Lospalluti M, Serio G, Carrel S, Dammacco F. Melanocyte tumor progression is associated with changes in angiogenesis and expression of the 67-kilodalton laminin receptor. Cancer 1993; 72:455–461.
68. Graham CH, Rivers J, Kerbel RS, Stankiewicz KS, White WL. Extent of vascularization as a prognostic indicator in thin (< 0.76 mm) malignant melanomas. Am J Pathol 1994; 145:510–514.
69. Saclarides TJ, Speziale NJ, Drab E, Szeluga DJ, Rubin DB. Tumor angiogenesis and rectal carcinoma. Dis Colon Rectum 1994; 37:921–926.
70. Maeda K, Chung Y-S, Takatsuka S, Ogawa Y, Sawada T, Yamashito Y, Onoda N, Kato Y, Nitta A, Arimoto Y, Kondo Y, Sowa M. Tumor angiogenesis as a predictor of recurrence in gastric carcinoma. J Clin Oncol 1995; 13:477–481.
71. Maeda K, Chung YS, Takatsuka S, Ogawa Y, Onoda N, Sawada T, Kato Y, Nitta A, Arimoto Y, Kondo Y, Sowa M. Tumor angiogenesis and tumor cell proliferation as prognostic indicators in gastric carcinoma. Br J Cancer 1995; 72:319–323.
72. Takebayashi Y, Akiyama S-I, Yamada K, Akiba S, Aikou T. Angiogenesis as an unfavorable prognostic factor in human colorectal carcinoma. Cancer 1996. In press.
73. Olivarez D, Ulbright T, DeRiese W, Foster R, Reister T, Einhorn L, Sledge G. Neovascularization in clinical stage A testicular germ cell tumor: prediction of metastatic disease. Cancer Res 1994; 54:2800–2802.
74. Vacca A, Ribatti D, Roncali L, Ranieri G, Serio G, Silvestris F, Dammacco F. Bone marrow angiogenesis and progression in multiple myeloma. Br J Haematol 1994; 87:503–508.
75. Li VW, Folkerth RD, Watanabe H, Yu C, Rupnick M, Barnes P, Scott RM, Black PM, Sallan SE, Folkman J. Microvessel count and cerebrospinal fluid basic fibroblast growth factor in children with brain tumors. Lancet 1994; 334:82–86.
76. Leon SP, Folkerth RD, Black PM. Microvessel density is a prognostic indicator for patients with astroglial brain tumors. Cancer 1996. In press.
77. Hollingsworth HC, Kohn EC, Steinberg SM, Rothenberg ML, Merino MJ. Tumor angiogenesis in advanced stage ovarian carcinoma. Am J Pathol 1995; 147:33–41.
78. Volm M, Koomagi R, Kaufmann M, Mattern J, Stammler G. Microvessel density,

expression of proto-oncogenes, and resistance-related proteins and incidence of metastases in primary ovarian carcinomas. Clin Exp Met 1996. In press.
79. Wiggins DL, Granai CO, Steinhoff MM, Calabresi P. Tumor angiogenesis as a prognostic factor in cervical carcinoma. Gynecol Oncol 1995; 56:353–356.
80. Bremer GL, Tiebosch ATMG, van der Putten HWHM, Schouten HJA, de Haan J, Arends J-W. Tumor angiogenesis: an independent prognostic parameter in cervical cancer. Am J Obstet Gynecol. In press.
81. Schlenger K, Hockel M, Mitze M, Schaffer U, Weikel W, Knapstein PG, Lambert A. Tumor vascularity—A novel prognostic factor in advanced cervical carcinoma. Gynecol Oncol 1995; 59:57–66.
82. Abulafia O, Triest WE, Sherer DM, Hansen CC, Ghezzi F. Angiogenesis in endometrial hyperplasia and stage I endometrial carcinoma. Obstet Gynecol 1995; 86: 479–485.
83. Jaeger TM, Weidner N, Chew K, Moore DH, Kerschmann RL, Waldman FM, Carroll PR. Tumor angiogenesis correlates with lymph node metastases in invasive bladder cancer. J Urol 1995; 154:59–71.
84. Bochner BH, Cote RJ, Weidner N, Groshen S, Chen S-C, Skinner DG, Nichols PW. Angiogenesis in bladder cancer: relationship between microvessel density and tumor prognosis. J Natl Cancer Inst 1995; 87:1603–1612.
85. Dickinson AJ, Fox SB, Persad RA, Hollyer J, Sibley GN, Harris AL. Quantification of angiogenesis as an independent predictor of prognosis in invasive bladder carcinomas. Br J Urol 1994; 74:762–766.
86. Kohno Y, Iwanari O, Kitao M. Prognostic importance of histologic vascular density in cervical cancer treated with hypertensive intraarterial chemotherapy. Cancer 1993; 72:2394–2400.
87. Zatterstrom UK, Brun E, Willen R, Kjellen E, Wennerberg J. Tumor angiogenesis and prognosis in squamous cell carcinoma of the head and neck. Head Neck 1995; 17:312–318.
88. Folkman J. Angiogenesis and its inhibitors. In: DeVita VT, Hellman S, Rosenberg SA, eds. Important Advances in Oncology. Philadelphia: J.B. Lippincott Co. 1985: 42–62.
89. Harris AL, Fox S, Bicknell R, Leek R, Relf M, LeJeune S, Kaklamanis L. Gene therapy through signal transduction pathways and angiogenic growth factors as therapeutic targets in breast cancer. Cancer 1994; 74(3 suppl):1021–1025.
90. Ingber D, Fujita T, Kishimoto S, Katsuichi S, Kanamaru T, Brem H, Folkman J. Synthetic analogues of fumagillin that inhibit angiogenesis and suppress tumor growth. Nature 1990; 348:555–557.
91. Gross JL, Herblin WF, Dusak BA, Czerniak P, Diamond M, Dexter DL. Modulation of solid tumor growth in vivo by bFGF. Proc Am Assoc Cancer Res 1990; 31:79 (abstr).
92. Kim KJ, Li B, Winer J, Armanini M, Gillett N, Phillips HS, Ferrara N. Inhibition of vascular endothelial growth factor-induced angiogenesis suppresses tumor growth in vivo. Nature 1993; 362:841–844.
93. Hori A, Sasada R, Matsutani E, Naito K, Sakura Y, Fujita T, Kozai Y. Suppression of solid tumor growth by immunoneutralizing monoclonal antibody against human basic fibroblast growth factor. Cancer Res 1991; 51:6180–6184.

94. Millauer B, Shawver LK, Plate KH, Risau W, Ullrich A. Glioblastoma growth inhibited in vivo by a dominant-negative Flk-1 mutant. Nature 1994; 367:576–579.
95. Brooks PC, Montgomery AMP, Rosenfeld M, Reisfeld RA, Hu T, Ilier G, Cheresh DA. Integrin alpha$_v$ beta$_3$ antagonists promote tumor regression by inducing apoptosis of angiogenic blood vessels. Cell 1994; 79:1157–1164.
96. O'Reilly MS, Holmgren L, Shing Y, Chen C, Rosenthal RA, Moses M, Lane WS, Cao Y, Sage EH, Folkman J. Angiostatin: a novel angiogenesis inhibitor that mediates the suppression of metastases by a Lewis lung carcinoma. Cell 1994; 79:315–328.
97. O'Reilley MS, Holmgren L, Chen K, Folkman J. Suppression of angiogenesis in mice by angiostatin inhibits murine and human primary tumor growth. Submitted.
98. Nicosia RF, Tchao R, Leighton J. Interactions between newly formed endothelial channels and carcinoma cells in plasma clot culture. Clin Exp Metastasis 1986; 4: 91–104.
99. Warren RS, Yuan H, Matli MR, Gillett NA, Ferrara N. Regulation by vascular endothelial growth factor of human colon cancer tumorigenesis in a mouse model of experimental liver metastasis. J Clin Invest 1995; 95:1789–1797.
100. Rak JW, Hegmann EJ, Lu C, Kerbel RS. Progressive loss of sensitivity to endothelium-derived growth inhibitors expressed by human melanoma cells during disease progression. J Cell Physiol 1994; 159:245–255.
101. Hamada J, Cavanaugh PG, Lotan O. Separable growth and migration factors for large-cell lymphoma cells secreted by microvascular endothelial cells derived from target organs for metastasis. Br J Cancer 1992; 66:349–354.
102. Folkman J. Angiogenesis and breast cancer. J Clin Oncol 1994; 12:441–443.
103. Pepper MS, Vassalli JD, Montesano R, Orci L. Urokinase type plasminogen activator is induced in migrating capillary endothelial cells. J Cell Biol 1987; 105:2535–2541.
104. Fox SB, Stuart N, Smith K, Brunner N, Harris AL. High levels of uPA and PA-1 are associated with highly angiogenic breast carcinomas. J Pathol 1993; 170(suppl): 388a.
105. Moscatelli D, Gross J, Rifkin D. Angiogenic factors stimulate plasminogen activator and collagenase production by capillary endothelial cells. J Cell Biol 1981; 91: 201a.
106. Dvorak HF. Tumors: wounds that do not heal. Similarities between tumor stroma generation and wound healing. N Engl J Med 1986; 315:1650–1659.
107. Folkman J, Klagsbrun M. Angiogenic factors. Science 1987; 235:442–447.
108. Polverini PJ, Leibovich SJ. Induction of neovascularization in vivo and endothelial proliferation in vitro by tumor associated macrophages. Lab Invest 1984; 51:635–642.
109. Guidi AJ, Fischer L, Harris JR, Schnitt SJ. Microvessel density and distribution in ductal carcinoma in situ of the breast. J Natl Cancer Inst 1994; 86:614–619.
110. Smith-McCune KK, Weidner N. Demonstration and characterization of the angiogenic properties of cervical dysplasia. Cancer Res 1994; 54:800–804.
111. Kandel J, Bossy-Wetzel E, Radvani F, Klagsburn M, Folkman J, Hanahan D. Neovascularization is associated with a switch to the export of bFGF in the multi-step development of fibrosarcoma. Cell 1991; 66:1095–1104.

112. Nguyen M, Watanabe H, Budson AE, Richie JP, Folkman J. Elevated levels of the angiogenic peptide basic fibroblast growth factor in urine of bladder cancer patients. J Natl Cancer Inst 1993; 85:241–242.
113. Dvorak HF, Brown LF, Detmar M, Dvorak AM. Vascular permeability factor/vascular endothelial growth factor, microvascular hyperpermeability, and angiogenesis. Am J Pathol 1995; 146:1029–1039.
114. Brown LF, Berse B, Jackman RW, Tognazzi K, Manseau EJ, Dvorak HF, Senger DR. Increased expression of vascular permeability factor (vascular endothelial growth factor) and its receptors in kidney and bladder carcinomas. Am J Pathol 1993; 143:1255–1262.
115. Brown LF, Berse B, Jackman RW, Tognazzi K, Manseau EJ, Senger DR, Dvorak HF. Expression of vascular permeability factor (vascular endothelial growth factor) and its receptors in adenocarcinomas of the gastrointestinal tract. Cancer Res 1993; 53:4727–4735.
116. Senger DR, Van De Water L, Brown LF, Nagy JA, Yeo K-T, Yeo T-K, Berse B, Jackman RW, Dvorak AM, Dvorak HF. Vascular permeability factor (VPF, VEGF) in tumor biology. Cancer Metastasis Rev 1993; 12:303–324.
117. Thompson WD, Campbell R, Evans T. Fibrin degradation and angiogenesis: quantitative analysis of the angiogenic response in the chick chorioallantoic membranes. J Pathol 1985; 145:27–37.
118. Toi M, Hoshina S, Takayanagi T, Tominaga T. Association of vascular endothelial growth factor expression with tumor angiogenesis and with early relapse in primary breast cancer. Jpn J Cancer Res 1994; 85:1045–1049.
119. Goto F, Goto K, Weindel K, Folkman J. Synergistic effects of vascular endothelial growth factor and basic fibroblast growth factor on the proliferation and cord formation of bovine capillary endothelial cells within collagen gels. Lab Invest 1993; 69:508–517.
120. Leibovich SJ, Polverini PJ, Fong TW, Harlow LA, Koch AE. Production of angiogenic activity by human monocytes requires an L-arginine/nitric oxide-synthase-dependent effector mechanism. Proc Natl Acad Sci U S A 1994; 91:4190–4194.
121. Laniado-Schwartzman M, Lavrovsky Y, Stotlz RA, Conners MS, Falck JR, Chauhan K, Abraham NG. Activation of nuclear factor kappa B and oncogene expression by 12(R)-hydroxyeicosatrienoic acid, an angiogenic factor in microvessel endothelial cells. J Biol Chem 1994; 269 (39):2432–2437.
122. Rastinejad F, Polverini PJ, Bouck NP. Regulation of the activity of a new inhibitor of angiogenesis by a cancer suppressor gene. Cell 1989; 56:345–355.
123. Bouck NP. Tumor angiogenesis: the role of oncogenes and tumor suppressor genes. Cancer Cells 1990; 2:179–185.
124. Zajchowski DA, Band V, Trask DK, Kling D, Connoly JL, Sager R. Suppression of tumor-forming ability and related traits in MCF-7 human breast cancer cells by fusion with immortal mammary epithelial cells. Proc Natl Acad Sci U S A 1990; 87:2314–2318.
125. Dameron KM, Volpert OV, Tainsky MS, Bouck N. Control of angiogenesis in fibroblasts by p53 regulation of thrombospondin-1. Science 1994; 265:1582–1584.
126. Folkman J. Angiogenesis in cancer,vascular, rheumatoid, and other disease. Nat Med 1995; 1:27–31.

127. Fidler IJ, Gersten DM, Hart IR. The biology of cancer invasion and metastasis. Adv Cancer Res 1978; 28:149–250.
128. Nicolson G. Cancer metastasis. Sci Am 1979; 240:66–76.
129. Weiss L. Biophysical aspects of the metastatic cascade. In: Weiss L, ed. Fundamental Aspects of Metastasis. Amsterdam: N. Holland, 1976:51–70.
130. Bemstein LR, Liotta LA. Molecular mediators of interactions with extracellular matrix components in metastasis and angiogenesis. Curr Opin Oncol 1994; 6:106–113.
131. Liotta L, Kleinerman J, Saidel G. Quantitative relationships of intravascular tumor cells, tumor vessels, and pulmonary metastases following tumor implantation. Cancer Res 1974; 34:997–1004.
132. Liotta L, Saidel G, Kleinerman J. The significance of hematogenous tumor cell clumps in the metastatic process. Cancer Res 1976; 36:889–894.
133. Nagy JA, Brown LF, Senger DR, Lanir N, Van de Water L, Dvorak AM, Dvorak HF. Pathogenesis of tumor stroma generation: a critical role for leaky blood vessels and fibrin deposition. Biochim Biophys Acta 1989; 948:305–326.
134. Sugino T, Kawaguchi T, Suzuki T. Stromal invasion is not essential to blood-borne metastais in mouse mammary carcinoma. In: Scientific Program Booklet of the Pathological Society of Great Britain and Ireland; 170th Meeting, January 1995; (abstr #161).
135. Smolin G. Hyundiuk RA. Lymphatic drainage from vascularized rabbit cornea. Am J Ophthalmol 1971; 72:147–151.
136. Folkman J. Angiogenesis. In: Verstraete M, Vermylen J, Lijnan R, Arnout J, eds. Thrombosis and Haemostasis. Leuven: Leuven University Press, 1987; 24:583–596.
137. Liotta LA, Stracke ML. Tumor invasion and metastasis: biochemical mechanisms. In: Lippman ME, Dickson RB, eds. Breast Cancer: Cellular and Molecular Biology. Boston: Kluwer Academic Publishers, 1988:223–238.
138. Brem S, Cotran R, Folkman J. Tumor angiogenesis: a quantitative method for histologic grading. J Natl Cancer Inst 1972; 48:347–356.
139. Folkman J, Watson K, Ingber D, Hanahan D. Induction of angiogenesis during the transition from hyperplasia to neoplasia. Nature 1989; 339:58–61.
140. Weidner N. The relationship of tumor angiogenesis and metastasis with emphasis on invasive breast carcinoma. In: Weinstein RS, ed. Adv Pathol Lab Med. Mosby Year Book, Chicago, 1992; 5:101–121.
141. Hall NR, Fish DE, Hunt N, Goldin RD, Guillou PJ, Monson JRT. Is the relationship between angiogenesis and metastasis in breast cancer real? Surg Oncol 1992; 1: 223–229.
142. Van Hoef MEHM, Knox WF, Dhesi SS, Howell A, Schor AM. Assessment of tumor vascularity as a prognostic factor in lymph node negative invasive breast cancer. Eur J Cancer 1993; 29A:1141–1145.
143. Miliaras D, Kamas A, Kalekou H. Angiogenesis in invasive breast carcinoma: is it associated with parameters of prognostic significance? Histopathology 1995; 26: 165–169.
144. Axelsson K, Ljung BME, Moore DH, Thor AD, Chew KL, Edgerton SM, Smith HS, Mayall BH. Tumor angiogenesis as a prognostic assay for invasive ductal carcinoma. J Natl Cancer Inst 1995; 87:997–1008.

145. Carnochan P, Briggs JC, Westbury G, Davies AJ. The vascularity of cutaneous melanoma: a quantitative histologic study of lesions 0.85–1.25 mm in thickness. Br J Cancer 1991; 64:102–107.
146. Leedy DA, Trune DR, Kronz JD, Weidner N, Cohen JI. Tumor angiogenesis, the p53 antigen, and cervical metastasis in squamous carcinoma. Otolaryngol Head Neck Surg 1994; 111:417–422.
147. Rutger JL, Mattox TF, Vargas MP. Angiogenesis in uterine cervical squamous cell carcinoma. Int J Gynecol Path 1995; 14:114–118.
148. van Diest PJ, Zevering JP, Zevering LC, Baak JPA. Prognostic value of microvessel quantitation in cisplatin treated Figo 3 and 4 ovarian cancer patients. Pathol Res Pract 1995; 191:25–30.
149. Siitonen SM, Haapasalo HK, Rantala IS, Helin HJ, Isola JJ. Comparison of different immunohistochemical methods in the assessment of angiogenesis: lack of prognostic value in a group of 77 selected node-negative breast carcinomas. Mod Pathol 1995; 8:745–752.
150. Goulding H, Rashid NFNA, Robertson JF, Bell JA, Elston CW, Blamey RW, Ellis IO. Assessment of angiogenesis in breast carcinoma: an important factor in prognosis? Hum Pathol 1995; 26:1196–1200.
151. Costello P, McCann A, Carney DN, Dervan PA. Prognostic significance of microvessel density in lymph node negative breast carcinoma. Hum Pathol 1995; 26: 1181–1184.
152. MacLennan GT, Bostwick DG. Microvessel density in renal cell carcinoma: lack of prognostic significance. Urology 1995; 46:27–30.
153. Tahan SR, Stein AL. Angiogenesis in invasive squamous cell carcinoma of the lip: tumor vascularity is not an indicator of metastatic risk. J Cutan Pathol 1995; 22: 236–240.
154. Dray TG, Hardin NJ, Sofferman RA. Angiogenesis as a prognostic marker in early head and neck cancer. Ann Otol Rhinol Laryngol 1995; 104:724–729.
155. Bamhill RL, Busam KJ, Berwick M, Blessing K, Cochran Aj, Elder DE, Fandrey K, Daraoli T, White WL. Tumor vascularity is not a prognostic factor for cutaneous melanoma [letter]. Lancet 1994; 344:1237–1238.
156. Kainz C, Speiser P, Wanner C, Obermair A, Tempfer C, Sliutz G. Reinthaller A, Breitenecker G. Prognostic value of tumor microvessel density in cancer of the uterine cervix stage IB to IIB. Anticancer Res 1995; 15:1549–1551.
157. DeYoung BR, Wick MR, Fitzgibbon JF, Sirgi KE, Swanson PE. CD31: an immunospecific marker for endothelial differentiation in human neoplasms. Appl Immunohistochem 1993; 1:97–100.
158. Longacre TA, Rouse RV. CD31: a new marker for vascular neoplasia. Adv Anat Pathol 1994; 1:16–20.
159. van de Rijn M, Rouse RV. CD34: a review. Appl Immunohistochem 1994; 2: 71–80.
160. Traweek ST, Kandalaft PL, Mehta P, Battifora H. The human hematopoietic progenitor cell antigen (CD34) in vascular neoplasia. Am J Clin Pathol 1991; 96: 25–31.
161. Schlingemann RO, Rietveld FJR, Kwaspen F, van de Kerkhof PCM, de Waal RMW, Ruiter DJ. Differential expression of markers for endothelial cells, pericytes,

and basal lamina in the microvasculature of tumors and granulation tissue. Am J Pathol 1991; 138:1335–1347.

162. Wang JM, Kumar S, Pye D, Haboubi N, Al-Nakib L. Breast carcinoma: comparative study of tumor vasculature using two endothelial-cell markers. J Natl Cancer Inst 1994; 86:386–388.
163. Wang JM, Kumar S, Pye D, van Agthoven AJ, Krupinski J, Hunter RD. A monoclonal antibody detects heterogeneity in vascular endothelium of tumors and normal tissues. Int J Cancer 1993; 54:363–370.
164. Watanabe II, Nguyen M, Schizer M. Basic fibroblast growth factor in human serum—a prognostic test for breast cancer. Mol Biol Cell 1992; 3:324a.
165. Nguyen M, Watanabe II, Budson AE. Elevated levels of an angiogenic peptide, basic fibroblast growth factor, in the urine of patients with a wide spectrum of cancers. J Natl Cancer Inst 1994; 86:356.
166. Li VW, Folkerth RD, Watanabe H, Yu C, Rupnick M, Barnes P, Scott RM, Black PM, Sallan SE, Folkman J. Microvessel count and cerebrospinal fluid basic fibroblast growth factor in children with brain tumors. Lancet 1994; 334:82–86.
167. Herlyn M, Clark WH, Rodeck U, Mancianti ML, Jambrosic J, Koprowski H. Biology of tumor progression in human melanocytes. Lab Invest 1987; 56:461–467.

29

The Prognostic and Diagnostic Value of Circulating Angiogenic Factors in Cancer Patients

Olaf A. J. Kerckhaert and Emile E. Voest
University Medical Center Utrecht, Utrecht, The Netherlands

I. INTRODUCTION

In the previous chapter, the prognostic value of tumor microvessel density was clearly demonstrated. Microvessel density reflects the net result of the balance between positive and negative regulators of angiogenesis. A large number of angiogenic factors are characterized, and antibodies against many of these peptides are now available. The generation of specific antibodies has facilitated a detailed analysis of the contribution of individual angiogenic factors to the malignant phenotype of cancers. Many studies have investigated the tissue expression level of (anti-)angiogenic factors and correlated this expression with tumor invasiveness, disease-free survival and overall survival. It is beyond the scope of this chapter to give an extensive overview of these studies. In general, tumors with high expression levels of angiogenic factors (e.g., vascular endothelial growth factor [VEGF], basic fibroblast growth factor [bFGF], matrix metalloproteinases [MMPs]) or low expression levels of inhibitors (thrombospondin, tissue inhibitors of metalloproteinases [TIMPs]) have a higher microvessel density, are locally more advanced, have a more aggressive behavior, and metastasize more frequently than tumors without this angiogenic phenotype. These immunohistochemical studies provide information on the angiogenic profile of a tumor. The expression level of factors involved in angiogenesis also may indicate which approach to use to inhibit angiogenesis. More specifically, the development of an anticancer treatment may be aimed at those proteins, which are overexpressed in tumors. The use of immunohistochemistry has limitations, however. Quantification of the expression level of markers on tissue sections is difficult and subjective. Therefore, investigators have looked for alternative methods to measure angiogenic factors. Several angiogenic factors are soluble and may enter the circulation. Measurement of soluble angiogenic factors may provide an objective and easy method to determine the angiogenic profile of a tumor. A number of enzyme-linked immunosorbent assays (ELISAs) are now commercially available to measure soluble angiogenic factors in various body fluids including serum, urine, and cerebrospinal fluid. These ELISAs are easy to handle and have a high sensitivity. Several angiogenic factors have been measured in urine and serum and analyzed for a possible prognostic value. The purpose of this chapter is to provide an overview of the clinical experience with the measurement of angiogenic factors in body fluids.

II. FIBROBLAST GROWTH FACTORS

Basic fibroblast growth factor (bFGF, FGF2) and acidic fibroblast growth factor (aFGF, FGF1) are among the most potent endothelial cell mitogens (1). Therefore they received substantial attention as markers of angiogenesis. The first study in this direction was performed in patients with bladder cancer. A significant difference in urine bFGF levels was found between patients with locally active disease, no evidence of disease, and metastatic bladder cancer (2). When compared with urine cytology, measurement of bFGF levels appeared to be more sensitive to detect cancer (sensitivity 81% vs 38%) than cytology, but less specific (specificity 64% vs 73%). The relationship between bladder cancer and bFGF was confirmed in an independent study, although the specificity and sensitivity of detecting bladder cancer by measuring urine bFGF was different (88% and 42%, respectively) (3). Acidic FGF was also analyzed as a prognostic and diagnostic tool in the detection of bladder cancer. In a large study, measurement of aFGF in urine had a sensitivity of 72% and a specificity of 91% to detect bladder cancer (4). The studies suggested that measurement of aFGF and bFGF in the urine of patients with bladder cancer is not sufficiently sensitive or specific to use as a screening method, but may have a place in monitoring the effectiveness of bladder cancer therapies. After these initial studies in patients with bladder cancer, bFGF was detected in the urine of patients with a variety of tumors (5). In a study of 76 patients with renal cell carcinoma, serum bFGF levels were significant higher in patients with disseminated cancer than in those with localized cancer (P = 0,0004) (6). Many studies have subsequently analyzed the value of measuring bFGF in urine and serum in a variety of cancers. Most of the published reports demonstrate a relationship between the progression or presence of cancer and elevated levels of bFGF (7–11).

Hemangiomas are benign vascular tumors characterized by rapid proliferation of endothelial cells in the first months of life followed by spontaneous involution in the years thereafter (12). Basic FGF is elevated during the rapid growth phase in these young children and decreases when hemangiomas involute either spontaneously or, in life-threatening situations, after treatment with steroids (13) or interferon $^{\alpha}$-2a (14, 15). This has led to the monitoring of bFGF levels in the urine of children during treatment of life-threatening hemangiomas. If bFGF levels fail to decrease during treatment with interferon$^{\alpha}$-2a, it is suggested that higher doses of interferon$^{\alpha}$-2a are needed to block the production of bFGF (14, 15). In addition, if bFGF is not detected in the urine, it may be argued whether treatment with interferon$^{\alpha}$-2a should be started.

Basic FGF was measured in the cerebrospinal fluid of 26 children and young adults with brain tumors and 18 controls (16). Basic FGF was detected in 62% of the patients with brain tumors and in none of the controls. The concentration of bFGF correlated with microvessel density of the tumors. However, serum bFGF levels do not necessarily correspond with the bFGF concentration in tumors (17). In contrast, serum and urine bFGF levels of sarcoma patients with advanced disease (n = 28) were not different from patients with a history of sarcoma but without evidence of disease (n = 15) (Voest, unpublished observations). This may suggest a limited contribution of bFGF to the progression of sarcomas. Interestingly, we easily detected bFGF in the urine of virtually all subjects, whereas bFGF in serum could only be detected in 14% of the subjects. The reason for this apparent preferential distribution of bFGF to the kidneys is unclear.

In summary, fibroblast growth factors may be released during both physiological and cancerous growth. As a consequence, the release of FGFs in body fluids lacks specificity and cannot be used as either a diagnostic tool or a screen test for cancer. The mechanism of clearance of bFGF is unclear and warrants further study. However, changes of bFGF in body fluids may have value as a therapy monitor.

III. VASCULAR ENDOTHELIAL GROWTH FACTOR

Vascular endothelial growth factor is one of the most important mediators of tumor angiogenesis. Because $VEGF_{165}$ and $VEGF_{121}$ are soluble isoforms, they may enter the circulation and become a marker of angiogenesis. Theoretically, the measurement of VEGF in serum (S-VEGF) has several limitations: a) S-VEGF is not specific for tumor angiogenesis and may be up-regulated by a variety of stimuli (chapter 14 for review); b) S-VEGF has a very short half-life (minutes); c) S-VEGF concentrations fluctuate significantly within one individual in time, (18). c) measurement of S-VEGF reflects the presence of $VEGF_{165}$ or

$VEGF_{121}$ and does not necessarily provide information on the presence of the other isoforms of VEGF; and e) serum levels of VEGF may merely reflect peripheral blood platelet numbers (19).

The observation that platelets release VEGF after the appropriate stimuli has important implications for the interpretation of S-VEGF levels. This is underlined by a study in which the S-VEGF levels of cancer patients during chemotherapy were a mirror image of platelet numbers (20). Plasma concentrations of VEGF were virtually undetectable. The nondetectable plasma concentrations are in line with the reported short half-life of VEGF when injected into the circulation. Platelets may have an important regulatory role in tumor angiogenesis, either by providing the tumor with VEGF or sequestering VEGF from sites of overproduction. How this process is regulated is currently under investigation (21). In spite of the aforementioned limitations, several studies have investigated the diagnostic value of S-VEGF in cancer patients. The first question was whether S-VEGF concentrations were elevated in cancer patients. Numerous studies in a variety of cancers have shown such an elevation (22–25). However, other studies did not establish a relationship between S-VEGF and the presence of cancer (7, 26). Next, the role of S-VEGF as a marker for disease progression was investigated. Some studies showed that S-VEGF correlated with stage of disease (7, 22), whereas in a study on patients with melanoma such a relationship could not be established (25).

The prognostic value of pretreatment S-VEGF was analyzed prospectively in patients with non-Hodgkin's lymphoma (27) small-cell lung cancer (28), and ovarian cancer (29). Data from these studies showed that a high pretreatment S-VEGF level was associated with poor outcome. This may suggest that VEGF facilitates tumor growth, which is in agreement with the observation that S-VEGF levels correlate with the growth rate of colorectal cancer (9).

Vascular endothelial growth factor was also analyzed in other body fluids. High concentrations of VEGF were found in both guinea pig and human tumor ascites fluids (18, 30). Accumulation of tumor ascites fluid might result from increased permeability of the blood vessels lining the peritoneal cavity because of VEGF production by tumor cells (31). High concentrations of VEGF were measured in glioblastoma and renal cyst fluid, suggesting that increased vascular permeability leads to cyst formation (26, 32). The high levels of VEGF suggest that VEGF has a role in the development of cysts and may allow novel strategies to treat ascites or cysts.

Recently VEGF was quantified in the urine of 261 patients, including 153 undergoing cytoscopic surveillance for bladder cancer and 108 with another advanced malignancy or a benign urological condition (33). Urinary VEGF was higher in patients undergoing cytoscopic surveillance for bladder cancer than in those with an advanced nonbladder malignancy ($P < 0.0001$) or a benign urological condition ($P = 0.004$). The sensitivity and specificity of urinary VEGF for diagnosing recurrent bladder cancer were 48% and 83%, respectively (n = 137). Furthermore, in 61 cases a correlation was established between urinary VEGF and stage T1 or less superficial bladder tumor recurrence rates ($r = 0.45$; $P < 0.0001$).

In conclusion, the measurement of VEGF in body fluids does not add to the current diagnostic tools in cancer patients. However, VEGF may be a valuable predictive factor in the follow-up of cancer patients, as suggestion that warrants further investigation.

IV. INTERLEUKIN 8

Interleukin 8 (IL8) is an angiogenic cytokine produced by tumor and inflammatory cells. It induces angiogenesis in the mouse cornea neovascularization assay and in the chick chorioallantoic membrane assay (34). To determine the prognostic role of IL8 in cancer patients, 53 consecutive sarcoma patients were monitored for IL8 in their urine and serum (Voest, unpublished observations). No significant differences were seen between urine IL8 levels of sarcoma patients with advanced disease and patients who were without evidence of disease (97 ± 264 pg/L and 20 ± 28 pg/L, respectively). Serum levels of IL8 were, on average, lower than urine levels. No differences in serum IL8 concentrations between both patient groups were seen (8 ± 22 pg/L and 7 ± 16 pg/L, respectively). This indicates that measurement of IL8 lacks the sensitivity and specificity required for a diagnostic marker. To determine whether IL8 could be used to monitor disease activity, sequential IL8 measurements were performed in a patient with angiosarcoma of the right humerus who underwent radiation therapy. Three months after completion of her treatment, there was no evidence of disease, and the extremely high IL8 levels at the start of treatment became undetectable (Fig. 1a). In comparison, levels of bFGF increased tenfold during radiation therapy, which may reflect tissue damage (Fig. 1b).

In conclusion, IL8 may play a role in the biological behavior of sarcomas. However, the lack of specificity and sensitivity of IL8 levels to detect cancer does not support a role for routine measurement of IL8 in the management of sarcoma patients.

V. PROTEASES AND PROTEASE INHIBITORS

During angiogenesis, two families of proteases—metalloproteinases and serine proteases—play a crucial role in the breakdown of the basement membrane and extracellular matrix (35). The degradation of extracellular matrix facilitates both

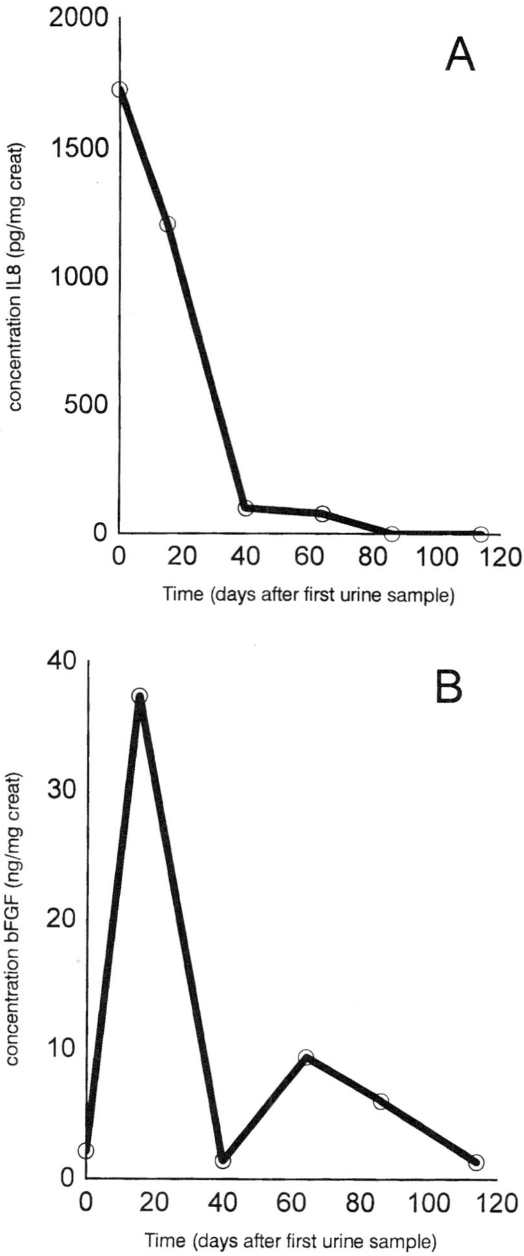

Figure 1 Changes in urine interleukin 8 (IL8) (**A**) and basic fibroblast growth factor (bFGF) (**B**) levels during successful treatment of a patient with an angiosarcoma of the right humerus. Treatment (radiation therapy) was started at day 0 and ended at day 20. At the end of follow-up (day 120), there was no evidence of disease.

endothelial cell movement and migration of other cell types, including tumor cells.

A. Metalloproteinases and Metalloproteinase Inhibitors

The value of measuring metalloproteinases (MMP) and their natural inhibitors, tissue inhibitors of metalloproteinases (TIMP) in body fluids in the diagnosis or follow-up of cancer patients remains to be determined. A limited number of studies have been published.

Patients with prostatic cancer (n = 40) had higher serum levels of TIMP-1 and collagenase and lower levels of TIMP-2 than control subjects (n = 56). Patients with metastatic cancer had significantly higher levels of collagenase than those without metastases. The combined information of serum TIMP-1 levels and collagenase levels was as sensitive as prostate-specific antigen as a marker of metastatic disease of prostate cancer (36). Metalloproteinase-2 levels are increased in serum of patients with colon and breast cancer (37). The belief that an imbalance between positive and negative regulators of angiogenesis is important for tumor progression is demonstrated by a study of 53 urothelial cancer patients in whom serum MMP-2 and TIMP-2 levels were measured. The mean MMP-2:TIMP-2 ratio in 31 patients with recurrence was significantly higher than that in 22 patients without recurrence. Multivariate analysis indicated that the ratio of serum levels of MMP-2 and TIMP-2 was an independent prognostic factor of recurrence. In addition, disease-free survival of patients with high MMP-2: TIMP-2 ratios was poor compared with that of patients with lower ratios (38, 39). The relevance of serum MMP-2 as a prognostic factor was further supported by a study in serous cystadenocarcinoma. Serum MMP-2 levels correlated with disease-free survival and reflected MMP-2 expression in tissue sections (40). Three molecular weight classes of MMPs, 72 kDa (MMP-2), 92 kDa (MMP-9), and high-molecular-weight (> or = 150 kDa) species, were measured in 68 urine specimens obtained from individuals with a variety of cancers and compared with 33 specimens obtained from healthy volunteers (41). The presence of biologically active MMP-2 ($P < 0.001$) or MMP-9 ($P = 0.002$) was an independent predictor of organ-confined cancer. The high-molecular-weight species ($P < 0.001$) was an independent predictor of metastatic cancer. These findings suggest that the evaluation of urinary MMPs may reflect disease status in patients with tumors, both within and outside the urinary tract.

B. Urokinase Plasminogen Activator System

Serum levels of urokinase-type plasminogen activator (u-PA) and its inhibitors, plasminogen activator inhibitor-1 and -2 (PAI-1, -2) were evaluated as a prognostic factor for malignancy in colorectal, gastric, head and neck squamous cell, and ovarian carcinoma (42–46). Although these results are not conclusive, most studies show an up-regulation of components of the plasminogen activation system in the serum of cancer patients. The soluble receptor for u-PA (suPAR) was also found in the blood of healthy individuals and in considerable amounts in ascites derived from patients with ovarian carcinoma (47–49). In a recent study in 87 ovarian cancer patients, the serum level of uPAR was increased ($P < 0.0001$), but a significant subset of carcinoma patients had overlapping uPAR values within the range of uPAR concentrations found in the healthy control values. Moreover, patients with high serum uPAR levels showed significantly worse prognosis in survival analysis ($P = 0.05$), but uPAR lost its significance in a direct comparison against FIGO (International Federation of Gynecology and Obstetrics) stage (50). Elevated plasma levels of uPAR also were seen in patients with non–small-cell lung cancer (51).

VI. MISCELLANEOUS

Repeated bladder instillations with bacille Calmette Guerin (BCG) are considered the standard treatment for superficial bladder cancer. Activation of the immune system with subsequent destruction of cancer cells is believed to be the mechanism of action. We have suggested that inhibition of angiogenesis may be an alternative mechanism of action of BCG (52). Bacille Calmette Guerin induces IL 12, which subsequently induces interferon gamma (53). Interferon gamma is a potent inducer of a novel angiogenesis inhibitor: interferon-inducible protein 10 (IP-10) (54). After treatment with BCG for transitional cell carcinoma, urine levels of the antiangiogenic protein IP-10 were increased. Future studies must determine whether levels of IP-10 are predictive of a response to BCG. However, the measurement of IP-10 in the urine of bladder cancer patients may serve as an example of a regulatory protein, which has potential value in the follow-up of patients.

The list of soluble factors that may be measured in the circulation is rapidly increasing. However, not only secreted factors may play a role in angiogenesis. It was reported that adhesion molecules are shed, released into the circulation, and have a regulatory effect on angiogenesis (55, 56). The predictive value of these soluble receptors in tumor progression and survival remains to be determined.

VII. CONCLUSION

In this chapter, we have summarized the findings from a large number of studies on angiogenic factors in patients with cancer. The experiences with measurement of a limited number of regulators of angiogenesis have shown both the possible merits of this approach and its limitations. In the future it may be possible to determine the angiogenic profile of a tumor and to use this profile to decide which type of angiogenesis inhibition may be best. For example, high levels of VEGF may suggest the use of anti-VEGF strategies, whereas high levels of MMPs may indicate the use of metalloproteinase inhibitors. Regulators of angiogenesis may be used in the follow-up of patients or as a marker of treatment efficacy. Examples are the measurement of bFGF in the urine of hemangioma patients or the production of IP-10 in the urine of patients with bladder cancer treated with BCG. The diagnostic use of angiogenic factors has limited value. Angiogenesis is not limited to tumor growth, and many factors, if not all, play a role in physiological angiogenesis. These early reports warrant further research to determine the true clinical value of an angiogenic tumor profile.

REFERENCES

1. Mason IJ. The ins and outs of fibroblast growth factors. Cell 1994; 78:547–552.
2. Nguyen M, Watanabe H, Budson AE, Richie JP, Folkman J. Elevated levels of the angiogenic peptide basic fibroblast growth factor in urine of bladder cancer patients. J Natl Cancer Inst 1993; 85:241–242.
3. O'Brien TS, Smith K, Cranston D, Fuggle S, Bicknell R, Harris AL. Urinary basic fibroblast growth factor in patients with bladder cancer and benign prostatic hypertrophy. Br J Urol 1995; 76:311–314.
4. Chopin DK, Caruelle JP, Colombel M, Palcy S, Ravery V, Caruelle D, Abbou CC, Barritault D. Increased immunodetection of acidic fibroblast growth factor in bladder cancer, detectable in urine. J Urol 1993; 150:1126–1130.
5. Nguyen M, Watanabe H, Budson AE, Richie JP, Hayes DF, Folkman J. Elevated levels of an angiogenic peptide, basic fibroblast growth factor, in the urine of patients with a wide spectrum of cancers. J Natl Cancer Inst 1994; 86:356–361.
6. Dosquet C, Coudert MC, Lepage E, Cabane J, Richard F. Are angiogenic factors, cytokines, and soluble adhesion molecules prognostic factors in patients with renal cell carcinoma? Clin Cancer Res 1997; 3:2451–2458.
7. Landriscina M, Cassano A, Ratto C, Longo R, Ippoliti M, Palazzotti B, Crucitti F, Barone C. Quantitative analysis of basic fibroblast growth factor and vascular endothelial growth factor in human colorectal cancer. Br J Cancer 1998; 78:765–770.
8. Dirix LY, Vermeulen PB, Pawinski A, Prove A, Benoy I, De Pooter C, Martin M, Van Oosterom AT. Elevated levels of the angiogenic cytokines basic fibroblast growth factor and vascular endothelial growth factor in sera of cancer patients. Br J Cancer 1997; 76:238–243.
9. Dirix LY, Vermeulen PB, Hubens G, Benoy I, Martin M, De Pooter C, Van Oosterom AT. Serum basic fibroblast growth factor and vascular endothelial growth factor and tumour growth kinetics in advanced colorectal cancer. Ann Oncol 1996; 7: 843–848.

10. Hsu PI, Chow NH, Lai KH, Yang HB, Chan SH, Lin XZ, Cheng JS, Huang JS, Ger LP, Huang SM, Yen MY, Yang YF. Implications of serum basic fibroblast growth factor levels in chronic liver diseases and hepatocellular carcinoma. Anticancer Res 1997; 17:2803–2809.
11. Meyer GE, Yu E, Siegal JA, Petteway JC, Blumenstein BA, Brawer MK. Serum basic fibroblast growth factor in men with and without prostate carcinoma. Cancer 1995; 76:2304–2311.
12. Takahashi K, Mulliken JB, Kozakewich HP, Rogers RA, Folkman J, Ezekowitz RA. Cellular markers that distinguish the phases of hemangioma during infancy and childhood. J Clin Invest 1994; 93:2357–2364.
13. Enjolras O, Riche MC, Merland JJ, Escande JP. Management of alarming hemangiomas in infancy: a review of 25 cases. Pediatrics 1990; 85:491–498.
14. Chang E, Boyd A, Nelson CC, Crowley D, Law T, Keough KM, Folkman J, Ezekowitz RA, Castle VP. Successful treatment of infantile hemangiomas with interferon-alpha-2b. J Pediatr Hematol Oncol 1997; 19:237–244.
15. Ezekowitz RA, Mulliken JB, Folkman J. Interferon alfa-2a therapy for life-threatening hemangiomas of infancy. N Engl J Med 1992; 326:1456–1463.
16. Li VW, Folkerth RD, Watanabe H, Yu C, Rupnick M, Barnes P, Scott RM, Black PM, Sallan SE, Folkman J. Microvessel count and cerebrospinal fluid basic fibroblast growth factor in children with brain tumours. Lancet 1994; 344:82–86.
17. Colomer R, Aparicio J, Montero S, Guzman C, Larrodera L, Cortes-Funes H. Low levels of basic fibroblast growth factor (bFGF) are associated with a poor prognosis in human breast carcinoma. Br J Cancer 1997; 76:1215–1220.
18. Kraft A, Weindel K, Ochs A, Marth C, Zmija J, Schumacher P, Unger C, Marme D, Gastl G. Vascular endothelial growth factor in the sera and effusions of patients with malignant and nonmalignant disease. Cancer 1999; 85:178–187.
19. Mohle R, Green D, Moore MA, Nachman RL, Rafii S. Constitutive production and thrombin-induced release of vascular endothelial growth factor by human megakaryocytes and platelets. Proc Natl Acad Sci U S A 1997; 94:663–668.
20. Verheul HM, Hoekman K, Luykx-de BS, Eekman CA, Folman CC, Broxterman HJ, Pinedo HM. Platelet: transporter of vascular endothelial growth factor. Clin Cancer Res 1997; 3:2187–2190.
21. Pinedo HM, Verheul HM, D'Amato RJ, Folkman J. Involvement of platelets in tumour angiogenesis? Lancet 1998; 352:1775–1777.
22. Salven P, Manpaa H, Orpana A, Alitalo K, Joensuu H. Serum vascular endothelial growth factor is often elevated in disseminated cancer. Clin Cancer Res 1997; 3: 647–651.
23. Takigawa N, Segawa Y, Fujimoto N, Hotta K, Eguchi K. Elevated vascular endothelial growth factor levels in sera of patients with lung cancer. Anticancer Res 1998; 18:1251–1254.
24. Linder C, Linder S, Munck-Wikland E, Strander H. Independent expression of serum vascular endothelial growth factor (VEGF) and basic fibroblast growth factor (bFGF) in patients with carcinoma and sarcoma. Anticancer Res 1998; 18:2063–2068.
25. Viac J, Schmitt D, Claudy A. Circulating vascular endothelial growth factor (VEGF) is not a prognostic indicator in malignant melanoma. Cancer Lett 1998; 125:35–38.
26. Los M, Aarsman CJ, Terpstra L, Wittebol-Post D, Lips CJM, Blijham GH, Voest

EE. Elevated ocular levels of vascular endothelial growth factor in patients with von Hippel-Lindau disease. Ann Oncol 1997; 8:1015–1022.

27. Salven P, Teerenhovi L, Joensuu H. A high pretreatment serum vascular endothelial growth factor concentration is associated with poor outcome in non-Hodgkin's lymphoma. Blood 1997; 90:3167–3172.
28. Salven P, Ruotsalainen T, Mattson K, Joensuu H. High pre-treatment serum level of vascular endothelial growth factor (VEGF) is associated with poor outcome in small-cell lung cancer. Int J Cancer 1998; 79:144–146.
29. Tempfer C, Obermair A, Hefler L, Haeusler G, Gitsch G, Kainz C. Vascular endothelial growth factor serum concentrations in ovarian cancer. Obstet Gynecol 1998; 92: 360–363.
30. Yeo KT, Wang HH, Nagy JA, Sioussat TM, Ledbetter SR, Hoogewerf AJ, Zhou Y, Masse EM, Senger DR, Dvorak HF. Vascular permeability factor (vascular endothelial growth factor) in guinea pig and human tumor and inflammatory effusions. Cancer Res 1993; 53:2912–2918.
31. Nagy JA, Herzberg KT, Dvorak JM, Dvorak HF. Pathogenesis of malignant ascites formation: initiating events that lead to fluid accumulation. Cancer Res 1993; 53: 2631–2643.
32. Takano S, Yoshii Y, Kondo S, Suzuki H, Maruno T, Shirai S, Nose T. Concentration of vascular endothelial growth factor in the serum and tumor tissue of brain tumor patients. Cancer Res 1996; 56:2185–2190.
33. Crew JP, O'Brien T, Bicknell R, Fuggle S, Cranston D, Harris AL. Urinary vascular endothelial growth factor and its correlation with bladder cancer recurrence rates. J Urol 1999; 161:799–804.
34. Koch AE, Polverini PJ, Kunkel SL, Harlow LA, DiPietro LA, Elner VM, Elner SG, Strieter RM. Interleukin-8 as a macrophage-derived mediator of angiogenesis. Science 1992; 258:1798–1801.
35. Chambers AF, Matrisian LM. Changing views of the role of matrix metalloproteinases in metastasis. J Natl Cancer Inst 1997; 89:1260–1270.
36. Baker T, Tickle S, Wasan H, Docherty A, Isenberg D, Waxman J. Serum metalloproteinases and their inhibitors: markers for malignant potential. Br J Cancer 1994; 70: 506–512.
37. Zucker S, Lysik RM, Zarrabi MH, Moll U. M(r) 92,000 type IV collagenase is increased in plasma of patients with colon cancer and breast cancer. Cancer Res 1993; 53:140–146.
38. Gohji K, Fujimoto N, Fuji A, Komiyama T, Okawa J, Nakajima M. Prognostic significance of circulating matrix metalloproteinase-2 to tissue inhibitor of metalloproteinases-2 ratio in recurrence of urothelial cancer after complete resection. Cancer Res 1996; 56:3196–3198.
39. Gohji K, Fujimoto N, Ohkawa J, Fujii A, Nakajima M. Imbalance between serum matrix metalloproteinase-2 and its inhibitor as a predictor of recurrence of urothelial cancer. Br J Cancer 1998; 77:650–655.
40. Garzetti GG, Ciavattini A, Lucarini G, Goteri G, de, Garbisa S, Masiero L, Romanini C, Graziella B. Tissue and serum metalloproteinase (MMP-2) expression in advanced ovarian serous cystoadenocarcinomas: clinical and prognostic implications. Anticancer Res 1995; 15:2799–2804.

41. Moses MA, Wiederschain D, Loughlin KR, Zurakowski D, Lamb CC, Freeman MR. Increased incidence of matrix metalloproteinases in urine of cancer patients. Cancer Res 1998; 58:1395–1399.
42. Huber K, Kirchheimer JC, Sedlmayer A, Bell C, Ermler D, Binder BR. Clinical value of determination of urokinase-type plasminogen activator antigen in plasma for detection of colorectal cancer: comparison with circulating tumor-associated antigens CA 19-9 and carcinoembryonic antigen. Cancer Res 1993; 53:1788–1793.
43. Rahr HB, Sorensen JV, Larsen JF, Jensen FS, Bredahl C. Plasminogen activators and plasminogen activator inhibitor before and after surgery in patients with and without gastric malignancy. Haemostasis 1995; 25:248–256.
44. Strojan P, Budihna M, Smid L, Vrhovec I, Skrk J. Urokinase-type plasminogen activator (uPA) and plasminogen activator inhibitor type 1 (PAI-1) in tissue and serum of head and neck squamous cell carcinoma patients. Eur J Cancer 1998; 34: 1193–1197.
45. Casslen B, Bossmar T, Lecander I, Astedt B. Plasminogen activators and plasminogen activator inhibitors in blood and tumour fluids of patients with ovarian cancer. Eur J Cancer 1994; 30A:1302–1309.
46. Ho CH, Chao Y, Lee SD, Chau WK, Wu CW, Liu SM. Diagnostic and prognostic values of plasma levels of fibrinolytic markers in gastric cancer. Thromb Res 1998; 91:23–27.
47. Ronne E, Pappot H, Grondahl-Hansen J, Hoyer-Hansen G, Plesner T, Hansen NE, Dano K. The receptor for urokinase plasminogen activator is present in plasma from healthy donors and elevated in patients with paroxysmal nocturnal haemoglobinuria. Br J Haematol 1995; 89:576–581.
48. Pedersen N, Schmitt M, Ronne E, Nicoletti MI, Hoyer-Hansen G, Conese M, Giavazzi R, Dano K, Kuhn W, Janicke F. A ligand-free, soluble urokinase receptor is present in the ascitic fluid from patients with ovarian cancer. J Clin Invest 1993; 92:2160–2167.
49. Chambers SK, Gertz REJ, Ivins CM, Kacinski BM. The significance of urokinase-type plasminogen activator, its inhibitors, and its receptor in ascites of patients with epithelial ovarian cancer. Cancer 1995; 75:1627–1633.
50. Sier CF, Stephens R, Bizik J, Mariani A, Bassan M, Pedersen N, Frigerio L, Ferrari A, Dano K, Brunner N, Blasi F. The level of urokinase-type plasminogen activator receptor is increased in serum of ovarian cancer patients. Cancer Res 1998; 58:1843–1849.
51. Pappot H, Hoyer-Hansen G, Ronne E, Hansen HH, Brunner N, Dano K, Grondahl-Hansen J. Elevated plasma levels of urokinase plasminogen activator receptor in non-small cell lung cancer patients. Eur J Cancer 1997; 33:867–872.
52. Poppas DP, Pavlovich CP, Folkman J, Voest EE, Chen X, Luster AD, O'Donnell MA. Intravesical bacille Calmette-Guerin induces the antiangiogenic chemokine interferon-inducible protein 10. Urology 1998; 52:268–275.
53. Voest EE, Kenyon BM, O'Reilly MS, Truitt G, D'Amato RJ, Folkman J. Inhibition of angiogenesis in vivo by interleukin 12. J Natl Cancer Inst 1995; 87:581–586.
54. Arenberg DA, Kunkel SL, Polverini PJ, Morris SB, Burdick MD, Glass MC, Taub DT, Iannettoni MD, Whyte RI, Strieter RM. Interferon-gamma-inducible protein 10 (IP-10) is an angiostatic factor that inhibits human non-small cell lung cancer

(NSCLC) tumorigenesis and spontaneous metastases. J Exp Med 1996; 184:981–992.

55. Koch AE, Halloran MM, Haskell CJ, Shah MR, Polverini PJ. Angiogenesis mediated by soluble forms of E-selectin and vascular cell adhesion molecule-1. Nature 1995; 376:517–519.
56. Wittig BM, Kaulen H, Thees R, Schmitt C, Knolle P, Stock J, Meyer zum Buschenfelde KH, Dippold W. Elevated serum E-selectin in patients with liver metastases of colorectal cancer. Eur J Cancer 1996; 32A:1215–1218.

30

Perspectives in Vascular Cancer Therapy

An Introduction

Geert H. Blijham
University Medical Center Utrecht, Utrecht, The Netherlands

I. INTRODUCTION

For the first time in more than 100 years, cancer mortality is falling. Between 1990 and 1995 in the United States the age-adjusted mortality rate of cancer decreased from 135 to 129.8 per 10^5 inhabitants (1). It is expected that this decrease will continue at a rate of 1% to 2% per year. Similar observations have been made in some western European countries.

The decline in cancer mortality is not the result of a reduction in the overall cancer incidence, which has been stable during the last 10 years. The relative contribution of lung cancer, however, is decreasing and this accounts for part of the reduction in overall mortality. Of equal importance is the reduced case fatality rate or, in other words, improved survival once the tumor has occurred (2). A better relative survival has been found for a number of tumors, including breast cancer, which may be the result of early detection or better treatment (3, 4). The exact contribution of better treatment is difficult to determine, but it is most likely that aggressive treatment for some uncommon tumors and adjuvant treatment for two of the most common cancers (breast and large bowel) have their impact on cancer-related mortality.

Important as these findings may be, they cannot take away the notion that the improvements are small and that many patients with cancer are still bound to die of their disease. Moreover, in the last 10 to 15 years very few effective cytotoxic drugs have become available, as is evidenced by the fact that paclitaxel was the first drug registered for the treatment of breast cancer in the last 20 years. This picture has changed with the clinical development of new topoisomerase inhibitors and spindle poisons such as the camptothecins, taxanes, and vinorelbine (5–7). It remains to be determined, however, whether these new agents will change the cure rate of the most common malignancies.

Given the apparent difficulty of improving the efficacy of directly cytotoxic therapy, attention has been focused on other ways to control abnormal growth. Molecular biology begins to provide tools to interfere with the mechanisms underlying uncontrolled growth, such as abnormal expression of growth factor receptors, deregulated pathways of signal transduction or apoptosis, and changes in the cell-cycle clock apparatus (8, 9). Progress is also being made in the fields of vaccination with gene-modified cells, with monoclonal antibodies recruiting and activating effector molecules and cells in the tumor and with inhibitors of the degradation of the matrix surrounding tumor cells (10, 11).

One of the most exciting prospects, however, is the clinical application of the concept that tumor growth and size are critically dependent on the formation and presence of blood vessels. Therapies based on this concept are often called "antiangiogenic." Their common denominator is not the inhibition of angiogenesis but the fact that they have the tumor-associated vasculature as their target. The term "vascular cancer therapy" perhaps better describes this new modality of clinical oncology.

II. VASCULAR CANCER THERAPY

The growth and survival of tumors is dependent on the presence of blood vessels (12). For example liver metastases from colorectal cancer initially are supported by portal venous blood, but beyond a critical size they begin to develop their own vascular system fed by the hepatic artery. Based on this notion, possibly the oldest form of vascular cancer therapy was developed: embolization of the branches of the hepatic artery that are responsible for this blood supply (13). This treatment has been tested in the clinic and indeed leads to objective responses, albeit generally of short duration. In case of liver metastases from a carcinoid tumor, it is still applied in selected cases.

Since the days of these early vascular therapies, enormous progress has been made in the understanding of the mechanisms underlying the formation of new vessels in and around growing tumors (14). This had lead to attempts to use the specific characteristics of this process as targets for therapy. Most of these new approaches target the endothelial cells and try to inhibit their proliferation and migration, either directly or indirectly, by interfering with growth factors and their receptors or with the relevant interactions with the surrounding matrix (15). Vascular cancer therapy is broader than these forms of antiangiogenesis and includes all interventions that target the tumor-associated microcirculation as a means to improve or deliver antitumor therapy. A summary is given in Table 1; the three other domains of vascular cancer apart from antiangiogenesis therapy will be briefly described.

The vessel wall is the gatekeeper for the influx of immune effector cells. There is evidence that within the tumor, the endothelial cells have a deficient expression of adhesion molecules for these effector cells, thereby allowing the tumor to escape from host-derived attack (16). Vascular cancer therapy may try to restore or even augment the ability of endothelial cells to selectively let effective immune cells (lymphocytes, monocytes, granulocytes) pass the gate to the tumor microenvironment.

Epitopes, that are (almost) exclusively present on endothelial cells involved in active angiogenesis can be used to bind monoclonal antibodies. These antibodies can be engineered in such a way that upon binding, they activate effector mechanisms leading to the destruction of the tumor microcirculation, or even tumor cells (17). Effector mechanisms include the coagulation cascade, the conversion of prodrugs to very potent cytotoxic agents, toxins, and killer cells. In experimental models, the localized activation of the coagulation cascade has been successful in obtaining tumor destruction (18).

If endothelial cells are able to circulate and embark in areas of active angiogenesis, they could be ideal vehicles for the local delivery of therapy. One possibility is the use of genetically modified endothelial cells carrying suicide genes (19). After administration of the prodrug, the innocent bystander effect will lead to effective but localized destruction of surrounding cells, including tumor cells. Also endothelial cells genetically modified to express specific epitopes could be transfused, setting the stage for the application of the endothelial cell-targeted

Table 1 Domains of Vascular Cancer Therapy

1. ANTI-ANGIOGENESIS
   Inhibition or prevention of tumor-induced outgrowth of new blood vessels leading to reduced growth rate or dormancy.
2. REVERSAL OF ANERGY
   Reversal of endothelial cell anergy to express adhesion molecules upon appropriate stimuli, leading to more effective host defense mechanisms.
3. VASCULAR TARGETING
   Destruction of tumor by targeting of killing or obstructing effector mechanisms to the tumor microcirculation.
4. ADOPTIVE ENDOTHELIAL CELL TRANSFER
   Targeted delivery of antitumor therapy by using the influx of endothelial cells in areas of tumor-associated angiogenesis.

therapies described above. In animal experiments, the capability of transfused endothelial cells to selectively home and survive in areas of active angiogenesis has been demonstrated as a first step in the exploration of this exciting new therapeutic modality (20).

III. CLINICAL APPLICATIONS

Of the four domains of vascular cancer therapy described, the one dealing with the inhibition of angiogenesis (antiangiogenesis) is certainly closest to clinical application. Agents have been identified that inhibit endothelial cell growth factors (e.g., vascular endothelial growth factor [VEGF] antagonists), induce apoptosis (e.g., α √ β3 antagonists, tumor necrosis factor [TNF]), inhibit proliferation (e.g., taxanes, statins, TNP-470), or inhibit migration (e.g., metalloproteinase inhibitors) (21). These agents will affect active angiogenesis and leave mature vessels resulting from earlier angiogenesis unaffected. Their main clinical application as single agents probably does not lie in the induction of massive tumor kill, but in the prevention of further tumor growth. For patients this is particularly important if they are in a stage of minimal tumor load, possibly below the level of detection. This is also the situation in which antiangiogenic agents are most likely to counteract successfully the activity of the tumor-derived inducers of angiogenesis.

Clinical trials should thus focus on adjuvant treatments for patients with micrometastases after surgery and radiotherapy or with minimal residual disease after obtaining complete remission with chemotherapy. Such trials should be comparative from the start and their clinical endpoint should be progression-free survival. The biological goal is to achieve a state of dormancy with subclinical tumor nodules that may actively proliferate but have an equal rate of apoptosis as the result of antiangiogenic therapy. This requires long-term, continuous treatment and, as a corollary, nontoxic agents and easy delivery systems. With this perspective, we and others are exploring the development of antiangiogenic gene therapy.

In growing tumors, vascularity and oxygenation are heterogeneously distributed. Radiotherapy and chemotherapy are most effective in areas of good perfusion and high oxygen tension and with actively dividing cells. Active angiogenesis is induced by hypoxia and can be expected to occur in other areas of the tumor. As a consequence antiangiogenesis and antitumor therapy, be it chemotherapy or radiotherapy, may at least be additive.

Also, direct interactions between these treatment modalities can be hypothesized. Chemotherapy could add to antiangiogenesis, either by killing dividing endothelial cells or by acting at the level of endothelial progenitor cells in the marrow. Furthermore, tumor cell kill by antitumor therapy may change an area with good oxygenation and mature vessels into an area of poor vascularization and hypoxia and thereby stimulate new angiogenic outbursts. Finally, the cytokinetic changes following tumor cell kill also may contribute to increased angiogenic activity.

Chemotherapy and radiotherapy on one hand and antiangiogenic therapy on the other may therefore be synergistic rather than additive. This hypothesis should be tested in phase II and phase III studies of chemotherapy or radiotherapy with or without angiogenesis inhibitors in patients with measurable disease with tumor response as a primary endpoint.

The combination of angiogenesis inhibitors with immunotherapy should be explored. With adoptive cell transfer or vaccination with genetically modified cells, it has become possible to provide the patient with tumor-specific effector cells (10). Endothelial cell anergy, that is the inability to express adhesion molecules upon appropriate stimuli, may constitute a formidable obstacle for these cells to exert their activity at the site of the tumor (22). Antiangiogenic agents, even if not able to fully suppress angiogenesis because of excessive proangiogenic factors, may at least partially reverse this anergy and enhance specific as well as aspecific immunotherapy. Trials to test this concept should be done, both in patients with measurable tumors (with response as an endpoint) and in the aduvant situation (with progression-free survival as the endpoint).

IV. FUTURE PERSPECTIVES

Interventions in the domains of vascular targeting and adoptive endothelial cell therapy are further away from the bedside, but they are being actively pursued in preclinical models (18, 20). The phage-display technique to generate antibodies with unique specificities and the possibilities of engineering these antibodies for specific therapeutic purposes will greatly improve our abilities in vascular targeting. Methodology to isolate cells with specific endothelial phenotypes from the peripheral blood and the development of effective gene transfer technology will both be instrumental in bringing adoptive endothelial cell therapy to the clinic. With these developments in vascular cancer therapy, we will finally be in a position in which angiogenesis truly becomes the tumor's Achilles' heel: It is needed for growth and metastasis but is also the common pathway for interventions that lead to its destruction.

REFERENCES

1. Cole P, Rodu B. Declining cancer mortality in the United States. Cancer 1996; 78: 2045–2048.
2. Mettlin CJ. New evidence of progress in the National Cancer Program. Cancer 1996; 78:2043–2044.

3. Garne JP, Aspegren K, Balldin G, Ranstam J. Increasing incidence of and declining mortality from breast carcinoma. Cancer 1997; 79:69–74.
4. Quinn M, Allen E. Changes in incidence of and mortality from breast cancer in England and Wales since introduction of screening. BMJ 1995; 311:1391–1395.
5. Dancey J, Eisenhauer EA. Current perspectives on camptothecins in cancer treatment. Br J Cancer 1996; 74:327–328.
6. Gelmon K. The taxoids: paclitaxel and docetaxel. Lancet 1994; 344:1267–1272.
7. Pinedo HM, Van Groeningen CJ. Vinorelbine: a horse of a different color? J Clin Oncol 1994; 9:1745–1747.
8. Kohl NE, Mosser SD, deSolms SJ, et al. Selective inhibition of *ras*-dependent transformation by a farnesytransferase inhibitor. Science 1993; 260:1934.
9. Lowe SW, Bodis S, McClatchey A. p53 Status and efficacy of cancer therapy in vivo. Science 1994; 266:807.
10. Scott AM, Cebon J. Clinical promise of tumour immunology. Lancet 1997; 349(suppl 2):19–22.
11. Brown PD, Giavazzi R. Matrix metalloproteinase inhibition—a review of antitumour activity. Ann Oncol 1995; 6:967–974.
12. Folkman J. What is the evidence that tumours are angiogenesis dependent? J Natl Cancer Inst 1990; 82:4–6.
13. Mitty HA, Warner RRP, Newman LH, et al. Control of carcinoid syndrome with hepatic artery embolization. Radiology 1985; 155:623.
14. Varner JA, Cheresh DA. Tumor angiogenesis and the role of vascular cell integrin $\alpha v\beta 3$. In: De Vita VT, Helman S, Rosenberg SA, eds. Important Advances in Oncology. Philadelphia: Lippincott-Raven, 1996:69–87.
15. Folkman J. Clinical applications of research on angiogenesis. New Engl J Med 1995; 33:1757–1763.
16. Griffioen AW, Damen CA, Martinotti S, Blijham GH, Groenewegen G. Endothelial ICAM-1 expression is suppressed in human malignancies: role of angiogenic factors. Cancer Res 1996; 56:1111–1117.
17. Burrows FJ, Thorpe P. Eradatication of large solid tumours in mice with an immunotoxin direct against tumor vasculature. Proc. Natl Acad Sci U S A 1993; 90:8996–9000.
18. Huang X, Molema G, King S, Watkins L, Edgington TS, Thorpe PE. Tumor infarction in mice by antibody-directed targeting of tissue factor to tumor vasculature. Science 1997; 275:547–550.
19. Huber BE, Austin EA, Good SS. In vivo antitumor activity of 5-fluorocytosine on human colorectal carcinoma cells genetically modified to express cytosine deaminase. Cancer Res 1993; 53:4619–4626.
20. Ojeifo JO, Forugh R, Paik S. Angiogenesis-directed implantation of genetically modified endothelial cells in mice. Cancer Res 1995; 55:2240–2244.
21. Harris AL. Antiangiogenesis for cancer therapy. Lancet 1997; 349(suppl 2):13–15.
22. Griffioen AW, Damen CA, Blijham GH, Groenewegen G. Tumor angiogenesis is accompanied by a decreased inflammatory response of tumor associated endothelium. Blood 1996; 88:667–673.

31

The Combination of Antiangiogenic Therapy with Cytotoxic Therapy

A Systems Approach

Beverly A. Teicher
Lilly Research Laboratories, Indianapolis, Indiana

I. INTRODUCTION

Cancer cure requires eradication of all malignant cells. Cancer growth, however, requires proliferation of malignant cells and normal cells. The several anticancer treatment modalities currently available including surgery, chemotherapy, radiation therapy, and immunotherapy target primarily the malignant cell. Research over the past 35 years has reinforced the Folkman's hypothesis that without the proliferation of normal cells, especially endothelial cells, a tumor cannot grow beyond the size of a colony (1). The consequence of this finding is that both the normal and malignant cells involved in tumor growth, as well as the chemical and mechanical signaling pathways that interconnect them, are valid targets for therapeutic intervention. The integration of therapeutics directed toward the vascular components, extracellular matrix components, stromal and infiltrating cells with classic cytotoxic anticancer therapies may be regarded as a systems approach to cancer treatment (2).

Although new noncytotoxic agents directed toward normal cells and extracellular enzymatic activities target processes critical to tumor growth, it is highly unlikely that treatment with these new agents alone will lead to tumor cure. The question of how to integrate these new therapeutic agents into existing cancer treatment regimens arises. Thus, by choosing multiple cellular and process targets for therapeutic attack, a systems approach to anticancer therapy may lead to the cure of systemic malignant disease.

II. PRECLINICAL THERAPEUTIC STUDIES: SMALL MOLECULES

Several studies have been reported using the Lewis lung carcinoma growing subcutaneously in C57BL mice with standard cytotoxic anticancer therapies along with one or more new agents directed toward the normal cellular and extracellular compartments of the tumor (3–9). The Lewis lung tumor is relatively resistant to many cancer therapies, and because this tumor metastasizes avidly to the lungs from subcutaneous implants, it is a suitable model for both primary and metastatic disease.

The angiostatic activity of several steroids was discovered some years ago; however, the mechanism by which these steroids inhibit vessel growth or produce regression of growing vessels is only now being elucidated (10–13). The most effective angiostatic steroid discovered was tetrahydrocortisol, which lacks the 4, 5 double bond in its A ring, and, for this reason, lacks all of the known functions of cortisone.

In 1983, Folkman, et al. (14) reported that heparin or a heparin fragment administered in combination with cortisone angiogenesis in the Chorioallantoic membrane (CAM) assay and inhibited the growth of several solid murine tumors. The same group found that β-cyclodextrin tetradecasulfate in combination with hydrocortisone was 100 to 1000 times more effective than heparin in combination with hydrocortisone in inhibiting capillary formation in the CAM assay and in preventing neovascularization induced by endotoxin in the rabbit cornea (15).

For tumor growth delay studies, tetrahydrocortisol (THC) and 14-sulfated-β-cyclodextrin 14(SO_4)βCD were prepared in a 14-day osmotic pump and implanted subcutaneously in the animals on day 4 after tumor cell implantation, by which time neovascularization of the tumors has begun (16, 17). Administration of minocycline intraperitoneal daily was also initiated on day 4 after tumor cell implantation and continued until day 18. Neither the 14-day continuous infusion of THC/14(SO_4)βCD nor daily intramuscular injection of minocycline for 2 weeks altered the growth of the Lewis lung carcinoma (Table 1). The three modulators administered together (THC/14(SO_4)βCD/minocycline) produced a modest tumor growth delay of 1.2 days in the Lewis lung carcinoma. Single-agent chemotherapy or radiation therapy was administered to the tumor-bearing animals beginning on day 7 when the tumors were about 100 mm^3. Each treatment agent was administered at a standard dosage and schedule.

The combination of the three modulators (THC/14(SO_4)βCD and minocycline) was most effective at increasing the response of the Lewis lung tumor to these cytotoxic therapies (Table 1). The tumor growth delay produced by the antitumor alkylating agents were increased by about 5.8-fold, 3.9-fold, 3.8-fold, and 2.3-fold for *cis*-diamminedichloroplatinum (CDDP), melphalan, and single and multiple doses of cyclophosphamide, respectively. Five of the 12 animals

Table 1 Growth Delay of the Lewis Lung Tumor Produced by Various Anticancer Treatments Alone or in Combination with β-Cyclodextrin Tetradecasulfate/Tetrahydrocorfisol, Minocycline or the Combination of Modulators

		Tumor growth delay, days[b]			
Treatment group	Dose[a]	Alone	+14(SO_4)βCD/THC	+Minocycline	+14(SO_4)βCD/THC/Mino
14(SO_4)βCD/THC	1000 mg/kg/125 mg/kg over 14 days		0.6 ± 0.3		
Minocycline	14 × 5 mg/kg		0.6 ± 0.3		
14(SO_4)βCD/THC/Mino	-as above-		1.2 ± 0.4		
CDDP	1 × 10 mg/kg	4.5 ± 0.3	2.2 ± 0.3	5.0 ± 0.3	26.2 ± 2.5
Melphalan	1 × 10 mg/kg	2.7 ± 0.3	1.1 ± 0.3	4.3 ± 0.3	10.5 ± 0.9
Cyclophosphamide	1 × 150 mg/kg	7.2 ± 0.4	16.2 ± 1.2	24.7 ± 2.7	27.6 ± 2.8
	3 × 150 mg/kg	21.5 ± 1.7	36.8 ± 3.4	45.2 ± 2.9[c]	48.8 ± 3.3[d]
Radiation	1 × 20 Gy	6.2 ± 0.5	8.3 ± 0.5	11.9 ± 1.4	13.8 ± 1.3
	5 × 3 Gy	4.4 ± 0.3	7.1 ± 0.7	7.8 ± 0.6	12.6 ± 1.2
Adriamycin	5 × 1.75 mg/kg	7.0 ± 0.6	—	9.8 ± 0.8	11.7 ± 1.2
Bleomycin	4 × 10 mg/kg	8.5 ± 0.6	—	12.0 ± 1.2	12.9 ± 1.3

[a] β-Cyclodextrin tetradecasulfate (1000 mg/kg) and tetrahydrocortisol (125 mg/kg) were administered in a 1.1 molar ratio by continuous infusion over 14 days in an Alzet osmotic pump from days 4–18 after tumor implant. Minocycline (5 mg/kg) was administered intraperitoneally on days 4–18 after tumor implant, *cis*-diammines dichlorplatinum (10 mg/kg), melphalan (10 mg/kg), and cyclophosphamide (150 mg/kg) were administered intraperitoneally on day 7 after tumor implant. Cyclophosphamide (150 mg/kg) was also administered on days 7, 9, and 11 after tumor implant. Radiation was delivered locally to the tumor-bearing limb as 20 Gy on day 7 or 3 Gy daily on days 7–11. Adriamycin (1.75 mg/kg) was administered intraperitoneally daily on days 7–11. Bleomycin (10 mg/kg) was administered intraperitoneally on days 6, 10, 13, and 16.

[b] Tumor growth delay is the difference in days for treated tumors to reach 500 mm^3 compared with untreated control tumors. Untreated control tumors reach 500 mm^3 in about 14 days. Mean of 15 animals ± SE.

[c] Four animals out of 12 were long-term survivors (> 120 days).

[d] Five animals out of 12 were long-term survivors (> 120 days).

were treated with the three-modulator combination and multiple doses of cyclophosphamide, respectively. Five of 12 of the animals treated with the three-modulator combination and multiple doses of cyclophosphamide were long-term survivors. The tumor growth delays produced by single-dose and multiple- dose radiation therapy were increased about 2.2-fold and 2.8-fold, respectively, in the presence of the three-modulator combination. The increases in tumor growth delay observed with adriamycin and bleomycin with the addition of the three modulators to the regimen were about 1.7-fold and 1.5-fold compared with the antitumor agents alone.

Untreated control animals bearing the Lewis lung tumors survived 21 to 25 days after tumor implantation and succumbed to disease metastatic to the lungs. The number and size of lung metastases in untreated and treated animals were scored on day 20 after tumor implant (Table 2). Treatment with THC/14(SO_4)βCD by continuous infusion from day 4 through day 18 after tumor implant did not alter the number of lung metastases nor the percent of large metastases observed in these animals. Treatment with minocycline or with the three-modulator combination (THC/14(SO_4)βCD/minocycline) over the same period had little effect on total number of metastases; however, only 40% to 50% of the metastases were large compared with about 70% in the untreated control animals. The cytotoxic antitumor treatments reduced the number of lung metastases in many cases to about one half the number observed in the untreated control animals. Treatment with THC/14(SO_4)βCD did not alter the lung metastases produced in animals treated with CDDP, melphalan, cyclophosphamide, or radiation therapy. The combination of minocycline with these cytotoxic therapies did not alter the number of lung metastases produced in animals treated with CDDP, melphalan, adriamycin, bleomycin, or radiation therapy; however, in animals treated with cyclophosphamide and minocycline, the number of lung metastases was reduced to 50% and 14% of those treated with single dose or multiple cyclophosphamide alone. The three-modulator combination (THC/14(SO_4)βCD and minocycline) along with the cytotoxic therapies was more effective against metastatic disease except when the cytotoxic therapy was radiation therapy to the primary tumor. In most cases, the number of lung metastases was reduced to about 50% of the number observed with the cytotoxic therapy alone, and the number of large metastases was 40% to 50% of those. The lowest number of large metastases was found in animals treated with cyclophosphamide and minocycline or the three-modulator combinations; in fact with multiple doses of cyclophosphamide in combination with minocycline, there were no large lung metastases present on day 20.

TNP-470, a synthetic derivative of fumagillin, an antibiotic with little antibacterial or antifungal activity but marked amebicidal activity (18, 19), is a potent inhibitor of endothelial cell migration (20), endothelial cell proliferation (21), and capillary tube formation (22). TNP-470 also inhibits angiogenesis, as demon-

Table 2 Numbers of Lung Metastases on Day 20 from Subcutaneous Lewis Lung Tumors After Various Anticancer Treatments or in Combination with β-Cyclodextrin Tetradecasulfate/Tetrahydrocortisol, Minocycline, or the Combination of Modulators

		Mean number of lung metastases (Number and % of vascularized metastases)[a]			
Treatment group	Dose[b]	Alone	$+14(SO_4)\beta CD/THC$	+Minocycline	$+14(SO_4)\beta CD/THC/Mino$
Untreated Controls		15 (10; 66%)			
$14(SO_4)\beta CD/THC$	1000 mg/kg/125 mg/kg over 14 days		14.5 (10; 69%)		
Minocycline	14 × 5 mg/kg			12 (5; 43%)	
$14(SO_4)\beta CD/$ THC/ Mino	-as above-				13 (6; 46%)
cis-diamminedichloro-platinum (CDDP)	1 × 10 mg/kg	12	15 (10: 67%)	10.5 (5; 48%)	6 (2.5; 39%)
Melphalan	1 × 10 mg/kg	8	8 (4; 48%)	6 (3; 50%)	5 (2.5; 47%)
Cyclophosphamide	1 × 150 mg/kg	6.5	6 (2; 32%)	3 (1; 33%)	4 (2; 44%)
	3 × 150 mg/kg	3.5	3 (0.5; 16%)	0.5 (0; 18%)	0.5 (0; 20%)
Radiation	1 × 20 Gy	8	7 (3; 40%)	8 (1; 25%)	7 (3; 46%)
	5 × 3 Gy	7	7 (2.5; 35%)	6.5 (2; 30%)	7 (3; 47%)
Adriamycin	5 × 1.75 mg/kg	8	—	7.5 (5; 63%)	5 (3; 57%)
Bleomycin	4 × 10 mg/kg	7	—	7 (4.5; 64%)	4 (2; 45%)

[a] The number of external lung metastases on day 20 after tumor implant were counted manually and scored as ≥ 3 mm^3 in diameter. The data are shown as the means from 6–12 pairs of lungs. Parentheses indicated the number of large (vascularized) metastases and percentage of the total number of metastases that were large.

[b] The schedules of drug administration were as shown under Table 1.

strated in chick CAM, the rabbit and rodent cornea (22). TNP-470 inhibits the growth of primary and metastatic murine tumors as well as human tumor xenografts (23–31). When administered to animals bearing the Lewis lung carcinoma subcutaneously on alternate days beginning on day 4 and continuing until day 18, TNP-470 was a moderately effective modulator of the cytotoxic therapies (Table 3). TNP-470 was most effective with melphalan, 1,3-bis(2-chloroethyl)-1-nitrosurea (BCNU), and radiation, increasing the tumor growth delay produced by these treatments 1.8- to 2.4-fold. TNP-470 administered with minocycline intraperitoneally daily on days 4–18 comprised a highly effective antiangiogenic agent combination. The increases in tumor growth delay produced by the modulator combination of TNP-470 and minocycline along with the cytotoxic therapies ranged from 2- to 4-fold. In the treatment group receiving TNP-470/minocycline and cyclophosphamide, approximately 40% of the animals were long-term survivors (>120 days). Each of the cytotoxic therapies (including radiation, which was delivered locally to the tumor-bearing limb) produced a reduction in the number of lung metastases found on day 20 (Table 4). Neither TNP-470, minocycline, nor the combination of antiangiogenic agents altered the number of lung metastases or the percentage of large (vascularized) lung metastases on day 20. The modulators did not alter the number of lung metastases from those obtained with the cytotoxic therapies, except in the case of cyclophosphamide, in which many animals treated with the drug and antiangiogenic agent combination had very few metastases on day 20, and most of those were very small.

The efficacy of the modulator combination of TNP-470/minocycline against the primary Lewis lung tumors is compared with that of other potential antiangiogenic modulator combinations in Table 5. The most effective combination with CDDP was $14(SO_4)\beta CD$/THC/minocycline, whereas with the other cytotoxic therapies each of the three antiangiogenic agent combinations were almost equally effective. Each of the three antiangiogenic agent combinations along with cyclophosphamide were highly effective, resulting in 40% to 50% long-term survivors. None of the antiangiogenic agent combinations alone was effective against metastatic disease, although in each case the percent of large metastases on day 20 was reduced (Table 6). There was a trend toward the combination of $14(SO_4)\beta CD$/THC/minocycline being the most effective antiangiogenic agents of cytotoxic therapies against metastatic disease.

In the data presented in Tables 3–6, antiangiogenic agent treatment was begun on day 4 when the primary tumor was palpable and continued through day 18 when the tumor had ''fully matured'' (16, 17). To determine the efficacy of the modulator combination against established disease, TNP-470 and minocycline were administered on different schedules, whereas the cytotoxic treatments remained as previously described (Table 7). The antiangiogenic agent administration schedule (days 4–11) began when the tumors were palpable and extended through the cytotoxic treatments; the second antiangiogenic agent schedule (days

Table 3 Growth Delay of the Lewis Lung Tumor Produced by Various Anticancer Treatments Alone or in Combination with Potential Antiangiogenic Modulators

Treatment group	Tumor growth delay, days[a]			
	Alone	+Minocycline[b]	+TNP-470	+TNP-470/MINO
—	—	1.2 ± 0.4	2.1 ± 0.4	1.8 ± 0.4
cis-diamminedichloro platinum (CDDP) (10 mg/kg)	4.5 ± 0.3	5.0 ± 0.3	6.0 ± 0.5	10.9 ± 0.8
Cyclophosphamide (3 × 150 mg/kg)	21.5 ± 1.7	32.4 ± 1.8	25.3 ± 2.2	44.8 ± 2.8[c]
Melphalan (10 mg/kg)	2.7 ± 0.3	4.3 ± 0.3	6.0 ± 0.5	8.5 ± 0.6
1,3-bis(a-chloroethyl)-1-nitrosurea (BCNU) (3 × 15 mg/kg)	3.6 ± 0.4	5.2 ± 0.4	6.3 ± 0.5	14.6 ± 1.0
X-rays (5 × 3 Gray)	4.4 ± 0.3	7.8 ± 0.6	10.6 ± 1.1	15.3 ± 1.2

[a] Tumor growth delay is the difference in days for treated tumors to reach 500 mm^3 compared with untreated control tumors. Untreated control tumors reach 500 mm^3 in about 14 days. Mean ± SE of 15 animals.

[b] Minocycline (10 mg/kg) was administered intraperitoneally daily on days 4–18; TNP-470 (30 mg/kg) was administered subcutaneously on alternate days for eight injections beginning on day 4; CDDP and melphalan were administered intraperitoneally on day 7. Cyclophosphamide and BCNU were administered intraperitoneally on days 7, 9, and 11. X-rays were delivered daily on days 7–11 locally to the tumor-bearing limb.

[c] Five of 12 long-term survivors (>180 days).

Table 4 Number of Lung Metastases on Day 20 from Subcutaneous Lewis Lung Tumors After Various Anticancer Therapies Alone or in Combination with Potential Antiangiogenic Modulators

Treatment group	Mean number of lung metastases (% large)			
	Alone	+ Minocycline	+ TNP-470	+ TNP-470/MINO
—	20 (62)	20 (50)	21 (51)	18 (54)
(CDDP) (10 mg/kg)	13 (58)	11 (48)	14.5 (34)	14 (50)
Cyclophosphamide (3 × 150 mg/kg)	12 (40)	6 (33)	6 (30)	2 (25)
Melphalan (10 mg/kg)	13 (48)	11 (50)	15 (47)	15 (45)
(BCNU) (3 × 15 mg/kg)	16 (53)	15 (38)	15.5 (45)	13 (38)
X-rays (5 × 3 Gray)	15 (40)	13 (30)	10 (40)	12 (42)

Abbreviations: *CDDP*, *cis*-diamminedichloroplatinum; *BCNU*, 1,3-bis(2-chloroethyl)-1-nitrosurea.

Table 5 Growth Delay of the Lewis Lung Tumor Produced by Various Anticancer Treatments Alone or in Combination with Potential Antiangiogenic Modulators

Treatment group	Tumor growth delay, days			
	Alone	+14(SO_4)βCD/THC/MINO	+14(SO_4)βCD/THC/TNP-470	+MINO/TNP-470
—	—	1.2 ± 0.4	1.5 ± 0.3	1.8 ± 0.4
CDDP (10 mg/kg)	4.5 ± 0.3	26.2 ± 2.5	10.6 ± 0.7	10.9 ± 0.8
Cyclophosphamide (3 × 150 mg/kg)	21.5 ± 1.7	48.8 ± 3.3 (5/12)[a]	49.2 ± 3.4 (6/12)[a]	44.8 ± 2.8 (5/12)[a]
Melphalan (10 mg/kg)	2.7 ± 0.3	10.5 ± 0.9	12.2 ± 1.4	8.5 ± 0.6
BCNU (3 × 15 mg/kg)	3.6 ± 0.4	9.8 ± 0.8	10.6 ± 1.1	14.6 ± 1.0
X-rays (5 × 3 Gy)	4.4 ± 0.3	12.6 ± 1.2	10.3 ± 0.9	15.3 ± 1.2

[a] Lived a normal lifespan (~2 years).

Abbreviations: *CDDP*, *cis*-diamminechloroplatinum; *BCNU*, 1,3-bis(2-chloroethyl)-1-nitrosurea.

Table 6 Number of Lung Metastases on Day 20 from Subcutaneous Lewis Lung Tumors After Various Anticancer Therapies Alone or in Combination with Potential Antiangiogenic Modulators

Treatment group	Mean number of lung metastases (% large)			
	Alone	+ $14(SO_4)\beta CD$/THC/MINO	+ $14(SO_4)\beta CD$/THC/TNP-470	+ MINO/TNP-470
—	20 (62)	17 (46)	18 (50)	18 (54)
CDDP (10 mg/kg)	13 (58)	8 (42)	15 (40)	14 (50)
Cyclophosphamide (3 × 150 mg/kg)	12 (40)	1 (0)	2 (50)	2 (25)
Melphalan (10 mg/kg)	13 (48)	7 (50)	15 (40)	15 (45)
BCNU (3 × 15 mg/kg)	16 (53)	14 (45)	14 (43)	13 (58)
X-rays (5 × 3 Gy)	15 (40)	9 (43)	11 (36)	12 (42)

Abbreviations: *CDDP*, *cis*-diamminechloroplatinum; *BCNU*, 1,3-bis(2-chloroethyl)-1-nitrosurea.

Table 7 Growth Delay of the Lewis Lung Tumor Produced by Various Anticancer Treatments Alone or in Combination with TNP-470 and Minocycline Administered on Various Schedules

Treatment group	Tumor growth delay, days TNP-1470 +Minocycline				
	Alone	Days 4–11	Days 7–11	Days 7–18	Days 4–18
—	—	1.4 ± 0.3	0.6 ± 0.3	0.9 ± 0.3	1.8 ± 0.4
Cyclophosphamide (3 × 150 mg/kg)	21.5 ± 1.7	37.1 ± 2.7	28.8 ± 2.4	32.1 ± 2.9	44.8 ± 2.8
BCNU (3 × 15 mg/kg)	3.6 ± 0.4	11.8 ± 1.4	10.4 ± 1.7	10.6 ± 1.5	14.6 ± 1.6
X-rays (5 × 3 Gy)	4.4 ± 0.3	10.4 ± 1.6	6.6 ± 1.2	6.7 ± 1.0	15.3 ± 1.7

Abbreviation: *BCNU*, 1,3-bis(2-chloroethyl)-1-nitrosurea.

7–11) allowed modulator administration during the same period as the cytotoxic therapies and the third antiangiogenic agent schedule (days 7–11) allowed initiation of modulator administration at the same time as initiation of the cytotoxic therapy and extended the modulators for 1 week after completion of the cytotoxic therapies. As would be expected, the most effective therapies were those begun on day 4 when the tumor burden was smallest. However, both the day 7–11 and day 7–18 modulator treatment schedule resulted in enhanced tumor growth delays compared with the cytotoxic therapies alone. In combination with cyclophosphamide, the antiangiogenic agent schedules beginning on day 4 resulted in 1.7- and 2.1-fold increased tumor growth delay and the antiangiogenic agent schedules beginning on day 7 resulted in 1.3- and 1.5-fold increased tumor growth delay compared with cyclophosphamide alone. On days 7, 9, and 11 BCNU along with the antiangiogenic agent schedules beginning on day 4 produced 3.3- and fourfold increases in tumor growth delay, whereas the antiangiogenic agent schedules beginning on day 7 produced a 2.9-fold increase in tumor growth delay. Finally, the antiangiogenic agent schedules beginning on day 4 resulted in 2.4- and 3.5-fold increases in tumor growth delay, whereas the antiangiogenic agent schedules beginning on day 7 resulted in a 1.5-fold increase in tumor growth delay. Varying the modulator administration schedules did not appear to affect response of the metastatic disease to the therapies (Table 8). Only in the case of cyclophosphamide was it evident that beginning the antiangiogenic agent administration on day 7 led to decreased efficacy of the therapy against metastatic disease.

A high soy food consumption has been suggested as a factor in the lower incidence of certain human cancers in Asians than in others (32–34). Genistein, a principal isoflavone in soybeans, is a potent inhibitor of the activity of tyrosine protein kinases such as epidermal growth factor receptors (35). Tyrosine phosphorylation is important in cell proliferation and transformation (36). Genistein specifically inhibits growth of *ras* oncogene-transfected NIH 3T3 cells (37) and diminishes the platelet-derived growth factor-induced c-*fos* and c-*jun* expression in CH310T1/2 fibroblasts. Genistein inhibited endothelial cell proliferation and in vitro angiogenesis at concentrations giving half-maximal inhibition at 5 and 150 μM, respectively (38). Suramin, which like heparin is a polysulfonated molecule, interferes with binding of many growth factors, including basic fibroblast growth factor (bFGF), to their receptors. Suramin is an inhibitor of angiogenesis, a suppressor of endothelial cell growth and migration (39–42). Elegant studies by Takano et al. (43) showed that suramin inhibited multiple control points of angiogenesis including those stimulated by b-FGF.

In tumor growth delay studies, genistein had some activity as a single agent, whereas suramin did not have a significant antitumor effect (Table 9). Two cytotoxic anticancer drugs, cyclophosphamide and adriamycin, were selected for the initial comparison of the potential of the various antiangiogenic treatments within a therapeutic regimen. Suramin and TNP-470/genistein were effective in increas-

Table 8 Number of Lung Metastases on Day 20 from Subcutaneous Lewis Lung Tumors After Various Anticancer Therapies Alone or in Combination with TNP-470 and Minocycline Administered on Various Schedules

	Mean number of lung metastases (% Large) TNP-470 + Minocycline				
Treatment group	Alone	Days 4–11	Days 7–11	Days 7–18	Days 4–18
—	20 (62)	17 (57)	20 (52)	20 (48)	18 (54)
Cyclophosphamide (3 × 150 mg/kg)	12 (40)	2 (25)	4 (18)	4 (28)	2 (25)
BCNU (3 × 15 mg/kg)	16 (53)	17 (41)	12 (42)	14 (25)	15 (45)
X-rays (5 × 3 Gy)	15 (40)	15 (38)	17 (34)	15 (38)	12 (42)

Abbreviation: *BCNU*, 1,3-bis(2-chloroethyl)-1-nitrosurea.

Table 9 Growth Delay of the Lewis Lung Tumor Produced by Potential Antiangiogenic Agents Alone or Along with a Standard Regimen of Cyclophosphamide or Adriamycin

	Tumor growth delay, days[a]		
Treatment group	Alone	+Cyclophosphamide[b]	+ Adriamycin
—	—	19.3 ± 1.7	5.3 ± 0.4
Suramin (20 mg/kg × 14)[c]	1.4 ± 0.3	31.5 ± 2.7[e]	6.6 ± 0.7
Genistein (100 mg/kg × 14)	2.4 ± 0.4[d]	23.5 ± 1.8	6.0 ± 0.6
TNP-470/Suramin	0.4 ± 0.3	25.7 ± 2.5[d]	6.6 ± 0.7
TNP-470/Genistein	1.9 ± 0.3	36.1 ± 2.8[e]	9.8 ± 1.1[e]
Mino/Suramin	0.5 ± 0.3	21.2 ± 1.8	6.6 ± 0.5
Mino/Genistein	2.4 ± 0.4[d]	21.3 ± 1.9	9.1 ± 0.9[d]
Suramin/Genistein	1.2 ± 0.3	19.6 ± 1.8	7.4 ± 0.5

[a] Tumor growth delay is the difference in days for treated tumors to reach 500 mm^3 compared with untreated control tumors. Untreated control tumors reach 500 mm^3 in about 14 days. Mean ± SE of 15 animals.

[b] Cyclophosphamide (150 mg/kg) was administered by intraperitoneal injection on days 7, 9, and 11 after tumor cell implantation. Adriamycin (1.75 mg/kg) was administered by intraperitoneal injection daily on days 7 through 11.

[c] Minocycline (10 mg/kg), suramin (20 mg/kg), and genistein (100 mg/kg) were administered intraperitoneally daily on days 4 to 18. TNP-470 (30 mg/kg) was administered subcutaneously on alternate days for eight injections, beginning on day 4.

[d] Significant tumor growth delay compared with untreated control or significantly increased tumor growth delay compared to cyclophosphamide or adriamycin; $P < 0.01$.

[e] $P < 0.005$.

Table 10 Number of Lung Metastases on Day 20 from Subcutaneous Lewis Lung Tumors Produced by Potential Antiangiogenic Agents Alone or Along with a Standard Regimen of Cyclophosphamide or Adriamycin

	Mean number of lung metastases (% large)		
Treatment group	Alone	+ Cyclophosphamide	+ Adriamycin
—	21 (63)	12 (40)	18 (39)
Suramin (20 mg/kg × 14)	19 (47)	5 (33)	15 (38)
Genistein (100 mg/kg × 14)	22 (41)	10 (29)	15 (40)
TNP-470/Suramin	23 (43)	7 (27)	14 (45)
TNP-470/Genistein	21 (60)	11.5 (33)	22 (49)
Mino/Suramin	21 (47)	9 (23)	16 (52)
Mino/Genistein	19 (53)	12 (35)	22 (32)
Suramin/Genistein	21 (54)	12 (40)	15 (40)

ing the tumor growth delay produced by cyclophosphamide. TNP-470/genistein and minocycline/genistein were effective in increasing the tumor growth delay produced by adriamycin.

None of the potential antiangiogenic agents, single or in two-agent combinations, reduced the number of lung metastases on day 20 in animals implanted subcutaneously with the Lewis lung tumor (Table 10). However, genistein significantly decreased the percent of large lung metastases (> 3 mm in diameter) potentially vascularized on day 20. Cyclophosphamide treatment decreased the number and percent of large lung metastases on day 20 from that in untreated controls. Suramin administered along with cyclophosphamide further decreased the number and percent of large lung metastases from treatment with cyclophosphamide. TNP-470/suramin produced significant decreases in the number of lung

Table 11 The Number of Intratumoral Blood Vessels as Determined by Immunohistochemistry in Lewis Lung Carcinoma Tumors After Treatment of the Animals with Various Potential Antiangiogenic Agents[a]

	1st exp.	2nd exp.	3rd exp.	Means ± SD
CD31				
Control	31.4	59.3	97.0	62.6 ± 39.6
TNP-470[b]	9.2	21.9	21.9	17.7 ± 14.6
TNP/Mino	7.6	39.7	33.7	27.0 ± 25.3
Suramin	11.0	23.2	41.2	25.1 ± 17.9
TNP/Suram	6.0	8.3	52.2	22.2 ± 28.6
Genistein	20.4	18.4	53.8	30.9 ± 21.8
TNP/Genistein	16.6	13.5	33.4	21.2 ± 15.5
Factor VIII				
Control	13.4	11.6	19.2	14.7 ± 6.9
TNP-470	3.5	7.1	7.1	5.9 ± 6.0
TNP/Mino	8.2	7.1	3.8	6.4 ± 4.9
Suramin	3.6	7.1	6.6	5.8 ± 4.0
TNP/Suram	6.2	5.3	7.9	6.5 ± 4.9
Genistein	12.9	9.5	6.1	9.5 ± 6.3
TNP/Genistein	6.9	4.0	9.9	6.9 ± 6.0

[a] Tumor tissue sections from paraffin-embedded blocks were deparaffinized and stained with monoclonal mouse antihuman endothelial cell antibody (CD31, DAKO Corp., Carpinteria, CA) or monoclonal mouse antihuman von Willebrand factor (Cell Biology, Boehringer, Mannheim) using Avidin-biotin complex (ABC) method (DAKO LSAB Kit, DAKO Corp., Carpinteria, CA). For the counting of blood vessels, the most vascular area of the tumor was located at low magnification, and vessels were counted on ten 200× fields. Data are the means of 10 high power fields at ×200.

[b] TNP-470 (30 mg/kg) was administered subcutaneously on alternate days—days 4 through 10. Minocycline (10 mg/kg), suramin (20 mg/kg), and genistein (100 mg/kg) were administered intraperitoneally, daily on days 4 through 10.

metastases when administered along with cyclophosphamide compared with cyclophosphamide alone. Treatment of the Lewis lung tumor-bearing animals with adriamycin as a single agent did not decrease the number of lung metastases on day 20 but did decrease the percent of lung metastases large enough to be vascularized on day 20 compared with untreated control animals (Table 10).

The number of intratumoral vessels in the Lewis lung carcinoma was determined by immunohistochemical staining with anti-CD31 or anti-factor VIII after treatment of the tumor-bearing animals with various potential antiangiogenic agents on days 4 through 10 after tumor cell implantation (Table 11). Each of the potential antiangiogenic therapies decreased the number of stainable intratumoral vessels to one half to one third of the number in the untreated control tumors. This effect was evident with both of the immunohistochemical stains. These data indicate that there are fewer stainable endothelial cells in the tumors of the animals treated with the potential antiangiogenic therapies, however, they do not address the issue of tumor blood flow or permeability.

III. MECHANISM(S) OF INTERACTION: TNP-470/ MINOCYCLINE

The antiangiogenic combination of TNP-470 and minocycline administered for 2 weeks did not alter the growth of the Lewis lung carcinoma, the EMT-6 mammary carcinoma, the 9L gliosarcoma or the FSaII fibrosarcoma (3, 4, 6, 8, 44–46). However, when TNP-470 and minocycline were added to treatment with cytotoxic anticancer therapies, tumor response was significantly increased. When C3H mice bearing the FSaIIC fibrosarcoma were treated with TNP-470/minocycline for 5 days before I.V. injection of the fluorescent dye Hoechst 33342, there was a shift toward greater brightness of the entire tumor cell population, so that the 10% brightest and the 20% dimmest cell subpopulations were composed of cells containing much more dye than the same subpopulations in the control tumor (Fig. 1) (3). The TNP-470/minocycline-treated tumors were more easily penetrated by the lipophilic dye (3). This was the first indication that TNP-470 and minocycline treatment might allow greater distribution of small molecules into tumors. To determine if TNP-470/minocycline affected cyclophosphamide tissue distribution, animals were injected intraperitoneally with [^{14}C]-cyclophosphamide (300 mg/kg) on day 8, then killed 6 hours later. Tissue levels of ^{14}C were determined (Fig. 2). An increased level of ^{14}C was noted in all of the tissues from TNP-470/minocycline-treated animals, except blood, compared with [^{14}C]-cyclophosphamide-only treated animals. The largest increases were: 2.6-fold in the tumor, 2.3-fold in the kidney, 3.2-fold in the heart, 5.6-fold in the gut, and 7.9-fold in skeletal muscle (4).

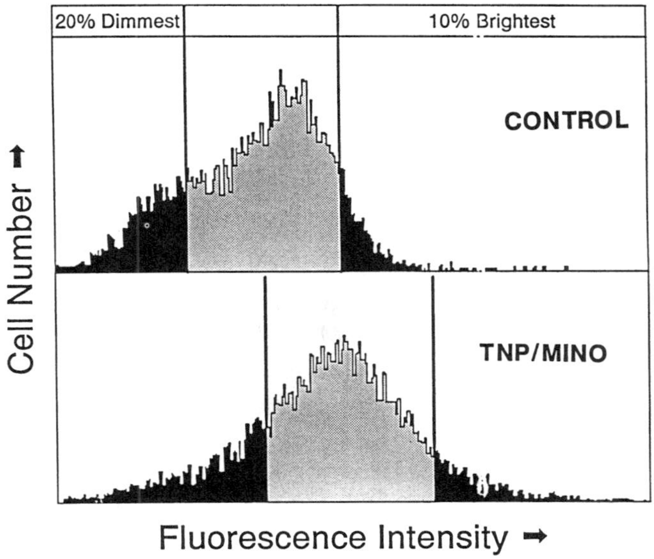

Figure 1 Fluorescence distribution in FSaIIC tumor cells after intravenous injection of tumor-bearing animals with Hoechst 33342 (2 mg/kg). The data shown are for an untreated control tumor and a tumor treated with TNP-470 (3 × 30 mg/kg, subcutaneously) and minocycline (5 × 10 mg/kg, intraperitoneally).

In a similar study, Lewis lung tumor-bearing mice, either pretreated with TNP-470/minocycline or untreated, were injected intraperitoneally with a single dose of CDDP (20 mg/kg) on day 8, then killed 6 hours later, and tissue levels of platinum (Pt) were determined (Fig. 3). There were increased levels of Pt in all of the tissues taken from animals treated with TNP-470/minocycline, except blood, compared with animals that were not pretreated. The largest increases were: 5.2-fold in the tumor, 3.8-fold in the gut, 3.0-fold in the skin, and 2.5-fold in the skeletal muscle (4).

Both cyclophosphamide (CTX) and CDDP are cytotoxic through formation of cross-links in cellular DNA. The DNA alkaline elution from tumors treated in vivo showed that there was increasing DNA cross-linking with increasing dose of CTX (Table 12). Treatment with CTX (300 mg/kg) alone resulted in a cross-linking factor of 4.7, whereas treatment with the same dose of CTX in animals pretreated with TNP-470/minocycline resulted in a cross-linking factor of 6.2, which extrapolates in equivalency to about 650 mg/kg of CTX. Increased DNA cross-linking also was detected with an increasing dose of CDDP. Treatment

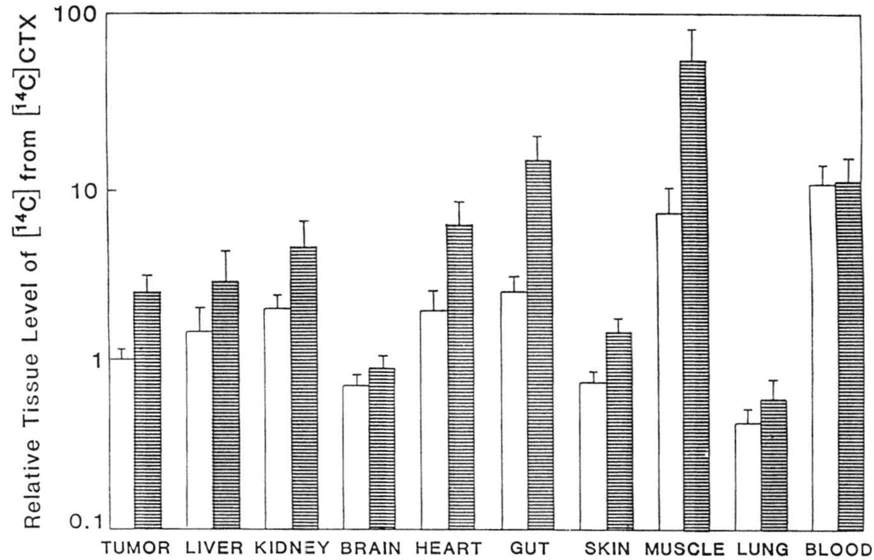

Figure 2 Relative tissue levels of ^{14}C from [^{14}C]-CTX in C57BL mice bearing Lewis lung tumors subcutaneously in the hind leg 6 hours after intraperitoneal injection of 300 mg/kg of the drug alone on day 8 (*open bar*) or after administration of the drug to animals treated with TNP-470 (30 mg/kg, subcutaneously) days 4, 6, 8 and minocycline (10 mg/kg, intraperitoneally) daily days 4–8 after tumor cell implantation (*solid bar*). Data are expressed relative to ^{14}C levels in the tumor in animals treated with the drug alone normalized to 1.0 per gram tissue.

with CDDP (20 mg/kg) alone resulted in a cross-linking factor of 2.0, whereas treatment with the same dose of CDDP in animals pretreated with TNP-470/minocycline resulted in a cross-linking factor of 8.9, which extrapolates in equivalency to about 85 mg/kg of CDDP (4).

The Lewis lung carcinoma growing subcutaneously in the hind leg of male C57BL mice is very hypoxic, having 92% of the pO_2 measurements of 5 mm Hg or lower as determined with a polarographic oxygen electrode (44). Administration of a perflubron emulsion (8 ml/kg) along with carbogen breathing increased the tumor oxygen level so that 82% of the pO_2 readings were 5 mm Hg or lower. Treating tumor-bearing animals with TNP-470 and minocycline daily beginning on day 4 after tumor cell implantation resulted in decreased hypoxia in the tumors on day 9 when pO_2 measurements were made. The percent of pO_2 readings of 5 mm Hg or lower in the tumors of the TNP-470/minocycline-treated animals was 75%, which upon administration of the perflubron emulsion along with carbogen breathing was reduced to 45%. Therapeutically, daily fractionated

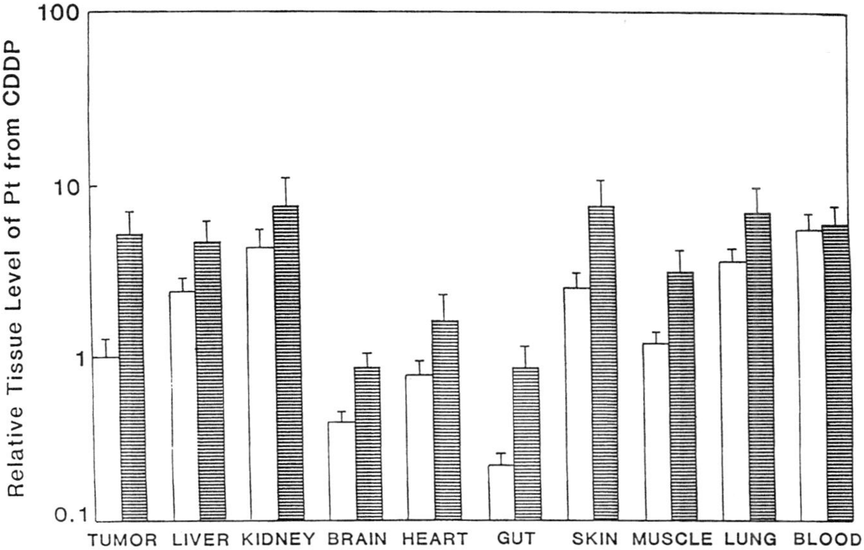

Figure 3 Relative tissue levels of platinum (Pt) from cis-diamminedichloroplatinum (II) (CDDP) in C57BL mice bearing Lewis lung tumors subcutaneously in the hind leg 6 hours after intraperitoneal injection of 20 mg/kg of the drug alone on day 8 (open *bar*) or after administration of TNP-470 (30 mg/kg, subcutaneously) on days 4, 6, 8, and minocycline (10 mg/kg, i.p.) daily days 4–8 after tumor cell implantation (*solid bar*). Data are expressed relative to Pt levels in the tumor in animals treated with the drug alone normalized to 1.0 per gram tissue.

radiation (2, 3 or 4 Gy × 5) was used as an oxygen-dependent cytotoxic modality. The radiation response of the tumors in TNP-470/minocycline-treated animals was greater than that in the untreated tumors (Fig. 4). The addition of carbogen breathing for 1 hour before and during radiation delivery further increased the radiation response so that overall there was a 2.2-fold increase in the tumor growth delay produced by the fractionated radiation in the animals treated with TNP-470/minocycline compared with untreated animals. Administration of the perflubron emulsion along with carbogen breathing before and during radiation delivery resulted in a 3.4-fold increase in tumor growth delay by the fractionated radiation regimens in the TNP-470/minocycline-treated animals compared with the tumor growth delay obtained with radiation alone. There was a linear relationship between decrease in the percent of pO_2 readings of 5 mm Hg or lower and tumor growth delay at each radiation dose, indicating that the diminution in tumor hypoxia produced by these treatments may be directly responsible for the increase in the effectiveness of the radiation therapy (Fig. 5).

Table 12 DNA Cross-Linking Factors from Lewis Lung Tumors by Alkaline Elution[a]

Treatment Group	DNA Cross-Linking Factor[b]
TNP-470/Minocycline	1.2
Cyclophosphamide:	
150 mg/kg	3.9
300 mg/kg	4.7
500 mg/kg	5.6
TNP-470/Minocycline/ Cyclophosphamide (300 mg/kg)	6.2
CDDP:	
10 mg/kg	1.7
20 mg/kg	2.0
30 mg/kg	2.8
TNP-470/Minocycline/CDDP (20 mg/kg)	8.9

[a] For DNA alkaline elution studies, Lewis lung carcinoma-bearing animals were treated with TNP-470 (30 mg/kg) subcutaneously on days 4, 6, and 8, with minocycline (10 mg/kg) intraperitoneally daily on days 4–8 and/or with cyclophosphamide (150, 300, or 500 mg/kg) intraperitoneally or CDDP (10, 20, or 30 mg/kg) intraperitoneally on day 8 after tumor cell implantation. [^{14}C]-Thymidine was administered intraperitoneally on days 7 and 8. The animals were sacrificed on day 9.

[b] A DNA cross-linking factor of 1.0 indicates no cross-links.

Abbreviation; *CDDP*, *cis*-diamminedichloroplatinum.

IV. PRECLINICAL THERAPEUTIC STUDIES: CYTOKINES

In addition to small molecules, the search for antiangiogenic substances has led to the discovery of proteins that inhibit various steps in the breakdown of the basement membrane (47, 48). These include naturally occurring proteins such as protamine (49); interferon (IFN)-α (50, 51); interferon-γ (52); platelet factor 4 (49, 53); tissue inhibitors of metalloproteinases (TIMPs) (54, 55); interleukin (IL)-12 (56–58); angiostatin (59); peptides derived from cartilages (60, 61); vitreous humor (62); smooth muscle (63); and aorta (63) as well as synthetic peptides such as synthetic laminin peptide (CDPG) YIGSR-NH_2 (64), somatostatin analogues such as somatoline (65) and antibodies such as MAb LM609 to human integrin $\alpha_v\beta_3$ (66–68).

Interleukin-12 is a naturally occurring cytokine that serves as a link between the innate and the cognate cellular immune systems (58, 69–71). It has the ability to act as a natural killer (NK) cell and a T-cell growth factor (72–74)

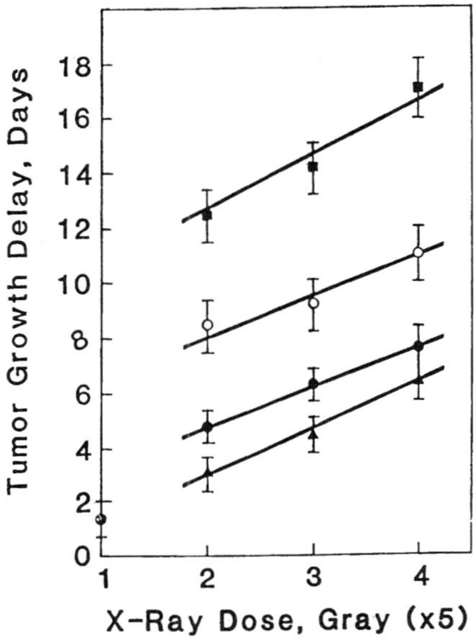

Figure 4 Growth delay of the Lewis lung carcinoma produced by daily fractionated radiation delivered in fractions of 2, 3, or 4 Gy locally to the tumor-bearing limb for 5 days on days 7–11 alone (*solid triangle*), in animals treated with TNP-470 (30 mg/kg, subcutaneously) on alternate days, and minocycline (10 mg/kg, intraperitoneally) daily on days 4–18 (*solid circle*), in animals treated with TNP-470/minocycline (as above) and allowed to breathe carbogen for 1 hour before and during radiation delivery (open circle), and in animals treated with TNP-470/minocycline (as above) and injected intravenously with the perflubron emulsion (8 ml/kg) and then allowed to breathe carbogen for 1 hour before and during radiation delivery (solid square). The points are the means of 15 animals and the bars are the S.E.M.

to enhance NK/lymphokine-activated killer (LAK) cell cytolytic activity (74–76), to augment cytolytic T-cell responses (75) and to induce secretion of cytokines, particularly IFN-γ from T and NK cells (77).

Interleukin-12 has been shown to induce tumor regression and rejection in a variety of murine tumor models when administered as a single agent (78–82). This tumor regression results from activation of immune mechanisms that involve IFN-γ, $CD4^+$, and $CD8^+$ cells (79, 80). Interleukin-12 has also been described as an antiangiogenic agent through the induction of interferon γ (56).

Both T and NK cells have been implicated as antitumor effector cells (83), and IFN-γ has been shown to have antitumor activity in animals (84, 85). Interleukin-12 has the potential to be used as an immunomodulatory cytokine in the therapy of malignancies (84, 86, 87), as well as in gene therapy (88, 89). Brunda

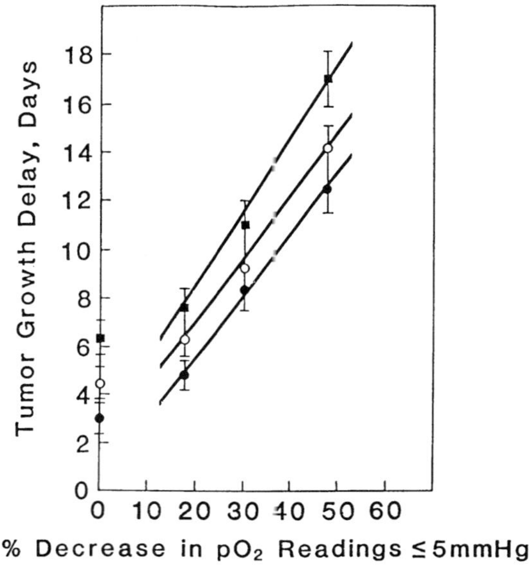

Figure 5 Relationship between decrease in the percent of tumor pO_2 readings of 5 mm Hg or lower and tumor growth delay at each radiation dose: 5 × 2 Gy (solid circle), 5 × 3 Gy (open circle), and 5 × 4 Gy (solid square). Points are the means of ten tumors. Bars = S.E.M.

et al. (79) have shown that systemic administration of murine IL-12 can slow, and in some cases inhibit, the growth of both established subcutaneous tumors in mice and experimental pulmonary or hepatic metastases of B16F10 murine melanoma, M5076 reticulum cell sarcoma, or RenCa renal cell adenocarcinoma and that local peritumoral injections of IL-12 can result in regression of established subcutaneous tumors. Based on results obtained using mice deficient in lymphocyte subsets and antibody depletion experiments, Brunda and colleagues concluded that the antitumor efficacy of IL-12 is mediated primarily through $CD8^+$ T cells (79, 90).

Interleukin-12 (rmIL-12) was found to be an active antitumor agent against the Lewis lung carcinoma. The antitumor activity relied on the rmIL-12 dose, the duration of treatment, and the tumor burden at the initiation of treatment. The effect of the schedule of rmIL-12 administration, both alone and with a 1-week regimen of fractionated radiation therapy (Table 13 and Fig. 6) or a 2-week regimen of fractionated radiation therapy (Table 14 and Fig. 7) was examined. Beginning treatment with rmIL-12 on day 2 after tumor cell implantation and treating for 5 days resulted in about 5 days of tumor growth delay, whereas begin-

Table 13 Growth Delay of the Lewis Lung Carcinoma and Number and Percent of Large Lung Metastases on Day 20 After Treatment with IL-12 and Fractionated Radiation Therapy Delivered Locally to the Tumor-Bearing Limb

Treatment group	Tumor growth delay, days[a]	Lung Metastases (% large)[b]
Control	—	25 (53)
IL-12 (45 μg/kg) intraperitoneally[c]		
days 2–6	4.9 ± 0.4	15 (43)
days 7–11	2.7 ± 0.3	16 (47)
days 2–11; 14–18	7.7 ± 0.5	8.5 (29)
days 7–11; 14–18	5.4 ± 0.4	9 (31)
days 14–18; 21–25	4.3 ± 0.4	16 (50)
days 21–25	0.3 ± 0.3	
5 × 2 Gy, days 7–11[d]	3.1 ± 0.4	17.5 (62)
5 × 3 Gy, days 7–11	4.3 ± 0.4	17 (53)
5 × 4 Gy, days 7–11	6.2 ± 0.6	17 (55)
IL-12 (45 μg/kg) intraperitoneally, days 2–6		
+ 5 × 2 Gy, days 7–11	6.8 ± 0.6	14 (27)
+ 5 × 3 Gy, days 7–11	7.8 ± 0.9	13 (35)
+ 5 × 4 Gy, days 7–11	10.0 ± 1.1	12 (39)
IL-12 (45 μg/kg) intraperitoneally, days 2–11; 14–18		
+ 5 × 2 Gy, days 7–11	8.7 ± 0.8	8 (40)
+ 5 × 3 Gy, days 7–11	11.2 ± 1.3	7 (35)
+ 5 × 4 Gy, days 7–11	16.1 ± 1.9	6 (33)
IL-12 (45 μg/kg) intraperitoneally, days 7–11; 14–18		
+ 5 × 2 Gy, days 7–11	6.9 ± 0.8	10 (24)
+ 5 × 3 Gy, days 7–11	12.5 ± 1.6	6 (30)
+ 5 × 4 Gy, days 7–11	19.8 ± 2.1	4 (27)
IL-12 (45 μg/kg) intraperitoneally, days 14–18; 21–25		
+ 5 × 2 Gy, days 7–11	4.2 ± 0.3	17 (39)
+ 5 × 3 Gy, days 7–11	7.4 ± 0.5	15 (32)
+ 5 × 4 Gy, days 7–11	10.6 ± 1.2	14 (23)
IL-12 (45 μg/kg) intraperitoneally, days 21–25		
+ 5 × 2 Gy, days 7–11	3.3 ± 0.3	19 (50)
+ 5 × 3 Gy, days 7–11	6.6 ± 0.4	18 (61)
+ 5 × 4 Gy, days 7–11	9.6 ± 1.0	16 (50)

[a] Tumor growth delay is the difference in days for treated tumors to reach 500 mm^3 compared with untreated control tumors. Untreated control tumors reach 500 mm^3 in 12.5 ± 0.3 days. Mean ± SE of 18 animals.

[b] The number of external lung metastases on day 20 after tumor implant as counted manually and scored as ≥3 mm in diameter. Data are the means from 6–12 pairs of lungs. Numbers in parentheses = number of large (vascularized) metastases.

[c] IL-12 was administered by intraperitoneal injection.

[d] Radiation therapy was delivered in fractions of 2, 3, or 4 Gy daily on days 7–11 locally to the tumor-bearing limb (100 rad/min; gamma cell 40).

Abbreviation; *IL*, interleukin.

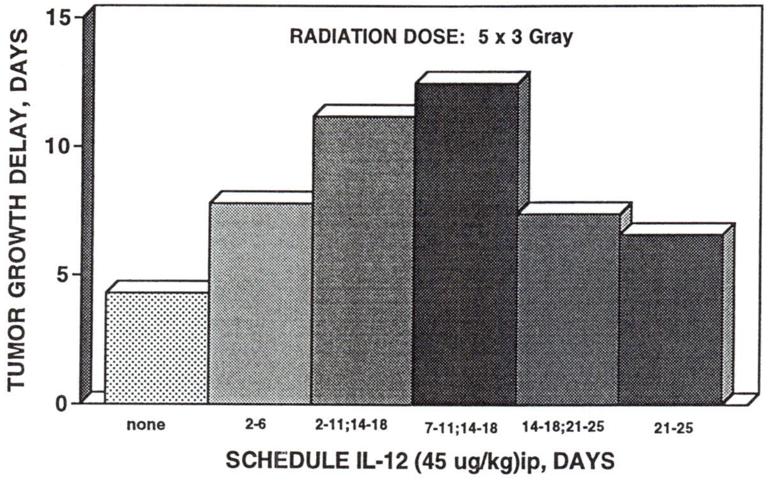

Figure 6 Growth delay of the Lewis lung carcinoma after treatment of the tumor-bearing animals with fractionated radiation therapy (2, 3, or 4 Gy) delivered locally to the tumor-bearing limb once per day on days 7 through 11 after tumor implantation alone or along with rm interleukin (IL)-12 (45 μg/kg, intraperitoneally) on days 2 through 6; days 2 through 11 and days 14 through 18; days 7 through 11 and days 14 through 18; days 14 through 18 and days 21 through 25, or days 21 through 25. Data are the means of three experiments ± S.E.M.

ning treatment with rmIL-12 on day 2 and treating for 10 days and then for 5 more days resulted in about 7.7 days of tumor growth delay (Table 13). Delaying the initiation of rmIL-12 treatment to day 7 after tumor cell implantation and treating for 5 days resulted in a tumor growth delay of about 2.7 days; extending that treatment to 10 injections increased the tumor growth delay to 5.4 days. Further delaying the initiation of rmIL-12 treatment until day 14 after tumor cell implantation and treating for 10 injections resulted in about 4.3 days of tumor growth delay. Finally, treating bulky disease with rmIL-12 for 5 days beginning on day 21 after tumor cell implantation did not alter tumor growth.

Fractionated radiation therapy in a 5-day regimen resulted in increasing tumor growth delay with increasing radiation dose (Table 13). Administering rmIL-12 for 5 days before radiation therapy resulted in an additive effect of the two treatments but did not increase the response of the tumor to the radiation therapy. Administration of rmIL-12 before during, and after radiation therapy resulted in a highly effective therapy that included an additive effect of the two therapies and dose modification of the radiation therapy with a dose modifying factor of 2. Administering rmIL-12 during and after fractionated radiation also

Table 14 Growth Delay of the Lewis Lung Carcinoma and Number and Percent of Large Lung Metastases on Day 20 After Treatment with IL-12 and 2 Weeks of Fractionated Radiation Therapy Delivered Locally to the Tumor-Bearing Limb.

Treatment Group	Tumor growth delay, days[a]	Lung metastases (% large)[b]
Control	—	25 (53)
10 × 2 Gy, days 7–11; 14–18[c]	4.1 ± 0.3	13 (32)
10 × 3 Gy, days 7–11; 14–18	5.1 ± 0.4	11 (38)
10 × 4 Gy, days 7–11; 14–18	8.9 ± 0.7	6 (27)
IL-12 (45 μg/kg) intraperitoneally, days 2–6[d]		
+ 10 × 2 Gy, days 7–11; 14–18	5.5 ± 0.4	7.5 (33)
+ 10 × 3 Gy, days 7–11; 14–18	7.6 ± 0.7	6 (30)
+ 10 × 4 Gy, days 7–11; 14–18	10.6 ± 0.9	5 (20)
IL-12 (45 μg/kg) intraperitoneally, days 7–11; 14–18		
+ 10 × 2 Gy, days 7–11; 14–18	7.2 ± 0.5	3.5 (43)
+ 10 × 3 Gy, days 7–11; 14–18	16.6 ± 1.3	2.5 (40)
+ 10 × 4 Gy, days 7–11; 14–18	28.9 ± 2.3	2 (50)
IL-12 (45 μg/kg) intraperitoneally, days 14–18; 21–25		
+ 10 × 2 Gy, days 7–11; 14–18	5.4 ± 0.5	10.5 (38)
+ 10 × 3 Gy, days 7–11; 14–18	11.1 ± 0.9	6 (42)
+ 10 × 4 Gy, days 7–11; 14–18	16.4 ± 1.1	5 (40)
IL-12 (45 μg/kg) intraperitoneally, days 21–25		
+ 10 × 2 Gy, days 7–11; 14–18	5.6 ± 0.4	15 (32)
+ 10 × 3 Gy, days 7–11; 14–18	7.7 ± 0.6	14 (52)
+ 10 × 4 Gy, days 7–11; 14–18	11.8 ± 1.1	6 (38)

[a] Tumor growth delay is the difference in days for treated tumors to reach 500 mm^3 compared with untreated control tumors. Untreated control tumors reach 500 mm^3 in 12.5 ± 0.3 days. Mean ± SE of 15 animals.

[b] The number of external lung metastases on day 20 after tumor implant as counted manually and scored as ≥3 mm in diameter. Data are the means from 6–12 pairs of lungs. Numbers in parentheses = number of large (vascularized) metastases.

[c] Radiation therapy was delivered in fractions of 2, 3, or 4 Gy daily on days 7–11 locally to the tumor-bearing limb (100 rad/min; gamma cell 40).

[d] IL-12 was administered by intraperitoneal injection.

Abbreviation; *IL*, interleukin.

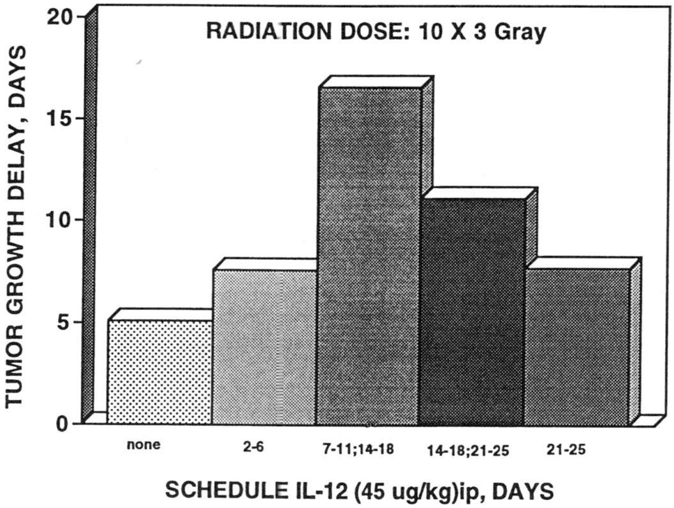

Figure 7 Growth delay of the Lewis lung carcinoma after treatment of the tumor-bearing animals with fractionated radiation therapy (2, 3, or 4 Gy) delivered locally to the tumor-bearing limb once per day on days 7 through 11 and days 14 through 18 after tumor implantation alone or along with rm interleukin (IL)-12 (45 μg/kg, intraperitoneally) on days 2 through 6; days 7 through 11 and days 14 through 18; days 14 through 18 and days 21 through 25, or days 21 through 25. Data are the means of three experiments ± S.E.M.

resulted in a highly effective therapeutic regimen, including an additive effect of the two therapies and a radiation dose modifying factor of 3. Delaying administration of rmIL-12 until 2 days or 1 week after completion of the radiation regimen resulted in less efficacious treatments than when the rmIL-12 was given concurrently and after the radiation therapy. Nevertheless, treatments in which the rmIL-12 was administered only after the radiation were as effective or more effective than radiation alone. Using 3 Gy (×5) as a representative radiation dose, there was a maximal 2.8-fold increase in tumor growth delay when rmIL-12 was administered during and after fractionated radiation therapy (Fig. 6). The efficacy of these regimens against systemic disease, represented by lung metastases, paralleled the effects observed in the primary tumor (Table 13). When rmIL-12 was administered before, during, and after radiation therapy or during and after radiation therapy, the numbers of lung metastases were decreased to 20% to 40% of the controls. The percent of large (vascularized) metastases was also decreased by treatment with rmIL-12.

When the fractionated radiation regimen was extended to 2 weeks, the results shown in Table 14 were obtained. Administration of rmIL-12 for 5 days before radiation therapy resulted in an additive effect of the two therapies, but no dose modification of the radiation occurred. Concurrent administration of rmIL-12 just before each of the ten radiation fractions formed a highly effective treatment regimen resulting in additivity of the two therapies and a radiation dose-modifying factor of 5. Administering rmIL-12 along with the second week of the fractionated radiation regimen and then for 5 days the week after radiation therapy also produced a highly effective treatment regimen, with an additive effect of the two therapies and a radiation dose-modifying factor of 2.7. When rmIL-12 administration was delayed until the completion of the radiation therapy, only a modest increase in tumor growth delay compared with radiation therapy alone was observed. Using the fractionated radiation regimen of 3 Gy ($\times$10) as a representative treatment, concurrent administration of rmIL-12 and radiation therapy resulted in a 3.3-fold increase in tumor growth delay compared with radiation therapy alone (Fig. 7). A reduction in the number of lung metastases was seen on day 20 with each of the 2-week radiation therapy regimens (Table 13). However, the treatment regimen including concurrent administration of rmIL-12 and radiation therapy that was most effective against the primary tumor was also most effective in decreasing the number of lung metastases on day 20.

Because treatment of rmIL-12 significantly decreased lung metastases after radiation therapy locally to the subcutaneous tumor-bearing limb, the Lewis lung carcinoma was implanted into each hind leg of mice; fractionated radiation therapy was then administered only to the right hind leg in the presence or absence of rmIL-12 treatment (Table 15). The presence of the second subcutaneous tumor in the animal did not alter the response of the treated tumor to the radiation therapy or the number or size of lung metastases on day 20. On days 7 through 11, radiation therapy to the tumor in the right hind leg resulted in a small but measurable tumor growth delay in the tumor in the left hind leg. Administration of rmIL-12 (45 or 4.5 μg/kg) on days 7 through 11 and days 14 through 18 along with fractionated radiation resulted in increased tumor growth delay in the irradiated subcutaneous tumor a response similar to rmIL-12 alone in the tumor in the contralateral limb and a significant decrease in the number and percent of large lung metastases when compared with radiation to the right tumor only. Two other schedules of rmIL-12, also to the same total dose of 450 μg/kg, were tested. rmInterleukin-12 (75 μg/kg) was administered on alternate days 7 through 18, or as two doses of 225 μg/kg on days 7 and 14 alone, or along with fractionated radiation therapy on days 7 through 11. Each of these schedules were less effective, as determined by each of the three experimental endpoints, than the rmIL-12 (45 μg/kg) on days 7 through 11 and 14 through 18 regimen.

Table 15 Growth Delay of the Lewis Lung Carcinoma in Animals Bearing Two Subcutaneous Tumors and Number and Percent Large Lung Metastases on Day 20 After Treatment with rmIL-12 and Fractionated Therapy Delivered Locally to the Subcutaneous Tumor in the Right Leg

Treatment group	Tumor Growth Delay, Days[a]		Lung metastases[b] (% large)
	Right (X-rays)	Left	
Control	—	—	24.5 (56)
5 × 2 Gy[c]	3.2 ± 0.4	—	17.5 (62)
5 × 3 Gy	4.3 ± 0.4	—	17 (53)
5 × 4 Gy	6.2 ± 0.6	—	17 (55)
5 × 2 Gy	3.1 ± 0.4	1.2 ± 0.3	18.5 (53)
5 × 3 Gy	4.0 ± 0.4	1.7 ± 0.3	14 (46)
5 × 4 Gy	5.8 ± 0.5	2.5 ± 0.3	13 (50)
IL-12 (4.5 μg/kg) days 7–11; 14–18[d]	3.6 ± 0.4		15 (33)
above + 5 × 2 Gy	5.9 ± 0.7	2.2 ± 0.3	5 (20)
above + 5 × 3 Gy	10.6 ± 0.9	3.0 ± 0.4	5 (17)
above + 5 × 4 Gy	15.6 ± 1.4	3.4 ± 0.4	1.5 (0)
IL-12 (45 μg/kg) days 7–11; 14–18	5.4 ± 0.4		7 (25)
above + 5 × 2 Gy	6.9 ± 0.7	4.5 ± 0.4	16 (24)
above + 5 × 3 Gy	14.3 ± 1.6	5.4 ± 0.4	5 (31)
above + 5 × 4 Gy	22.7 ± 1.9	5.9 ± 0.5	3 (19)
IL-12 (75 μg/kg) days 7, 9, 11, 14, 16, 18	1.5 ± 0.3		14 (32)
above + 5 × 2 Gy	6.0 ± 0.4	3.5 ± 0.3	95 (45)
above + 5 × 3 Gy	12.4 ± 1.3	4.6 ± 0.4	9 (29)
above + 5 × 4 Gy	17.6 ± 1.6	4.9 ± 0.4	8 (27)
IL-12 (225 μg/kg) days 7 and 14	3.0 ± 0.3		14.5 (29)
above + 5 × 2 Gy	6.9 ± 0.7	2.9 ± 0.3	10.5 (30)
above + 5 × 3 Gy	7.8 ± 0.8	3.4 ± 0.3	10 (26)
above + 5 × 4 Gy	10.0 ± 1.0	3.6 ± 0.4	6 (24)

[a] Tumor growth is the difference in days for treated tumors to reach 500 mm^3 compared with untreated control tumors. Untreated control tumors reach 500 mm^3 in about 14 days. Mean ± SE of 18 animals.

[b] The number of external lung metastases on day 20 after tumor implant as counted manually and scored as ≥ 3 mm in diameter. Data are the means from 6–12 pairs of lungs. Numbers in parentheses = number of large (vascularized) metastases.

[c] Radiation therapy was delivered in fractions of 2, 3, or 4 Gy daily on days 7–11 locally to the tumor-bearing limb (100 rad/min; gamma cell 40).

[d] IL-12 was administered by intraperitoneal injection.

Abbreviation: *IL*, interleukin.

rmInterleukin-12 was also found to be an active antitumor agent in the MB-49 bladder carcinoma. The antitumor activity depended on IL-12 dose, the duration of treatment, and the tumor burden at the initiation of treatment (Table 16). When IL-12 treatment was initiated on day 4 (tumor volume approximately 30 mm^3), there was no statistically significant difference in the tumor growth delay produced by IL-12 (0.45 μg/kg or 4.5 μg/kg) administered for 5 or 11 doses. However, when IL-12 (45 μg/kg) was administered to the animals for 11 doses, the tumor response was significantly greater than that obtained with the 5-dose regimen. Delaying IL-12 treatment until day 10, when the tumors were approximately 200 mm^3 in volume, resulted in decreased tumor growth delay so that only the highest dose of IL-12 (45 μg/kg) produced a significant tumor response. The number of lung metastases in these animals on day 20 was significantly decreased, but only at the highest dose of IL-12 (45 μg/kg), and the percent of large (vascularized) lung metastases was not different from that seen in the controls.

In the design of treatment regimens including systemic administration of IL-12 and chemotherapy, two major issues were: (a) possible damage of the IL-12 target T cells by the chemotherapy thus ablating the IL-12 effect and (b)

Table 16 Tumor Growth Delay and Number and Size of Lung Metastases in Animals Bearing the MB-49 Bladder Carcinoma Treated with rmIL-12 on different schedules

Treatment group	Total rmIL-12 dose, μg	Tumor growth delay, days[a]	No. lung metastases (% large)
Controls		—	22 (44%)
daily days 4 → 8 after tumor implantation			
rmIL-12 (1 μg)	5	7.3 ± 1.2	12 (38%)
rmIL-12 (0.1 μg)	0.5	5.9 ± 0.9	17 (35%)
rmIL-12 (0.01 μg)	0.05	3.8 ± 0.6	18.5 (46%)
daily days 4 → 14 after tumor implantation			
rmIL-12 (1 μg)	11	10.9 ± 1.5	8 (42%)
rmIL-12 (0.1 μg)	1.1	5.7 ± 0.9	14 (35%)
rmIL-12 (0.01 μg)	0.11	4.3 ± 0.6	18 (42%)
daily days 7 → 11 and 14 → 18 after tumor implantation			
rmIL-12 (0.1 μg)	1	4.5 ± 0.7	—
daily days 10 → 14 after tumor implantation			
rmIL-12 (1 μg)	5	3.2 ± 0.6	9 (43%)
rmIL-12 (0.1 μg)	0.5	1.6 ± 0.3	14 (45%)
rmIL-12 (0.01 μg)	0.05	1.5 ± 0.3	16 (47%)

[a] Tumor growth is the difference in days for treated tumors to reach 500 mm^3 compared with untreated control tumors. Untreated control tumors reach 500 mm^3 in about 14 days. Mean ± SE of 18 animals.

increased toxicity of the combination therapy. Therefore, IL-12 was studied over a dosage range—0.45, 4.5, and 45 μg/kg—with the chemotherapy and on schedules before, after, and overlapping with the chemotherapy. Each of the chemotherapeutic agents studied, adriamycin, cyclophosphamide, and 5-fluorouracil, were active antitumor agents against the MB-49 bladder carcinoma (Table 17). Interleukin-12 treatment did not increase the toxicity of the chemotherapy. There was increased anticancer activity when IL-12 administration was added to treatment with each chemotherapeutic agent. The increased tumor response relied on IL-12 dose and schedule with overlapping therapy producing the greatest effect (Table 17). Adriamycin (1.75 mg/kg) on days 7 through 11 produced 10.8 days of tumor growth delay. However, the greatest tumor growth delay was obtained with extended IL-12 treatment, days 4 through 14 combined with adriamycin, which resulted in 23.4 days of tumor growth delay. Cyclophosphamide (100 mg/kg) administered on days 7, 9, and 11 produced 8.0 days of tumor growth delay. When IL-12 was administered along with cyclophosphamide on the longer schedule, days 4 through 14, a tumor growth delay of 21.7 days was produced. 5-Fluorouracil (30 mg/kg) administered on days 7 through 11 produced 6.2 days of tumor growth delay. Interleukin-12 treatment extended to days 4 through 14 along with 5-fluorouracil resulted in 16.5 days of tumor growth delay. Shorter-duration treatment with IL-12 before or after chemotherapy regimens was less effective in all treatment groups (Table 17). Interestingly, administering IL-12 (45 μg/kg) simultaneously with the chemotherapy and then again on days 14 through 18 was not a very effective combination therapy (Table 17).

Interleukin-12 included in the therapeutic regimen greatly increased the efficacy against metastatic disease (Table 17). The highest dose of IL-12, 45 μg/kg, was most effective against metastasis to the lungs. Unlike tumor growth delay, the combinations with adriamycin, cyclophosphamide, or 5-fluorouracil were similar at all schedules evaluated. In combination with adriamycin or 5-fluorouracil, there was little impact of IL-12 administration on the percent of lung metastases 3 mm in diameter or larger indicating that these treatments were not altering the growth pattern of the metastases. However, IL-12 in combination with cyclophosphamide did decrease the percent of large lung metastases, indicating that the growth rate of the metastases was slowed.

The B16 melanoma is a highly metastatic murine solid tumor that grows more slowly than the MB-49 bladder carcinoma, thus providing a convenient model in which to address the question of cycling IL-12 administration with cytotoxic therapy. Several schedules of rmIL-12 and cyclophosphamide were tested in which rmIL-12 administration was initiated after cyclophosphamide therapy in a manner that overlapped the terminal portion of the chemotherapy regimen or that started 2 days after the completion of the chemotherapy regimen and extended for 1, 2, or 3 weeks (Table 18). Cyclophosphamide (125 mg/kg) was administered for one course (days 7, 9, and 11) or for two courses (days 7,

Table 17 Tumor Growth Delay and Number and Size of Lung Metastases in Animals Bearing the MB-49 Bladder Carcinoma Treated with rmIL-12 and an Anticancer agent

Treatment group	Tumor growth delay, days[a]	No. lung metastases,[b] (% large)
Controls	—	22 (44%)
Adriamycin (1.25 mg/kg) Days 7 → 11		
alone	10.8 ± 1.2	18 (42%)
+ rmIL-12 (45 μg/kg) days 4 → 8	17.1 ± 2.0	7.5 (33%)
+ rmIL-12 (4.5 μg/kg) days 4 →8	15.0 ± 1.7	15 (37%)
+ rmIL-12 (0.45 μg/kg) days 4 → 8	14.6 ± 1.6	17 (38%)
+ rmIL-12 (45 μg/kg) days 4 → 14	23.4 ± 3.7	8 (38%)
+ rmIL-12 (4.5 μg/kg) days 4 → 14	15.1 ± 1.8	11.5 (38%)
+ rmIL-12 (0.45 μg/kg) days 4 → 14	13.8 ± 1.7	12 (38%)
+ rmIL-12 (45 μg/kg) days 7 → 11, 14 →18	12.8 ± 1.7	—
+ rmIL-12 (45 μg/kg) days 10 → 14	14.8 ± 1.4	5 (42%)
+ rmIL-12 (4.5 μg/kg) days 10 → 14	13.6 ± 1.4	12 (46%)
+ rmIL-12 (0.45 μg/kg) days 10 → 14	13.0 ± 1.3	14 (41%)
Cyclophosphamide (100 mg/kg) Days 7, 9, 11		
alone	8.0 ± 0.8	12 (38%)
+ rmIL-12 (45 μg/kg) days 4 → 8	17.0 ± 1.7	3 (17%)
+ rmIL-12 (4.5 μg/kg) days 4 → 8	15.6 ± 1.6	4 (38%)
+ rmIL-12 (0.45 μg/kg) days 4 → 8	15.0 ± 1.3	3.5 (28%)
+ rmIL-12 (45 μg/kg) days 4 → 14	21.7 ± 3.3	4 (21%)
+ rmIL-12 (4.5 μg/kg) days 4 → 14	16.5 ± 1.8	5 (23%)
+ rmIL-12 (0.45 μg/kg) days 4 → 14	14.3 ± 1.5	6 (28%)
+ rmIL-12 (45 μg/kg) days 7 → 11, 14 → 18	12.8 ± 1.6	—
+ rmIL-12 (45 μg/kg) days 10 → 14	17.6 ± 1.9	1.5 (50%)
+ rmIL-12 (4.5 μg/kg) days 10 → 14	14.6 ± 1.7	5 (33%)
+ rmIL-12 (0.45 μg/kg) days 10 → 14	12.7 ± 1.2	8 (27%)
5-fluorouracil (30 mg/kg) Days 7 → 11		
alone	6.2 ± 0.7	17 (42%)
+ rmIL-12 (45 μg/kg) days 4 → 8	12.3 ± 1.1	10 (25%)
+ rmIL-12 (4.5 μg/kg) days 4 → 8	11.9 ± 1.0	11.5 (39%)
+ rmIL-12 (0.45 μg/kg) days 4 → 8	10.2 ± 0.9	16 (38%)
+ rmIL-12 (45 μg/kg) days 4 → 14	16.5 ± 1.8	10 (27%)
+ rmIL-12 (4.5 μg/kg) days 4 → 14	11.0 ± 1.0	13.5 (35%)
+ rmIL-12 (0.45 μg/kg) days 4 → 14	8.5 ± 0.7	19 (39%)
+ rmIL-12 (45 μg/kg) days 7 → 11, 14 → 18	7.1 ± 0.6	—
+ rmIL-12 (45 μg/kg) days 10 → 14	11.2 ± 1.1	11 (43%)
+ rmIL-12 (4.5 μg/kg) days 10 → 14	9.2 ± 0.9	21 (44%)
+ rmIL-12 (0.45 μg/kg) days 10 → 14	9.1 ± 0.9	22 (41%)

[a] Tumor growth is the difference in days for treated tumors to reach 500 mm^3 compared with untreated control tumors. Untreated control tumors reach 500 mm^3 in about 14 days. Mean ± SE of 18 animals.

[b] The number of external lung metastases on day 20 post-tumor implant as counted manually and scored as ≥ 3 mm in diameter. Data are the means from 6–12 pairs of lungs. Numbers in parentheses = number of large (vascularized) metastases.

Table 18 Growth Delay of the B16 Melanoma and Number and Size of Lung Metastases on Day 30 Produced by Treatment with IL-12 and/or Cyclophosphamide

Treatment group	Tumor growth delay, days	Lung metastases (% large)
Controls		
IL-12 (45 μg/kg), intraperitoneally		
days 10–14	4.6 ± 0.4	8 (21)
days 14–18	5.1 ± 0.4	10 (23)
days 10–14; 18–22	6.4 ± 0.5	3 (25)
days 14–18; 21–25	6.3 ± 0.5	10 (23)
days 14–18; 21–25; 28–32	6.8 ± 0.5	8 (44)
IL-12 (4.5 μg/kg), intraperitoneally		
days 10–14	2.1 ± 0.3	11 (24)
days 10–14; 18–22	3.2 ± 0.3	16 (27)
Cyclophosphamide (125 mg/kg), intraperitoneally		
days 7, 9, 11	16.8 ± 1.4	3.5 (31)
days 7, 9, 11; 28, 30, 32	28.5 ± 2.1	3.5 (29)
CTX + IL-12 (45 μg/kg)		
CTX, days 7, 9, 11 + IL–12, d 10–14	25.8 ± 2.7	2.5 (27)
CTX, days 7, 9, 11 + IL-12, d 14–18	19.0 ± 1.6	3.5 (43)
CTX, days 7, 9, 11 + IL-12, d 14–18; 21–25	30.9 ± 2.5	2 (0)
CTX, days 7, 9, 11 + IL-12, d 14–18; 21–25; 28–32	33.4 ± 2.1	1 (0)
CTX, days 7, 9, 11 + IL-12, d 14–18; 21–25 + CTX, d 28, 30, 32 + IL-12, d 35–39	40.0 ± 2.2	1 (0)
CTX + IL-12 (4.5 μg/kg)		
CTX, days 7, 9, 11 + IL-12, days 14–18; 21–25	23.2 ± 1.3	6 (17)
CTX, days 7, 9, 11 + IL-12, days 14–18; 21–25; 28–32	23.7 ± 1.7	2.5 (0)
CTX, days 7, 9, 11 + IL-12, days 14–18; 21–25 + CTX days 28, 30, 32 + IL-12, days 35–39	28.2 ± 1.9	2 (25)
Cyclophosphamide (62 mg/kg) intraperitoneally days 7, 9, 11; 15, 17, 19	6.8 ± 0.5	6 (50)
CTX, days 7, 9, 11 + IL-12 (45 μg/kg) days 10–14 + CTX, days 15, 17, 19 + IL-12 (45 μg/kg) days 18–22	11.6 ± 1.0	0.5 (8)
CTX, days 7, 9, 11 + IL-12 (4.5 μg/kg) days 10–14 + CTX, days 15, 17, 19 + IL-12 (4.5 μg/kg) days 18–22	9.1 ± 0.8	4.5 (22)

[a] Tumor growth is the difference in days for treated tumors to reach 500 mm^3 compared with untreated control tumors. Untreated control tumors reach 500 mm^3 in about 14 days. Mean ± SE of 18 animals.
[b] The number of external lung metastases on day 20 after tumor implant as counted manually and scored as ≥ 3 mm in diameter. Data are the means from 6–12 pairs of lungs. Numbers in parentheses = number of large (vascularized) metastases.
Abbreviations: *IL*, interleukin; *CTX*, cyclophosphamide.

9, 11, 28, 30, and 32). Both rmIL-12 and cyclophosphamide were active antitumor agents against the B16 melanoma. The tumor growth delay produced by rmIL-12 depended on the dose and duration of treatment. Administration of 45 μg/kg of rmIL-12 was more effective than administration of 4.5 μg/kg of rmIL-12. Administration of rmIL-12 for 2 weeks was more effective than administration of rmIL-12 for 1 week. However, administration of rmIL-12 for 3 weeks did not increase the tumor response further. Greater tumor growth delay resulted when the 5-day rmIL-12 regimen was administered overlapping with the terminal portion of the chemotherapy treatment than if a 2-day break was allowed from completion of the cyclophosphamide treatment to initiation of the rmIL-12 administration. Extending the rmIL-12 administration to 2 weeks (ten injections) resulted in a highly effective therapeutic regimen with a tumor growth delay of about 31 days. Adding a third week of rmIL-12 administration to that regimen increased the tumor growth delay by only 2.4 days. When the dose of rmIL-12 was decreased to 4.5 μg/kg, the tumor growth delays observed with the combination regimens were decreased to 23 to 24 days which was significantly greater than cyclophosphamide alone. Administration of two courses of cyclophosphamide on days 7, 9, and 11 and again on days 28, 30, and 32 produced a tumor growth delay of about 28.5 days. When rmIL-12 (45 μg/kg) was administered between and after completion of the cyclophosphamide courses, a tumor growth delay of 40 days resulted that was greater than expected for additivity for the two therapies. When the same treatment regimen was carried out with the lower dose of rmIL-12 (4.5 μg/kg), the tumor growth delay observed was about 28 days. To explore the effect of cyclophosphamide dose and schedule, a total dose of 375 mg/kg of cyclophosphamide, administered as three injections of 125 mg/kg alone, was divided into six injections of 62 mg/kg administered over two courses (Table 18). Decreasing the dose intensity of the cyclophosphamide resulted in a decrease in the tumor growth delay from 16.8 days for 3 × 125 mg/kg of cyclophosphamide to 6.8 days for 6 × 62 mg/kg of cyclophosphamide. Administering the rmIL-12 (4.5 μg/kg or 45 μg/kg) between and after the chemotherapy treatment resulted in additivity of the two therapies.

The efficacy of rmIL-12 and rmIL-12 and cyclophosphamide combinations against B16 melanoma metastatic to the lungs depended on the day of treatment initiation, dose of rmIL-12, and duration of treatment (Table 18). Beginning treatment with rmIL-12 on day 10 when the tumor burden was lower was more effective in reducing the number and percent of large lung metastases than were rmIL-12 treatment regimens beginning later. In general, treatment regimens including two courses of cyclophosphamide were more effective. The rmIL-12 treatment regimens decreased both the number of lung metastases on day 30 and significantly decreased the percent of lung metastases that were large enough to be undergoing angiogenesis.

In all of the combination treatment regimens of IL-12 with chemotherapy, there was a significant effect on disease metastatic to the lungs with each of the tumors studied. Interleukin-12 has been described as an antiangiogenic agent (56). The antiangiogenic activity of IL-12 appears to be due to the induction of interferon-γ by the cytokine (56). Although the mechanism by which interferon-γ exerts antiangiogenic effects remains unelucidated, several studies have shown that the interferons inhibit production of matrix metalloproteinases (91–94). Gohji et al. (91) found that incubation of human KG-2 renal cell carcinoma cells with interferon-β or -γ suppressed transcription of the 72-kDa gelatinase gene and, hence, production of gelatinase activity. These inhibitory effects of interferons were independent of their antiproliferative effects. Treatment of KG-2 cells with interferon-β or -γ significantly inhibited cell invasion through reconstituted basement membrane toward chemoattractants produced by kidney fibroblasts. The inhibitory activity of interferons was specific to the KG-2 cells as gelatinase activity by various fibroblasts was unaffected. In human A2058 melanoma cells, Hujanen et al. (92) found that interferon-β and -γ were potent regulators of both M_r 72,000 and M_r 92,000 type-IV collagenase/gelatinase A and B genes, showing biphasic and parallel effects on mRNA levels of both enzymes, depending on the treatment time. They also found that the M_r 72,000 metalloproteinase/gelatinase A was the predominant basement membrane-degrading type-IV collagenase in the A2058 human melanoma cell line. Norioka et al. (93) found that interferon-γ alone and in combination with IL-1 inhibited the proliferation of human umbilical vein endothelial cells stimulated with bFGF in culture. Local administration of interferon-γ inhibited bFGF and stimulated angiogenesis in mouse skin. Interferon-γ, especially in combination with IL-1, down-regulated expression of bFGF receptor on the endothelial cells. On the other hand, Hiscox et al. (94) found that IL-12 directly inhibited the attachment of the human colon cancer cell lines HRT18, HT29, and HT115 to Matrigel. Interleukin-12 did not affect the growth of these colon carcinoma cell lines. Flow cytometry, Western analysis, and immunohistochemistry showed an up-regulation of E-cadherin cell-surface adhesion molecules. These direct effects of IL-12 on colon cancer cells suggest a potentially important role for IL-12 in metastasis. Therefore, administration of IL-12 may act as an antiangiogenic agent directly or indirectly by preventing invasion and extravasation of tumor cells through vasculature and by preventing angiogenic activity in implanted metastatic tumor cells.

The immune basis of IL-12 activity would suggest that combining IL-12 with other therapies that enhance immune response could potentiate the antitumor activity of IL-12. The combination of IL-12 with IL-2, a cytokine with a similar pharmacological profile, was found to be no more effective than the optimal dose of IL-12 alone (90, 95). It was hypothesized that this outcome may have resulted from the substantially increased toxicity associated with IL-12/IL-2 combination therapy (90); however, pulse IL-2 along with IL-12 was less toxic and more efficacious (95). The combination of IL-12 with monocyte-colony stimulating factor (M-CSF), a macrophage activator and growth factor, was synergistic, especially with local fractionated radiation therapy (96). These results concur and extend those of Lu et al. (97) that M-CSF is effective in enhancing the response of the Lewis lung carcinoma to radiation therapy. Macrophages are present in tumors (98), have a significant role in antigen presentation and lymphocyte activation, and have been identified as a primary source of endogenous IL-12 (90, 99). They produce a variety of other inflammatory cytokines, such as TNF-α, IL-1, and interferon (INF)-α, β as well as oxygen radicals and other cytostatic and cytolytic factors. Macrophage-colony stimulating factor augments many of these antitumor functions (100).

V. CONCLUSION

The molecules described herein as antiangiogenic and antimetastatic agents represent a wide variety of molecular structures with a wide variety of biological effects and targets. Most often these agents have been generally classified as antiangiogenic or antimetastatic by their effects in an in vitro bioassay system. The diversity in this group of molecules gives strength to the potential of this approach in therapeutic applications. The biological and biochemical pathways involved in angiogenesis are numerous and redundant. It is likely that there are many angiogenic factors and many pathways of invasion; therefore, it is likely that blockade of more than one pathway related to angiogenesis or invasion will be necessary to effect the natural progress of a malignant disease.

The vasculature forms the first barrier to penetration of molecules into tumors. Although the antiangiogenic agent treatments administered in these studies did not inhibit angiogenesis in these tumors completely, the vasculature present in the treated tumors may be impaired compared to control tumors. Overall, the best speculation is that the main targets for the antiangiogenic agents are extracellular matrix processes or tumor endothelial cells and that inhibition or impairment of these nonmalignant functions can improve therapeutic responses when used in combination with cytotoxic therapies. The incorporation of antiangiogenic agents and antimetastatic agents into therapeutic regimens represents an important challenge. The successful treatment of cancer requires the eradication of all malignant cells and treatment with cytotoxic therapies. The compatibility of antiangiogenic therapy and anti-invasion agents with cytotoxic chemotherapeutic agents is not obvious (101).

The goal of the addition of any noncytotoxic potentiator to a therapeutic regimen is to take a *good* therapy and, without additional toxicity, "push" it to cure. Cyclophosphamide is a *good* drug against the Lewis lung carcinoma, although no long-term survivors of animals bearing Lewis lung carcinoma are achieved with cyclophosphamide treatment alone. Adding antiangiogenic agents to treatment of this tumor with cyclophosphamide produced a cure rate of 40% to 50%, meaning that both the primary and metastatic disease has been eradicated in these animals. Cures were achieved only when the antiangiogenic treatments extended from days 4 to 18 after Lewis lung tumor implantation. The results obtained with the addition of antiangiogenic agents to cytotoxic anticancer therapies in in vivo models of established solid tumors have been very positive and provide direction for future clinical trials including these antiangiogenic agents. Two conclusions may be drawn. First, combinations of antiangiogenic or antimetastatic agents evoke a greater effect on tumor response to therapy than does treatment with single agents of these classes. Second, treatment with antiangiogenic agents or antimetastatic agents can interact in a positive way with cytotoxic therapies.

The early phases of the clinical testing (phase I & II) of antiangiogenic therapies should be performed with the highest degree of science possible. In addition to pharmacokinetic studies of the test agent, patients' blood and urine levels of angiogenic markers and tumor markers should be monitored. Ideally, a noninvasive measurement of endothelial cells metabolic activity could be devised. In lieu of that, a noninvasive measurement of tumor metabolic activity such as positron emission tomography of [^{18}F]fluorodeoxyglucose may be useful in elucidating a biological effect of these new agents in established disease. In terms of traditional clinical response criteria, stable disease may be considered a response over the relatively short time frame of many phase I clinical protocols (102).

The true strength of antiangiogenic therapies may be in their use in combination with traditional cytotoxic therapies in which they will add a new dimension to anticancer treatment options.

REFERENCES

1. Folkman J. Tumor angiogenesis: therapeutic implications. New Engl J Med 1971; 285:1182–1186.
2. Teicher B. A systems approach to cancer therapy (antiangiogenics + standard cytotoxics' mechanism(s) of interaction). Cancer Metastasis Rev 1996; 15:247–272.
3. Teicher BA, Holden SA, Ara G, Alvarez Sotomayor E, Huang ZD, Chen Y-N, Brem H. Potentiation of cytotoxic cancer therapies by TNP-470 alone and with other antiangiogenic agents. Int J Cancer 1994; 57:920–925.
4. Teicher BA, Dupuis NP, Robinson M, Emi Y, Goff D. Antiangiogenic treatment (TNP-470/minocycline) increases tissue levels of anticancer drugs in mice bearing Lewis lung carcinoma. Oncology Res 1995; 7:237–243.
5. Teicher BA, Alvarez Sotomayor E, Huang ZD, Ara G, Holden S, Khandekar V, Chen Y-N. β-Cyclodextrin tetradecasulfate/tetrahydrocortisol ± minocycline as modulators of cancer therapies *in vitro* and *in vivo* against primary and metastatic Lewis lung carcinoma. Cancer Chemother Pharmacol 1993; 33:229–238.

6. Teicher BA, Holden SA, Ara G, Northey D. Response of the FSaII fibrosarcoma to antiangiogenic modulators plus cytotoxic agents. Anticancer Res 1993; 13:2101–2106.
7. Alvarez Sotomayor E, Teicher BA, Schwartz GN, Holden SA, Menon K, Herman TS, Frei III E. Minocycline in combination with chemotherapy or radiation therapy *in vitro* and *in vivo*. Cancer Chemother Pharmacol 1992; 30:377–384.
8. Teicher BA, Alvarez Sotomayor E, Huang ZD. Antiangiogenic agents potentiate cytotoxic cancer therapies against primary and metastatic disease. Cancer Res 1992; 52:6702–6704.
9. Teicher BA, Holden SA, Chen Y-N, Ara G, Korbut TT, Northey D. CAI:effects on cytotoxic therapies *in vitro* and *in vivo*. Cancer Chemother Pharmacol 1994; 34:515–522.
10. Folkman J, Klagsbrun M. Angiogenic factors. Science 1987; 235:442–447.
11. Ingber D, Folkman J. Inhibition of angiogenesis through modulation of collagen metabolism. Lab Invest 1988; 59:44–51.
12. Folkman J, Ingber DE. Angiostatic steroids: method of discovery and mechanism of action. Ann Surg 1987; 206:374–383.
13. Ingber DE, Madri JA, Folkman J. A possible mechanism for inhibition of angiogenesis by angiostatic steroids: induction of capillary basement membrane dissolution. Endocrinology 1986; 119:1768–1775.
14. Folkman J, Langer R, Lingardt R, Haudenschild C, Taylor S. Angiogenesis inhibition and tumour regression caused by heparin or a heparin fragment in the presence of cortisone. Science 1983; 221:719–725.
15. Folkman J, Weisz PB, Joullie MM, Li WW, Ewing WR. Control of angiogenesis with synthetic heparin substitutes. Science 1989; 243:1490–1493.
16. Grunt TW, Lametschwadtner A, Karrer K, Staindl O. The angioarchitecture of the Lewis lung carcinoma in laboratory mice. Scand Electron Microsc 1986; 11:557–574.
17. Grunt TW, Lametschwadtner A, Karrer K. The characteristic structural feature of the blood vessels of the Lewis lung carcinoma. Scand Electron Microsc 1986; 11: 575–589.
18. Killough JH, Magill GB, Smith RC. The treatment of amebiasis with fumagillin. Science 1952; 115:71–72.
19. Katznelson H, Jamieson CA. Control of nosema disease of honeybees with fumagillin. Science 1952; 115:70–71.
20. Brem H, Ingber D, Blood CH, Bradley D, Urioste S, Folkman J. Suppression of tumor metastasis by angiogenesis inhibition. Surg Forum 1991; 42:439–441.
21. Ingber D, Fujita T, Kishimoto S, Sudo K, Kanamaru T, Brem H, Folkman J. Synthetic analogues of fumagillin that inhibit angiogenesis and suppress tumour growth. Nature 1990; 348:555–557.
22. Kusaka M, Sudo K, Fujita T, Marui S, Itoh F, Ingber D, Folkman J. Potent antiangiogenic action of AGM-1470: comparison to the fumagillin parent. Biochem Biophys Res Commun 1991; 174:1070–1076.
23. Brem H, Folkman J. Analysis of experimental antiangiogenic therapy. J Pediatr Surg 1993; 28:445–451.
24. Takayamiya Y, Friedlander RM, Brem H, Malick A, Martuza RL. Inhibition of

angiogenesis and growth of human nerve sheath tumors by AGM-1470. J Neurosurg 1993; 78:470–476.

25. Brem H, Gresser I, Grossfeld J, Folkman J. The combination of antiangiogenic agents to inhibit primary tumor growth and metastasis. J Pediatr Surg 1993; 28: 445–451.
26. Kamei S, Okada H, Inoue Y, Yoshioka T, Ogawa Y, Toguchi H. Antitumor effects of angiogenesis inhibitor TNP-470 in rabbits bearing VX-2 carcinoma by arterial administration of microspheres and oil solution. J Pharmacol Exper Ther 1993; 264:469–474.
27. Yamaoka M, Yamamoto T, Masaki T, Ikeyama S, Sudo K, Fujita T. Inhibition of tumor growth and metastasis of rodent tumors by the angiogenesis inhibitor O-(Chloroacetyl-carbamoyl)fumagillin (TNP-470; AGM-1470). Cancer Res 1993; 53: 4262–4267.
28. Toi M, Yamamoto Y, Imazawa T, Takayanagi T, Akutsu K, Tominaga T. Antitumor effect of the angiogenesis inhibitor AGM-1470 and its combination effect with tamoxifen in DMBA induced mammary tumors in rats. Int J Oncol 1993; 3:525–528.
29. Yamaoka M, Yamamoto T, Ikeyama S, Sudo K, Fujita T. Angiogenesis inhibitor TNP-470 (AGM-1470) potently inhibits the tumor growth of hormone-independent human breast and prostate carcinoma cell lines. Cancer Res 1993; 53:5233–5236.
30. Schoof DD, Obando JA, Cusack JC Jr, Goedegebuure PS, Brem H, Eberlein TJ. The influence of angiogenesis inhibitor AGM-1470 on immune system status and tumor growth in vitro. Int J Cancer 1993; 55:630–635.
31. Yanase T, Tamura M, Fujita K, Kodama S, Tanaka K. Inhibitory effect of angiogenesis inhibitor TNP-470 in rabbits bearing VX-2 carcinoma by arterial administration of microspheres and oil solution. Cancer Res 1993; 53:2566–2570.
32. Setchell KDR, Borriello SP, Kirk DN, Axelson M. Nonsteroidal estrogens of dietary origin: possible role in hormone-dependent disease. Am J Clin Nutr 1984; 40:569–578.
33. Barnes S, Grubbs C, Setchell KDR, Carlson J. Soybeans inhibit mammary tumor in models of breast cancer. In: Pariza M, AR Liss, eds. Mutagens and carcinogens in the diet. New York: Wiley-Liss, 1990:239–253.
34. Messina M, Barnes S. The role of soy products in reducing risk of cancer. J Natl Cancer Inst 1991; 83:541–546.
35. Akiyama T, Ishida J, Nakawaga S, Ogawara H, Watanabe S, Itoh N, Shibuya M Fukami Y. Genistein, a specific inhibitor of tyrosine-specific protein kinases. J Biol Chem 1987; 262:5592–5595.
36. Hunter T, Cooper JA. Protein-tyrosine kinase. Ann Rev Biochem 1985; 54:897–930.
37. Okura A, Arakawa H, Oka H, Yoshinari T, Monden Y. Effect of genistein on topoisomerase activity and on the growth of [Val12] Ha-*ras*-transformed NIH 3Y3 cells. Biochem Biophys Res Commun 1988; 157:183–189.
38. Fotsis T, Pepper M, Adlercreutz H, Fleischmann G, Hase T, Montesano R, Schweigerer L. Genistein, a dietary-derived inhibitor of *in vitro* angiogenesis. Proc Natl Acad Sci U S A 1993; 90:2690–2694.
39. Takano S, Gately S, Neville M, Herblin WF, Gross JL, Brem S. Suramin, an inhib-

tor of angiogenesis, suppresses endothelial cell growth, migration and plasminogen activator activity. Proc Amer Assoc Cancer Res 1993; 34:74.
40. Danesi R, Del Bianchi S, Soldani P, Campagni A, La Rocca RV, Myers CE, Paparelli A, Del Tacca M. Suramin inhibits bFGF-induced endothelial cell proliferation and angiogenesis in the chick chorioallantoic membrane. Br J Cancer 1993; 68: 932–938.
41. Stein CA, LaRocca RV, Thomas R, McAtee N, Myers CE. Suramin: an anticancer drug with a unique mechanism of action. J Clin Oncol 1989; 7:499–508.
42. Yayon A, Klagsbrun M. Autocrine transformation by chimeric signal peptide-basic fobroblast growth factor: reversal by suramin. Proc Natl Acad Sci U S A 1990; 87:5346–5350.
43. Takano S, Gately S, Neville ME, Herblin WF, Gross JL, Engelhard H, Perricone M, Eidsvoog K, Brem S. Suramin, an anticancer and angiosuppressive agent, inhibits endothelial cell binding of basic fibroblast growth factor, migration, proliferation, and induction of urokinase-type plasminogen activator. Cancer Res 1994; 54:2654–2660.
44. Teicher BA, Dupuis N, Kusumoto T, Robinson MF, Liu F, Menon K, Coleman CN. Antiangiogenic agents can increase tumor oxygenation and response to radiation therapy. Radiat Oncol Invest 1995; 2:269–276.
45. Teicher BA, Holden SA, Dupuis NP, Kakeji Y, Ikebe M, Emi Y, Goff D. Potentiation of cytotoxic therapies by TNP-470 and minocycline in mice bearing EMT-6 mammary carcinoma. Breast Cancer Res Treat 1995; 36:227–236.
46. Teicher BA, Holden SA, Ara G, Dupuis N, Liu F, Yuan J, Ikebe M, Kakeji Y. Influence of an anti-angiogenic treatment on 9L gliosarcoma: oxygenation and response to cytotoxic therapy. Int J Cancer 1995; 61:732–737.
47. Terranova VP, Hujanen ES, Martin GR. Basement membrane and the invasive activity of metastatic tumor cells. J Natl Cancer Inst 1986; 77:311–316.
48. Tryggvason K, Hoyhtya M, Salo T. Proteolytic degradation of extracellular matrix in tumor invasion. Biochim Biophys Acta 1987; 907:191–217.
49. Taylor S, Folkman J. Protamine is an inhibitor of angiogenesis. Nature 1982; 297: 307–312.
50. Groopman JE, Scadden DT. Interferon therapy for Kaposi sarcoma associated with the acquired immunodeficiency syndrome (AIDS). Ann Int Med 1989; 110:335–337.
51. White CW, Sondheimer HM, Crouch EC, Wilson H, Fan LL. Treatment of pulmonary hemangiomatosis with recombinant interferon alfa-2a. Med Intell 1989; 18: 1197–1200.
52. Strieter RM, Kunkel SL, Arenberg DA, Burdick MD, Polverini PJ. Interferon γ-inducible protein 10 (IP-10), a member of the C-X-C chemokine family, is an inhibitor of angiogenesis. Biochem Biophys Res Commun 1995; 210:51–57.
53. Kolber DL, Knisely TL, Maione TE. Inhibition of development of murine melanoma lung metastases by systemic administration of recombinant platelet factor 4. J Natl Cancer Inst 1995; 87:304–309.
54. Stetler-Stevenson WG, Krutzsch HC, Liotta LA. Tissue inhibitor of metalloproteinase (TIMP-2). A new member of the metalloproteinase inhibitor family. J Biol Chem 1989; 264:17374–17378.
55. Welgus HG, Stricklin GP. Human skin fibroblast collagenase inhibitor. Compara-

tive studies in human connective tissues, serum, and amniotic fluid. J Biol Chem 1983; 258:12259–12264.
56. Voest EE, Kenyon BM, O'Reilly MS, Truitt G, D'Amato RJ, Folkman J. Inhibition of angiogenesis *in vivo* by interleukin 12. J Natl Cancer Inst 1995; 87:581–586.
57. Kerbel RS, Hawley RG. Interleukin 12: newest member of the antiangiogenesis club. J Natl Cancer Inst 1995; 87:557–558.
58. Banks RE, Patel PM, Selby PJ. Interleukin 12: a new clinical player in cytokine therapy. Br J Cancer 1995; 71:655–659.
59. O'Reilly MS, Holmgren L, Shing Y, Chen C, Rosenthal RA, Moses M, Lane WS, Cao Y, Sage EH, Folkman J. Angiostatin: a novel angiogenesis inhibitor that mediates the suppression of metastases by a Lewis lung carcinoma. Cell 1994; 79: 315–328.
60. Lee A, Langer R. Shark cartilage contains inhibitors of tumor angiogenesis. Science 1983; 221:1185–1187.
61. Moses MA, Sudhalter J, Langer R. Identification of an inhibitor of neovascularization from cartilage. Science 1990; 248:1408–1410.
62. Taylor CM, Weiss JB. Partial purification of a 5.7K glycoprotein from bovine vitreous which inhibits both angiogenesis and collagenase activity. Biochem Biophys Res Commun 1985; 133:911–916.
63. DeClerck YA. Purification and characterization of a collagenase inhibitor produced by bovine vascular smooth muscle cells. Arch Biochem Biophys 1988; 265: 28–37.
64. Sakamoto N, Iwahana M, Tanaka NG, Osada Y. Inhibition of angiogenesis and tumor growth by a synthetic laminin peptide, CDPGYIGSR-NH_2. Cancer Res 1991; 51:903–906.
65. Bogden AE, Taylor JE, Moreau J-P, Coy DH, LePage DJ. Response of human lung tumor xenografts to treatment with a somatostatin analogue (somatuline). Cancer Res 1990; 50:4350–4365.
66. Brooks PC, Clark RA, Cheresh DA. Requirement of vascular integrin $\alpha_v\beta_3$ for angiogenesis. Science 1994; 264:569–573.
67. Brooks PC, Montgomery AMP, Rosenfeld M, Reisfeld RA, Hu T, Klier G, Cheresh DA. Integrin $\alpha_v\beta_3$ antagonists promote tumor regression by inducing apoptosis of angiogenic blood vessels. Cell 1994; 79:1157–1164.
68. Cheresh DA. Human endothelial cells synthesize and express an Arg-Gly-Asp-directed adhesion receptor involved in attachment to fibrinogen and von Willebrand factor. Proc Natl Acad Sci U S A 1987; 84:6471–6475.
69. Gazzinelli RT, Hieny S, Wynn TA, Wolf S, Sher A. Interleukin 12 is required for the T-lymphocyte-independent induction of interferon γ by an intracellular parasite and induces resistance in T-cell-deficient hosts. Proc Natl Acad Sci U S A 1993; 90:6115–6119
70. Locksley RM. Interleukin 12 in host defense against microbial pathogens. Proc Natl Acad Sci U S A 1993; 90:5879–5880.
71. Robertson M, Ritz J. Interleukin 12: basic biology and potential applications in cancer treatment. Oncologist 1996; 1:88–97.
72. Gately MK, Desai B, Wolitzky AG, Quinn PM, Dwyer CM, Podlaski FJ, Familletti PC, Sinigaglia F, Chizzonite R, Gubler U, Stern AS. Regulation of human lympho-

cyte proliferation by a heterodimeric cytokine, IL-12 (cytotoxic lymphocyte maturation factor). J Immunol 1991; 147:874–882.
73. Perussia B, Chan SH, D'Andres A, Tsuji K, Santoli D, Pospisil M, Young D, Wolf SF, Trinchieri G. Natural killer (NK) cell stimulatory factor of IL-12 has differential effects on the proliferation of TCR-$\alpha\beta^+$, TCR-$\gamma\delta^+$ T lymphocytes, and NK cells. J Immunol 1992; 149:3495–3502.
74. Robertson MJ, Soiffer RJ, Wolf SF, Manley TJ, Donahue C, Young D, Herrmann SH, Ritz J. Responses of human natural killer (NK) cells to NK cell stimulatory factor (NKSF): cytolytic activity and proliferation of NK cells are differentially regulated by NKSF. J Exp Med 1992; 175:779–788.
75. Gately MK, Wolitzky AG, Quinn PM, Chizzonite R. Regulation of human cytolytic lymphocyte responses by interleukin-12. Cell Immunol 1992; 143:127.
76. Naume B, Gately M, Espevik T. A comparative study of IL-12 (cytotoxic lymphocyte maturation factor)-, IL-2-, and IL-7-induced effects on immunomagnetically purified CD56$^+$ NK cells. J Immunol 1992; 148:2429–2436.
77. Chan SH, Perussia B, Gupta JW, Kobayashi M, Pospisil M, Young HA, Wolf SF, Young D, Clark SC, Trinchieri G. Induction of interferon γ production by natural killer cell stimulatory factor: characterization of the responding cells and synergy with other inducers. J Exp Med 1991; 173:869–879.
78. Brunda M, Luistro L, Rumennik L, Wright R, Dvorozniak M, Aglione A, Wigginton J, Wiltrout R, Hendrzak J, Palleroni A. Antitumor activity of interleukin 12 in preclinical models. Cancer Chemother Pharmacol 1996; 38:S16–S21.
79. Brunda MJ, Luistro L, Warrier RR, Wright RB, Hubbard BR, Murphy M, Wolf SF, Gately MK. Antitumor and antimetastatic activity of Interleukin-12 against murine tumors. J Exp Med 1993; 178:1223–1230.
80. Nastala CL, Edington HD, McKinney TG, Tahara H, Nalesnik MA, Brunda MJ, Gately MK, Wolf SF, Schreiber RD, Storkus WJ, Lotze MT. Recombinant IL-12 administration induces tumor regression in association with IFN-γ production. J Immunol 1994; 153:1697–1706.
81. Noguchi Y, Richards EC, Chen Y-T, Old LJ. Influence of interleukin 12 on p53 peptide vaccination against established Meth A sarcoma. Proc Natl Acad Sci USA 1995; 92:2219–2223.
82. Fujiwara H, Hamaoka T. Antitumor and antimetastatic effects of interleukin 12. Cancer Chemother Pharmacol 1996; 38:S22–S26.
83. Kedar E, Klein E. Cancer immunotherapy: are the results discouraging? Can they be improved? Adv Cancer Res 1992;59:245.
84. Seder RA, Gazzinelli R, Sher A, Paul WE. Interleukin 12 acts directly on CD4+ T cells to enhance priming for interferon γ production and diminishes interleukin 4 inhibition of such priming. Proc Nat Acad Sci USA 1993; 90:10188–10192.
85. Yoshida A, Koide Y, Uchijima M, Yoshida TO. IFN-γ induces IL-12 mRNA expression by a murine macrophage cell line, J774. Biochem Biophys Res Commun 1994; 198:857–861.
86. Gately MK, Warrier RR, Honasoge S, Carvajal DM, Faherty DA, Connaughton SE, Anderson TD, Sarmiento U, Hubbard BR, Murphy M. Administration of recombinant IL-12 to normal mice enhances cytolytic lymphocyte activity and induces production of IFN-γ in vivo. Int Immunol 1994; 6:157–167.

87. Zeh III HJ, Hurd S, Storkus WJ, Lotze MT. Interleukin-12 promotes the proliferation and cytolytic maturation of immune effectors: implications for the immunotherapy of cancer. J Immunother 1993; 14:155–161.
88. Caruso M, Pham-Nguyen K, Kwong Y, Xu B, Kosai K, Finegold M, Woo S, Chen S. Adenovirus-mediated interleukin-12 gene therapy for metastatic colon carcinoma. Proc Natl Acad Sci USA 1996; 93:11302–11306.
89. Nishimura T, Watanabe K, Yahata T, Ushaku L, Ando K, Kimura M, Saiko I, Uede T, Habu S. Application of interleukin 12 to antitumor cytokine and gene therapy. 1996; 38:S27–S34.
90. Brunda MJ. Interleukin-12. J Leukoc Biol 1994; 55:280–288.
91. Gohji K, Fidler I, Tsan R, Radinsky R, von Eschenbach A, Tsuruo T, Nakajima M. Human recombinant interferons-beta and -gamma decrease gelatinase production and invasion by human KG-2 renal-carcinoma cells. Int J Cancer 1994; 58: 380–384.
92. Hujanen ES, Väisänen A, Zheng A, Tryggvason K, Turpeenniemi-Hujanen. Modulation of M_r 72,000 and M_r 92,000 type-IV collagenase (gelatinase A and B) gene expression by interferons alpha and gamma in human melanoma. Int J Cancer 1994; 58:582–586.
93. Norioka K, Mitaka T, Mochizuki Y, Hara M, Kawagoe M, Nakamura H. Interaction of Interleukin-1 and Interferon-γ on fibroblast growth factor-induced angiogenesis. Jpn J Cancer Res 1994; 85:522–529.
94. Hiscox S, Hallett MB, Puntis MCA, Jiang WG. Inhibition of cancer cell motility and invasion by interleukin-12. Clin Exp Metastasis 1995; 13:396–404.
95. Wigginton JM, Komschlies KL, Back TC, Franco JL, Brunda MJ, Wiltrout RH. Administration of Interleukin-12 with pulse Interleukin-2 and the rapid and complete eradication of murine renal carcinoma. J Natl Cancer Inst 1996; 88:38–43.
96. Teicher BA, Ara G, Menon K, Schaub RG. *In vivo* studies with interleukin-12 alone and in combination with monocyte-colony stimulating factor and/or fractionated radiation therapy. Int J Cancer 1995; 65:80–84.
97. Lu L, Shen R-N, Lin Z-H, Aukerman SL, Ralph P, Broxmeyer HE. Anti-tumor effects of recombinant human macrophage colony-stimulating factor, alone or in combination with local irradiation, in mice inoculated with Lewis lung carcinoma cells. Int J Cancer 1991; 47:143–147.
98. Bonta IL, Ben-Efraim S. Involvement of inflammatory mediators in macrophage antitumor activity. J Leukoc Biol 1993; 54:613–626.
99. Wolf SF, Sieburth D, Sypek J. Interleukin 12: a key modulator of immune function. Stem Cells 1994; 12:154–168.
100. Munn DH, Cheung NK. Antibody-dependent antitumor cytotoxicity by human monocytes cultured with recombinant macrophage colony-stimulating factor: induction of efficient antibody mediated antitumor cytotoxicity not detected by isotope release assays. J Exp Med 1989; 170:511–526.
101. Gasparini G, Harris AL. Clinical importance of the determination of tumor angiogenesis in breast carcinoma: much more than a new prognostic tool. J Clin Oncol 1995; 13:765–782.
102. Toppmeyer D. Phase I trial design and methodology. In: Teicher B, ed. Anticancer Drug Development: Preclinical Screening, Clinical Trial and Approval. New Jersey: The Humana Press, 1997:227–247.

32
Targeting the Vasculature of Solid Tumors

Philip E. Thorpe and Sophia Ran
The University of Texas Southwestern Medical Center, Dallas, Texas

I. INTRODUCTION

Vascular targeting agents (VTA) are broadly defined as drugs that bind selectively to components of the vasculature of a disease site and locally affect the vasculature in a manner that produces a therapeutic effect at the disease site. In this chapter, we will restrict the disease to cancer, but it is important to emphasize that VTA might be constructed for use in arthritis, psoriasis, atherosclerosis, ocular neovascularization, and other diseases in which modifying the behavior of the vasculature (for example, by targeting a steroid) would be expected to attenuate the disease.

The types of VTA discussed in this chapter are immunoconjugates consisting of an antibody directed against a tumor endothelial cell antigen, linked to an effector molecule that causes thrombosis of the tumor vessels and tumor infarction. The effectors are ricin A-chain, which kills the tumor endothelial cells and induces platelet adhesion on the injured vessels, or a genetically engineered form of the human coagulation-initiating protein, tissue factor, which directly induces thrombotic occlusion of the vessels. Other effector mechanisms can also be used: for example, the drug CM101, a bacterial polysaccharide, targets tumor neovasculature and triggers a complement-activated inflammatory attack on the tumor vasculature by host leukocytes, leading to thrombosis and hemorrhage within the tumor and tumor necrosis (1–3).

Vascular targeting agents have several advantages over other types of anticancer drugs (4, 5). First, vascular endothelial cells are directly accessible to VTA in the blood, whereas drugs that act on tumor cells themselves have to permeate into the tumor (6). Entry of drugs into tumors is hindered by rises in interstitial pressure within the tumor core that oppose the influx of molecules in the fluid flow from the blood and restrict the process of drug entry to the comparatively slow process of diffusion (7, 8). Second, the vascular endothelial cells, which are the target for VTA, are genetically stable, normal cells unlikely to acquire mutations that render them drug resistant. In contrast, tumor cells, which are the target for most anticancer drugs, often become drug resistant (9). Third, VTAs have an inherent amplification mechanism in their action. Damage to the endothelial cells of a tumor vessel can cause complete cessation of blood flow through the vessel and the death of the thousands of tumor cells that were depending on that vessel for oxygen and nutrients (10). Fourth, VTAs should be of use in treating numerous types of solid tumors because most have similar vessels expressing similar markers.

Vascular targeting agents are conceptually different from drugs that inhibit angiogenesis. Inhibitors of angiogenesis prevent vascular endothelial cell remodeling while having little or no effect on vasculature where remodeling is not taking place (11, 12). These drugs inhibit tumor growth in regions of neovascularization but do not prevent tumor growth along existing vascular tracts or tumor survival in regions of the tumor served by mature, nonproliferating vessels. Angiogenesis inhibitors are most effective against tumors and metastases where angiogenesis is occurring vigorously; they are less effective against large tumors having a more established vasculature. Giving the drug for prolonged periods is essential to drive quiescent tumor endothelium into division as the tumor tries to revascularize zones of necrosis that occur naturally or that are created by earlier courses of the drug. In contrast, VTA are designed to induce platelet activation and coagulation of blood in vessels where division is taking place *and* where it is not. This broadens the effect on the tumor because most vessels are affected and because blood flow is halted in tumor vessels upstream of the thrombosed vessels, even if they lack the target marker. The action of the VTA is, therefore, less influenced by regional differences in vessels and better suited to the treatment of larger tumors. The downside, of course, is that VTA are riskier to use than angiogenesis inhibitors because any mistargeting to the vasculature of normal tissues could result in toxic side effects.

II. DIFFERENCES BETWEEN TUMOR AND NORMAL BLOOD VESSELS

For vascular targeting to succeed in the clinic, antibodies are required that bind to cell-surface markers that are unique to, or up-regulated in, vascular endothelial cells in human tumors. Numerous anatomical, morphological, and behavioral differences between tumor blood vessels and normal ones have been documented (reviewed in 10, 13, 14). Tumor blood vessels are often tortuous, highly variable in diameter with blind endings, and have fenestrations that increase vascular permeability (10). Progressive tumor growth necessitates the development of new blood vessels (angiogenesis) to meet the nutritional needs of the expanding tumor mass. Angiogenesis takes place by a multistage process (12) in which endothelial cells in a postcapillary venule degrade their underlying basement membrane, migrate toward the angiogenic stimulus, proliferate, form into tubes, lay down a new basement, and anastomose with an existing vessel so that blood flow is initiated. Thus, during neovascularization, migration of endothelial cells could expose previously occult abluminal proteins (15) or could require the synthesis of new molecules that mediate tissue degradation or cellular locomotion. Similarly, because endothelial cells in solid tumors proliferate at a rate 50 to 200 times higher than do endothelial cells in normal tissues (10, 16, 17), proliferation-linked determinants could serve as markers for tumor endothelium (10). Tumor-derived angiogenic growth factors such as basic fibroblast growth factor (bFGF) and vascular endothelial growth factor (VEGF) could directly induce new cell-surface molecules on local vascular elements or themselves serve as markers after binding to receptors on tumor endothelial cells (18) (see below). The hypoxic and acidic conditions within solid tumors also could directly induce the expression of new endothelial markers, or may do so indirectly by stimulating VEGF production (19, 20).

Other possible inducing agents of tumor vascular endothelial cell antigens are inflammatory or immunoregulatory cytokines, including interleukin (IL)-1, tumor necrosis factor (TNF), and IL-6, which are synthesized by many tumors, most notably melanoma and Hodgkin's disease (21–23). For example, E-selectin and vascular cellular adhesion molecule-1 (VCAM-1) are present in the vasculature of Hodgkin's and other solid tumors, but not in that of noninflamed normal tissues (23, 24). Finally, procoagulant changes are common on the endothelium of solid tumors and lead to the expression of such molecules as tissue factor, which is ordinarily absent from normal endothelium (25).

III. VALIDATION OF THE VASCULAR TARGETING APPROACH IN MICE EXPRESSING MHC CLASS II ANTIGEN

A. Proof of Concept in Mouse Model

We first set out to demonstrate the principle of vascular targeting in a mouse model (26, 27). A murine neuroblastoma cell line, transfected with the murine interferon *gamma* (IFN) gene (C1300 Muγ) was injected subcutaneously into nude mice. The IFN secreted by the tumor cells induced the expression of class II antigens of the major histocompatibility complex on the tumor vascular endothelial cells. Vascular endothelial cells in normal mouse tissues do not express class II antigens unless activated by IFN-γ, and so the class II antigen acted as a tumor vasculature specific marker in this model.

B. Targeting Ricin A-Chain to the Tumor Vasculature

Immunotoxins, prepared by linking the A-chain of the toxin ricin to monoclonal antibodies, selectively kill cells expressing the relevant target antigens at their surfaces by irreversibly inactivating ribosomes and inhibiting protein synthesis (28). A single intravenous injection of an anti-class II ricin A-chain immunotoxin into mice bearing large (≥ 1 cm in diameter solid tumors induced a potent, dose-dependent antitumor effect (Fig. 1). Tumors regressed, usually completely, although in all cases mice later relapsed with a progressively growing tumor at the original site of tumor growth. In contrast, an antitumor immunotoxin directed against the class I antigens of the tumor allograft only destroyed those tumor

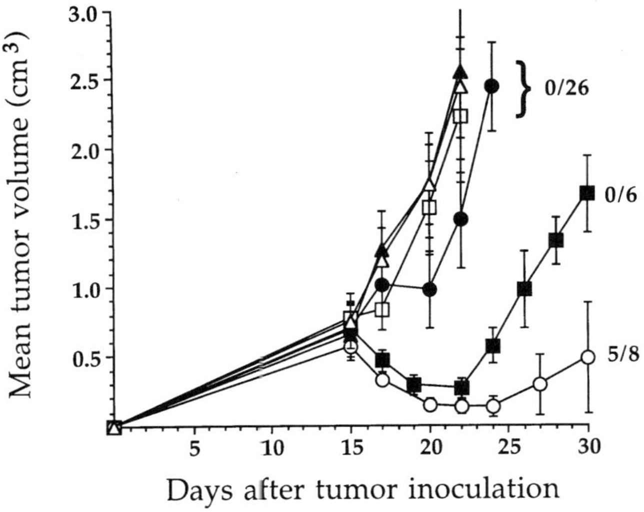

Figure 1 Regressions of solid tumors in mice induced by antitumor endothelial cell immunotoxin. C1300 Muγ tumor-bearing mice were given intravenous injections of 40 μg of anti-class II.dgA (solid square) directed against the tumor endothelial cells or 100 μg of anti-class I.dgA (solid circle) directed against the tumor cell themselves. Other mice received a combination of 20 μg anti-class II.dgA plus 50 μg anti-class I.dgA (open circle), 100 μg of an isotype-matched control immunotoxin (open triangle), 100 μg of anti-class II antibody (open square), or phosphate buffered saline (solid triangle). Error bars indicate the standard error of the mean. Also indicated: number of permanent complete remissions.

cells close to blood vessels and had little effect on tumor growth. The vascular targeting and direct tumor cells targeting approaches were complementary as, when both immunotoxins were used in combination, improved antitumor effects were achieved: 60% of animals treated with the combination cleared their tumors and remained disease free (Fig. 1).

A study of the time courses of the events in the tumors of mice treated with the anti-class II immunotoxin confirmed that tumor necrosis was secondary to intravascular thrombosis. The first loss of endothelial cells occurred about 2 hours after injection of the immunotoxin. Degeneration of the endothelial cell layer induced platelet adhesion and fibrin deposition. By 6 hours, many blood vessels in the tumor were occluded with thrombi and were stripped of their endothelial cell lining. At this time, the tumor cells were morphologically unchanged. By 24 hours, all vessels contained mature thrombi and the surrounding tumor cells had pyknotic nuclei. By 48 hours, widespread tumor necrosis had occurred, followed by autolysis and the physical collapse of the tumor mass.

C. Targeting Truncated Tissue Factor to the Tumor Vasculature

The same mouse model has been used to demonstrate antitumor effect of targeting human tissue factor (TF) to tumor endothelium (29). Tissue factor is the major initiator of the coagulation cascade (30). Cells typically in contact with plasma, including vascular endothelial cells, are devoid of TF under normal circumstances, whereas fibroblasts, smooth muscle cells, and epithelia, which are outside the blood, have TF incorporated into their plasma membranes (31–33). Blood coagulation is normally triggered at sites of injury when factor VIIa in the blood comes in contact with tissue factor on these extravascular tissues. The tissue factor: VIIa complex then rapidly activates factors IX and X by limited proteolysis, which leads to formation of thrombin and the fibrin clot (31).

The recombinant, truncated form of tissue factor (tTF) lacks the cytosolic and transmembrane domains and has only one hundred-thousandth of the factor X-activating activity of native TF, despite its retained ability to bind factor VIIa (34, 35). This is because the tTF: VIIa complex is soluble and does not associate with plasma membranes. Membrane association is required for the coagulation cascade to proceed, because phospholipids (mainly phosphatidylserine [PS]) in the lipid membrane provide the organizational surface upon which the coagulation complexes assemble (36). However, when the directing antibody delivers tTF to the tumor endothelial cell surface, it regains thrombogenic activity (29).

To target TF to tumor vasculature, a bispecific antibody was constructed. One arm of the bispecific antibody recognized the MHC class II antigen and the other was directed against a noninhibitory epitope on tTF. The antibody was mixed with tTF before injection, thus creating a complex termed a ‘‘coaguli-

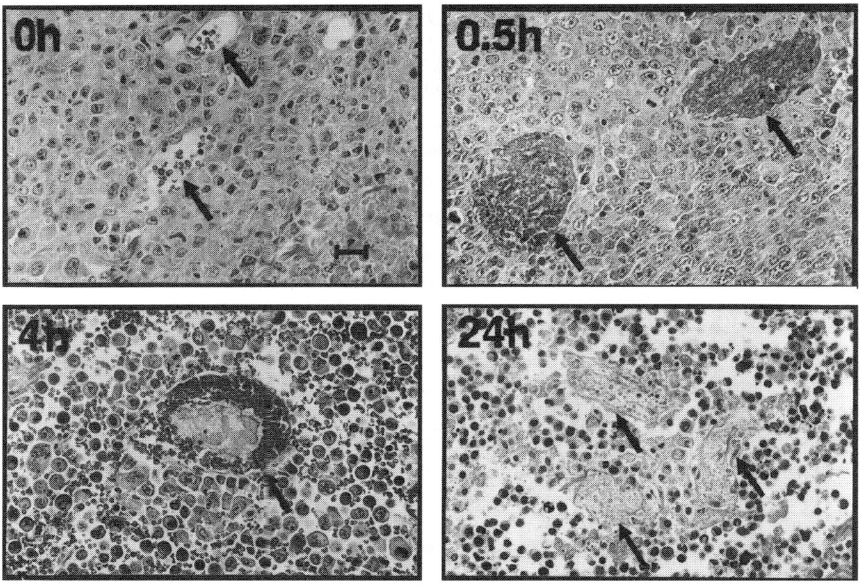

Figure 2 Time course of vascular thrombosis and tumor necrosis after administration of antitumor endothelial cell coaguligand. **Top left**. Before injection, the blood vessels are intact and the tumor cells are normal. **Top right**. 0.5 Hours after injection of coaguligand, blood vessels throughout the tumor are thrombosed. **Bottom left**. 4 Hours after injection, the tumor cells begin to separate from one another and develop pyknotic nuclei. **Bottom right**. 24 Hours after injection, advanced necrosis is apparent throughout the tumor. *Arrows* show blood vessels.

gand.'' When mice bearing large tumors (0.8 cm in diameter) were injected with anticlass II-coaguligand, thrombosis of tumor vasculature (Fig. 2) followed by dramatic tumor regressions was observed (Fig. 3). Thirty-eight percent of treated animals showed complete tumor regressions (Fig. 4) and a further 24% showed more than 50% tumor shrinkage (29).

D. Comparison of Immunotoxins and Coaguligands as Vascular Targeting Agents

The magnitude of the antitumor effect in the class II model was similar for the ricin A-chain immunotoxin and the tTF coaguligand. One difference between the two agents was the speed at which they induced thrombosis of tumor vessels. The coaguligand induced thrombosis in less than 30 minutes, whereas the immunotoxin took 6 hours to achieve the same effect. A second difference between

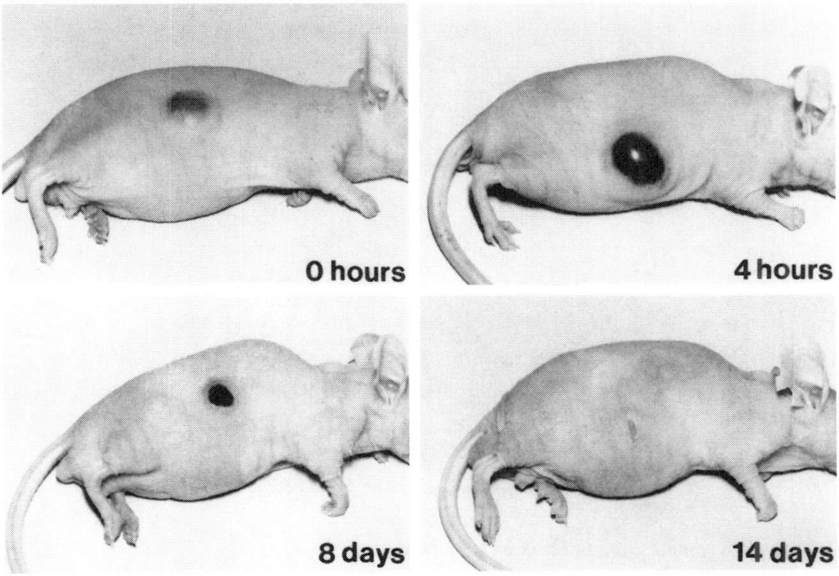

Figure 3 Gross appearance of subcutaneous tumors after treatment with antitumor endothelial cell coaguligand. At the time of treatment (0 hours) the tumor was pink, indicating florid vascularization. After 4 hours, the tumor appeared bruised and blackened. Over the next 8 days the tumor collapsed. By day 14, only fibrous scar tissue was visible in many of the mice.

the immunotoxin and the coaguligand is that they have different toxic side effects. The immunotoxin caused a lethal destruction of class II-expressing gastrointestinal epithelium unless antibiotics were given to suppress class II induction by intestinal bacteria. The coaguligand caused no gastrointestinal damage, as expected, because of the absence of clotting factors outside of the blood, but caused coagulopathies in mice occasionally when administered at high dosages. Coaguligand treatment may be preferable if the target antigen in the tumor vasculature is also expressed on normal tissues outside the blood, as cross-reactivity of immunotoxins with normal tissues can lead to unacceptable toxicities (37).

One major advantage of coaguligands over immunotoxins is that coaguligands can be made completely of human origin, making immune reactions in patients unlikely. Therefore, coaguligands can be administered to attack the primary tumor, and then repeated treatments can be given to act on any metastases that grow to the point where they become dependent on a blood supply. The use of tTF as the effector also offers other advantages: it is fully functional as a

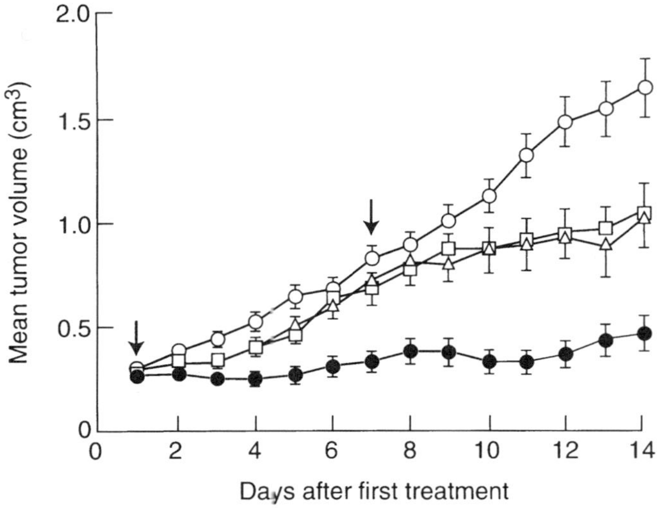

Figure 4 Regressions of solid tumors in mice induced by targeting tissue factor to tumor endothelial cells. C1300 Muγ Tumor-bearing mice were given two intravenous injections of 12.5 μg of human truncated tissue factor (tTF) complexed with 15 μg of a bispecific antibody directed against class II on tumor endothelial cells (*solid circle*). Other mice received intravenous injections of equivalent doses of tTF alone (*open square*), a control coaguligand directed against an irrelevant antigen (*open triangle*) or phosphate buffered saline (*open circle*). *Arrows* indicate days of injection. Each group contained 12 to 27 mice. Points represent mean tumor volume per group ± SEM.

coagulant in rodents, enabling a realistic evaluation of the construct in animal tumor models; neither free tTF nor antibody-conjugated moiety is functional in the absence of acidic membrane phospholipids, thereby preventing nonspecific blood coagulation; and it is expected to cause tumor-restricted thrombosis because tumor vasculature is predisposed toward coagulation (38) whereas normal vasculature is not (39).

IV. TARGETING VCAM-1 AND E-SELECTIN EXPRESSED ON THE VESSELS OF HODGKIN'S TUMOR IN MICE

A. VCAM-1 and E-Selectin Are Markers of Tumor Vasculature

Vascular cell adhesion molecule-1 and E-selectin are inducible endothelial cell adhesion molecules that play a role in the recruitment of leukocytes into sites of inflammation (40–42). E-selectin expression is induced by IL-1 and TNF, whereas VCAM-1 expression is induced by IL-1, TNF, and IL-4 (24, 43–45).

E-selectin and VCAM-1 are moderately to strongly expressed on the vascular endothelium of tumors having significant leukocytic infiltrates, in particular Hodgkin's disease (23, 24) non–small-cell lung carcinoma (46), breast carcinoma (47, 48), and nasopharyngeal carcinomas (49). The antigens are either induced by cytokines released by the infiltrating host cells or by cytokines released by the tumor cell themselves.

E-selectin is absent from vessels in normal human tissues apart from those in lymph nodes and tonsil (44). Vascular cell adhesion molecule-1 is absent from vessels in normal tissues apart from thyroid, testis, and tonsil and is present on activated macrophages and dendritic cells (43). Thus, both markers are largely restricted to tumor vessels and provide a basis for targeting of VTA.

We have recently explored the possibility of targeting VCAM-1 and E-selectin expressed on the vasculature of human Hodgkin's lymphoma (50). The mouse model of Hodgkin's disease was established by implanting L540cy lymphoma cells (derived from an end-stage patient) subcutaneously into immunodeficient mice. This xenograft shows all hallmarks of the human disease, including the expression of inflammatory cytokines and up-regulation of VCAM-1 and E-selectin on tumor vasculature. Immunohistochemical studies demonstrated the presence of both markers on vessels of the Hodgkin's tumor and the absence of E-selectin from all normal organs. In rodents, constitutive expression of VCAM-1 is confined to a few vessels in the heart and lungs. The constitutive expression of VCAM-1 in normal organs is apparently not induced by inflammatory cytokines as it is found in the control and tumor-bearing mice. Up-regulation of the expression of VCAM-1 and E-selectin on murine tumor vasculature is presumably induced by non–species-specific cytokines secreted by the L540 tumor cells.

B. Thrombotic and Antitumor Effects of Anti-VCAM-1 Coaguligand in L540 Tumor Model

To deliver tissue factor to Hodgkin's tumor vasculature, a coaguligand was constructed, consisting of rat IgG against murine VCAM-1 chemically linked to tTF. Intravenous injection of 20 μg of anti-VCAM-1 · tTF caused a profound thrombosis in 40% to 70% of the tumor blood vessels. As shown in Figure 5, within 4 hours of injection of coaguligand, the majority of blood vessels were thrombosed, containing occlusive platelet aggregates, packed erythrocytes, and fibrin. In several regions, erythrocytes had spilled into the tumor interstitium. By 24 hours, the blood vessels were still occluded and extensive hemorrhage was evident in the intratumoral region. Tumor cells had separated from one another and had pyknotic nuclei. By 72 hours, advanced necrosis was evident throughout the tumor. Necrosis was even present in the central region where the vessels do not originally express VCAM-1. Thromboses were confined to tumoral vessels: thromboses were not observed in the peritumoral vascular network.

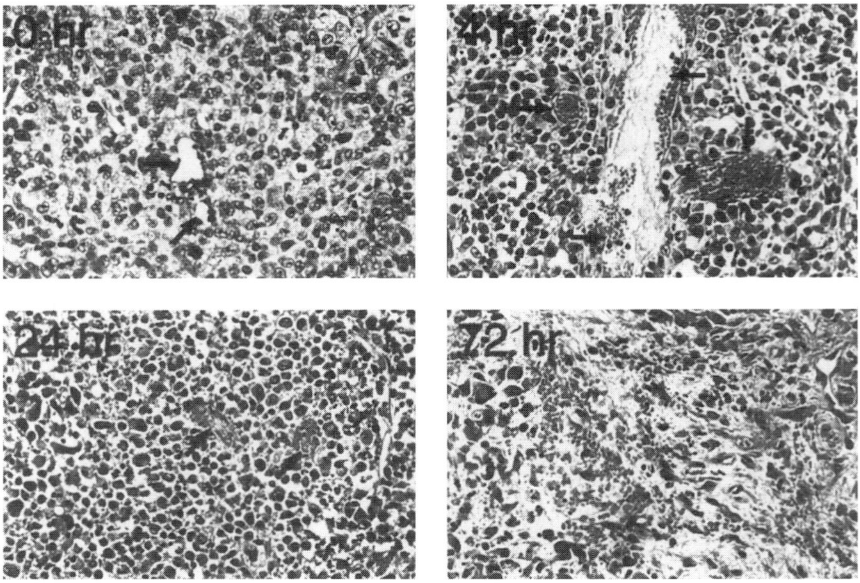

Figure 5 Time course of thrombosis of L540 tumor vasculature after injection of anti-VCAM-1 · tTF. 0, 4, 24, and 72 hours represent time after injection. At time 0, tumor cells are viable and blood vessels are intact. Note lack of thrombosis or hemorrhages in the untreated tumor. At 4 hours, many blood vessels are packed with erythrocytes and clots. Vascular walls are damaged, allowing leakage of erythrocytes into interstitial spaces. By 24 hours, tumor cells have separated from each other and are undergoing pyknosis and cytolysis. At 72 hours, areas of advanced necrosis are observed. *Arrows* indicate blood vessels.

Vasculature of the heart and lungs in all tumor-bearing animals was resistant to the thrombotic action of the coaguligand despite the localization of the conjugate to VCAM-1-positive vessels of both normal organs (Fig. 6). Localization of the construct in vivo was determined by two different detecting antibodies: antibody specific to rat IgG and the 10H10 antibody, specific for human TF. The staining by both antibodies completely overlapped, demonstrating the presence of intact coaguligand on vessels of tumor, heart, and lungs, and lack of reactivity in any other tissue. These experiments show that binding of coaguligand to VCAM-1 on normal vasculature in heart and lung does not induce coagulation, and that tumor vasculature provides additional factors to support coaguligand's action.

The antitumor activity of anti-VCAM-1 · tTF coaguligand was determined in mice bearing 0.3 to 0.4 cm^3 L540 tumors. The drug was administered intrave-

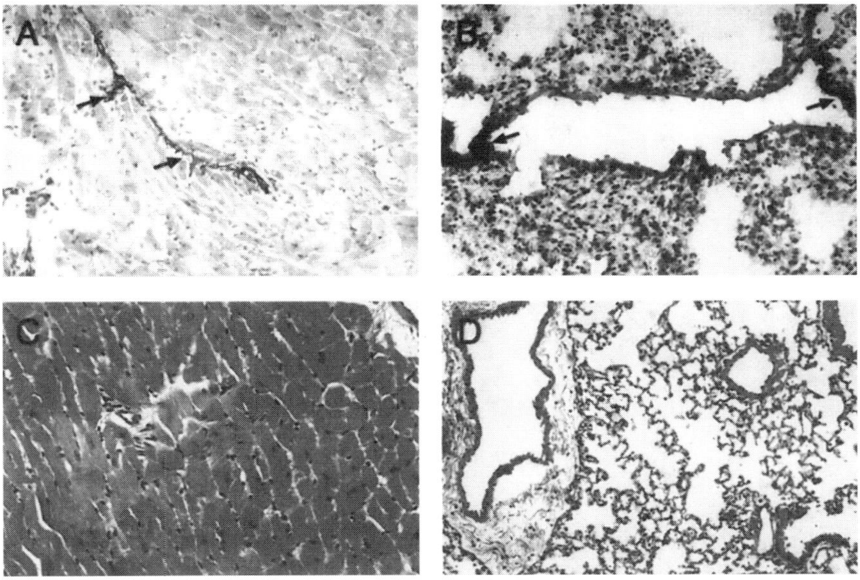

Figure 6 Lack of thrombosis of VCAM-1-expressing blood vessels in heart and lung after injection of anti-VCAM-1·tTF. Immunohistochemical detection of coaguligand bound to vessels in heart (**A**) and lung (**B**). Histology of heart (**C**) and lung (**D**) showing no thrombosis of vessels induced by coaguligand.

nously three times at intervals of 4 days. The pooled results from three separate experiments are shown in Figure 7. The mean tumor volume of anti-VCAM-1 · tTF-treated mice was significantly reduced at 21 days of treatment ($P < 0.001$) in comparison to all other groups. Nine of 15 mice treated with the specific coaguligand showed more than 50% reduction in tumor volume. The effect was specific because unconjugated tTF, control immunoglobulin-G (IgG) coaguligand, and a mixture of free anti-VCAM-1 antibody and tTF did not affect tumor growth. No toxicity was observed in mice treated with anti-VCAM-1·tTF coaguligand, as was determined by daily measurements of body weight, appearance, and physical activity. This is consistent with our observations that thrombotic activity of the specific coaguligand is restricted to the tumor site.

C. Tumor Endothelium Expresses PS on the Luminal Surface Where It Can Support the Activity of Coaguligands

The lack of thrombosis induced by anti-VCAM-1 · tTF in VCAM-1-positive normal vessels suggested that normal vessels might lack an ancillary molecule

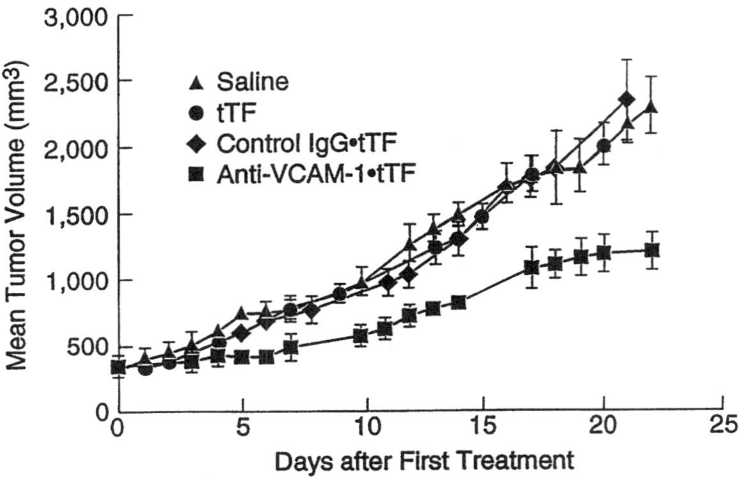

Figure 7 Retardation of growth of L540 tumors in mice treated with anti-VCAM-1·truncated tissue factor (tTF). L540 tumor-bearing mice were injected intravenously with either saline, 20 μg of anti-VCAM-1 · tTF, 4 μg of unconjugated tTF, or 20 μg of control IgG · tTF. Injections were repeated on days 4 and 8 after the first treatment. Tumors were measured daily. Mean tumor volume and S.D. of 8 mice per group are shown.

that was needed to support the coaguligand's action. We postulated that the ancillary molecule might be (PS), which is known to participate in thrombotic reactions (51–54). This notion is supported by our finding that the coaguligand's activity was diminished in the presence of annexin V in vitro. We reasoned that normal vessels might segregate PS to the cytosolic side of the membrane, whereas tumor vessels might express PS on the external luminal side.

To test this hypothesis, we determined the biodistribution of specific anti-PS monoclonal IgM (55) in L540 tumor-bearing mice. Anti-PS antibody specifically bound to the majority of L540 tumor blood vessels but not to vessels in normal organs, including VCAM-1-positive vessels in the heart and lung (Fig. 8). Similar results were obtained in mice bearing HT29 colonic tumors or H358 lung carcinoma. A mouse monoclonal IgM antibody against another acidic phospholipid, cardiolipin, did not localize to any organ, confirming the specificity of the detection by anti-PS IgM. No detection of either IgM was observed if frozen sections were treated by acetone, probably because the lipid was extracted by the organic solvent. We conclude that PS is exposed on the external surface of vascular endothelial cells in tumors but not in normal tissues. In the absence of PS surface exposure, anti-VCAM-1 · tTF binds to VCAM-1-positive vessels in heart and lungs but cannot induce coagulation. In contrast, VCAM-1-expressing

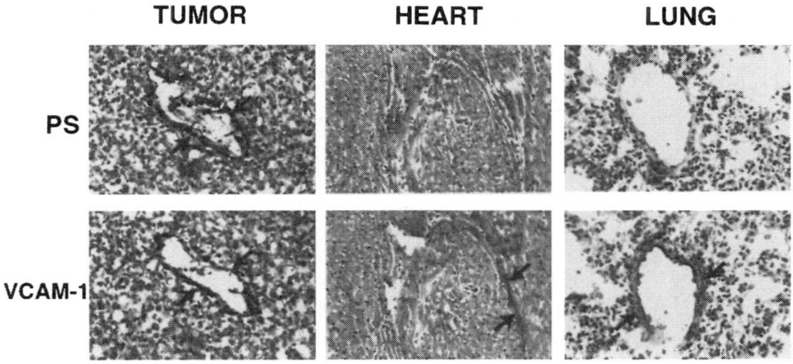

Figure 8 Coincident expression of phosphatidylserine (PS) on VCAM-1-expressing vessels in L540 tumors. Lack of expression of PS on vessels in heart and lung. L540 tumor-bearing mice were injected intravenously with 20 μg of anti-PS antibody and, 10 minutes later, were anesthetized and exsanguinated. Tumor and normal organs were snap-frozen. Serial frozen sections were stained with either anti-mouse IgM-HRP or with anti-VCAM-1 antibody. **Upper panels**. Anti-PS antibody localizes to tumor blood vessels but not to vessels in the heart and lungs. **Lower panel**. Tumor vessels coexpress VCAM-1 and PS, whereas vessels in heart and lungs express VCAM-1 but not PS.

vessels in the tumor show coincident expression of surface PS. This enables endothelium-bound coaguligand to activate coagulation factors and to locally induce formation of thrombi.

Phosphatidylserine expression on the surface of tumor vessels probably explains the switch to a prothrombotic phenotype that has been observed in numerous studies (38, 39, 56). Phosphatidylserine is normally segregated to the inner surface of the plasma membrane bilayer by an ATP-dependent aminophospholipid translocase (57). An increase in intracellular Ca^{2+} resulting from cell activation or perturbation activates a phospholipid scramblase to cause a rapid bidirectional movement of phospholipid between leaflets resulting in the exposure of PS at the cell surface (58). Ca^{2+} entry is caused by endothelial cell activation by cytokines, injury, and apoptosis, all of which have been observed to occur in the tumor environment.

The requirement for coincident expression of the target molecule and PS on tumor endothelium is of particular importance for the development of coaguligands. None of the known markers of tumor vasculature is completely absent from normal organs (59). This, however, may not disqualify these proteins as potential targets, as coaguligand activity is restricted to the tumor environment. Normal vessels are known to maintain the fibrinolytic status through numerous mechanisms (60–62), including segregation of PS to the inner side of the membrane (51). As shown in our studies, this fibrinolytic status is preserved, even on vessels in the heart and lung that constitutively express the endothelial cell activation marker, VCAM-1 (Fig. 6). Thus, coaguligands directed against VCAM-1 and E-selectin may be selective thrombotic agents for the treatment of solid tumors.

V. ANTIBODIES TO HUMAN TUMOR VASCULATURE

The perfect antibody for vascular targeting of solid tumors would: (a) recognize a cell-surface antigen that is present on a high proportion of tumor vascular endothelial cells in diverse solid tumors; (b) show no cross-reactivity with endothelial cells, or other cells, in normal tissues. The search for tumor vasculature-specific antibodies is a relatively young field and, to date, no antibodies have been found that meet both criteria. However, a number of antibodies have been reported to recognize antigens that show preferential expression in tumor vascular endothelial cells. The most promising of these antigens are reviewed below.

A. Endoglin

TEC-11 is a mouse monoclonal antibody of the IgM class that recognizes endoglin (63). Endoglin is an essential component of the TGF-β receptor system on human endothelial cells, binding transforming growth factor (TGF)-β1 and TGF-β3 with high affinity (Kd = 50 pM) (64). It is a dimeric glycoprotein composed of two 95 kDa disulfide-linked subunits whose primary sequence is known (65) and against which monoclonal antibodies have previously been raised (66–69). Endoglin is expressed on human endothelial cells, fetal syncytiotrophoblast (67), some macrophages (68), immature erythroid cells (69), and some leukemic and hemopoietic cell lines (69). Its expression on dermal endothelium is up-regulated in several chronic inflammatory skin lesions (70).

TEC-11 stained vascular endothelial cells in a panel of frozen sections of miscellaneous human malignant tumors moderately to strongly (63). Typically, 80% to 100% of vessels that stained with anti-von Willebrand factor antibody were stained with TEC-11. Endothelial cells of normal human tissues demonstrated weak immunoreactivity with TEC-11 under the same conditions. The exceptions were adrenals, placenta, and lymphoid organs in which the endothelial cells showed moderate staining.

The explanation for the more intense staining of endothelial cells in malignant tumors appears to be that endoglin is a proliferation-linked marker. Endothelial cells in malignant tissues other than B-cell lymphomas proliferate at rates up to 50 to 200 times faster than do endothelial cells in most normal tissues (16). The evidence that endoglin levels are proliferation linked derives from observations that subconfluent human umbilical vein endothelial cells (HUVEC) bind

TEC-11 strongly and homogeneously, and that when cells attain confluence and cease division, their TEC-11 binding falls to approximately one fifth of the level on dividing cells (63).

An immunotoxin prepared by linking TEC-11 to ricin A-chain was 3000-fold more potent at killing subconfluent, dividing HUVEC than it was at killing confluent, nondividing HUVEC (63). The greater sensitivity of dividing HUVEC to the drug can be attributed partly to the greater level of expression of endoglin on dividing HUVEC and partly to a difference in the routing of the drug after it binds to cell surface (63). Although nondividing HUVEC degrade the immunotoxin (presumably in lysosomes), dividing HUVEC internalize the drug by a pathway that avoids degradation and that favors A-chain translocation to the cytosol, where the A-chain has its toxic action.

A significant antitumor effect on an antiendoglin immunotoxin has been demonstrated recently in a mouse model of human breast carcinoma, MCF-7 (71, 72). Tumor-bearing mice were treated either with the antiendoglin immunotoxin, a mixture of unconjugated deglycosylated ricin A toxin and antiendoglin antibody or a conjugate of irrelevant antigen specificity. Only antiendoglin-treated mice showed a complete regression of the tumors, observed in the majority of the mice as long as they lived (more than 100 days). No apparent toxicity was reported in these studies, indicating that quiescent endothelial cells in normal tissues were unharmed by the immunotoxin, although they express endoglin at low levels. In contrast, dividing endothelial cells in the tumor, which express higher levels of endoglin, were effectively killed.

A monoclonal antibody, E-9, is an IgG1 that was raised against cultured HUVEC and detects an endoglin-like molecule (73, 74). E-9 shows very similar staining of endothelial cells in malignant and normal tissues to that described above for TEC-11, except that the endothelium of placenta does not stain with E-9. It is possible that there are epitope differences between endoglin in different locations, and that E-9 and TEC-11 distinguish between these.

B. VEGF and VEGF-Receptor Complex

Vascular endothelial growth factor, also known as vascular permeability factor (VPF), is a dimeric Mr 34000-42000 glycoprotein that is secreted by many tumor cells in response to hypoxia (19). The molecule is an endothelial cell-specific chemotactic factor and mitogen and enhances vascular permeability, all of which are important in the neovascularization of solid tumors (75). Two endothelial cell-surface receptors, VEGFR-1 (Flt-1) and VEGFR-2 (Flk-1/KDR) have been established as the mediators of the angiogenic responses of VEGF. Polyclonal antibodies to the amino terminus of VEGF intensely stain the endothelial cells in frozen sections of tumors, as well as the tumor cells themselves. In contrast, endothelial cells in normal tissue more than 0.5 mm away from the tumor did not stain (18). Vascular endothelial growth factor mRNA is localized to tumor cells and is absent from endothelial cells. By contrast, the mRNA for the VEGFR-1 and VEGFR-2 are mainly restricted to endothelium (75) and are up-regulated on tumor endothelium (20, 76, 77). These findings indicate that VEGF synthesized by the tumor cells is secreted and binds to VEGF receptors on adjacent endothelial cells. Thus, within the tumor microenvironment, the high concentration of both VEGF and its receptors leads to an accumulation of VEGF-receptor complex on the tumor endothelium.

The pivotal role for VEGF in tumor neovascularization can be demonstrated by blocking antibodies against VEGFR-2, which inactivate this receptor, disrupt ongoing angiogenesis and prevent malignant human keratinocyte invasion (78). Tumor angiogenesis and tumor growth also can be suppressed by VEGF-neutralizing antibodies (79–81), soluble receptors constructs (82, 83), and anti-VEGF-directed antisense strategies (84, 85). Overexpression of VEGF receptors on the tumor endothelium has been used to target VEGF conjugates with a truncated form of diphtheria toxin (86, 87). The VEGF-toxin construct was selectively toxic to endothelial cells in vitro and inhibited tumor growth in vivo by inducing vascular injury followed by hemorrhagic necrosis of the tumor mass (87).

Our laboratory generated and characterized six monoclonal antibodies to VEGF, the VEGF-receptor complex, or both (88). Five of the monoclonal antibodies did not interfere with the binding of VEGF to its receptor, whereas one (2C3) blocked this interaction. The 2C3 antibody prevented binding of VEGF to VEGFR-2, blocked VEGF-induced permeability in vivo, and significantly suppressed tumor growth in three different mice models (88a). The nonblocking antibodies recognized VEGF in association with Flk-1 in in vitro assays and stained blood vessels of human and rodent tumors. Three of these antibodies (3E7, GV39M, 11B5) show excellent specificity for tumor vessels after injection into tumor-bearing mice (Fig. 9) and are candidates for targeting or imaging tumor vasculature in humans.

C. Endosialin

Monoclonal antibody FB5 of the IgG2a isotype was raised against cultured human fetal fibroblasts and detects a novel cell-surface antigen, endosialin (89). Endosialin has a molecular mass of 165 kDa that is made up of a 95-kDa core polypeptide and several highly sialyated O-linked oligosaccharides. FB5 detects endothelial cells in about two thirds of human tumors, whereas normal blood vessels and other adult tissues lacked detectable endosialin. There was considerable variability between tumors in the number of FB5-positive vessels, ranging from a small subset of capillaries to virtually the entire capillary bed. No discernible parameter distinguished the degree of FB5 reactivity within the tumor. FB5

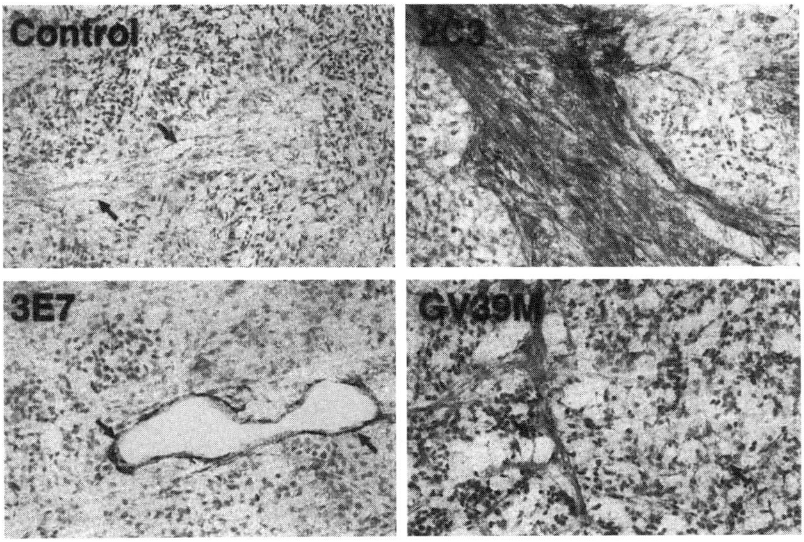

Figure 9 In vivo localization of 2C3, GV39M, and 3E7 antibodies to tumor vessels of NCI-H358 lung carcinoma xenograft. Biotinylated anti-VEGF or control IgG antibodies (100 μg) were injected into immunodeficient mice bearing human tumor xenograft. Twenty-four hours later, the mice were sacrificed and perfused, and the tumors were removed. Frozen sections of the tumors were stained for the presence of the injected antibody using standard immunohistochemical techniques. Representative sections of tumor are shown. *Arrows* indicate blood vessels.

also reacted with cultured fibroblasts and neuroblastoma cell lines. No reactivity was detected against other tumor types or with HUVEC, even after activation with cytokines. FB5 is rapidly internalized into endosialin-expressing cells and so is a candidate for the vascular targeting of agents such as ricin A-chain that have intracellular sites of action.

D. Fibronectin ED-B Domain

Monoclonal antibody BC-1, raised against fibronectin from the culture medium of SV-40-transformed human fibroblasts, reacts with an isoform of fibronectin that is present in the stroma of fetal and neoplastic tissues and in vessels in sites of angiogenesis (90). The epitope recognized by BC-1 lies within the ED-B sequence of fibronectin. BC-1 stained 38% of human tumors tested, including breast carcinoma (91, 92), hepatocellular carcinoma (93), colorectal carcinoma (94), and skin cancers (95). In almost all the positive tumors, BC-1 staining was confined to the tumor interstitium surrounding tumor cell nests and to the vascular intima. In normal adult tissues, BC-1 staining was limited to the superficial synovial cells, the intima of some ovarian vessels, scattered areas of the ovarian interstitium, and isolated areas of the basement membranes of the celomic epithelium, and to the areas of the myometrium.

An immunohistochemical study of the glioblastoma multiform and anaplastic astrocytoma demonstrated intense BC-1 staining of the cytoplasm of endothelial cells, whereas there was no staining associated with the tumor cells (96), suggesting that the BC-1-positive fibronectin isoform may be produced in the tumor vascular endothelial cells themselves. Administration of technetium 99m-labeled BC-1 antibody to patients with brain tumors resulted in high uptake at the tumor site where it identified an area of peripheral tumor growth (97). In contrast, the uptake in bone marrow, liver, and spleen was very low, suggesting that the ED-B fibronectin is specifically associated with immature malignant vessels (95).

Recently, single-chain Fv antibody fragments specific for ED-B domain have been isolated using phage display libraries and combinatorial mutagenesis (98). One of the fragments (L19) bound to the ED-B variant with the extremely high affinity of 54 pM (99). When administrated to nude mice bearing syngeneic teracarcinoma, 20% of the injected L19 fragment localized to the tumor (98). These results demonstrate that although tumor vasculature represents a small fraction of the total tumor mass, high affinity antibodies to selectively expressed markers can efficiently target tumors in vivo.

E. $\alpha_v\beta_3$ Integrin

The monoclonal antibody, LM609, recognizes the integrin $\alpha_v\beta_3$, a marker of angiogenic vascular tissue (100). After induction of angiogenesis, endothelial cells enter the cell cycle and express increased levels of $\alpha_v\beta_3$. LM609 antagonizes the binding of the endothelial cells through their $\alpha_v\beta_3$ integrins to extracellular matrix components. The cells fail to receive a signal from the extracellular matrix and undergo apoptosis (101).

The $\alpha_v\beta_3$ integrin is expressed on blood vessels in human wound granulation tissue but not in normal skin, and it shows a fourfold increase in expression during angiogenesis on the chick chorioallantoic membrane (CAM) (100). Similar induction of the $\alpha_v\beta_3$ expression was observed on the neovasculature of human breast carcinoma (102), melanoma (103), and various epithelial cancers (104). LM609 inhibited tumor-induced and bFGF-induced angiogenesis on the CAM after intravenous injection (101). Likewise, the disruption of $\alpha_v\beta_3$ integrin–ligand interaction by peptides mimicking the binding site on the ligand (105) results in apoptosis of tumor vasculature and suppression of tumor growth. This effect can be enhanced by combining anti-integrin-and antitumor-specific therapies. Lode et al. (106) showed that simultaneous administration of integrin antagonist and antitumor-IL-2 fusion protein induced tumor regressions and eradicated hepatic metastases, whereas monotherapy was only partially effective.

In addition to direct therapy, anti-integrin peptides have been used to deliver cytotoxic drugs to tumor endothelium (107). It has been shown in this study that coupling of α_v integrin-binding peptide to the anticancer drug, doxorubicin, enhanced the efficacy of the drug against breast cancer xenografts and reduced its toxicity to normal organs (107).

F. Prostate-Specific Membrane Antigen

As the name suggests, the expression of prostate-specific membrane antigen (PSMA) was originally thought to be exclusively restricted to the epithelial cell membrane of the prostate (108, 109). It is a good candidate for prostate-specific targeting therapies, because it is expressed on a high proportion of prostate cancers (110), and the expression is increased in metastatic disease. However, it now appears that antibodies to PSMA also react strongly with the vascular endothelium in a wide range of carcinomas, including lung, colon, and breast (111, 112) but do not react with normal endothelium. The reason why tumor endothelium should express PSMA, which is an enzyme (a gamma glutamyl hydrolase), is currently unknown. Antibodies against the extracellular domain of PSMA (111, 113) are promising vehicles for vascular targeting of a wide variety of cancers.

G. TIE-1, TIE-2, Angiopoietin-1, and Angiopoietin-2

TIE-1 and TIE-2 are receptor tyrosine kinases that are specifically expressed in developing vascular endothelial cells (114). Their expression is low in mature vessels and becomes up-regulated in growing blood vessel endothelial cells during tumor angiogenesis and wound healing (115, 116). Gene knock-out studies in mice indicate that TIE-1 is involved in forming intact functional (nonleaky) vessels and that TIE-2 is involved in vascular remodeling to provide more branches and larger and smaller vessels (117). One of the ligands for TIE-2, angiopoietin-1, is believed to have a stabilizing action on endothelium in sites of vascular remodeling (118, 119). Its naturally occurring antagonist, angiopoietin-2, binds to TIE-2 with similar affinity but blocks the activity of the receptor (120). Recent studies suggest that angiopoietin-2 is responsible for regression of vessels at vascular remodeling sites. Angiopoietin-2 may, paradoxically, promote tumor angiogenesis by opening up the endothelium to the angiogenic effects of VEGF (121). Because of the up-regulation of TIE-1, TIE-2, and its ligands in sites of tumor angiogenesis and vascular remodeling, antibodies to these proteins, or angiopoietin-1 or -2 themselves, could provide a means of targeting tumor vessels selectively.

VI. NEW TECHNOLOGIES FOR IDENTIFYING TUMOR ENDOTHELIAL ANTIGENS

Powerful new techniques for searching for tumor endothelial cell markers are being developed. Jacobson and colleagues (122) described a method for extracting endothelial cell luminal membrane proteins from solid tumors. The method involves perfusing an organ containing a tumor with cationic colloidal silica. The silica binds to the luminal membrane of the endothelial cells. The silica coating is then stabilized by overcoating it with a polyanion. The tumor is then surgically separated from the normal tissue, homogenized, and the silica-coated membranes sedimented by density centrifugation. Two-dimensional gel electrophoresis is then used to compare the proteins extracted from tumor vessels with those from normal vessels. Proteins present only in tumor endothelium are then isolated and sequenced or are used to raise specific monoclonal antibodies. Preliminary results indicate that at least 20 new proteins (or ones differing in their glycosylation patterns) can be detected in the endothelium of lung tumors in rats.

A second very promising technique has been described by Pasqualini and Ruoslahti (123). They injected phage display peptide libraries intravenously into mice and subsequently recovered and amplified those phage that homed selectively to blood vessels in the brain. Phage having thirteenfold selectivity for the brain were isolated. Peptides from these phage were coated onto glutaraldehyde-fixed red cells and were found to localize selectively in the brain. Analogous techniques using phage antibody display libraries or aptameric libraries could be useful for identifying new luminal markers on tumor endothelium.

VII. CONCLUSION

The final design of a VTA will depend on how specific the antibody moiety is for tumor endothelium. If one has an antibody that shows perfect, or nearly perfect, specificity for tumor endothelial cells, the effector moiety should be one that is active on both dividing and nondividing cells. Protein synthesis inhibitory toxins, such as ricin and *Pseudomonas* exotoxin, lend themselves to this purpose because they have very high potency and often excellent specificity as immunotoxins (124). Vascular leak syndrome, which is the dose-limiting side effect with immunotoxins (124), may not be a problem because the doses that need to be administered to saturate an antigen on tumor endothelial cells are likely to be much lower than for a relatively inaccessible extravascular target. Truncated TF would also be an excellent choice of effector moiety, as it induces coagulation of plasma equally efficiently from the surface of dividing and nondividing endothelial cells. Alpha emitters also lend themselves to vascular targeting because the entire energy of the α-particle would be delivered to the single endothelial cell that has internalized it, leading to high potency and fewer effects on bystander cells.

However, it seems likely that tumor vasculature markers will be expressed on the vasculature of at least some normal or inflamed tissues, albeit at reduced levels. Since both ricin A-chain and tTF have the potential to display very potent effects when targeted to dividing and nondividing cells, it is critical to assess whether cross-reactivity with endothelium in normal tissues can be tolerated. There are a number of reasons why some cross-reactivity might be tolerated. Firstly, the level of target antigen expression in normal endothelium may be below a threshold level required to bind sufficient immunotoxin or coaguligand to initiate endothelial cell killing or coagulation. Secondly, normal quiescent endothelium does not support coaguligand's action, even if the cells express the target marker at high density (50). This appears to be due to the absence of ancillary molecules, such as PS, on the outer surface of quiescent endothelial cells. In contrast, endothelial cells in tumors externalize PS that promotes assembly of the coagulation complexes and, therefore, support coagulation (50). Thirdly, the internalization route of a given immunotoxin may differ between dividing endothelial cells in tumors and quiescent endothelial cells in normal tissues, rendering the latter refractory to the toxic effects of the immunotoxin. This may be the case for the antiendoglin immunotoxin, TEC-11.ricin A-chain. Fourthly, there is little vascular redundancy in solid tumors because tumor cell proliferation and viability are rate-limited by the supply of oxygen and nutrients. Therefore, tumor cell killing may occur under conditions in which normal tissues survive.

In the event of unacceptable cross-reactivities of antitumor vasculature antibodies precluding the use of toxins or coagulation proteins as effector molecules, agents such as short-path radioisotopes or chemotherapeutic drugs, which have selectivity for dividing cells, should be considered in vascular targeting strategies to minimize damage to normal tissues.

A further possibility would be to use antibodies to target cytotoxic cells (as opposed to drugs) to tumor vasculature. A bispecific antibody recognizing both a tumor endothelial cell marker and a cytotoxic leukocyte antigen could theoretically cause an inflammatory reaction in tumor vessels. Alternatively, cytokines or chemokines targeted to tumor endothelial cells are amenable to genetic modification in situ (125), so it may also be possible to use antibodies to target DNA into tumor endothelial cells and confer proinflammatory, immunoregulatory, or tumor growth-regulatory activities upon them.

ACKNOWLEDGMENTS

We would like to thank Drs. Francis Burrows and Elaine Derbyshire for help in writing this manuscript, and Ms. Karen Schiller for excellent secretarial assistance.

REFERENCES

1. Thurman GB, Russel BA, York GE, Wang Y-F, Page DL, Sundell HW, Hellerqvist CG. Effects of group B Streptococcus toxin on long-term survival of mice bearing transplanted Madison lung tumors. J Cancer Res Clin Oncol 1994; 120:479–484.
2. Hellerqvist CG, Thurman GB, Page DL, Wang Y-F, Russell BA, Montgomery CA, Sundell HW. Antitumor effects of GBS toxin: a polysaccharide exotoxin from group B beta-hemolytic streptococcus. J Cancer Res Clin Oncol 1993; 120:63–70.
3. Thurman GB, Page DL, Wamil BD, Wilkinson LE, Kasami M, Hellerqvist CG. Acute inflammatory changes in subcutaneous microtumors in the ears of mice induced by intravenous CM101 (GBS toxin). J Cancer Res Clin Oncol 1996; 122(9): 549–553.
4. Denekamp J. Vascular attack as a therapeutic strategy for cancer. Cancer Met Rev 1990; 9:267–282.
5. Burrows FJ, Thorpe PE. Vascular targeting—a new approach to the therapy of solid tumors. Pharmacol Ther 1994; 64:155–174.
6. Kennel SJ, Falcioni R, Wesley JW. Microdistribution of specific rat monoclonal antibodies to mouse tissues and human tumor xenografts. Cancer Res 1991; 51: 1529–1536.
7. Jain RK. Transport of molecules in the tumor interstitium. Cancer Res 1987; 47: 3039–3051.
8. Jain RK. Transport of molecules across tumor vasculature. Cancer Metastasis Rev 1987; 6:559–594.
9. Morrow CS, Cowan KH. Mechanisms of antineoplastic drug resistance. In: DeVita VT, Hellman S, Rosenberg SA, eds. Cancer: Principles and Practice of Oncology. Philadelphia: J.B. Lippincott Company, 1993:340–348.
10. Denekamp J. Vascular attack as a therapeutic strategy for cancer. Cancer Metastasis Rev 1990; 9(3):267–282.
11. Folkman J, Shing Y. Angiogenesis. J Biol Chem 1992; 267:10931–10934.
12. Folkman J. Angiogenesis and its inhibitors. In: DeVita VT, Hellman S, Rosenberg SA, eds. Important Advances in Oncology, Part I. Philadelphia: J.B. Lippincott Company, 1985:42–62.
13. Dvorak HF, Nagy JA, Dvorak AM. Structure of solid tumors and their vasculature: implications for therapy with monoclonal antibodies. Cancer Cells 1991; 3:77–85.
14. Jain RK. Determinants of tumour blood flow: a review. Cancer Res 1988; 48:2641–2658.
15. Gospodarowicz D, Greenburg G, Vlodavsky I, Alvarado J, Johnson LK. The identification and localization of fibronectin in cultured corneal endothelial cells: cell surface polarity and physiological implications. Exp Eye Res 1979; 29:485–509.
16. Denekamp J, Hobson B. Endothelial cell proliferation in experimental tumours. Br J Cancer 1982; 461:711–720.
17. Hobson B, Denekamp J. Endothelial proliferation in tumours and normal tissues: continuous labelling studies. Br J Cancer 1984; 49:405–413.
18. Dvorak HF, Sioussat TM, Brown LF, Berse B, Nagy JA, Sotrel A, Manseau EJ, Vandewater L, Senger DR. Distribution of vascular permeability factor (vascular

endothelial growth factor) in tumors—concentration in tumor blood vessels. J Exp Med 1991; 174:1275–1278.

19. Shweiki D, Itin A, Soffer D, Keshet E. Vascular endothelial growth factor induced by hypoxia may mediate hypoxia-initiated angiogenesis. Nature 1992; 359:843–845.
20. Plate KH, Breier G, Weich HA, Risau W. Vascular endothelial growth factor is a potential tumour angiogenesis factor in human gliomas in vivo. Nature 1992; 359: 845–848.
21. Jucker M, Abts H, Li W, Schlinder R, Merz H, Gunther A, von Kalle C, Schaadt M, Diamantstein T, Feller AC, Krueger GRF, Kiehl V, Blankenstein T, Tesch H. Expression of interleukin-6 and interleukin-6 receptor in Hodgkin's disease. Blood 1991; 77:2413–2418.
22. Burrows FJ, Haskard DO, Hart IR, Marshall JF, Selkirk S, Poole S, Thorpe PE. Influence of tumor-derived interleukin-1 on melanoma-endothelial cell interactions in vitro. Cancer Res 1991; 51:4768–4775.
23. Ruco LP, Pomponi D, Pigott R, Stoppacciaro A, Monardo F, Uccini S, Boaraschi D, Tagliabue A, Santoni A, Dejana E, Mantovani A, Baroni CD. Cytokine production (IL-a alpha, IL-1 beta, and TNF alpha) and endothelial cell activation (ELAM-1 and HLA-DR) in reactive lymphadenitis, Hodgkin's disease, and in non-Hodgkin's lymphomas. Am J Pathol 1990; 137(5):1163–1171.
24. Cotran RS, Gimbrone MA, Bevilacqua MP, Mendrick DL, Pober JS. Induction and detection of a human endothelial activation antigen in vivo. J Exp Med 1986; 164: 661–666.
25. Contrino J, Hair G, Kreutzer DL, Rickles FR. In situ detection of tissue factor in vascular endothelial cells: correlation with the malignant phenotype of human breast disease. Nat Med 1996; 2:209–215.
26. Burrows FJ, Watanabe Y, Thorpe PE. A murine model for antibody-directed targeting of vascular endothelial cells in solid tumors. Cancer Res 1992; 52:5954–5962.
27. Burrows FJ, Thorpe PE. Eradication of large solid tumors in mice with an immunotoxin directed against tumor vasculature. Proc Natl Acad Sci U S A 1993; 90:8996–9000.
28. Vitetta ES, Thorpe PE, Uhr JW. Immunotoxins: magic bullets or misguided missiles? Immunol Today 1993; 14:148–154.
29. Huang X, Molema G, King S, Watkins L, Edgington TS, Thorpe PE. Tumor infarction in mice by antibody-directed targeting of tissue factor to tumor vasculature. Science 1997; 275(5299):547–550.
30. Ruf W, Edgington TS. Structural biology of tissue factor, the initiator of thrombogenesis in vivo. FASEB J 1994; 8:385–390.
31. Wilcox JN, Smith KM, Schwartz SM, Gordon D. Localization of tissue factor in the normal vessel wall and in the atherosclerotic plaque. Proc Natl Acad Sci U S A 1989; 86:2839–2843.
32. Drake TA, Morrissey JH, Edgington TS. Selective cellular expression of tissue factor in human tissues: implications for disorders of hemostatis and thrombosis. Am J Pathol 1989; 134:1087–1097.
33. Fleck RA, Rao LVM, Rapaport SI, Varki N. Localization of human tissue factor

antigen by immunostaining with monospecific, polyclonal anti-human tissue factor antibody. Thromb Res 1990; 59:421–437.

34. Ruf W, Rehemtulla A, Edgington TS. Phospholipid-independent and-dependent interactions required for tissue factor receptor and cofactor function. J Biol Chem 1991; 266:2158–2166.
35. Ruf W, Kalnik MW Lund-Hansen T, Edgington T. Characterization of factor VII association with tissue factor in solution. J Biol Chem 1991; 266:15719–15725.
36. Schafer AI. Coagulation cascade: an overview. In: Loscalzo J, Schafer AI, eds. Thrombosis and Hemorrhage. Boston: Blackwell Scientific Publications, 1994:3–12.
37. Gould BJ, Borowitz MJ, Groves ES, Carter PW, Anthony D, Weiner LM, Frankel AE. Phase I study of an anti-breast cancer immunotoxin by continuous infusion: report of a targeted toxic effect not predicted by animal studies. J Natl Cancer Inst 1989; 81:775–781.
38. Nawroth P, Handley D, Matsueda G, De Waal R, Gerlach H, Blohm D, Stem D. Tumor necrosis factor/cachectin-induced intravascular fibrin formation in meth A fibrosarcomas. J Exp Med 1988; 168(2):637–647.
39. Zacharski LR, Memoli VA, Ornstein DL, Rousseau SM, Kisiel W, Kudryk BJ. Tumor cell procoagulant and urokinase expression in carcinoma of the ovary. J Natl Cancer Inst 1993; 85(15):1225–1230.
40. Munro JM, Pober JS, Cotran RS. Tumor necrosis factor and interferon-gamma induce distinct patterns of endothelial activation and associated leukocyte accumulation in skin of Papio anubis. Am J Pathol 1989; 135:121–133.
41. Pelletier RP, Ohye RG, Vanbuskirk A, Sedmak DD, Kincade P, Ferguson RM, Orosz CG. Importance of endothelial VCAM-1 for inflammatory leukocytic infiltration in vivo. J Immunol 1992; 149:2473–2481.
42. Rice GE, Munro JM, Bevilacqua MP. Inducible cell adhesion molecule 110 (INCAM-110) is an endothelial receptor for lymphocytes. A CD11/CD18-independent adhesion mechanism. J Exp Med 1990; 171:1369–1374.
43. Rice GE, Munro JM, Corless C, Bevilacqua MP. Vascular and nonvascular expression of INCAM-110: a target for mononuclear leukocyte adhesion in normal and inflamed human tissues. Am J Pathol 1991; 138(2):385–393.
44. Kuzu I, Bicknell R, Fletcher CDM, Gatter KC. Expression of adhesion molecules on the endothelium of normal tissue vessels and vascular tumors. Lab Invest 1993; 69(3):322–328.
45. Fries JWU, Williams AJ, Atkins RC, Newman W, Lipscomb MF, Collins T. Expression of VCAM-1 and E-selectin in an in vivo model of endothelial activation. Am J Pathol 1993; 143:725–737.
46. Staal-van den Brekel AJ, Thunnissen FBJM, Buurman WA, Wouters EFM. Expression of E-selectin, intercellular adhesion molecule (ICAM)-1 and vascular cell adhesion molecule (VCAM)-1 in non-small-cell lung carcinoma. Virchows Arch 1996; 428:21–27.
47. Charpin C, Bergeret D, Garcia S, Andrac L, Martini F, Horschowski N, Choux R, Lavaut MN. ELAM selectin expression in breast carcinoma detected by automated and quantitative immunohistochemical assays. Int J Oncol 1998; 12(5):1041–1048.

48. Charpin C, Garcia S, Andrac L, Horschowski N, Choux R, Lavaut MN. VCAM (IGSF) adhesion molecule expression in breast carcinomas detected by automated and quantitative immunocytochemical assays. Hum Pathol 1998; 29(9):896–903.
49. Ruco LP, Stoppacciaro A, Uccini S, Breviano F, Dejana E, Gallo A, DeVincentis M, Pileri S, Nicholls JM, Barens CD. Expression of intercellular adhesion molecule-1 and vascular cell adhesion molecule-1 in undifferentiated nasopharyngeal carcinoma (lymphoepithelioma) and in malignant epithelial tumors. Hum Pathol 1994; 25:924–928.
50. Ran S, Gao B, Duffy S, Watkins L, Rote N, Thorpe PE. Infarction of solid Hodgkin's tumors in mice by antibody-directed targeting of tissue factor to tumor vasculature. Cancer Res 1998; 58(20):4646–4653.
51. Williamson P, Schlegel RA. Back and forth. The regulation and function of transbilayer phospholipid movement in eukaryotic cells. Mol Membr Biol 1994; 11(4): 199–216.
52. Dachary-Prigent J, Toti F, Satta N, Pasquet JM, Uzan A, Freyssinet JM. Physiopathological significance of catalytic phospholipids in the generation of thrombin. Semin Thromb Hemost 1996; 22(2):157–164.
53. Ortel TL, Devore-Carter D, Quinn-Allen M, Kane WH. Deletion analysis of recombinant human factor V. Evidence for a phosphatidylserine binding site in the second C-type domain. J Biol Chem 1992; 267(6):4189–4198.
54. Bevers EM, Rosing J, Zwaal RF. Membrane phospholipids are the major determinant of the binding site for factor X activating and prothrombinase complexes at the surface of human platelets. Agents Actions Suppl 1986; 20:69–75.
55. Rote NS, Ng AK, Dostal-Johnson DA, Nicholson SL, Siekman R. Immunologic detection of phosphatidylserine externalization during thrombin-induced platelet activation. Clin Immunol Immunopathol 1993; 66(3):193–200.
56. Donati MB. Cancer and thrombosis: from Phlegmasia alba dolens to transgenic mice. Thromb Haemost 1995; 74(1):278–281.
57. Julien M, Tournier JF, Tocanne JF. Basic fibroblast growth factor modulates the aminophospholipid translocase activity present in the plasma membrane of bovine aortic endothelial cells. Eur J Biochem 1995; 230(1):287–297.
58. Zhao J, Zhou Q, Wiedmer T, Sims PJ. Level of expression of phospholipid scramblase regulates induced movement of phosphatidylserine to the cell surface. J Biol Chem 1998; 273(12):6603–6606.
59. Thorpe PE, Burrows FJ. Antibody-directed targeting of the vasculature of solid tumors. Breast Cancer Res Treat 1995; 36(2):237–251.
60. Wu KK, Thiagarajan P. Role of endothelium in thrombosis and hemostasis. Annu Rev Med 1996; 47:315–331.
61. Benedict C, Pakala R, Willerson J. Endothelial-dependent procoagulant and anticoagulant mechanisms. Tex Heart Inst J 1994; 21:86–90.
62. Mosher DF. Blood coagulation and fibrinolysis: an overview. Clin Cardiol 1990; 4(suppl 6):VI5–11.
63. Burrows FJ, Derbyshire EJ, Tazzari PL, Amlot P, Gazdar AF, King SW, Letarte M, Vitetta ES, Thorpe PE. Endoglin is an endothelial cell proliferation marker that is upregulated in tumor vasculature. Clin Cancer Res 1995; 1:1623–1634.

64. Cheifetz S, Bellon T, Cales C, Vera S, Bernabeu C, Massague J, Letarte M. Endoglin is a component of the transforming growth factor-beta receptor system in human endothelial cells. J Biol Chem 1992; 267:19027–19030.
65. Gougos A, Letarte M. Primary structure of endoglin an RGD-containing glycoprotein of human endothelial cells. J Biol Chem 1990; 265:8361–8364.
66. Gougos A, Letarte M. Identification of a human endothelial cell antigen with monoclonal antibody 44G4 produced against a pre-B leukemic cell line. J Immunol 1988; 141:1925–1933.
67. Gougos A, St. Jacques S, Greaves A, O'Connell PJ, d'Apice AJF, Buhring HJ, Bernabeu C, Vanmourik JA, Letarte M. Identification of distinct epitopes of endoglin, an RGD-containing glycoprotein of endothelial cells, leukemic cells and syncitiotrophoblasts. Int Immunol 1992; 4:83–92.
68. O'Connell PJ, McKenzie A, Fisicaro N, Rockman SP, Pearse MJ, d'Apice AJF. Endoglin: a 180-kD endothelial cell and macrophage restricted differentiation molecule. Clin Exp Immunol 1992; 90:154–159.
69. Buhring HJ, Muller CA, Letarte M, Gougos A, Saalmuller A, van Agthoven AJ, Busch FW. Endoglin is expressed on a subpopulation of immature erythroid cells or normal bone marrow. Leukemia 1991; 5:841–847.
70. Westphal JR, Willems HW, Schalkwijk CJ, Ruiter DJ, deWaal RM. A new 180-kDa dermal endothelial cell activation antigen: in vitro and in situ characteristics. J Invest Dermatol 1993; 100:27–34.
71. Seon BK, Matsuno F, Haruta Y, Kondo M, Barcos M. Long-lasting complete inhibition of human solid tumors in SCID mice by targeting endothelial cells of tumor vasculature with antihuman endoglin immunotoxin. Clin Cancer Res 1997; 3:1031–1044.
72. Matsuno F, Haruta Y, Kondo M, Tsai H, Barcos M, Seon BK. Induction of lasting complete regression of preformed distinct solid tumors by targeting the tumor vasculature using two new anti-endoglin monoclonal antibodies. Clin Cancer Res 1999; 5:371–382.
73. Wang JM, Kumar S, Pye D, Vanagthoven AJ, Krupinski J, Hunter RD. A monoclonal antibody detects heterogeneity in vascular endothelium of tumours and normal tissues. Int J Cancer 1993; 54:363–370.
74. Letarte M, Greaves A, Vera S. CD105 endoglin cluster report. In: Schlossman SF, Boumsell L, Gilks W, Harlan J, Kishimoto T, Morimoto C, Ritz J, Shaw S, Silverstein T, Tedder T, Todd R, eds. Leukocyte Typing V: White Cell Differentiation Antigens. Oxford: Oxford University Press, 1995.
75. Senger DR, Vandewater L, Brown LF, Nagy JA, Yeo K-T, Yeo T-K, Berse B, Jackman RW, Dvorak AM, Dvorak HF. Vascular permeability factor (VPF, VEGF) in tumor biology. Cancer Metastasis Rev 1993; 12:303–324.
76. Brown LF, Berse B, Jackman RW, Tognazzi K, Manseau EJ, Senger DR, Dvorak HF. Expression of vascular permeability factor (vascular endothelial growth factor) and its receptors in adenocarcinomas of the gastrointestinal tract. Cancer Res 1993; 53:4727–4735.
77. Brown LF, Berse B, Jackman RW, Tognazzi K, Manseau EJ, Dvorak HF, Senger DR. Vascular permeability factor (vascular endothelial growth factor) and its receptors in kidney and bladder carcinoma. Am J Pathol 1993; 143:1255.

78. Skobe M, Rockwell P, Goldstein N, Vosseler S, Fusenig NE. Halting angiogenesis suppresses carcinoma cell invasion. Nature Med 1997; 3(11):1222–1227.
79. Kim KJ, Li B, Winer J, Armanini M, Gillett N, Phillips HS, Ferrara N. Inhibition of vascular endothelial growth factor-induced angiogenesis suppresses tumour growth in vivo. Nature 1993; 362(6423):841–844.
80. Presta LG, Chen H, O'Connor SJ, Chisholm V, Meng YG, Krummen L, Winkler M, Ferrara N. Humanization of an anti-vascular endothelial growth factor monoclonal antibody for the therapy of solid tumors and other disorders. Cancer Res 1997; 57(20):4593–4599.
81. Asano M, Yukita A, Matsumoto T, Kondo S, Suzuki H. Inhibition of tumor growth and metastasis by an immunoneutralizing monoclonal antibody to human vascular endothelial growth factor/vascular permeability factor 121. Cancer Res 1995; 55(22):5296–5301.
82. Aiello LP, Pierce EA, Foley ED, Takagi H, Chen H, Riddle L, Ferrara N, King GL, Smith LE. Suppression of retinal neovascularization in vivo by inhibition of vascular endothelial growth factor (VEGF) using soluble VEGF-receptor chimeric proteins. Proc Natl Acad Sci U S A 1995; 92(23):10457–10461.
83. Lin P, Sankar S, Shan S, Dewhirst MW, Polverini PJ, Quinn TQ, Peters KG. Inhibition of tumor growth by targeting tumor endothelium using a soluble vascular endothelial growth factor receptor. Cell Growth Differ 1998; 9(1):49–58.
84. Millauer B, Shawver LK, Plate KH, Risau W, Ullrich A. Glioblastoma growth inhibited in vivo by a dominant-negative Flk-1 mutant. Nature 1994; 367(6463): 576–579.
85. Saleh M, Stacker SA, Wilks A. Inhibition of growth of C6 glioma cells in vivo by expression of antisense vascular endothelial growth factor sequence. Cancer Res 1996; 56(2):393–401.
86. Ramakrishnan S, Olson TA, Bautch VL, Mohanraj D. Vascular endothelial growth factor-toxin conjugate specifically inhibits KDR/flk-1-positive endothelial cell proliferation in vitro and angiogenesis in vivo. Cancer Res 1996; 56(6):1324–1330.
87. Olson TA, Mohanraj D, Roy S, Ramakrishnan S. Targeting the tumor vasculature: inhibition of tumor growth by a vascular endothelial growth factor-toxin conjugate. Int J Cancer 1997; 73(6):865–870.
88. Brekken RA, Huang X, King SW, Thorpe PE. Vascular endothelial growth factor as a marker of tumor endothelium. Cancer Res 1998; 58(9):1952–1959.
88a. Brekken RA. Cancer Res. In press.
89. Rettig WJ, Garinchesa P, Healey JH, Su SL, Jaffe EA, Old LJ. Identification of endosialin, a cell surface glycoprotein of vascular endothelial cells in human cancer. Proc Natl Acad Sci U S A 1992; 89:10832–10836.
90. Carnemolla B, Balza E, Siri A, Zardi L, Nicotra MR, Bigotti A, Natali PG. A tumor-associated fibronectin isoform generated by alternative splicing of messenger RNA precursors. J Cell Biol 1989; 108:1139–1148.
91. Kaczmarek J, Castellani P, Nicolo G, Spina B, Allemanni G, Zardi L. Distribution of oncofetal fibronectin isoforms in normal, hyperplastic and neoplastic human breast tissues. Int J Cancer 1994; 59(1):11–16.
92. D'Ovidio MC, Mastracchio A, Marzullo A, Ciabatta M, Pini B, Uccini S, Zardi L, Ruco LP. Intratumoral microvessel density and expression of ED-A/ED-B

sequences of fibronectin in breast carcinoma. Eur J Cancer 1998; 34(7):1081–1085.

93. Matsui S, Takahashi T, Oyanagi Y, Takahashi S, Boku S, Takahashi K, Furukawa K, Arai F, Asakura H. Expression, localization and alternative splicing pattern of fibronectin messenger RNA in fibrotic human liver and hepatocellular carcinoma. J Hepatol 1997; 27(5):843–853.
94. Hauptmann S, Zardi L, Siri A, Carnemolla B, Borsi L, Castellucci M, Klosterhalfen B, Hartung P, Weis J, Stocker G, Haubeck HD, Kirkpatrick CJ. Extracellular matrix proteins in colorectal carcinomas. Expression of tenascin and fibronectin isoforms. Lab Invest 1995; 73(2):172–182.
95. Karelina TV, Eisen AZ. Interstitial collagenase and the ED-B oncofetal domain of fibronectin are markers of angiogenesis in human skin tumors. Cancer Detect Prev 1998; 22(5):438–444.
96. Castellani P, Viale G, Dorcaratto A, Nicolo G, Kaczmarek J, Querze G, Zardi L. The fibronectin isoform containing the ED-B oncofetal domain: a marker of angiogenesis. Int J Cancer 1994; 59:612–618.
97. Mariani G, Lasku A, Balza E, Gaggero B, Motta C, Di Luca L, Dorcaratto A, Viale GA, Neri D, Zardi L. Tumor targeting potential of the monoclonal antibody BC-1 against oncofetal fibronectin in nude mice bearing human tumor implants. Cancer 1997; 80(12 suppl):2378–2384.
98. Viti F, Tarli L, Giovannoni L, Zardi L, Neri D. Increased binding affinity and valence of recombinant antibody fragments lead to improved targeting of tumoral angiogenesis. Cancer Res 1999; 59(2):347–352.
99. Pini A, Viti F, Santucci A, Camemolla B, Zardi L, Neri P, Neri D. Design and use of a phage display library. Human antibodies with subnanomolar affinity against a marker of angiogenesis eluted from a two-dimensional gel. J Biol Chem 1998; 273(34):21769–21776.
100. Brooks PC, Clark RA, Cheresh DA. Requirement of vascular integrin alpha v beta 3 for angiogenesis. Science 1994; 264:569–571.
101. Brooks PC, Montgomery AMP, Rosenfeld M, Reisfeld RA, Hu T, Klier G, Cheresh DA. Integrin alpha V beta 3 antagonists promote tumor regression by inducing apoptosis of angiogenic blood vessels. Cell 1994; 79:1157–1164.
102. Gasparini G, Brooks PC, Biganzoli E, Vermeulen PB, Bonoldi E, Dirix LY, Ranieri G, Miceli R, Cheresh DA. Vascular integren alpha(V)beta 3: a new prognostic indicator in breast cancer. Clin Cancer Res 1998; 4(11):2625–2634.
103. Ruegg C, Yilmaz A, Bieler G, Bamat J, Chaubert P, Lejeune FJ. Evidence for the involvement of endothelial cell integrin alpha V beta 3 in the disruption of the tumor vasculature induced by TNF and IFN-gamma. Nature Med 1998; 4(4):408–414.
104. Max R, Gerritsen RR, Nooijen PT, Goodman SL, Sutter A, Keilholz U, Ruiter DJ, De Waal RM. Immunohistochemical analysis of integrin alpha V beta 3 expression on tumor-associated vessels of human carcinomas. Int J Cancer 1997; 71(3):320–324.
105. Pasqualini R, Koivunen E, Ruoslahti E. Alpha V integrins as receptors for tumor targeting by circulating ligands. Nat Biotechnol 1997; 15(6):542–546.
106. Lode HN, Moehler T, Xiang R, Jonczyk A, Gillies SD, Cheresh DA, Reisfeld RA.

Synergy between an antiangiogenic integrin alpha V antagonist and an antibody-cytokine fusion protein eradicates spontaneous tumor metastases. Proc Natl Acad Sci U S A 1999; 96(4):1591–1596.

107. Arap W, Pasqualini R, Ruoslahti E. Cancer treatment by targeted drug delivery to tumor vasculature in a mouse. Science 1998; 279(5349):377–380.
108. Horoszewicz JS, Kawinski E, Murphy GP. Monoclonal antibodies to a new antigenic marker in epithelial cells and serum of prostatic cancer patients. Anticancer Res 1987; 7:927–936.
109. Israeli RS, Powell CT, Fair WR, Heston WDW. Molecular cloning of a complementary DNA encoding a prostate-specific membrane antigen. Cancer Res 1993; 53: 227–230.
110. Wright GL Jr, Haley C, Beckett ML, Schelhammer PF. Expression of prostate-specific antigen in normal, benign, and malignant prostate tissues. Urol Oncol 1995; 1:18–28.
111. Liu H, Moy P, Kim S, Xia Y, Rajasekaran A, Navarro V, Knudsen B, Bander NH. Monoclonal antibodies to the extracellular domain of prostate-specific membrane antigen also reacts with tumor vascular endothelium. Cancer Res 1997; 57:3629–3634.
112. Silver DA, Pellicer I, Fair WR, Heston WDW, Cordon-Cardo C. Prostate-specific membrane antigen expression in normal and malignant human tissues. Clin Cancer Res 1997; 3:81–85.
113. Murphy GP, Greene TG, Tino WT, Boynton AL, Holmes EH. Isolation and characterization of monoclonal antibodies specific for the extracellular domain of prostate specific membrane antigen. J Urol 1998; 160:2396–2401.
114. Partanen J, Armstrong E, Makela TP, Korhonen J, Sandberg M, Renkonen R, Knuuitila S, Huebner K, Alitalo K. A novel endothelial cell surface receptor tyrosine kinase with extracellular epidermal growth factor homology domains. Mol Cell Biol 1992; 12:1698–1707.
115. Kaipainen A, Vlaykova T, Hatva E, Bohling T, Jekunen A, Pyrhonen S, Alitalo K. Enhanced expression of the tie receptor tyrosine kinase messenger RNA in the vascular endothelium metastatic melanomas. Cancer Res 1994; 54:6571–6577.
116. Korhonen J, Partanen J, Armstrong E, Vaahtokari A, Elenius K, Jalkanen M, Alitalo K. Enhanced expression of the tie receptor kinase in endothelial cells during neovascularization. Blood 1992; 80:2548–2555.
117. Sato TN, Tozawa Y, Deutsch U, Wolburg-Buchholz K, Fujiwara Y, Gendron-Maguire M, Gridley T, Wolburg H, Risau W, Qin Y. Distinct roles of the receptor tyrosine kinases Tie-1 and Tie-2 in blood vessel formation. Nature 1995; 376:70–74.
118. Davis S, Aldrich TH, Jones PF, Acheson A, Compton DL, Jain V, Ryan TE, Bruno J, Radziejewski C, Maisonpierre PC, Yancopoulos GD. Isolation of angiopoietin-1, a ligand for the TIE2 receptor, by secretion-trap expression cloning. Cell 1996; 87:1161–1169.
119. Suri C, Jones PF, Patan S, Bartunkova S, Maisonpierre PC, Davis S, Sato TN, Yancopoulos GD. Requisite role of angiopoietin-1, a ligand for the TIE2 receptor, during embryonic angiogenesis. Cell 1996; 87:1171–1180.
120. Maisonpierre PC, Suri C, Jones PF, Bartunkova S, Wiegand SJ, Radziejewski C,

Compton D, McClain J, Aldrich TH, Papadopoulos N, Daly TJ, Davis S, Sato TN, Yancopoulos GD. Angiopoietin-2, a natural antagonist for Tie2 that disrupts in vivo angiogenesis. Science 1997; 277:55–60.

121. Stratmann A, Risau W, Plate KH. Cell-type specific expression of angiopoietin-1 and angiopoietin-2 suggests a role in glioblastoma angiogenesis. Am J Pathol 1998; 153:1459–1466.

122. Jacobson BS, Stolz DB, Schnitzer JE. Identification of endothelial cell-surface proteins as targets for diagnosis and treatment of disease. Nat Med 1996; 2:482–484.

123. Pasqualini R, Ruoslahti E. Organ targeting in vivo using phage display peptide libraries. Nature 1996; 380:364–366.

124. Vitetta ES, Uhr JW, Thorpe PE. Immunotoxin therapy. In: DeVita VT Jr, Hellman S, Rosenberg SA, eds. Cancer: Principles and Practice of Oncology. J.B. Lippincott Company, 1993:2624–2636.

125. Nabel EG, Plantz G, Nabel GJ. Site-specific gene expression in vivo by direct gene transfer into the arterial wall. Science 1990; 249:1285–1288.

33

Combining Antivascular Approaches with Radiotherapy

A Perspective

Juliana Denekamp
Umeå University, Umeå, Sweden

Poor tumor vasculature has been perceived as a problem for effective radiotherapy for decades. It results in abnormal oxygen gradients, with cells in solid tumors having a lower average pO_2, and some cells being virtually hypoxic. Acute hypoxia confers an enormous degree of tumor-specific radioprotection. It can reduce tumor cell kill at a curative radiation dose by a factor of 1 million or more. Chronic hypoxia, by contrast, can sensitize cells to radiation because of the attendant loss of cellular energy reserves. This makes them less able to perform enzymatic repair of DNA lesions. The balance between acute and chronic hypoxia will determine the overall response. Much effort has been invested in attempts to manipulate the vascular network and tumor blood flow to selectively increase tumor radiosensitivity.

Antiangiogenesis and other vascular targeting strategies have the intention of worsening the tumor blood supply. They seek to minimize vessel growth or even to cause vessel occlusion or regression. This may carry with it the induction of higher levels of tumor cell hypoxia. If these two approaches are to be combined with a curative intent, the details and the sequencing are likely to be crucial. Because radiotherapy is already effective in curing many localized cancers, the addition of antiangiogenic methods to gain an extra 2 or 3 decades of cell kill in the primary tumor could have a major impact on overall cure rates. It could also provide a more effective treatment for disseminated disease, changing palliation to cure. If it increases chronic hypoxia, it could lead to radiosensitization. However, if it coincidentally increased acute hypoxia, it would cause far more cells to survive the radiotherapy. The balance is not predictable at present and could increase or decrease the overall cure rates currently achievable with radiotherapy alone. Thus, it is important to consider the interplay of these strategies. It is a combination of therapies with considerable promise, but it will have to be approached with caution.

I. INTRODUCTION

The allied fields of antiangiogenesis and vascular attack have evolved during the last 25 years. Substances produced by tumor cells that will stimulate endothelial proliferation, migration, and basement membrane degradation to allow capillary buds to be produced have been identified. Most of this volume deals with the current status of antiangiogenesis. The essence of the concept was that solid tumors cannot expand without developing a new network of vessels to support them and provide their nutritional requirements. Therefore, it was argued that if vessel growth can be inhibited, the growth of tumors can be arrested, the aim being cytostasis, not cytotoxicity. Arresting vessel growth could, in theory, arrest tumor growth. Since the first crude tumor extracts of TAF were shown to have vessel-growth-promoting activity (1), a whole science and industry has developed, with the isolation of many stimulating factors and inhibitors, some of which are now showing clinical promise. At the same time, several other approaches have evolved that also relate to the poor tumor microcirculation (Table 1).

This new concept of antiangiogenesis required the development of different assays for detecting both angiogenic and antiangiogenic substances. The screening assays have usually been sites of new vessel ingrowth into a normally avascular area. The main models are the developing fertilized egg (chorioallantoic membrane [CAM] assay) and the cornea. The addition of angiogenic factors causes a dense capillary ingrowth, which can then be used to test whether it can be blocked by the inhibitors. Some of the inhibitors of vessel growth identified in these assays have subsequently demonstrated considerable antitumor effectiveness when administered to mice bearing solid tumors. They have not resulted merely in the cessation of tumor growth, but have led to tumor regression or even complete tumor eradication (2, 3, 4). This unexpected advantage beyond what was predicted is, of course, very encouraging, but in the next phase, before translating this into patient benefit, it is important to understand why it is so effective. Is another unsuspected mode of damage also involved, and if so what is it? Or could it be an artifact of the animal models that have been used (5)? As with radiotherapy, the answer to these questions could influence both the clinical implementation of existing drugs and the search for more effective strategies (6).

Table 1 Illustration of the Novel Strategies in Cancer Treatment That Are Related to the Inadequate Tumor Microcirculation and the Abnormal Microenvironment

Approach	Proposed Mechanism	Examples
Antiagiogenesis	• Block the growth factors that stimulate endothelial cell division, migration,and tube formation • Prevent further expansion of the vascular network • Cytostatic action	Protamine Heparin + cortisone Fumagillin analogues Suramin Thrombospondin Angiostatin Endostatin Thalidomide
Vascular targeting	• Attack immature proliferating endothelial cells to kill them or alter their function • Cause vessels to collapse, occlude, or hemorrhage • Cytotoxic action	Hyperthermia Hyperglycemia Photodynamic therapy Flavone acetic acid Xanthenone acetic acid Misonidazole Endotoxin Interferons Interleukins Tumor necrosis factor Vinca alkaloids Combretastatin Ab against vascular endothelial growth factor
Bioreductive drugs	• Use hypoxia for preferential bioreduction of a nontoxic prodrug to a toxic product	Mitomycin C Porfiromycin Metronidazole Pimonidazole Tirapazamine EO9
pH-dependent cytotoxicity	• Preferential localization, uptake, or toxicity in regions of low pH	Hyperthermia Meta-iodobenzylguanidine Nigericin and chemotherapy

One might expect that, if the process of angiogenesis is blocked, expansion of the tumor mass would be prevented and maturation of the vessels should occur. Tumor growth might then stabilize if a perfect balance between cell production and cell loss could be re-established. However, the metabolizing mass of the existing tumor would still need the pre-existing neovascular network. This differs greatly from the corneal assay used to find these drugs. There, if the abnormal exogenous signals for vessel growth are blocked and there is no functional need for the newly formed vessels, the vessels can regress and the tissue can revert to its original avascular characteristics.

Because tumor regression does occur, I conclude that these antiangiogenic agents have some additional activity. They cannot merely be blocking endothelial cell proliferation, unless the endothelium in tumors differs from that in developing normal tissues, for example, if it cannot mature and become quiescent. This anomaly is rarely discussed, but it is important. We should consider whether another mechanism is also involved and linked to, but functionally separate from, the agent's blockade of the proliferative activity of the endothelial cells.

Many drugs, when investigated in detail, have been shown to have more than one mechanism of action (7–9). Perhaps the same is true for those that have been found by screening for antiangiogenic activity. If this is so, the dose-response relationships for the multiple modes of action need to be understood before effective translation of the exciting preclinical results into clinical benefit can occur. Many other breakthroughs in cancer research have failed at this hurdle, because they were assumed to have only one mode of action and were, therefore, administered to patients in a way that did not allow for the unsuspected underlying alternative mechanism (5–9).

II. THE INTERDEPENDENCE OF ENDOTHELIAL CELL AND TUMOR CELL PROLIFERATION

The growth of tumors is not, as was once assumed, totally out of control. It is under a different form of control that is largely influenced by the microvasculature. Human tumors vary widely in their volume doubling times, ranging from a week to almost a year. There is a smaller range of tumor cell cycle times or potential doubling times (Tpot). The advent of antibodies that recognize BrdUrd incorporated into DNA has made it possible to estimate the Tpot of cells within thousands of human tumors. This technique is based on the uptake of this precursor of DNA synthesis in preparation for mitosis, allowing the fraction of cells in S to be determined, which is called the labeling index (LI). It is now possible to measure the movement of cells through the S phase between injection and biopsy (10). This allows the measurement of Tpot, which is the reciprocal of the birth rate. It measures the time for the cell number to double, taking into account that not all cells are actively contributing to the proliferating pool. In many tumor types, the median Tpot is between 4 and 7 days, when all stromal and tumor cells are measured together, as in a flow cytometer. This is 2 to 100 times faster than the volume doubling times. However, when more selective histochemical techniques are used to identify only the tumor cells, the median Tpot is even shorter (2 to 3 days). Indeed, within most human tumors there are "hot spots," where the tumor cells are doubling as fast as 1 to 1.5 days.

This very rapid tumor cell production does not translate into equally rapid volume doubling times because the vascular network does not expand rapidly enough to maintain an adequate nutrient supply. Many of the cells produced are pushed down the nutrient gradient and die of nutrient depletion. Extensive cell loss is known to occur in most carcinomas, with 90% to 99% of the additional cells produced dying and being lost from the tumor volume.

III. ENDOTHELIAL PROLIFERATION RATES

Normal blood vessels in the mature animal are quiescent, with very little wear and tear and requiring very little replacement. Thus, there is a very slow rate of cell turnover (11). The labeling index of endothelial cells is usually in the range 0.01% to 0.1%, corresponding to a turnover time of months, or even years. Endothelial cell proliferation is equally slow in a wide range of normal tissues and does not seem to be correlated with the turnover time of the parenchymal cells of the organ. It is similar in the fast turnover tissues such as intestinal villi, moderate turnover tissues such as skin, and in the more quiescent tissues such as brain, kidney, and lung.

Tumor neovasculature, in contrast, is lined by rapidly proliferating endothelial cells that have LI values of 1% to 30%, that is, 10 to 1000 times higher than in normal vessels (11–20). The high LI values in tumor endothelium appear to be independent of the size of the tumors. They are similar in lung micrometastases and tumors approaching 0.5 g, that is, a few percent of the body mass in mice. They are also in the same range in the much larger tumors in patients. There is a rough correlation in mice between endothelial LI and tumor volume doubling times, so it is perhaps not surprising that the LI values in humans seem, on average, to be about half of those seen in the mice. (Human tumors have much longer volume doubling times than those in mice.) If the endothelial LI values are compared only with the more slowly growing mouse tumors, they are very similar, and the range in human and murine tumors totally overlaps. Fewer data are available for normal tissues, but an average ratio of tumor to normal endothelial LI values of 10 to 45 has been detected in the human comparisons of colon and breast and the tumors arising in them. These are the same as, or slightly lower than, the differential in mice, and are still impressive (11–20).

IV. VASCULAR TARGETING AS AN ALTERNATIVE CONCEPT

When this large and very reproducible difference in endothelial cell proliferation between all solid tumors and all normal tissues was first recognized, it was proposed as a new target for cytotoxic therapies (14). The main difference from the antiangiogenic strategy was that it aimed to kill the proliferating endothelial cells in order to cause edema and coagulation, resulting in cessation of blood flow and starvation of the tumor cells. The target cells were the same (proliferating endothelium), but the concept was based on cytotoxicity, not cytostasis. When the search for possible ways of exploiting this began in the mid-80s, it was quickly recognized that the immature proliferating endothelial cells showed functional abnormalities that could supplement, or even be more important than, their proliferation characteristics as a target. To distinguish vascular mediated damage from direct tumor cell kill required experiments that would look for vascular occlusion and the resultant characteristic pattern of patchy ischemic necrosis. Many existing and novel forms of therapy included an element, within their effects on murine tumors, that involved vascular mediated injury (7, 8). Specific agents known to occlude the blood vessels, such as hyperthermia, photodynamic therapy, tumor necrosis factor (TNF), flavone acetic acid (FAA), the vinca alkaloids, and Combretastatin have been shown to cause considerable tumor regression or long delays in regrowth, even after single doses (21, 22). Some of these are summarized in Table 1 and described in more detail elsewhere (7, 8). Although the philosophies and the proposed mechanism of action of the two approaches, antiangiogenesis and vascular targeting, are conceptually different, there is considerable overlap in the results achieved. Both result in ischemic tumor necrosis, regression, and delay in regrowth.

V. COMBINING ANTIVASCULAR STRATEGIES WITH RADIOTHERAPY

Radiation oncology is one of the oldest branches of cancer treatment. It is second only to surgery in its effectiveness in eradicating localized tumors. It contributes to a significant fraction of tumor cures, whether used alone or in combination with surgery or systemic therapies. The cure rate is 95% in some tumor sites and stages, but only 1% to 5% in others. These variations occur both because of the differences in the intrinsic and micro-environmentally determined radioresistance of the tumor cells and the limitations placed on the total dose by the sensitivity of different adjacent normal tissues. The use of radiation as a combined modality with surgery is increasing, resulting in better organ conservation than surgery alone, better cosmetic results, and improved quality of life. Combining radiation with systemic therapies such as chemotherapy is also increasing so that the chance of cure can be extended to more disseminated disease, with radiation being one of two main tools used for the localized tumor, and chemotherapy for the distant disease. It is in this area that combinations with the newly emerging antivascular strategies might be the most attractive.

Most existing chemotherapy and most current efforts to develop new anticancer strategies are aimed at the control of cell proliferation and its disturbance in transformed malignant vs normal cells. If the therapy is systemic and reaches all proliferating cells, the fastest dividing normal cells in the body, for instance, those in bone marrow, hair follicles, and intestinal crypts, will always limit the dose that can be given. Unless there is an additional reason for tumor selectivity, these organs will continue to be dose limiting, no matter how novel or ingenious the new approach to blocking or damaging cells through stages in the proliferative cell cycle. The poor vasculature and the associated pathological nutrient gradients may provide this new differential. They should no longer be viewed only as a problem for the oncologist, although they do limit the access of conventional cytotoxic drugs and influence the effectiveness of radiotherapy.

VI. RADIOTHERAPY AND ITS DEPENDENCE ON THE MICROVASCULAR ARCHITECTURE

The microvascular architecture in tumors consists of cuffs of cells, often 5 to 10 cells wide around each capillary, with areas of necrosis developing if the intercapillary distances get larger than 100 to 150 microns. This is illustrated in Figure 1, a photomicrograph of a mouse mammary tumor. The hypoxic cells have been stained by the nitroimidazole marker, NITP, which has a theophylline side chain that is detectable with an antibody. This staining occurs when NITP is bound within the cell after bioreductive metabolism, which only takes place in low oxygen concentrations (23). This corded pattern around capillaries has been known as a characteristic feature of solid tumors for many years (24), although new techniques are only now emerging to allow its quantitative study (25, 26). The oxygen gradient resulting from this inadequate structure has been the focus of much radiobiological research. Some of these concepts are illustrated in Figure 2, which shows the change in the oxygenation of cells in the successive layers around a capillary and the way that radiosensitivity changes by a factor of 3 over the oxygen range that is relevant in vivo. The abnormally low oxygen gradient in tumors can confer hypoxic radioresistance, which is, unfortunately, specific for the tumor as normal tissues are all well oxygenated. In vitro, it can readily be shown that three times as much radiation dose is needed to kill an equivalent number of cells if they are irradiated after an abrupt change to pure nitrogen instead of air (Fig. 3a). Although this factor of 3 does not seem to be a very large dose ratio, it can translate into a 40 million-fold difference in the fraction of oxic and hypoxic cells that can survive a potentially curative single dose because of the exponential nature of the cell killing process (Fig. 3a). The presence of even a minor subset of hypoxic cells, for example, 10%, can give almost as much protection against large doses of radiation as it would if the whole

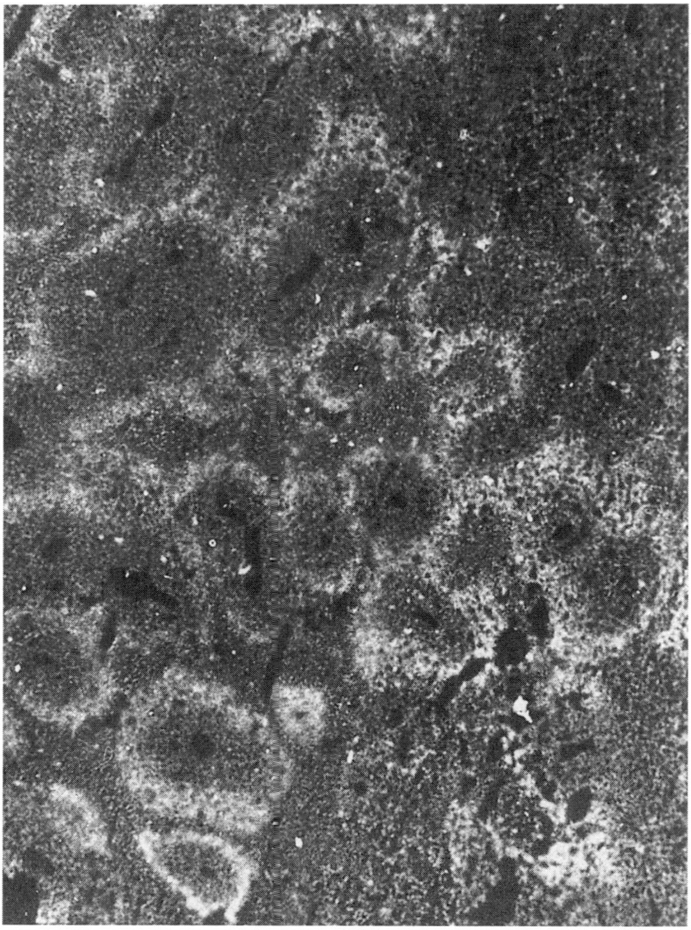

Figure 1 Photomicrograph of CaNT, an experimental mouse mammary carcinoma, taken from an animal that had been injected with the nitroimidazole, NITP. The bright rings, which are 100–200 μm in diameter, show the biochemically active but hypoxic cells around many of the capillaries. The distribution of hypoxia is heterogeneous even within this small area of a single tumor. (Photograph kindly provided by Dr. Richard Hodgkiss.)

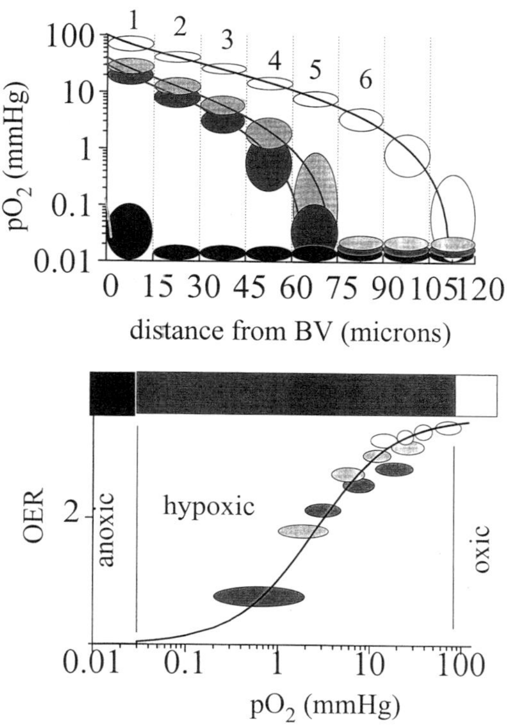

Figure 2 Illustration of the oxygen gradients around individual capillaries and the radiobiological consequence. The top panel shows the average cellular oxygenation of successive cell layers around capillaries in which the blood pO_2 is 100, 40, 30, or 0.1 mm Hg. This represents arterial or venous blood flowing through tumor vessels and those with almost no flow. The numbers above the columns indicate the relative number of cells in successive cell rings, assuming cylindrical symmetry. The lower panel shows the relative radiosensitivity of the first four cell layers around the three vessels with flowing blood. (Redrawn from Waites et al., 1998.)

population was anoxic. These radioresistant cells can only regrow the tumor after a subcurative dose of radiation if their nutrient status improves and they are rescued from starvation. This process is commonly called reoxygenation. In curative radiotherapy, large single doses are never given. Instead, a series of daily doses of about 2 Gy are used to benefit from the sensitization resulting from reoxygenation between the daily fractions (Figure 3c). It was the adoption of appropriate fractionated schedules that transformed early radiotherapy from a merely palliative treatment to a curative modality. The outcome of the total schedule of treatment depends critically on the reoxygenation characteristics of the individual tumor

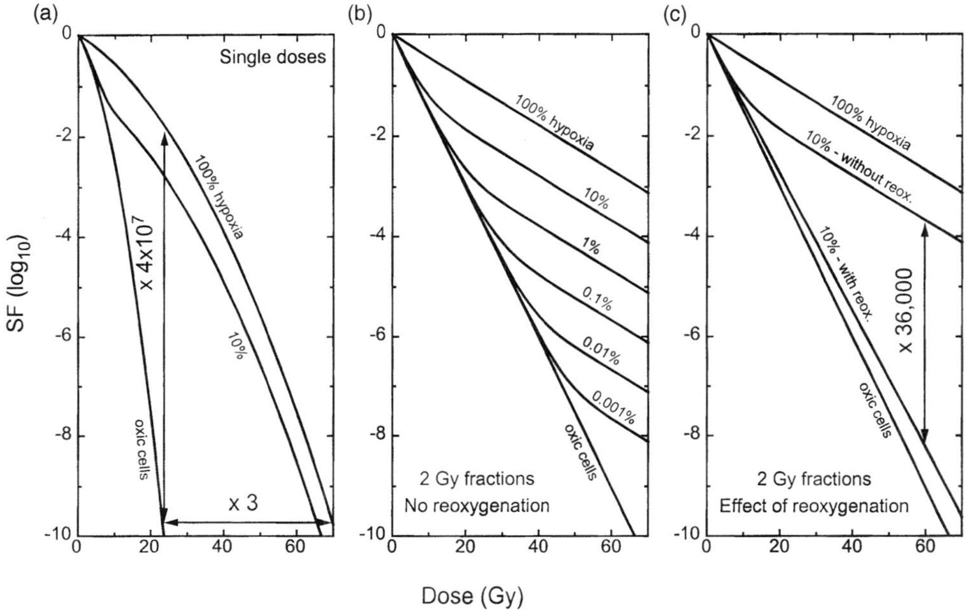

Figure 3 Schematic cell survival curves show how the threefold resistance conferred by acute hypoxia translates into an enormous effect on the ratio of surviving cells, i.e., 40 million-fold resistance for single doses. **a**. Ninety percent of the cells being well oxygenated does little to reduce this effect ratio. Panel **b** shows the same dominant effect of acute hypoxia with daily 2-Gy fractions if there is no reoxygenation. Panel **c** illustrates how effective reoxygenation (back to 10% before each fraction) can almost abolish the effect of hypoxic resistance. Prevention of this reoxygenation would increase the surviving fraction by a factor of 36,000 at 60 Gy.

(Figure 3c). Unfortunately, the reoxygenation pattern is a very difficult thing to measure, even in experimental tumors.

VII. SPATIAL AND TEMPORAL HYPOXIA

Two forms of hypoxia are recognized:

Chronic hypoxia: a progressive reduction in oxygen as cells born close to blood vessels push their neighbors further away. These hypoxic cells gradually become deprived of all other nutrients, and their energy charge eventually drops when anaerobic glycolysis exhausts the glucose supply. These cells will be resistant if they are hypoxic, but they will retain their intracellular energy charge.

However, when their energy charge falls, they may become biochemically restricted in their DNA repair capacity. This will offset or even reverse the hypoxic resistance. Eventually, they die of starvation.

Acute hypoxia: tumor vessels often close temporarily, or there is a transient reduction in the content of erythrocytes carrying oxygen (i.e., plasma flow). The result is that all the cells around those vessels become temporarily more hypoxic for a period of seconds, minutes, or a few hours. If the duration of hypoxia is less than 30 minutes, it will not be long enough for them to become energy depleted. Such cells will, therefore, be very radioresistant. If this form of ischemia lasts more than an hour, the energy charge will fall and all the cells will eventually die.

VIII. SUBSTRUCTURE TO THE CELL SURVIVAL CURVE AND ITS CONSEQUENCES

For many years the two forms of hypoxia have been assumed to confer equal radioresistance. Many in vitro studies have demonstrated the 2.5- to 3.0-fold increase in dose needed in hypoxic conditions compared to air, which is illustrated in Figures 2 and 3. Because the effect of oxygen is known to involve ultrarapid free radical chemistry (all complete within a microsecond), it has been common practice to expose the hypoxic cells to reduced oxygen tensions for only a short period. This usually is done for a few minutes before and during the irradiation and the cells are left undisturbed as far as other nutrients are concerned, and they are returned to air after the irradiation. However, several studies have shown a difference in the response of acutely hypoxic cells in a good nutrient environment compared with those that have been severely deprived of both oxygen and glucose for long periods until their high energy phosphate reserves become depleted (27, 28). Such starved hypoxic cells become much more sensitive, apparently because they lose their biochemical ability for enzymatic repair of DNA damage. Thus a balance must occur between the chemical redox protection resulting from hypoxia and the sensitization that develops as biochemical repair competence disappears.

We have recently undertaken theoretical studies that model the response of cells in tumors under different conditions and exposed to different fractionation regimes (29–31). The details of the response to low doses have gone unrecognized until recently because of the technical difficulties of investigating this region where little cell kill occurs after single small doses. Any effects, however, will be greatly magnified in fractionated experiments, as the effect is raised to the power (e.g., 35) corresponding to the number of fractions. New techniques and new experimental designs have, over the last decade, revealed a complex substructure to the response of cells to clinically relevant low doses, both in vivo and in vitro (32–34). Untreated, naive cells are now recognized as being initially very sensitive to radiation, but a small dose of about 0.1 to 0.2 Gy seems to act as a stress signal. The cell apparently responds by generating more DNA repair enzymes, which it then uses to remove the damage inflicted by the radiation. This adaptation to genotoxic damage has been termed ''inducible repair.'' The extent of this inducible repair varies from one cell line to another, resulting in different inherent radiosensitivities as they are expressed in the therapeutic dose range of 1.5 to 2.5 Gy.

We have shown that this substructure may provide a therapeutic window during which hypoxia can even act as a radiosensitizer (35). At very low doses of radiation, for example 0.5 Gy, the inducible repair has been triggered in oxic

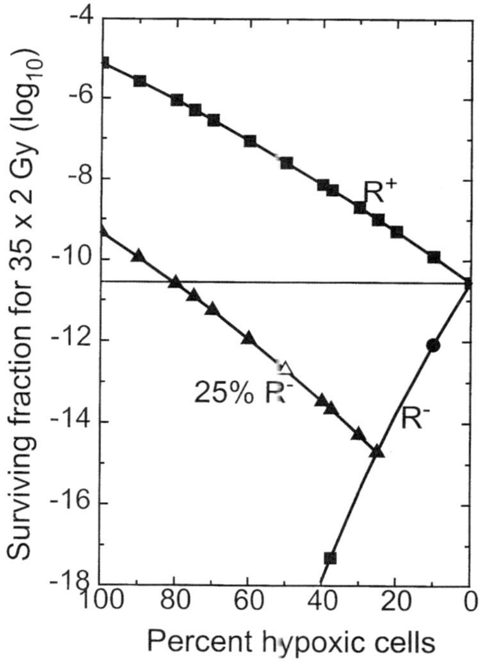

Figure 4 Schematic illustration of the difference in the radioresistance of hypoxic cells if they are biochemically repair competent, R^+, or repair incompetent, R^-. (The hypoxic fraction has been assumed to stay constant at each fraction). The horizontal line represents the response of a well oxygenated population. Acute hypoxia(R^+) confers resistance. Chronic hypoxia (R^-) dramatically increases the cell kill. An hypoxic tumor containing 25% R^+ and 25% R^- (shown by the *open triangle*) would still have 2 decades of extra cell kill compared to the oxic population.

(normal) cells but not in hypoxic (tumor) cells. This can lead to a reversal of their radiosensitivities.

Furthermore, we now interpret the earlier experimental data in energy-deprived cells as showing that chronic hypoxia can prevent the normal response to stress (36). The net outcome of the balance between chemical protection by acute hypoxia and loss of biochemical protection by prolonged hypoxia differs from one cell line to another. However, all chronically hypoxic cells could be much more sensitive than acutely hypoxic cells, and even more sensitive than oxic cells at all dose levels. This is an heretical and startling conclusion!

Figure 4 shows how acutely hypoxic cells would decrease the cell kill but chronically hypoxic cells would increase it. Both forms of hypoxia are known to coexist, but the usual mixture could still result in more efficient cell kill in the partially hypoxic tumors than in the oxic normal tissues. Indeed the very presence of chronic hypoxia may provide the reason why tumors are curable at doses that are tolerated by oxic normal tissues (37). This illustrates the importance of reconsidering the entire database in the light of any new experimental data (in this case the demonstration of inducible repair).

These theoretical studies have emphasized the important possibility that the two well-recognized types of hypoxic cells may behave in totally different ways. Acute hypoxia is certainly radioprotective, but chronic hypoxia can act as an overall radiosensitizer. The relative magnitude of these two competing effects is linked to the intrinsic radioresistance through the capacity for inducible repair (37).

IX. COMBINING ANTIVASCULAR APPROACHES WITH RADIOTHERAPY

This potential difference between acute and chronic hypoxia is an important new concept when we consider the details of the possible interplay of antivascular approaches and radiosensitivity. If there is a risk of accidentally increasing the fraction of hypoxic cells, the duration of hypoxia and the associated depletion of other nutrients may be crucial. Accidental induction of an increase in chronic hypoxia should be beneficial in certain tumor types, whereas induction of more acutely hypoxic cells at the time of irradiation certainly will not be helpful.

To consider the combination of antiangiogenic agents with radiotherapy, the main concern must be what influence the antiangiogenic agent may have on the oxygen gradients in direction, magnitude, and duration.

If expansion of the vessel network is simply arrested, but the existing network remains functional, the oxygen gradients and the overall radioresistance are likely to remain unchanged. A new balance should be established in which one cell is lost by starvation for every new cell born, if there is not net growth.

By contrast, if the vessels are also partially damaged, flow may be reduced and the overall oxygenation in the tumor diminished. In this case, the gradients will change. A partial and temporary reduction in flow for just a few hours could be serious enough to kill the cells previously in a critical condition near the bottom of the nutrient gradient. Those closest to the capillary might be able to survive the temporary reduction. If flow and oxygenation then improved, the diffusion distance would expand and encompass the surviving cells in the shrunken cord within a higher range on the oxygen gradient, that is, reoxygenation would occur. The radiosensitivity of the survivors would increase temporarily until cell proliferation restored the original balance, which would probably occur within a few days.

Some antivascular therapies seem to create large areas of necrosis with cords of tumor cells around the few vessels that are still patent. Thus the treatment seems to kill *all* the cells around those of the vessels that are most susceptible to the treatment, but it leaves areas where the vessels and their dependent cells seem much less affected (38). In this case, the cell kill from such an agent would be merely additive. The surviving portions of the tumor would be expected to have the same overall radiosensitivity, but the viable cell burden would have diminished, making the tumor easier to cure with radiotherapy. If the cord diameter around the vessels that remain patent diminishes, the cells may be temporarily reoxygenated until cell proliferation restores the original cord diameter and the corresponding oxygen gradients.

Figure 3b shows the potential influence of varying the percentage of hypoxic cells between treatments in a fractionated schedule. Anything that increases the reoxygenation between fractions will have a beneficial influence on the cell kill. Anything that inadvertently reduces the extent of natural reoxygenation easily could be detrimental. It could even counterbalance 2 or 3 decades of cell kill from the antivascular agent.

Thus, it is very important to know what effect each of the antiangiogenic and vascular targeting strategies has on the blood flow through the vessels that remain patent. Does it simply prevent expansion of the network? Does it completely eliminate some vessels, without affecting others? Or does it make the flow through the remaining network better or worse? So far, this has not been investigated in any detail with antiangiogenic or vascular targeted agents.

The identification of blood flow alterations has been one of the main means by which the previously unsuspected vascular-mediated component of action has been detected from agents like the interleukins, interferon, TNF, hyperthermia, and photodynamic therapy (7, 8). If it transpires that an increased level of acute hypoxia accompanies the action of antiangiogenic strategies, then it would be worthwhile to consider combining bioreductive drugs, or drugs that are more effective in acidic conditions in the overall design of a curative approach. The new markers to identify hypoxic cells, such as NITP, EF5, and Pimonidazole (23) that have emerged from the field of bioreductive drug design also may be important in the linking of advances in antiangiogenesis and radiation oncology. So far, relatively few studies have been reported of the combination of antiangiogenic or vascular-targeted therapies with radiotherapy or chemotherapy (39–44). Such studies need to be linked to measurements of hypoxia and flow changes introduced by the antivascular agents, or to histological assessments to determine the contributions of the two forms of injury.

ACKNOWLEDGMENTS

This work was supported by the Umeå Lions Cancer Research Fund and the Swedish Cancerfonden. I am grateful to my colleagues, Richard Hodgkiss, Anthony Waites, and Alexandru Dasu for assistance with the illustrations.

REFERENCES

1. Folkman J, Merler E, Abernathy C, Williams G. Isolation of a tumor factor responsible for angiogenesis. J Exp Med 1971; 133:275–288.
2. Ingber D, Fujita T, Kishimoto S, Sudo K, Kanamaru T, Brem H, Folkman J. Synthetic analogues of fumagillin that inhibit angiogenesis and suppress tumor growth. Nature 1990; 348:555–557.
3. O'Reilly MS, Holmgren L, Shing Y, Chen C, Rosenthal RA, Moses M, Lane WS, Cao YH, Sage EH, Folkman J. Angiostatin: a novel angiogenesis inhibitor that mediates the suppression of metastases by a Lewis lung-carcinoma. Cell 1994; 79:315–328.
4. O'Reilly MS, Boehm T, Shing Y, Fukai N, Vasios G, Lane WS, Flynn E, Birkhead JR, Olsen BR, Folkman J. Endostatin: an endogenous inhibitor of angiogenesis and tumor growth. Cell 1997; 88:277–285.
5. Denekamp J. The choice of experimental models in cancer research: the key to ultimate success or failure? NMR Biomed 1992; 5:234–237.
6. Denekamp J. Quality control of the translation of the laboratory research into clinical practice. Proceeds of the International Atomic Energy Agency and the International Society for Radiologic Oncology, Vienna May 8–9, 1995. Vienna: International Atomic Energy Agency, 1997:181–194.
7. Denekamp J. Review article: angiogenesis, neovascular proliferation and vascular pathophysiology as targets for cancer therapy. Br J Radiol 1993; 66:181–196.
8. Moore JV, West DC, eds. Vasculature as a target for anti-cancer therapy. Proceedings of the 16th L.H. Gray Conference. Int J Radiat Biol 1991; 60:1–421.
9. Tannock IF. Treatment of cancer with radiation and drugs. J Clin Oncol 1996; 14: 3156–3174.
10. Begg AC, McNally NJ, Shrieve D, Kärcher H. A method to measure the duration of DNA synthesis and the potential doubling time from a single sample. Cytometry 1985; 6:620–626.

11. Hobson B, Denekamp J. Endothelial proliferation in tumors and normal tissues: continuous labeling studies. Br J Cancer 1984; 49:405–413.
12. Tannock IF. Population kinetics of carcinoma cells, capillary endothelial cells and fibroblasts in a transplanted mouse mammary tumour. Cancer Res 1970; 20:2470–2476.
13. Gunduz N. Cytokinetics of tumor and endothelial cells and vascularisation of lung metastases in C3H/He mice. Cell Tissue Kinet 1981; 14:343–363.
14. Denekamp J. Endothelial cell proliferation as a novel approach to targeting tumor therapy. Br J Cancer 1982; 45:136–139.
15. Denekamp J, Hobson B. Endothelial cell proliferation in experimental tumors. Br J Cancer 1982; 46:711–720.
16. Fox BS, Gatter KC, Bicknell R, Going JJ, Stanton P, Cooke TG, Harris AL. Relationship of endothelial cell proliferation to tumor vascularity in human breast cancer. Cancer Res 1993;53:4161–4163.
17. Vartanian RK, Weidner N. Correlation of intratumoral endothelial cell proliferation with microvessel density (tumor angiogenesis) and tumor cell proliferation in breast carcinoma. Am J Pathol 1994; 144:1188–1194.
18. Vermeulen PB, Verhoeven D, Hubens G, Van Marck E, Goovaerts G, Huyghe M, Bruijn EA, Van Oosterom AT, Dirix LY. Microvessel density, endothelial cell proliferation and tumor cell proliferation in human colorectal adenocarcinomas. Ann Oncol 1995; 6:59–64.
19. Vermeulen PB, Dirix LY, Van Marck E, Van Oosterom AT. High endothelial cell proliferation index and high microvessel density in vascular hotspots suggest an active angiogenic process in human colorectal adenocarcinomas. Br J Cancer 1996; 74:1506–1510.
20. Vermeulen PB, Dirix LY, Libura J, Vanhoolst IF, Van Marck E, Van Oosterom AT. Correlation of the fractions of proliferating tumor and endothelial cells in breast and colorectal adenocarcinoma is independent of tumor histiotype and microvessel density, Microvasc Res 1997; 54:88–92.
21. Hill SA, Williams KB, Denekamp J. Vascular collapse after flavone acetic acid: a possible mechanism of its anti-tumor action. Eur J Cancer Clin Oncol 1989; 25: 1419–1424.
22. Dark GG, Hill SA, Prise VE, Tozer GM, Pettit GR, Chaplin DJ. Combretastatin A-4, an agent that displays potent and selective toxicity toward tumor vasculature. Cancer Res 1997; 57:1829–1834.
23. Hodgkiss RJ, Wardman P. The measurement of hypoxia in tumours. In: Radiation Science: Of Molecules, Mice and Men. Denekamp J, Hirst DG, eds. Br J Radiol 1992; Report 24:104–109.
24. Thomlinson RH, Gray LH. The histological structure of some human lung cancers and the possible implications for radiotherapy. Br J Cancer 1955; 9:539–549.
25. Stone HB, Brown JM, Phillips TL, Sutherland RM. Oxygen in human tumors: correlations between methods of measurement and response to therapy. Summary of a workshop held November 19–20, 1992, at the National Cancer Institute, Bethesda, Maryland. Radiat Res 1993; 136:422–434.
26. Rijken PF, Bernsen HJ, van der Kogel AJ. Application of an image analysis system to the quantitation of tumor perfusion and vascularity in human glioma xenografts. Microvasc Res 1995; 50:141–153.

27. Kwok TT, Sutherland RM. The radiation response of cells recovering after chronic hypoxia. Radiat Res 1989; 119:261–270.
28. Gerweck LE, Seneviratne T, Gerweck KK. Energy status and radiobiological hypoxia at specified oxygen concentrations. Radiat Res 1993; 135:69–74.
29. Waites A, Rojas A, Denekamp J. Are current concepts of hypoxia and radioresistance inadequate? Radiother Oncol. Submitted.
30. Dasu A, Denekamp J. New insights into factors influencing the clinically relevant oxygen enhancement ratio. Radiother Oncol 1998; 46:269–277.
31. Denekamp J, Dasu A, Waites A. Vasculature and microenvironmental gradients: the missing links in novel approaches to cancer therapy? Adv Enzyme Regul 1998; 38: 281–299.
32. Joiner MC, Denekamp J, Maughan RL. The use of top-up experiments to investigate the effects of very small doses per fraction in mouse skin. Int J Radiat Biol 1986; 49:565–580.
33. Palcic B, Jaggi B. The use of solid-state image sensor technology to detect and characterize live mammalian cells growing in tissue culture. Int J Radiat Biol 1986; 50:345–352.
34. Joiner MC, Marples B, Johns H. The response of tissues to very low doses per fraction: a reflection of induced repair? Cancer Res 1993; 130:27–40.
35. Dasu A, Denekamp J. Superfractionation as an hypoxic cell radiosensitiser: the choice of an optimum dose per fraction. Int J Radiat Oncol Biol Phys 1998; 42(4): 705–709.
36. Dasu A, Denekamp J. Superfractionation as a potential hypoxic cell radiosensitiser: prediction of an optimum dose per fraction. Int J Radiat Oncol Biol Phys 1999; 43(5):1083–1094.
37. Dasu A, Denekamp J. Inducible repair and intrinsic radiosensitivity: a complex but predictable relationship. Radiat Res 2000; 153(3):279–288.
38. Denekamp J, Dasu A. Inducible repair and the two forms of tumour hypoxia—time for a paradigm shift. Acta Oncol 1999; 38(7):903–918.
39. Gorski DH, Mauceri HJ, Salloum RM, Gately S, Hellman S, Beckett MA, Sukhatme VP, Soff GA, Kufe DW, Weichselbaum RR. Potentiation of the antitumor effect of ionizing radiation by brief concomitant exposures to angiostatin. Cancer Res 1998; 58:5686–5689.
40. Hill SA, Denekamp J. Histology as a method for determining thermal gradients in heated tumours. Br J Radiol 1982; 55:651–656.
41. Kakeji Y, Teicher BA. Preclinical studies of the combination of angiogenic inhibitors with cytotoxic agents. Invest New Drugs 1997; 15:39–48.
42. Li L, Rojiani A, Siemann DW. Targeting the tumor vasculature with combretastatin A-4 disodium phosphate: effects on radiation therapy. Int J Radiat Oncol Biol Phys 1998; 42:899–903.
43. Mauceri HJ, Hanna NN, Beckett MA, Gorski DH, Staba MJ, Stellato KA, Bigelow K, Heimann R, Gately S, Dhanabal M, Soff GA, Sukhatme VP, Kufe DW, Weichselbaum RR. Combined effects of angiostatin and ionizing radiation in antitumour therapy. Nature 1998; 394:287–291.
44. Teicher BA, Holden SA, Ara G, Korbut T, Menon K. Comparison of several antiangiogenic regimens alone and with cytotoxic therapies in the Lewis lung carcinoma. Cancer Chemother Pharmacol 1996; 38:169–177.

34
Antiangiogenic Gene Therapy

Jaap C. Reijneveld and Emile E. Voest
University Medical Center Utrecht, Utrecht, The Netherlands

I. INTRODUCTION

Angiogenesis is critical to tumor growth and metastasis (1, 2). Several lines of preclinical evidence have demonstrated beyond doubt that inhibition of angiogenesis is a valuable addition to the currently used anticancer treatment modalities. It is important to realize that tumor cells are not directly affected by antiangiogenic therapy. Tumor cells will be kept in a state of dormancy characterized by a balance between proliferation and apoptosis of tumor cells (3). Tumor growth will occur when the concentration of angiogenesis inhibitor drops below a certain threshold level. This implies that suppression of angiogenesis should be continuous and should not occur during a short period. For example, interleukin 12 (IL-12) is a very potent inhibitor of angiogenesis in the mouse corneal neovascularization assay in which basic fibroblast growth factor (bFGF) is the angiogenic stimulus (4, 5). The antiangiogenic effect of IL-12 is mediated by interferon gamma (IFNγ). Interleukin-12 induces a continuous release of IFNγ into the circulation, which is essential for complete inhibition in the mouse corneal neovascularization assay. If IFNγ is administered as daily bolus injections, it is rapidly cleared from the circulation and not detectable within 12 hours (4). The bolus injections result in only 50% inhibition of neovascularization in the mouse cornea. However, when IFNγ is administered through an implanted pump at half the dose of the bolus injection, the inhibition of angiogenesis is complete and comparable to the effect of IL-12 (Fig. 1). This experiment indicates the importance of a continuous antiangiogenic environment.

The limited clinical experience with angiogenesis inhibitors showed rapid clearance of the drugs from the circulation (6, 7). To circumvent this problem,

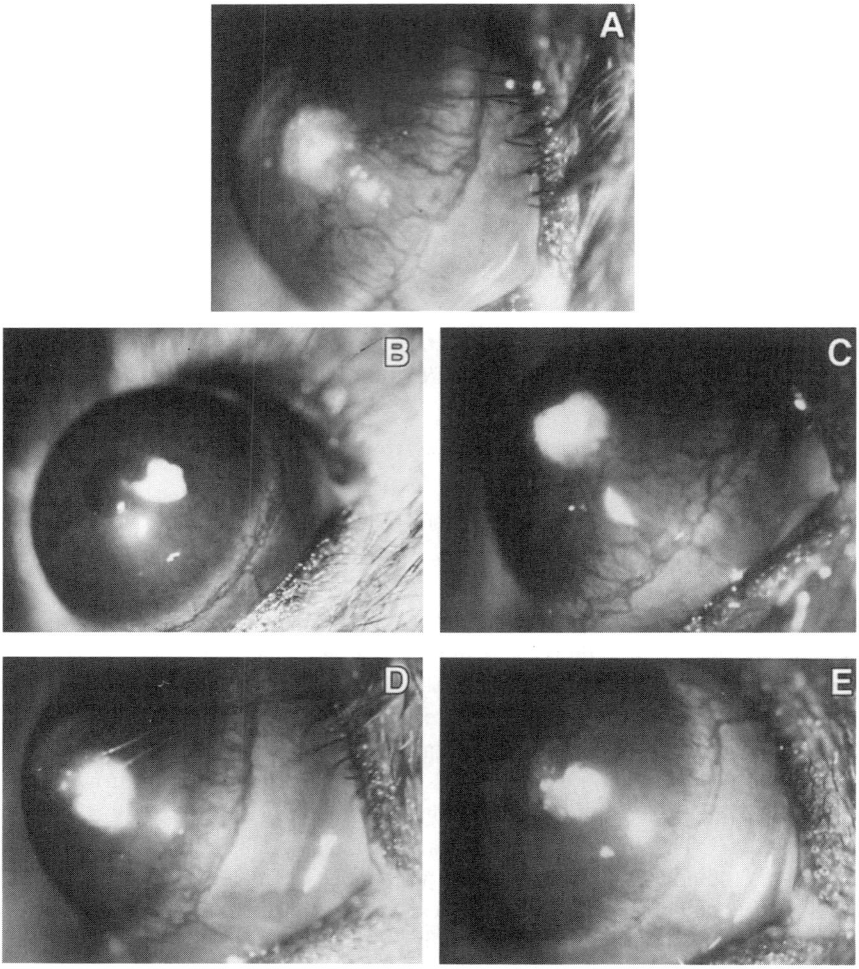

Figure 1 The conceptual basis of antiangiogenic gene therapy. In the mouse cornea neovascularization assay bFGF induces extensive neovascularization (A). Treatment of mice with IL-12, which induces a sustained release of interferon gamma, completely inhibits angiogenesis in this model (B). Blocking antibodies against interferon gamma antagonize the inhibitory effect of IL 12 (C). Bolus injections of sublethal concentrations interferon gamma result only in a partial inhibition of angiogenesis (D). Continuous infusion of interferon gamma (at half the concentration of interferon gamma used in the bolus injections) results in complete inhibition of angiogenesis (E).

clinical trials have been initiated with angiogenesis inhibitors administered by continuous infusion.

Another way to change the half-life of a drug is to alter the structure of the drug so that it will be cleared more slowly. This is a cumbersome procedure because the mechanism through which the angiogenesis inhibitors act at the molecular level is often unknown. Changes in the molecular structure may render the drug inactive.

A novel but logical approach to the problem is the use of gene transfer systems (8–10). Most angiogenesis inhibitors are endogenous proteins (e.g., thrombospondin and platelet factor 4) or split products from endogenous proteins (e.g., angiostatin and endostatin). The cDNAs of these inhibitors are characterized and may be used in gene transfer systems.

II. GENE THERAPY

Gene therapy was originally developed for the treatment of genetic diseases. The mutated gene underlying the disease was compensated by adding a normally functioning gene. Examples of this approach are gene therapy protocols for patients with cystic fibrosis, adenosine deaminase deficiency, or hemophilia (11–15). These early studies showed the feasibility of gene transfer in patients and generated enthusiasm for the concept of gene therapy. The clinical proof of successful gene transfer extended the use of gene therapy to other, nonhereditary diseases. The majority of the current gene therapy trials involve cancer patients (16). The treatment strategies that have evolved include immunotherapy, the protection of bone marrow during chemotherapy by introduction of a drug-resistance gene into marrow stem cells, and the use of vectors that express factors capable of killing tumor cells. Several gene transfer systems are now available (Table 1) (17).

Currently, the most potent gene transfer vectors are derived from natural viruses, including murine retroviruses, human adenoviruses, adeno-associated vi-

Table 1 Currently Used Gene Transfer Systems

Viral gene transfer systems	Nonviral gene transfer systems
Adenovirus	Naked DNA
Adeno-associated virus	Liposomes
Retrovirus	
Herpes virus	
Lentivirus	

rus, and herpes simplex virus (17). The majority of approved gene transfer protocols involve retroviral vectors. However, the use of adenovirus-derived vectors increases rapidly. Therefore, we will focus on these two vector systems.

A. The Retrovirus Vector System

The retrovirus-derived vector system uses the retrovirus' unique capacity to integrate its genome into the chromosomal DNA of the host cell. The vectors are derived from murine retroviruses that are crippled by deletion of the viral genes and only retain the sequences required for packaging and integration. The therapeutic gene replaces the viral genes, often in combination with a selectable marker (mostly a gene that renders the infected cell resistant to such drugs as neomycin or hygromycin B). These defective viruses can only be propagated in special packaging cell lines that synthesize the viral proteins required by the virus to replicate and to be packaged. The defective vector viruses produced in the packaging cells can be used to deliver the gene of interest to the target cell. To date, retroviral vectors are the most useful gene transfer vehicles for achieving stable integration of foreign DNA into the target cell. However, the use of retroviral vectors is limited or troubled by the insert capacity (< 8 kilobases [kb]), inactivation by serum complement, the achievable titers, difficult large-scale production, generation of replication-competent retroviruses, and a limited host range. Improved retroviral vectors are being constructed that may solve the above-mentioned problems and increase the applicability of the system for gene therapy strategies.

B. The Adenovirus Vector System

A viral vector system that has attracted much attention in recent years is the adenoviral vector system. Human adenoviruses (Ads) have a linear DNA genome of approximately 35 kb. After infection of a target cell, the first viral gene to be expressed is the E1 gene. This gene encodes a set of proteins that can activate the transcription of the viral genes required for the viral DNA replication and packaging. In the adenovirus vectors used to date, the E1 region of the virus is replaced by the gene of interest. These vectors are replication deficient, as they lack the E1 region and, therefore, cannot activate the other viral genes required for replication. The E1-deleted adenoviral vectors can only be propagated in special helper cell lines that express the E1 gene products, such as 293 (18) and PER C6 cells (19). In addition, some recombinant adenoviral vectors (rAdVs) are also deprived of E3 or E4 sequences to increase the amount of heterologous sequences that can be accommodated in the vector. None of the Ad E3 gene products are required for replication in cultured cells. The E3-encoded proteins do, however, play an important role in Ads multiplication in vivo, as they protect infected cells from being eradicated by the host's immune response. The Ad E4 gene products are required for replication. E1- and E4-deleted Ads can only be propagated in E1 and E4 expressing helper cell lines (20).

Gene transfer vectors derived from Ads have a number of features that make them particularly useful for gene transfer purposes: (a) the biology of Ads is characterized in detail, (b) the virus is extremely efficient in introducing its DNA into the host cell, (c) Ads can infect a wide variety of dividing and nondividing cells and have a broad host range, and (d) the virus can be produced in large quantities with relative ease. In contrast to retroviruses, Ads do not integrate into the host cell genome.

Currently, two major problems are associated with the use of rAdVs: the generation of replication-competent adenoviruses (RCA) and the host-defense reactions against treatment with adenovirus. The major cause of RCA production is homologous recombination between overlapping sequences from the recombinant vector and the adenovirus constructs in the helper cells. Thus, generation of RCA should be prevented by elimination of sequence homology between the vector DNA and the Ads sequences in the genome of the helper cells. This has been realized by the construction of new adenovirus vectors from which all E1-encoding sequences are deleted and by the development of helper cells that contain E1-encoding sequences only (19). The host-defense reactions against treatment with adenovirus are caused by the strong immunogenicity of the virus particle and by the expression of adenovirus genes that reside in the E1-deleted vectors, resulting in a cytotoxic T-cell (CTL) response against the transduced cells. In vivo administration of Ads particles triggers the development of neutralizing antibodies by the host. As a result, a subsequent administration of the virus will be less effective or completely ineffective. Currently, much effort is put into the development of improved adenoviral vectors with extended deletions (21). These vectors are expected to be less immunogenic, and that they will allow prolonged expression of the transferred gene.

III. CHOICES TO BE MADE FOR SUCCESSFUL ANTIANGIOGENIC GENE THERAPY

By outlining the different gene transfer systems, it becomes clear that choices have to be made to develop antiangiogenic gene therapy (Table 2). The first question to be answered is, which angiogenesis inhibitor is most suitable for this type of treatment? This may depend on the intended application. If an attempt is made to prevent local recurrence of a tumor and there is no danger of growth of distant metastases (e.g., brain tumors), the creation of a local antiangiogenic environment may be sufficient. Proteins may be selected that require expression on the cell membrane or have a high affinity for the extracellular matrix. For

Table 2 Choices to be Made in Antiangiogenic Gene Therapy

Angiogenesis inhibitor:	Local or systemic control
	Size of insert
Gene transfer system:	Viral or nonviral
	Single or repeated treatment
Treatment:	In vivo or ex vivo
Duration of control:	Temporary or long-term
Target cell:	Specific or nonspecific

example, the expression of a dominant-negative Flk-1 receptor on cell membranes inhibits angiogenesis, but is unlikely to provide systemic control (22, 23). The angiogenesis inhibitor, thrombospondin, may serve as another example of a protein with high affinity for the extracellular matrix and, therefore, unlikely to give systemic control of angiogenesis (24). Because most cancer patients die of metastatic disease, it may be important to induce systemic control of angiogenesis. Angiostatin and endostatin are examples of an angiogenesis inhibitor that circulates and suppresses angiogenesis of dormant avascular metastases (25–28).

The size of the corresponding cDNA will be an important factor in the choice of gene transfer system. Nonviral gene transfer systems can accommodate unrestricted cDNA sizes, whereas viral gene transfer systems have a maximal capacity depending on the recombinant virus used. The ideal form of antiangiogenic gene therapy achieves long-term production of an angiogenesis inhibitor by a single injection of recombinant virus. In mice, intravenous injections of rAdV results primarily in infection of hepatocytes. It may be attractive to use hepatocytes to produce large amounts of an inhibitor. Angiostatin is a fragment of plasminogen, which is made exclusively by hepatocytes. It may be beneficial to introduce the angiostatin cDNA, into hepatocytes to obtain sufficient production of angiostatin.

Targeting the recombinant virus to a specific cell may increase the production of specific antiangiogenic proteins. Unfortunately, such targeting to specific cells or organs still has technical limitations. To overcome this problem, the first gene therapy protocols used ex vivo gene transfer systems. Cells of interest (mostly lymphocytes and fibroblasts) are isolated from the patient, transduced in vitro under optimal conditions, and reinfused or reimplanted in the patient. This allows careful monitoring of the transfection efficacy and subsequent protein production. However, the procedure is laborious, requires extensive safety measures, and is limited to a small number of cell types that may be isolated and subsequently survive in culture. In the next sections, the experience with ex vivo and in vivo antiangiogenic gene therapy will be discussed.

IV. EX VIVO ANTIANGIOGENIC GENE THERAPY FOR CANCER

Several growth factor receptor tyrosine kinases have been implicated in angiogenesis, including receptors for epidermal, fibroblast, and platelet-derived growth factors, as well as the receptors Flk-1/KDR, Flt-1, Tie-2, and Tie-1 (29). Endothelial cells express Flk-1/KDR and Flt-1, receptors for vascular endothelial growth factor (VEGF), which are up-regulated in the tumor vasculature (30). Vascular endothelial growth factor is an endothelial cell-specific mitogen that is considered one of the most important angiogenic factors. Millauer and coworkers studied the contribution of Flk-1 to tumor angiogenesis using a dominant-negative methodology in vivo (22, 23). Their strategy involved the introduction of a truncated Flk-1 receptor, which lacks the kinase domain, into cells that express the wild-type receptor. The mutant receptor associates with the wild-type receptor on ligand binding, thus preventing activation of tyrosine kinase activity. For this purpose, a retroviral vector carrying the truncated Flk-1 receptor cDNA was constructed. Coimplantation of virus-producing cells together with various types of tumor cells into athymic mice resulted in the formation of very small tumors relative to those produced from tumor cells implanted alone. The same approach also reduced the growth of glioma cells implanted intracerebrally into Fisher 344 rats and increased the survival times. In all cases, impaired tumor growth coincided with a reduced blood vessel density. Apparently, angiogenesis was inhibited and, as a consequence, this reduced tumor growth. It was concluded that expression of truncated Flk-1 reduced tumor growth by inhibiting endothelial cell proliferation. Kong and colleagues (31) used the same approach, constructing an adenoviral vector carrying the cDNA of a secreted form of the extracellular domain of the Flt-1 receptor. Ex vivo transfection of only 30% of tumor cells resulted in effective suppression of the growth of subcutaneously implanted tumors in mice, whereas transfection had no effect on in vitro growth rates.

Tanaka and coworkers (32) monitored the effect of viral vector-mediated introduction of a modified platelet factor 4 (PF4) cDNA on angiogenesis and tumor growth. Platelet factor 4 (PF4), a 70-amino acid protein that is normally found in alpha granules of platelets, is a potent inhibitor of endothelial proliferation in vitro and angiogenesis in vivo. Intratumoral administration of recombinant PF4 results in significant inhibition of tumor growth; however, sustained exposure to the protein is necessary for maximum effect (33–35). Tanaka et al. constructed retroviral and adenoviral vectors encoding a secreted form of PF4 (sPF4). Glioma cells were transduced ex vivo and implanted in animals. The viral vector-mediated sPF4 transduction mediated endothelial cell proliferation in vitro and resulted in hypovascular tumors that grow slowly in vivo (32). Similar studies were performed with constructed retroviral and adenoviral vectors encoding angiostatin (36). Mitogen-stimulated proliferation of endothelial cells infected ex vivo with an angiostatin-expressing RADV was significantly inhibited. Transduction of glioma cells with these viral vectors had no effect on the growth in vitro. However, the growth of rat glioma cells in vivo was significantly inhibited after transduction with the adenoviral and retroviral vectors. Histological examination revealed that the tumors transduced by the angiostatin-expressing vectors contained more apoptotic cells and fewer blood vessels than the control tumors.

Another example of ex vivo antiangiogenic gene therapy was described by Ojeiffo and colleagues (37). Human umbilical vein endothelial cells (HUVEC) were infected with the LacZ marker gene and intravenously injected in tumor-bearing animals. The authors found that a portion of the injected HUVECs were incorporated in the vasculature of tumors. The observation that ''foreign'' endothelial cells homed to a tumor and took part in the formation of new blood vessels may open up a different way of using antiangiogenic gene therapy. Endothelial cells may be loaded with suicide genes (herpes simplex thymidine kinase [HSVtk]) and allowed to incorporate into capillaries. Herpes simplex virus tyrosine kinase can convert ganciclovir into a nucleoside analogue that will cause DNA chain termination that results in endothelial cell death. Because normal cells lack the HSVtk gene, they are unaffected by ganciclovir treatment. The death of only a few endothelial cells in newly formed capillaries may cause a cascade of effects leading to the destruction of the vascular architecture. Targeting the tumor vasculature is a very effective method of inducing regression of established tumors (38). This approach does not require long-term expression of the transgene, which is a distinct advantage given the short lifespan of transduced genes. However, it may be difficult to isolate sufficient endothelial cells from a patient to perform this study in a clinical setting. It has been reported that progenitor endothelial cells exist that may be isolated and used to target sites of angiogenesis (39).

These studies indicate that gene therapy with angiogenesis inhibitors is feasible. One limitation of these early ''proof of principle'' studies is the necessity of ex vivo transduction with recombinant viruses.

V. IN VIVO ANTIANGIOGENIC THERAPY OF CANCER

The clinical applications of antiangiogenic gene therapy will depend on its success in preclinical models mimicking the clinical situation. Preferably, in experimental models, the transgene should be administered in vivo by a gene transfer system to nonmalignant cells. This is a more realistic model and resembles the clinical situation in which patients are at risk for local or systemic recurrence of the tumor after successful surgery, radiation therapy, or chemotherapy.

Tanaka et al. (32, 36) used local injections of rAdVs carrying either PF4 or angiostatin in pre-established subcutaneous and intracerebral tumors. Tumor-associated angiogenesis was inhibited and animal survival was prolonged. Griscelli et al. (40) demonstrated that a single intratumoral injection of rAdV with cDNA encoding for angiostatin dramatically inhibits tumor growth and intratumoral angiogenesis in two pre-established subcutaneous tumor models.

These studies suggest that angiostatin is produced in a biologically active form by in vivo transduction of tumor cells with an angiostatin cDNA containing RADV. Further proof of the feasibility of in vivo antiangiogenic gene therapy comes from studies modulating endothelial cell receptor expression. Adenoviral-mediated transfer of a truncated Flt-1 receptor suppressed tumor growth in three different experimental tumor models. Regional administration of the rAdV yielded a more extensive inhibition of tumor growth in two of the three models (31). To explore the therapeutic potential of blocking the Tie-2 pathway, Lin and co-workers constructed an rAdV containing a soluble Tie-2 receptor. Administration of this vector in mice with two different pre-established subcutaneous tumors resulted in a significant inhibition of the growth rate and metastatic potential of both tumors (41).

Although the above-mentioned studies demonstrate the feasibility of in vivo antiangiogenic gene therapy using recombinant viruses, it is a misconception that recombinant retro- and adenoviruses will easily infect any nondividing primary cell type. Fibroblasts and endothelial cells are very hard to infect. In addition to the high viral concentrations needed for infection, the short lifespan of transgene expression is a severe limitation. Expression of the transgene may be present from weeks to months. As discussed earlier, the immune system of the host recognizes virus proteins and removes infected cells very effectively. However, to suppress angiogenesis, a continuous, sustained, and prolonged production of angiogenesis inhibitors is required. These criteria have to be met to have a treatment with clinical value. Improvement of the gene transfer systems may ultimately overcome the problems and will allow the use of in vivo gene therapy to inhibit angiogenesis.

VI. CONCLUSIONS

There is a sound scientific rationale for antiangiogenic gene therapy. Ex vivo and in vivo experimental antiangiogenic gene therapy studies have shown the feasibility of this approach. Clinical applications of this novel treatment modality, however, require improved gene transfer systems and sustained transgene expression.

REFERENCES

1. Hanahan D, Folkman J. Patterns and emerging mechanisms of the angiogenic switch during tumorigenesis. Cell 1996; 86:353–364.
2. Folkman J. Angiogenesis in cancer, vascular, rheumatoid and other disease. Nat. Med. 1995; 1:27–31.
3. Holmgren L, O'Reilly MS, Folkman J. Dormancy of micro-metastases: balanced proliferation and apoptosis in the presence of angiogenesis suppression. Nat Med 1995; 1:149–153.
4. Voest EE, Kenyon BM, O'Reilly MS, Truitt G, D'Amato RJ, Folkman J. Inhibition of angiogenesis in vivo by interleukin 12. J Natl Cancer Inst 1995; 87:581–586.
5. Kenyon BM, Voest EE, Chen CC, Flynn E, Folkman J, D'Amato RJ. A model of angiogenesis in the mouse cornea. Invest Ophthalmol Vis Sci 1996; 37:1625–1632.
6. Auerbach W, Auerbach R. Angiogenesis inhibition: a review. Pharmacol Ther 1994; 63:265–311.
7. Kuiper RAJ, Schellens JHM, Beijnen JH, Blijham GH, Voest EE. Clinical research on antiangiogenic therapy. Pharmacol Res 1999, in press.
8. Hitt MM, Addison CL, Graham FL. Human adenovirus vectors for gene transfer into mammalian cells. Adv Pharmacol 1997; 40:137–206.
9. Nabel EG, Simari R, Yang Z, San H, Nabel GJ. In vivo gene transfer: a biological tool. Ann N Y Acad Sci 1997; 811:289–292.
10. Mulligan RC. The basic science of gene therapy. Science 1993; 260:926–932.
11. Connelly S, Kaleko M. Gene therapy for hemophilia A. Thromb Haemost 1997; 78: 31–36.
12. Wagner JA, Gardner P. Toward cystic fibrosis gene therapy. Annu Rev Med 1997; 48:203–216.
13. Fallaux FJ, Hoeben RC, Briet E. State and prospects of gene therapy for the hemophilias. Thromb Haemost 1995; 74:266–273.
14. Blaese RM, Culver KW, Miller AD, Carter CS, Fleisher T, Clerici M, Shearer G, Chang L, Chiang Y, Tolstoshev P, Greenblatt JJ, Rosenberg SA, Klein M, Berger M, Mullen CA, Ramsey WJ, Muul L, Morgan RA, Anderson WF. T lymphocyte-directed gene therapy for ADA-SCID: initial trial results after 4 years. Science 1995; 270:475–480.
15. Bordignon C, Notarangelo LD, Nobili N, Ferrari G, Casorati G, Panina P, Mazzolari E, Maggioni D, Rossi C, Servida P, Gene therapy in peripheral blood lymphocytes and bone marrow for ADA-immunodeficient patients. Science 1995; 270:470–475.
16. Roth JA, Cristiano RJ. Gene therapy for cancer: what have we done and where are we going? J Natl Cancer Inst 1997; 89:21–39.
17. Crystal RG. Transfer of genes to humans: early lessons and obstacles to success. Science 1995; 270:404–410.
18. Graham FL, Smiley J, Russell WC, Nairn R. Characteristics of a human cell line transformed by DNA from adenovirus type 5. J Gen Virol 1977; 36:59–72.
19. Fallaux FJ, Bout A, van der Velde I, van den Wollenberg DJ, Hehir KM, Keegan

J, Auger C, Cramer SJ, van Ormondt H, van der Eb AJ, Valerio D, Hoeben RC. New helper cells and inactivated early region 1-deleted adenoviral vectors prevent generation of replication-competent adenovirus. Hum Gene Ther 1998; 9:1909–1917.

20. Voest EE, Aarsman CJM, Blijham GH. Telomere shortening in microvascular endothelial cells: implications for tumor angiogenesis in the elderly (abstr). Proc Am Assoc Cancer Res 1998; 2576.
21. Wang Q, Finer MH. Second-generation adenovirus vectors. Nat Med 1996; 2:714–716.
22. Millauer B, Longhi MP, Plate KH, Shawver LK, Risau W, Ullrich A, Strawn LM. Dominant-negative inhibition of Flk-1 suppresses the growth of many tumor types in vivo. Cancer Res 1996; 56:1615–1620.
23. Millauer B, Shawver LK, Plate KH, Risau W, Ullrich A. Glioblastoma growth inhibited in vivo by a dominant-negative Flk-1 mutant. Nature 1994; 367:576–579.
24. Dameron KM, Volpert OV, Tainsky MA, Bouck N. Control of angiogenesis in fibroblasts by p53 regulation of thrombospondin-1. Science 1994; 265:1582–1584.
25. O'Reilly MS, Holmgren L, Chen C, Folkman J. Angiostatin induces and sustains dormancy of human primary tumors in mice. Nat Med 1996; 2:689–692.
26. O'Reilly MS, Holmgren L, Shing Y, Chen C, Rosenthal RA, Moses M, Lane WS, Cao Y, Sage EH, Folkman J. Angiostatin: a novel angiogenesis inhibitor that mediates the suppression of metastases by a Lewis lung carcinoma. Cell 1994; 79:315–328.
27. O'Reilly MS, Boehm T, Shing Y, Fukai N, Vasios G, Lane WS, Flynn E, Birkhead JR, Olsen BR, Folkman J. Endostatin: an endogenous inhibitor of angiogenesis and tumor growth. Cell 1997; 88:277–285.
28. Boehm T, Folkman J, Browder T, O'Reilly MS. Anti-angiogenic therapy of experimental cancer does not induce acquired drug resistance. Nature 1998; 390:404–407.
29. Mustonen T, Alitalo K. Endothelial receptor tyrosine kinases involved in angiogenesis. J Cell Biol 1995; 129:895–898.
30. Plate KH, Breier G, Millauer B, Ullrich A, Risau W. Up-regulation of vascular endothelial growth factor and its cognate receptors in a rat glioma model of tumor angiogenesis. Cancer Res 1993; 53:5822–5827.
31. Kong HL, Hecht D, Song W, Kovesdi I, Hackett NR, Yayon A, Crystal RG. Regional suppression of tumor growth by in vivo transfer of a cDNA encoding a secreted form of the extracellular domain of the flt-1 vascular endothelial growth factor receptor. Hum Gene Ther 1998; 10:823–833.
32. Tanaka T, Manome Y, Wen P, Kufe DW, Fine HA. Viral vector-mediated transduction of a modified platelet factor 4 cDNA inhibits angiogenesis and tumor growth. Nat Med 1997; 3:437–442.
33. Sharpe RJ, Byers HR, Scott CF, Bauer SI, Maione TE. Growth inhibition of murine melanoma and human colon carcinoma by recombinant human platelet factor 4. J Natl Cancer Inst 1990; 82:848–853.
34. Maione TE, Gray GS, Hunt AJ, Sharpe RJ. Inhibition of tumor growth in mice by an analogue of platelet factor 4 that lacks affinity for heparin and retains potent angiostatic activity. Cancer Res 1991; 51:2077–2083.
35. Hersh EM, Wiggins CE, Crook LL, Bonnem EM. Phase I study of recombinant

platelet factor 4 (rPF4) in patients with metastatic melanoma and renal cell carcinoma (abstr). Proc Am Soc Clin Oncol 1995; 14:488.

36. Tanaka T, Cao Y, Folkman J, Fine H. Viral vector-targeted antiangiogenic gene therapy utilizing an angiostatin complementary DNA. Cancer Res 1998; 58:3362–3369.
37. Ojeifo JO, Forough R, Paik S, Maciag T, Zwiebel JA. Angiogenesis-directed implantation of genetically modified endothelial cells in mice. Cancer Res 1995; 55:2240–2244.
38. Burrows FJ, Thorpe PE. Eradication of large solid tumors in mice with an immunotoxin directed against tumor vasculature. Proc Natl Acad Sci U S A 1993; 90:8996–9000.
39. Asahara T, Murohara T, Sullivan A, Silver M, van der Zee R, Li T, Witzenbichler B, Schatteman G, Isner JM. Isolation of putative progenitor endothelial cells for angiogenesis. Science 1997; 275:964–967.
40. Griscelli F, Li H, Bennaceur-Griscelli A, Soria J, Opolon P, Soria C, Perricaudet M, Yeh P, Lu H. Angiostatin gene transfer: inhibition of tumor growth in vivo by blockage of endothelial cell proliferation associated with a mitosis arrest. Proc Natl Acad Sci U S A 1998; 95:6367–6372.
41. Lin P, Buxton JA, Acheson A, Radziejewski C, Maisonpierre PC, Yancopoulos GD, Channon KM, Hale LP, Dewhirst MW, George SE, Peters KG. Antiangiogenic gene therapy targeting the endothelium-specific receptor tyrosine kinase Tie2. Proc Natl Acad Sci U S A 1998; 95:8829–8834.

Index

About the Editors

EMILE E. VOEST is a Professor of Medical Oncology and Head of the Department of Internal Medicine, Division of Medical Oncology, and Codirector of the Research Institute "Oncology and Developmental Biology," University Medical Center, Utrecht, The Netherlands. The research program of the Division of Medical Oncology is devoted to angiogenesis research and early clinical trials with antivascular agents. Dr. Voest is a former Fellow of the Dutch Cancer Society and a member of the American Association for Cancer Research, the European Society for Medical Oncology, the American Society of Clinical Oncology, and the Dutch Association for Oncology. He received the M.D. (1985) and Ph.D. (1993) degrees from the Utrecht University School of Medicine, The Netherlands.

PATRICIA A. D'AMORE is a Senior Scientist at the Schepens Eye Research Institute, a Professor of Ophthalmology and Pathology, and the Jules & Doris Stein Research to Prevent Blindness Professor, Harvard Medical School, Boston, Massachusetts. She received the B.A. degree from Regis College, Weston, Massachusetts, the M.B.A. degree from Northeastern University, Boston, and the Ph.D. degree from Boston University.

ISBN 0-8247-0264-6

90000

9 780824 702649